T0250112

Acute Respiratory Distress Syndrome

LUNG BIOLOGY IN HEALTH AND DISEASE

Executive Editor

Claude Lenfant

Former Director, National Heart, Lung, and Blood Institute
National Institutes of Health
Bethesda, Maryland

1. Immunologic and Infectious Reactions in the Lung, *edited by C. H. Kirkpatrick and H. Y. Reynolds*
2. The Biochemical Basis of Pulmonary Function, *edited by R. G. Crystal*
3. Bioengineering Aspects of the Lung, *edited by J. B. West*
4. Metabolic Functions of the Lung, *edited by Y. S. Bakhle and J. R. Vane*
5. Respiratory Defense Mechanisms (in two parts), *edited by J. D. Brain, D. F. Proctor, and L. M. Reid*
6. Development of the Lung, *edited by W. A. Hodson*
7. Lung Water and Solute Exchange, *edited by N. C. Staub*
8. Extrapulmonary Manifestations of Respiratory Disease, *edited by E. D. Robin*
9. Chronic Obstructive Pulmonary Disease, *edited by T. L. Petty*
10. Pathogenesis and Therapy of Lung Cancer, *edited by C. C. Harris*
11. Genetic Determinants of Pulmonary Disease, *edited by S. D. Litwin*
12. The Lung in the Transition Between Health and Disease, *edited by P. T. Macklem and S. Permutt*
13. Evolution of Respiratory Processes: A Comparative Approach, *edited by S. C. Wood and C. Lenfant*
14. Pulmonary Vascular Diseases, *edited by K. M. Moser*
15. Physiology and Pharmacology of the Airways, *edited by J. A. Nadel*
16. Diagnostic Techniques in Pulmonary Disease (in two parts), *edited by M. A. Sackner*
17. Regulation of Breathing (in two parts), *edited by T. F. Hornbein*
18. Occupational Lung Diseases: Research Approaches and Methods, *edited by H. Weill and M. Turner-Warwick*
19. Immunopharmacology of the Lung, *edited by H. H. Newball*
20. Sarcoidosis and Other Granulomatous Diseases of the Lung, *edited by B. L. Fanburg*
21. Sleep and Breathing, *edited by N. A. Saunders and C. E. Sullivan*
22. *Pneumocystis carinii* Pneumonia: Pathogenesis, Diagnosis, and Treatment, *edited by L. S. Young*
23. Pulmonary Nuclear Medicine: Techniques in Diagnosis of Lung Disease, *edited by H. L. Atkins*
24. Acute Respiratory Failure, *edited by W. M. Zapol and K. J. Falke*

For information on volumes 25–182 in the *Lung Biology in Health and Disease* series, please visit www.informahealthcare.com

183. Acute Exacerbations of Chronic Obstructive Pulmonary Disease, *edited by N. M. Siafakas, N. R. Anthonisen, and D. Georgopoulos*

184. Lung Volume Reduction Surgery for Emphysema, *edited by H. E. Fessler, J. J. Reilly, Jr., and D. J. Sugarbaker*

185. Idiopathic Pulmonary Fibrosis, *edited by J. P. Lynch III*

186. Pleural Disease, *edited by D. Bouros*

187. Oxygen/Nitrogen Radicals: Lung Injury and Disease, *edited by V. Vallyathan, V. Castranova, and X. Shi*

188. Therapy for Mucus-Clearance Disorders, *edited by B. K. Rubin and C. P. van der Schans*

189. Interventional Pulmonary Medicine, *edited by J. F. Beamis, Jr., P. N. Mathur, and A. C. Mehta*

190. Lung Development and Regeneration, *edited by D. J. Massaro, G. Massaro, and P. Chambon*

191. Long-Term Intervention in Chronic Obstructive Pulmonary Disease, *edited by R. Pauwels, D. S. Postma, and S. T. Weiss*

192. Sleep Deprivation: Basic Science, Physiology, and Behavior, *edited by Clete A. Kushida*

193. Sleep Deprivation: Clinical Issues, Pharmacology, and Sleep Loss Effects, *edited by Clete A. Kushida*

194. Pneumocystis Pneumonia: Third Edition, Revised and Expanded, *edited by P. D. Walzer and M. Cushion*

195. Asthma Prevention, *edited by William W. Busse and Robert F. Lemanske, Jr.*

196. Lung Injury: Mechanisms, Pathophysiology, and Therapy, *edited by Robert H. Notter, Jacob Finkelstein, and Bruce Holm*

197. Ion Channels in the Pulmonary Vasculature, *edited by Jason X.-J. Yuan*

198. Chronic Obstructive Pulmonary Disease: Cellular and Molecular Mechanisms, *edited by Peter J. Barnes*

199. Pediatric Nasal and Sinus Disorders, *edited by Tania Sih and Peter A. R. Clement*

200. Functional Lung Imaging, *edited by David Lipson and Edwin van Beek*

201. Lung Surfactant Function and Disorder, *edited by Kaushik Nag*

202. Pharmacology and Pathophysiology of the Control of Breathing, *edited by Denham S. Ward, Albert Dahan, and Luc J. Teppema*

203. Molecular Imaging of the Lungs, *edited by Daniel Schuster and Timothy Blackwell*

204. Air Pollutants and the Respiratory Tract: Second Edition, *edited by W. Michael Foster and Daniel L. Costa*

205. Acute and Chronic Cough, *edited by Anthony E. Redington and Alyn H. Morice*

206. Severe Pneumonia, *edited by Michael S. Niederman*

207. Monitoring Asthma, *edited by Peter G. Gibson*

208. Dyspnea: Mechanisms, Measurement, and Management, Second Edition, *edited by Donald A. Mahler and Denis E. O'Donnell*

209. Childhood Asthma, *edited by Stanley J. Szefler and Sφren Pedersen*

210. Sarcoidosis, *edited by Robert Baughman*
211. Tropical Lung Disease, Second Edition, *edited by Om Sharma*
212. Pharmacotherapy of Asthma, *edited by James T. Li*
213. Practical Pulmonary and Critical Care Medicine: Respiratory Failure, *edited by Zab Mosenifar and Guy W. Soo Hoo*
214. Practical Pulmonary and Critical Care Medicine: Disease Management, *edited by Zab Mosenifar and Guy W. Soo Hoo*
215. Ventilator-Induced Lung Injury, *edited by Didier Dreyfuss, Georges Saumon, and Rolf D. Hubmayr*
216. Bronchial Vascular Remodeling in Asthma and COPD, *edited by Aili Lazaar*
217. Lung and Heart–Lung Transplantation, *edited by Joseph P. Lynch III and David J. Ross*
218. Genetics of Asthma and Chronic Obstructive Pulmonary Disease, *edited by Dirkje S. Postma and Scott T. Weiss*
219. *Reichman and Hershfield's* Tuberculosis: A Comprehensive, International Approach, Third Edition (in two parts), *edited by Mario C. Raviglione*
220. Narcolepsy and Hypersomnia, *edited by Claudio Bassetti, Michel Billiard, and Emmanuel Mignot*
221. Inhalation Aerosols: Physical and Biological Basis for Therapy, Second Edition, *edited by Anthony J. Hickey*
222. Clinical Management of Chronic Obstructive Pulmonary Disease, Second Edition, *edited by Stephen I. Rennard, Roberto Rodriguez-Roisin, Gérard Huchon, and Nicolas Roche*
223. Sleep in Children, Second Edition: Developmental Changes in Sleep Patterns, *edited by Carole L. Marcus, John L. Carroll, David F. Donnelly, and Gerald M. Loughlin*
224. Sleep and Breathing in Children, Second Edition: Developmental Changes in Breathing During Sleep, *edited by Carole L. Marcus, John L. Carroll, David F. Donnelly, and Gerald M. Loughlin*
225. Ventilatory Support for Chronic Respiratory Failure, *edited by Nicolino Ambrosino and Roger S. Goldstein*
226. Diagnostic Pulmonary Pathology, Second Edition, *edited by Philip T. Cagle, Timothy C. Allen, and Mary Beth Beasley*
227. Interstitial Pulmonary and Bronchiolar Disorders, *edited by Joseph P. Lynch III*
228. Chronic Obstructive Pulmonary Disease Exacerbations, *edited by Jadwiga A. Wedzicha and Fernando J. Martinez*
229. Pleural Disease, Second Edition, *edited by Demosthenes Bouros*
230. Interventional Pulmonary Medicine, Second Edition, *edited by John F. Beamis, Jr., Praveen Mathur, and Atul C. Mehta*
231. Sleep Apnea: Implications in Cardiovascular and Cerebrovascular Disease, Second Edition, *edited by T. Douglas Bradley and John Floras*
232. Respiratory Infections, *edited by Sanjay Sethi*
233. Acute Respiratory Distress Syndrome, Second Edition, *edited by Augustine M. K. Choi*

The opinions expressed in these volumes do not necessarily represent the views of the National Institutes of Health.

Acute Respiratory Distress Syndrome
Second Edition

Edited by

Augustine M. K. Choi

Brigham and Women's Hospital
Harvard Medical School
Boston, Massachusetts, USA

informa
healthcare

New York London

Informa Healthcare USA, Inc.
52 Vanderbilt Avenue
New York, NY 10017

© 2010 by Informa Healthcare USA, Inc.
Informa Healthcare is an Informa business

No claim to original U.S. Government works

10 9 8 7 6 5 4 3 2 1

International Standard Book Number-10: 1-4200-8840-8 (Hardcover)
International Standard Book Number-13: 978-1-4200-8840-3 (Hardcover)

This book contains information obtained from authentic and highly regarded sources. Reprinted material is quoted with permission, and sources are indicated. A wide variety of references are listed. Reasonable efforts have been made to publish reliable data and information, but the author and the publisher cannot assume responsibility for the validity of all materials or for the consequence of their use.

No part of this book may be reprinted, reproduced, transmitted, or utilized in any form by any electronic, mechanical, or other means, now known or hereafter invented, including photocopying, microfilming, and recording, or in any information storage or retrieval system, without written permission from the publishers.

For permission to photocopy or use material electronically from this work, please access www.copyright.com (http://www.copyright.com/) or contact the Copyright Clearance Center, Inc. (CCC) 222 Rosewood Drive, Danvers, MA 01923, 978-750-8400. CCC is a not-for-profit organization that provides licenses and registration for a variety of users. For organizations that have been granted a photocopy license by the CCC, a separate system of payment has been arranged.

Trademark Notice: Product or corporate names may be trademarks or registered trademarks, and are used only for identification and explanation without intent to infringe.

Library of Congress Cataloging-in-Publication Data

Acute respiratory distress syndrome. – 2nd ed. / edited by Augustine M.K. Choi.
    p. ; cm. – (Lung biology in health and disease ; 233)
    Includes bibliographical references and index.
    ISBN-13: 978-1-4200-8840-3 (hardcover : alk. paper)
    ISBN-10: 1-4200-8840-8 (hardcover : alk. paper)   1. Respiratory distress syndrome, Adult.   I. Choi, Augustine M. K.   II. Series: Lung biology in health and disease ; v. 233.
    [DNLM: 1. Respiratory Distress Syndrome, Adult.   2. Systemic Inflammatory Response Syndrome. W1 LU62 v.233 2009 / WF 140 A183453 2009]
    RC776.R38A2795   2009
    616.2′4–dc22
                                                                                              2009025997

For Corporate Sales and Reprint Permissions call 212-520-2700 or write to: Sales Department, 52 Vanderbilt Avenue, 16th floor, New York, NY 10017.

Visit the Informa Web site at
www.informa.com

and the Informa Healthcare Web site at
www.informahealthcare.com

Foreword

The first modern description of what has come to be known as the acute respiratory distress syndrome (ARDS) appeared more than 40 years ago (1). It is interesting to review the rich history of ARDS and the context in which this new concept in critical care emerged.

At the time we observed our first patients, the use of mechanical ventilators was rare except in immediate postoperative period. Very few patients, nonsurgical and non-traumatic, with severe insults to the respiratory system received mechanical ventilation in order to gain time for survival. Available ventilations of the era were crude and could not deliver high inflation pressures. In those days only the venerable Engstrom respirator used in the polio era could provide the option of positive end-expiratory pressure (PEEP) and a few emerging volume-cycled devices that were coming onto the scene, for example, Emerson, Ohio, and Bennett Series.

Our first report included 12 patients. Seven survived (mean age 27.5 years). Common features in these patients were the requirement of high-inspired oxygen fractions and high inflation pressures. Tissue from autopsies revealed hyperemic lungs and hyaline membrane formation. A surfactant abnormality was identified in the two patients that we studied for this condition.

Our second article in 1971 described the principles of treatment, course, and prognosis factors influencing prognosis in patients (2). In this article, we added the concept of stratification of lung injury severity by the degree of oxygen transfer impairment (2).

At first the concept of the ARDS received criticism from experts in the field (3,4). Later a revision of the original definition in concept was offered by one of the critics (5).

The following four decades have brought advances in the knowledge of the mechanisms of lung injury, that is, oxidative proteolytic, mediated surfactant destruction and damage, etc. Important advances in principles of management have resulted from controlled clinical trials. The major advance in management has been the use of low tidal volume ventilation and the limitations in the inspiratory pressures in hope of avoiding barotrauma during the early management and recovery phase of ARDS.

We learned fairly early on that the survival in ARDS is approximately 40–50%. This has been improving with requirements in treatment and more disciplined respiratory mechanical ventilation, including the employment of concepts of mitigating barotrauma (6).

The prevalence of ARDS in the United States has been the subject of considerable debate. The best estimates are 100,000 to 150,000 patients per year are dependent on definition and selection criteria, including the separation of ARDS from less severe states of acute lung injury by oxygen transfer criteria (7).

Although a surfactant abnormality was part of the original concept of ARDS, and numerous studies have suggested the use of a variety of agents ranging from native surfactant to semisynthetic surfactant. The true role of surfactant therapy in the prevention and/or treatment of ARDS has not been established. Corticosteroids have been considered both useful and of no value in ARDS.

Certainly thousands of lives have been saved as a result of conceptualization of ARDS and refinements in understandings in pathogenesis and treatment. The present volume with 50 authors, all experts in the field, represents the very latest in the ever-changing field in critical care medicine that has been dubbed ARDS.

References

1. Ashbaugh DG, Bigelow DB, Petty TL, et al. Acute respiratory distress in adults. Lancet 1967; 2;319–323.
2. Petty TL, Ashbaugh DG. The adult respiratory distress syndrome: clinical features, factors influencing prognosis, and principles of management. Chest 1971; 60;233–239.
3. Murray JF. The adult respiratory distress syndrome, ARDS (may it rest in peace). Am Rev Respir Dis 1975; 111;716–718.
4. Petty TL. The adult respiratory distress syndrome (confessions of a lumper). Am Rev Respir Dis 1975; 111;713–715.
5. Murray JF, Matthay MA, Luce JM, et al. An expanded definition of the adult respiratory distress syndrome. Am Rev Respir Dis 1988; 138;720–723.
6. The ARDS Network. Ventilation with lower tidal volumes as compared with traditional tidal volumes for acute lung injury and acute respiratory distress syndrome. N Engl J Med 2000; 342;1301–1308.
7. Bernard GR, Artigas A, Brigham KL, et al. The American-European Consensus Conference on ARDS: definitions, mechanisms, relevant outcomes, and clinical trials coordination. Am J Respir Crit Care Med 1994; 149;818–824.

Thomas L. Petty
Denver, Colorado, U.S.A.

Introduction

The series of monographs Lung Biology in Health and Disease has had a long interest in acute respiratory distress syndrome (ARDS). Although the titles of the many monographs that cover this topic have varied over the years, the "spirit" and intent of these volumes has been very consistent, namely, to provide the most timely and excellent information of what has been learned from basic and clinical research, with a goal to improve care of patients suffering from ARDS. A review of the names of the editors and authors of the successive monographs provides a who's who of scientists and clinicians working on this difficult and very severe lung disease.

The first monograph titled *Acute Respiratory Failure*, edited by Warren M. Zapol and Konrad J. Falke, appeared in 1985. Suffice it to compare the table of contents of the 1985 volume with this new monograph titled *Acute Respiratory Distress Syndrome*, edited by Dr. Augustine Choi, to capture the changes in the understanding of ARDS. It remains one of the most serious diseases, a reaction to a myriad of injuries to the lung. Although treatment has improved, the death rate remains very significant and patients who do survive suffer a long and complicated course of recovery.

In the mid-1950s Dr. Julius H. Comroe, with much foresight, conceptualized modern lung biology and predicted in the last Foreword he wrote for this series of monographs (Volume 23) that it would help to attract "imaginative, creative and perceptive young scientists to attack ... difficult problems (of the lung)."

ARDS remains a very difficult problem. However, Dr. Choi has selected some of the best research scientists and clinicians working on ARDS, and in turn they have presented progress and new therapeutic approaches that will certainly benefit patients as well as stimulate further research. For this, I am very grateful to Dr. Choi and his authors for the opportunity to present this volume to the readership of this series of monographs.

Claude Lenfant, MD
Vancouver, Washington, U.S.A.

Preface

According to the American Lung Association, the incidence of acute respiratory distress syndrome (ARDS) is reaching toward 71 per 100,000 persons in the United States. Screenings of medical and surgical patients confirm the significant incidence and mortality. Onset of ARDS develops quickly, often within 24 to 48 hours of the injury or illness and overall mortality rates are nearly 50% of all cases. In patients who survive, recovery is a long process, with normal lung function resuming 6 to 12 months after the patient's initial victory.

There is currently no comprehensive book available to the clinician that gathers in one place the significant advances that have occurred since publication of Michael Matthay's 2003 *Acute Respiratory Distress Syndrome*. Lung clinicians and researchers, pulmonary and critical physicians, and all scientists working in lung disease require a single source guide to prediction and management of ARDS and treatment of the patient. This book will be a comprehensive review of both clinical and experimental paradigms of ARDS.

This new edition will review the current state-of-the-art paradigms and tenets in the field of ARDS. It is paramount to update the previous edition as the field continues to evolve with advancements with significant implications in patient care and treatment of ARDS. The chapters will address important aspects of both pathophysiology and pathogenesis of ARDS. Pathogenesis itself will be discussed in both experimental and clinical studies before discussion of pathogenesis of ventilator-induced lung injury and sepsis/septic-induced lung injury.

Much progress has also been noted in various forms of therapy. Although the overall effectiveness of many therapies remain a topic of debate in competing studies, the latest methods are thoroughly presented including glucocorticoid therapy, surfactant therapy, prone position, forms of mechanical ventilation (invasive and noninvasive), and current research in the use of mesenchymal stem cells.

This edition covers new topics in addition to the important topics covered previously. These new areas have blossomed markedly in the past five years that warrant new chapters for this book, particularly predictive factors including gene expression profiling and biomarkers, and chemokines and cytokines in ARDS. Over 60% of ARDS patients develop nosocomial pulmonary infections and a new chapter is devoted to host defense mechanisms and infection prevention. We have also added key new chapters on the management of the ARDS patient, including cell-based therapy, fluid management in ARDS, and nonpulmonary and nonsepsis management. Additionally, chapters covering transfusion-related acute lung injury, vascular endothelium leakage, and the long-term clinical outcomes have been added to ensure the best in patient management and care.

Augustine M. K. Choi

Contributors

Antonio Anzueto   South Texas Veterans Health Care System, Audie L. Murphy Division, and The University of Texas Health Science Center at San Antonio, San Antonio, Texas, U.S.A.

Rebecca M. Baron   Department of Medicine, Division of Pulmonary and Critical Care, Brigham and Women's Hospital, Boston, Massachusetts, U.S.A.

Laurent Brochard   Réanimation Médicale, INSERM U 492 and Hopital Henri Mondor, Université Paris 12, Créteil, France

Roy G. Brower   Pulmonary and Critical Care Medicine, Johns Hopkins University, Baltimore, Maryland, U.S.A.

Carolyn S. Calfee   Pulmonary and Critical Care Medicine and Cardiovascular Research Institute, University of California, San Francisco, California, U.S.A.

Eddie T. Chiang   Department of Medicine, Section of Pulmonary and Critical Care Medicine, Pritzker School of Medicine, University of Chicago, Chicago, Illinois, U.S.A.

Augustine M. K. Choi   Division of Pulmonary and Critical Care Medicine, Brigham and Women's Hospital, Harvard Medical School, Boston, Massachusetts, U.S.A.

David C. Christiani   Department of Medicine, Pulmonary and Critical Care Unit, Massachusetts General Hospital, Harvard Medical School, and Department of Environmental Health, Harvard School of Public Health, Boston, Massachusetts, U.S.A.

Benedict C. Creagh-Brown   Department of Critical Care Medicine, Imperial College School of Medicine, Royal Brompton Hospital, London, U.K.

Timothy W. Evans   Department of Critical Care Medicine, Imperial College School of Medicine, Royal Brompton Hospital, London, U.K.

Carol Feghali-Bostwick   Division of Pulmonary, Allergy and Critical Care Medicine, University of Pittsburgh School of Medicine, Pittsburgh, Pennsylvania, U.S.A.

James A. Frank   University of California, San Francisco VA Medical Center, San Francisco, California, U.S.A.

Ognjen Gajic   Department of Medicine, Division of Pulmonary and Critical Care, Mayo Clinic, Rochester, Minnesota, U.S.A.

Joe G. N. Garcia   Department of Medicine, Section of Pulmonary and Critical Care Medicine, Pritzker School of Medicine, University of Chicago, Chicago, Illinois, U.S.A.

Luciano Gattinoni   Ospedale Maggiore Policlinico, Milan, Italy

Michelle Ng Gong   Department of Medicine, Critical Care Medicine, Montefiore Medical Center, and Department of Epidemiology and Population Health, Albert Einstein College of Medicine, Bronx, New York, U.S.A.

Philip C. Goodman   Radiology/Cardiac and Thoracic Imaging, Duke University Medical Center, Durham, North Carolina, U.S.A.

Naveen Gupta   Department of Medicine, Division of Pulmonary and Critical Care, University of Pittsburgh School of Medicine, Pittsburgh, Pennsylvania, U.S.A.

Estelle S. Harris   Divisions of Respiratory and Critical Care Medicine and General Internal Medicine, Department of Medicine, University of Utah, Salt Lake City, Utah, U.S.A.

Judie Howrylak   Division of Pulmonary and Critical Care Medicine, Brigham and Women's Hospital, Harvard Medical School, Boston, Massachusetts, U.S.A.

Yumiko Imai   Department of Physiology and Pharmacology, Akita University School of Medicine, Akita, Japan

Michael P. Keane   Department of Medicine, St Vincent's University Hospital and University College Dublin, Dublin, Ireland and Department of Medicine, University of Virginia, Charlottesville, Virginia, U.S.A.

Emer Kelly   Department of Medicine, St Vincent's University Hospital and University College Dublin, Dublin, Ireland and Department of Medicine, University of Virginia, Charlottesville, Virginia, U.S.A.

Lester Kobzik   Department of Pathology, Brigham & Women's Hospital, Harvard Medical School and Harvard School of Public Health, Boston, Massachusetts, U.S.A.

Gabriel D. Lang   Department of Medicine, Section of Pulmonary and Critical Care Medicine, Pritzker School of Medicine, University of Chicago, Chicago, Illinois, U.S.A.

Jae-Woo Lee   Department of Anesthesiology, University of California, San Francisco, California, U.S.A.

James F. Lewis   University of Western Ontario and St. Joseph's Health Center, Ontario, Canada

Mark R. Looney   Department of Medicine, Division of Pulmonary and Critical Care, University of California, San Francisco, California, U.S.A.

Thomas R. Martin   Veteran's Affairs Puget Sound Health Care System, and Division of Pulmonary and Critical Care Medicine, Department of Medicine, University of Washington School of Medicine, Seattle, Washington, U.S.A.

Michael A. Matthay   Pulmonary and Critical Care Medicine and Cardiovascular Research Institute, University of California, San Francisco, California, U.S.A.

Gustavo Matute-Bello   Division of Pulmonary and Critical Care Medicine, Department of Medicine, University of Washington School of Medicine, Seattle, Washington, U.S.A.

Danielle Morse   Division of Pulmonary and Critical Care Medicine, Brigham and Women's Hospital, Harvard Medical School, Boston, Massachusetts, U.S.A.

Marc Moss   Division of Pulmonary Sciences and Critical Care Medicine, University of Colorado Health Sciences Center, Denver, Colorado, U.S.A.

Margaret J. Neff   Division of Pulmonary and Critical Care, Harborview Medical Center, University of Washington, Seattle, Washington, U.S.A.

Mark A. Perrella   Department of Medicine, Division of Pulmonary and Critical Care; and Newborn Medicine, Brigham and Women's Hospital, Boston, Massachusetts, U.S.A.

Desirée M. Quiñones   Hospital del Maestro Avenida Domenech, Hato Rey, Puerto Rico

Todd W. Rice   Division of Allergy, Pulmonary and Critical Care Medicine, Department of Medicine, Vanderbilt University School of Medicine, Nashville, Tennessee, U.S.A.

Matthew T. Rondina   Divisions of Respiratory and Critical Care Medicine and General Internal Medicine, Department of Medicine, University of Utah, Salt Lake City, Utah, U.S.A.

Gordon D. Rubenfeld   Program in Trauma, Emergency, and Critical Care, Department of Critical Care, Sunnybrook Health Sciences Centre, University of Toronto, Toronto, Ontario, Canada

Hansjörg Schwertz   Division of Vascular Surgery, Department of Surgery, University of Utah, Salt Lake City, Utah, U.S.A.

Lynette Sholl   Department of Pathology, Brigham and Women's Hospital, Harvard Medical School, Boston, Massachusetts, U.S.A.

Arthur S. Slutsky   Keenan Research Center at the Li Ka Shing Knowledge Institute of St. Michael's Hospital and the University of Toronto, Toronto, Ontario, Canada

Roger G. Spragg   University of California, San Diego, and Medicine Service, San Diego VA Medical Center, San Diego, California, U.S.A.

Robert M. Strieter   Department of Medicine, St Vincent's University Hospital and University College Dublin, Dublin, Ireland and Department of Medicine, University of Virginia, Charlottesville, Virginia, U.S.A.

B. Taylor Thompson   Pulmonary and Critical Care Unit, Department of Medicine, Massachusetts General Hospital and Harvard Medical School, Boston, Massachusetts, U.S.A.

Franco Valenza   Dipartimento di Anestesiologia, Rianimazione e Scienze Dermatologiche, Fondazione Ospedale Maggiore Policlinico, Mangiagalli e Regina Elena – IRCSS, Università degli Studi di Milano, Milan, Italy

Lorraine B. Ware   Division of Allergy, Pulmonary and Critical Care Medicine, Department of Medicine, Vanderbilt University, Nashville, Tennessee, U.S.A.

Andrew S. Weyrich   Division of Respiratory and Critical Care Medicine, Department of Medicine, and the Program in Human Molecular Biology and Genetics, University of Utah, Salt Lake City, Utah, U.S.A.

Arthur P. Wheeler Division of Allergy, Pulmonary and Critical Care Medicine, Department of Medicine, Vanderbilt University School of Medicine, Nashville, Tennessee, U.S.A.

Guy A. Zimmerman Division of Respiratory and Critical Care Medicine, Department of Medicine, and the Program in Human Molecular Biology and Genetics, University of Utah, Salt Lake City, Utah, U.S.A.

Contents

Foreword Thomas L. Petty .... *vii*
Introduction Claude Lenfant .... *ix*
Preface .... *xi*
Contributors .... *xiii*

1. Definitions and Clinical Risk Factors *1*
   Marc Moss and B. Taylor Thompson

2. Epidemiology of Acute Lung Injury: A Public Health Perspective *17*
   Gordon D. Rubenfeld and Margaret J. Neff

3. Radiographic Findings of the Acute Respiratory Distress Syndrome *31*
   Philip C. Goodman and Desirée M. Quiñones

4. Pulmonary Pathology of ARDS: Diffuse Alveolar Damage *46*
   Lester Kobzik and Lynette Sholl

5. Pathogenesis of Acute Lung Injury: Experimental Studies *59*
   Rebecca M. Baron and Mark A. Perrella

6. Pathogenesis of Acute Lung Injury: Clinical Studies *72*
   Benedict C. Creagh-Brown and Timothy W. Evans

7. Apoptosis in the Pathogenesis and Resolution of Acute Lung Injury *93*
   Gustavo Matute-Bello and Thomas R. Martin

8. Pathogenesis of Ventilator-Induced Lung Injury *109*
   Franco Valenza, James A. Frank, Yumiko Imai, and Arthur S. Slutsky

9. Sepsis in the Acute Respiratory Distress Syndrome:
   Treatment Implications *146*
   Arthur P. Wheeler and Todd W. Rice

10. Transfusion-Related Acute Lung Injury *171*
    Mark R. Looney and Ognjen Gajic

11. Mechanisms of Fibroproliferation in Acute Lung Injury *184*
    Danielle Morse and Carol Feghali-Bostwick

12. Current Approaches and Recent Advances in the Genetic
    Epidemiology of Acute Lung Injury/Acute Respiratory
    Distress Syndrome *196*
    Michelle NG Gong and David C. Christiani

13. **Gene Expression Profiling and Biomarkers in ARDS** *220*
    Judie Howrylak and Augustine M. K. Choi

14. **Resolution of Alveolar Edema: Mechanisms and Relationship to
    Clinical Acute Lung Injury** *237*
    Lorraine B. Ware and Michael A. Matthay

15. **Lung Vascular Dysfunction and Repair in Acute Lung Injury:
    Role of the Endothelial Cytoskeleton** *262*
    Gabriel D. Lang, Eddie T. Chiang and Joe G. N. Garcia

16. **Surfactant Therapy in the Acute Respiratory Distress Syndrome** *287*
    Roger G. Spragg and James F. Lewis

17. **Prone Position in ARDS** *313*
    Antonio Anzueto and Luciano Gattinoni

18. **Mechanical Ventilation in the Acute Respiratory Distress Syndrome** *335*
    Roy G. Brower and Laurent Brochard

19. **Fluid Therapy and Hemodynamic Monitoring in Acute Lung Injury** *359*
    Carolyn S. Calfee, Naveen Gupta, and Michael A. Matthay

20. **Pathogenesis of Sepsis and Sepsis-Induced Acute Lung Injury** *369*
    *Estelle S. Harris, Matthew T. Rondina, Hansjörg Schwertz, Andrew S. Weyrich,
    and Guy A. Zimmerman*

21. **Cell-Based Therapy for Acute Lung Injury and Acute Respiratory
    Distress Syndrome** *420*
    Naveen Gupta, Jae-Woo Lee, and Michael A. Matthay

22. **Chemokines and Cytokines in ARDS** *432*
    Michael P. Keane, Emer Kelly, and Robert M. Strieter

Index *447*

1
Definitions and Clinical Risk Factors

MARC MOSS
Division of Pulmonary Sciences and Critical Care Medicine, University of Colorado Health Sciences Center, Denver, Colorado, U.S.A.

B. TAYLOR THOMPSON
Pulmonary and Critical Care Unit, Department of Medicine, Massachusetts General Hospital and Harvard Medical School, Boston, Massachusetts, U.S.A.

I. Introduction

The acute respiratory distress syndrome (ARDS) is characterized by increased permeability of the alveolar-capillary membrane, diffuse alveolar damage, the accumulation of proteinaceous interstitial and intra-alveolar edema, and the presence of hyaline membranes. These pathological changes are accompanied by physiological alterations including severe hypoxemia, an increase in the mean pulmonary dead-space fraction, and a decrease in pulmonary compliance. ARDS is a relatively common diagnosis in patients who require mechanical ventilation for greater than 24 hours. In a population-based cohort study of 21 hospitals over a 16-month period of time, 21% of patients who required mechanical ventilation for more than 24 hours met established criteria for ARDS (1). A European survey of 132 intensive care units similarly demonstrated that 18% of mechanically ventilated patients had ARDS (2). Economically, ARDS patients account for a disproportionately higher amount of hospital resources due to their prolonged intensive care unit and hospital length of stays. In one observational study, ARDS patients who required mechanical ventilation for at least seven days represented only 6% of intensive care unit (ICU) admissions yet comprised 33% of all ICU patient days and 24% of all hospital charges among ICU patients (3).

Because ARDS is a syndrome and not a disease, patients are defined as having ARDS when they meet predetermined diagnostic criteria. Potential goals for these diagnostic criteria are to identify patients with a specific clinical entity for epidemiological purposes and to select patients who will respond to ARDS-specific therapies. The diagnostic criteria used to define ARDS have evolved over time. In this chapter, we will discuss the evolution of the definition of ARDS and the continued need for modifications of the present diagnostic criteria. We will also review a variety of demographic and clinical factors that are associated with alterations in the susceptibility and mortality associated with ARDS.

II. The Definition of ARDS

The first official description of ARDS was reported in 1967 and consisted of a case series of 12 patients with the acute onset of dyspnea, tachypnea, severe hypoxemia, chest radiographic abnormalities, and decreased static respiratory system compliance (4).

With the increased availability of pulmonary artery catheterization in ICUs, ARDS was recognized as a noncardiogenic form of pulmonary edema, characterized by the accumulation of both protein and cells in the alveoli in the presence of normal left atrial pressures. Subsequently, several ARDS definitions were used in the early 1980s that required at least four basic clinical features, three of which were based on physiological and radiographic criteria adapted from this original case series: hypoxemia (varying severity), decreased respiratory system compliance, and chest radiographic abnormalities (often of an ill-defined type and degree). The fourth diagnostic criterion was usually the documentation of a pulmonary artery occlusion pressure of 18 mm Hg or less using a pulmonary artery catheter (5–9).

When the mortality associated with ARDS did not appear to improve during the 1980s, the possibility was raised that the requirement of all four of these criteria biased the understanding of ARDS and contributed to the negative results of several therapeutic trials for ARDS (10). One concern was that these strict diagnostic criteria that required placement of a pulmonary artery catheter only identified patients with severe ARDS and a very poor prognosis (11). The requirement for pulmonary artery catheterization could also delay the diagnosis of ARDS (12). Because approximately 50% of patients develop ARDS within the first 24 hours of meeting an at-risk diagnosis, delaying the administration of a therapy in order to insert a pulmonary artery catheter may diminish the chance for a successful therapeutic intervention (13). More recently, large clinical trials have demonstrated that a pulmonary artery catheter does not improve outcome for a variety of critically ill patients including patients with ARDS (14,15).

The older diagnostic criteria of ARDS also lack specificity. For example, patients with vasculitis and alveolar hemorrhage meet the diagnostic criteria for ARDS, yet the pathogenesis of this disorder is different from ARDS (11). In addition, patients with an elevated pulmonary artery occlusion pressure are excluded, although these patients may have lung injury in addition to either hypervolemia or congestive heart failure (either systolic or diastolic). Several investigators postulated that the differences in reported epidemiological data, such as mortality rates, could be attributed to inconsistent cutoff values for the hypoxemia criteria and variations in the interpretation of other diagnostic considerations (6). It was also recognized that these diagnostic criteria defined ARDS as an all-or-none phenomenon. The presentation of ARDS includes a continuum of radiographic and arterial blood gas abnormalities, and any single cutoff value for the definition of ARDS is arbitrary. Therefore, the identification of several gradations or categories of acute lung injury that have prognostic or therapeutic implications would be beneficial.

A. The Murray Lung Injury Score

Newer ARDS definitions emerged in an attempt to improve both the sensitivity and specificity of the diagnostic criteria by including early and limited cases of ARDS while still excluding patients who did not truly have diffuse alveolar damage, the histologic correlate of acute lung injury (11,16). In 1988, Murray and colleagues proposed a lung injury score that was based on four components (chest radiograph, hypoxemia, positive end-expiratory pressure, and respiratory system compliance), two of which (chest radiograph and hypoxemia) must be available for all patients (7) (Table 1). Each component is assigned a score of 1 to 4. The final value is obtained by dividing the aggregate sum by the number of available components, and three categories of lung injury are defined. A final score of

Table 1 The Lung Injury Score

Chest roentgenogram score	
No alveolar consolidation	0
Alveolar consolidation in one quadrant	1
Alveolar consolidation in two quadrants	2
Alveolar consolidation in three quadrants	3
Alveolar consolidation in four quadrants	4
Hypoxemia score	
$Pao_2/Fio_2 \geq 300$	0
Pao_2/Fio_2 225–299	1
Pao_2/Fio_2 175–224	2
Pao_2/Fio_2 100–174	3
$Pao_2/Fio_2 < 100$	4
Respiratory system compliance score (when ventilated) (mL/cm H_2O)	
≥ 80	0
60–79	1
40–59	2
20–39	3
19	4
Positive end-expiratory pressure score (when ventilated) (cm H_2O)	
≤ 5	0
6–8	1
9–11	2
12–14	3
≥ 15	4
Final value[a]	
No lung injury	0
Acute lung injury	0.1–2.5
Severe injury (ARDS)	>2.5

[a]Obtained by dividing aggregate sum by number of components used.

zero equals no lung injury, 0.1 to 2.5 constitutes mild to moderate lung injury, and >2.5 is defined as ARDS. The authors also recommended that this scoring system be used only in patients with specific diagnoses, such as sepsis and trauma. In addition, the placement of a pulmonary artery catheter and measurement of a pulmonary capillary occlusion pressure were not required.

B. The American-European Consensus Conference

Subsequently, the American-European Consensus Conference (AECC) on ARDS was convened with a major goal of bringing "clarity and uniformity to the definition of ARDS" (17). The diagnostic criteria for ARDS proposed by this committee were $Pao_2/Fio_2 \leq 200$, bilateral infiltrates on chest radiograph that need not be diffuse, and pulmonary artery occlusion pressure ≤ 18 mm Hg or no clinical evidence of left atrial hypertension when a pulmonary artery catheter was not used. The spectrum of disease severity was also expanded to include patients with milder hypoxemia. This definition, which includes

Table 2 Recommended Criteria for Acute Lung Injury and Acute Respiratory Distress Syndrome

	Timing	Oxygenation	Chest radiograph	Pulmonary artery wedge pressure
ALI criteria	Acute onset	$Pao_2/Fio_2 \leq$ 300 mm Hg (regardless of PEEP level)	Bilateral infiltrates seen on frontal chest radiograph	$\leq$18 mm Hg when measured or no clinical evidence of left atrial hypertension
ARDS criteria	Acute onset	$Pao_2/Fio_2 \leq$ 200 mm Hg (regardless of PEEP level)	Bilateral infiltrates seen on frontal chest radiograph	$\leq$18 mm Hg when measured or no clinical evidence of left atrial hypertension

patients with ARDS, was called acute lung injury (ALI), and the diagnostic criteria were similar except the Pao_2/Fio_2 ratio was $\leq$300 (Table 2).

To determine the accuracy of the Murray lung injury score and the AECC definition, the diagnostic criteria for these two new definitions were compared to the previous definition of ARDS that required all four diagnostic criteria (16). Both definitions maintained a high degree of accuracy (>90%) for those ICU patients with a clearly defined at-risk diagnosis for the development of ARDS. Therefore, it is likely that the lung injury score and the AECC definition actually identify a patient population similar to the older strict definitions of ARDS for those patients with clearly defined at-risk diagnoses.

The members of the AECC reconvened to clarify some questions concerning their diagnostic criteria for ARDS. They acknowledged that the theoretical differentiation of ARDS from ALI based on severity of hypoxemia had not established two separate entities with different clinical associations and prognoses. In regard to the chest radiographic criteria, the committee stated that the "bilateral infiltrates" should be consistent with pulmonary edema, even if mild or patchy in nature. Opacities that were not considered appropriate for the radiographic criteria for ALI/ARDS include pleural effusions, pleural thickening, pulmonary masses or nodules, chronic scarring, volume loss, lobar collapse, plate-like atelectasis if the surrounding borders are sharp, extrathoracic opacities, and subcutaneous air. The AECC committee also commented on the difficulty in excluding hydrostatic or cardiogenic causes as the sole cause for pulmonary edema. They acknowledged the lack of a perfect cutoff value of the pulmonary artery occlusion pressure that would differentiate the hydrostatic pulmonary edema from permeability pulmonary edema (ARDS). However, no alterations in this controversial diagnostic criterion were recommended. The original AECC definition did not set a time limit for the word "acute," but clearly ARDS needs to be differentiated from interstitial lung diseases that develop over weeks to months (17). Based on the results of one epidemiological study demonstrating that all patients developed ARDS by seven days of meeting the at-risk diagnosis, the length of time for the development of ARDS was defined as being less than seven days from the time of onset of their critical illness.

C. The Delphi Definition of ARDS

In 2005, Ferguson and colleagues used a formal consensus-building process called the Delphi technique in an attempt to further improve upon the accuracy of the AECC

Table 3 The Delphi Definition of ARDS[a]

Defining characteristic	Operational definition
1 Hypoxemia	$Pao_2/Fio_2 < 200$ mm Hg with PEEP ≥ 10
2 Acute onset	Rapid onset in <72 hr
3 Radiographic abnormalities	Bilateral airspace disease involving ≥ 2 quadrants on frontal chest X-ray
4 Noncardiogenic in origin	No clinical evidence of congestive heart failure (including use of pulmonary artery catheter and/or echo if clinically indicated)
5 Decreased lung compliance	Static respiratory system compliance <50 mL/cm H_2O (with patient sedated, tidal volume of 8 mL/kg, ideal body weight, PEEP ≥ 10)
6 Predisposition	Direct and/or indirect factor associated with lung injury

[a] ARDS is indicated by the presence of criteria 1–4 and one of 5 or 6.

definition of ARDS (18). The goal of this process was to reduce bias and improve the operating characteristics of the selected diagnostic criteria. A group of 11 opinion leaders first identified several defining characteristics of ARDS, and then refined and reduced these criteria through a pooled and anonymous feedback system. The end result were slightly different diagnostic criteria from the AECC definition including a definition of hypoxemia that required a Pao_2/Fio_2 ratio of ≤ 200 mm Hg with a PEEP of ≥ 10, the documentation of a predisposing risk factor for the development of ARDS, and the reinsertion of a decreased static respiratory system compliance (Table 3).

III. Persistent Problems and Controversies Involving the Definition of ARDS

In spite of these several attempts to develop diagnostic criteria for ARDS, fundamental problems still remain. Esteban and colleagues determined the validity of the AECC diagnostic criteria against autopsy results in 382 patients who died while in the ICU (19). Patients were considered to fulfill the pathological diagnosis of ARDS if they had diffuse alveolar damage defined as the presence of hyaline membranes plus at least one of the following criteria: alveolar type I or endothelial cell necrosis, edema, organizing interstitial fibrosis, or prominent alveolar type II cell proliferation. A total of 127 (33%) of the decedents met the AECC diagnostic criteria, and 112 (29%) met the pathological diagnosis. The sensitivity and specificity of the AECC definition using the pathological diagnosis as the gold standard was 75% and 84%, respectively. The accuracy of the AECC definition did not improve when only the 284 patients with risk factors were included. The most common pathological findings in those patients who met the AECC criteria for ARDS but did not fulfill the pathological diagnosis of ARDS were pneumonia, pulmonary hemorrhage, and pulmonary edema. Conversely, the clinical diagnoses of the patients who met the pathological criteria for ARDS but did not meet the AECC clinical criteria were again pneumonia and pulmonary edema. A Brazilian study examining the results of only 22 autopsy studies again confirmed the relative inaccuracy of the AECC definition (20). Studying a subset of 138 decedents from the previously cited Esteban data, the diagnostic accuracy of the lung injury score and the recently developed Delphi definition were determined and compared to the AECC diagnostic criteria (21). Unfortunately, these two additional definitions of ARDS also did not accurately identify patients with pathological evidence of ARDS. The sensitivity for the diagnosis of ARDS was similar for all three definitions. However, the specificity of the lung injury score and the Delphi definition were significantly better than the AECC definition.

The chest radiographic criteria used to define ARDS also remain problematic. When 21 established investigators reviewed 28 randomly selected chest radiographs from intubated patients with a Pao_2/Fio_2 of <300, there was considerable variability in their interpretations of whether the films were consistent with ARDS (22). Other studies have also demonstrated a similar lack of consistency in chest radiographs scores when using the four-point radiographic criteria from the Murray lung injury score (16,23). Importantly, formal training in the interpretation of chest radiographs for the diagnosis of ARDS can improve the inter-rater reliability between investigators (24). After a standardized session during which physicians refined the standards and rules they would apply to the radiographic interpretation, their inter-rater reliability in regard to identification of chest radiographs consistent with ARDS was nearly perfect. Therefore, formal training in radiographic interpretation among investigators would decrease the heterogeneity of patients enrolled in clinical trials for ARDS.

There is also controversy surrounding the specific hypoxemia criteria included in the definition of ARDS. Individual or institutional variations in mechanical ventilator strategy could impact the incidence of ARDS/ALI in an ICU or medical center. Increasing the level of positive end-expiratory pressure (PEEP) alone may improve the Pao_2 and directly alter the Pao_2/Fio_2 ratio. Several studies have demonstrated that up to 50% of patients who meet the hypoxemia criteria for ARDS without PEEP will significantly improve their oxygenation with higher levels of PEEP, and subsequently may no longer meet the hypoxemia criteria for ARDS (25,26). As a result, a PEEP requirement of 12 cm H_2O was included in the hypoxemia criteria in the Delphi definition in order to exclude these patients as being diagnosed with ARDS (18). However, it is presently unclear what specific level of PEEP should be included in the definition and whether the inclusion of a PEEP requirement results in the identification of a more homogeneous group of ARDS patients.

Finally, in order to differentiate ARDS from hydrostatic (cardiogenic/volume overload) pulmonary edema, the AECC consensus definition includes either a pulmonary artery occlusion pressure of ≤18 mm Hg or no clinical evidence of left atrial hypertension. Some patients who meet clinical criteria for ARDS may have a pulmonary capillary occlusion pressure that is above the selected cutoff value of 18 mm Hg. In the ARDS network pulmonary artery catheter trial, 29% of ALI patients had a pulmonary artery occlusion pressures that exceeded the traditionally accepted threshold of 18 mm Hg (14). In addition, there are no specific recommendations by the AECC committee about what constitutes clinical signs of an elevated left atrial pressure. Depending on the specific diagnostic criteria used to define clinical left atrial hypertension, between 5% and 30% of patients meeting chest radiograph and hypoxemia criteria may be excluded from a formal diagnosis of ARDS (27).

Despite these concerns, the present diagnostic criteria of the AECC definition have proven to be extremely useful in regard to clinical trial design. Importantly, patients who meet the present AECC definition of ARDS respond to specific therapies that are associated with improvement of their outcome including a 25% reduction in mortality with the use of a low tidal volume ventilatory strategy and a significant reduction in ventilator free days with the use of a fluid conservative strategy (28,29).

IV. Future Directions

The identification of an accurate diagnostic or prognostic marker for diffuse alveolar damage and ARDS would significantly improve the ability to diagnose patients with ARDS and improve our understanding of this syndrome. As described in several other chapters in this volume, ARDS is associated with the initiation and propagation of an intense inflammatory cascade involving myriad inflammatory cells and mediators that result in injury to the alveolar-capillary barrier. The most likely source of a biochemical marker for ARDS would be obtained either from the peripheral blood, urine, or possibly from endotracheal tube aspirate of edema fluid. Numerous studies have attempted to identify a clinically useful biochemical marker for ARDS (30). Although much has been learned about the pathogenesis of ARDS from these studies, there is presently no clearly identified biochemical marker for ARDS.

Measurements of pulmonary vascular permeability or the accumulation of extravascular lung water also has promise as diagnostic or prognostic biomarkers for ARDS. Positron emission tomography can measure protein flux between intravascular and extravascular components of the lung (31,32). Using this technique, ARDS patients have been reported to have increased pulmonary vascular permeability (PVP) when compared to normal controls (31). The ability of PVP measurements to diagnose ARDS has also been examined. In this study, these noninvasive techniques were utilized in an attempt to differentiate patients with ARDS from those with commonly confused diagnoses such as congestive heart failure and pneumonia (32). Though PVP was significantly higher in ARDS patients when compared to those with congestive heart failure, they were not different from measurement of PVP in patients with pneumonia, both in the regions with infiltrate and in radiographically normal areas (32). In addition, the accumulation of extravascular lung water can be measured in critically ill patients using a thermistor-tipped arterial catheter and a technologically advanced rapid-response processor. In one study of patients with severe sepsis, patients who met criteria for ARDS had significantly higher levels of extravascular lung water when compared to severe sepsis patients without lung injury (33). Further investigation is needed before these noninvasive measures of PVP or invasive measures of extravascular lung water would be incorporated into the formal definition of ARDS.

Finally, the distinction between ALI and ARDS has not proven to be very useful clinically. Based on the work of Gattinoni and colleagues, there is a subset of ARDS patients who have a predominance of lung edema and therefore a greater potential to recruit alveoli (34). This subset of patients might actually benefit from the use of higher levels of PEEP. Creating reliable and feasible diagnostic criteria that accurately identify this subset of patients may prove to be an important method of risk-stratifying patients with ARDS and identifying those patients that would clinically benefit from the use of higher levels of PEEP.

V. Clinical Risk Factors for the Development of ARDS

Since its initial description, ARDS has been noted to occur in patients with a variety of diagnoses. The specific patients that are at risk for the development of ARDS were

Table 4 Incidence of ARDS Among Patients with Specific At-Risk Diagnoses

At-risk diagnosis	Incidence rates, 1980–1981 (Fowler series) (%)	Incidence rates, 1982 (Pepe series) (%)	Incidence rates, 1983–1985 (Hudson series) (%)
Sepsis		38	41
Aspiration of gastric contents	36	30	22
Pulmonary contusion		17	22
Hypertransfusion	5	24	36
Multiple fractures	5	8	11
Near drowning		66	33
Cardiopulmonary bypass	2		
Burns	2		

better defined in the 1980s, when Fowler and colleagues identified and monitored all patients who required mechanical ventilation with one of eight different conditions, including cardiopulmonary bypass, burns, bacteremia, hypertransfusion, multiple long bone or pelvic fractures, disseminated intravascular coagulation, severe pneumonia, and aspiration of gastric contents (5). In total, 88 patients developed ARDS, with an incidence ranging from 1.7% after cardiopulmonary bypass to 35.6% with pulmonary aspiration (Table 4). Pepe and colleagues performed a similar study and followed patients with a variety of diagnoses, including sepsis syndrome, aspiration of gastric contents, pulmonary contusion, hypertransfusion, and multiple fractures (9). The incidence of ARDS among these at-risk diagnoses ranged from 8% for major fractures to 38% with sepsis syndrome (Table 4). Both of these studies also reported that patients with multiple at-risk diagnoses were at a markedly increased risk for developing ARDS. Several years later, Hudson and colleagues reported similar incidences for the development of ARDS in critically ill patients (13).

As these epidemiological studies revealed, the majority of patients who are at increased risk for the development of ARDS can be classified into three common categories: pneumonia, nonpulmonary sepsis, and aspiration of gastric contents. In one large population cohort study, pneumonia, severe sepsis, and witnessed aspiration accounted for 93% of the patients who developed ALI (46%, 36%, 11%, respectively) (1). Major trauma was the fourth most common diagnosis associated with the development of ALI yet only responsible for 7% of these patients (1). Additional studies have identified secondary factors that were associated with an increased risk for the development of ARDS in trauma patients including long bone fractures, chest trauma, and the requirement of blood transfusion during resuscitation (35). The combination of abdominal and extremities injuries was also independently associated with the development of ARDS (36). More recently, patients following pulmonary resection surgery were reported to be at increased risk for the development of ARDS. In a study of 1139 patients who underwent lung surgery, 3.9% of the patients developed ALI or ARDS on average four days postoperatively (37). Over half of the operations were performed on patients with lung cancer. Because lung surgery is a relatively common procedure, this relatively low percentage still represented nearly one new ARDS patient every two months from pulmonary resection at a single institution.

Other investigators have suggested alternative methods of categorizing the various at-risk diagnoses including whether the lung injury occurs through direct (primary) or indirect (secondary) mechanisms (38–40). There are diverse causes of direct injury, including pneumonia, aspiration of gastric contents, and smoke inhalation. The etiologies of indirect lung injury are even more heterogeneous and include such diagnoses as nonpulmonary sepsis and multiple long bone or pelvic fractures. The importance of this differentiation between direct and indirect injury is supported by different respiratory mechanics and responsiveness to PEEP between these two groups of ARDS patients. In addition, CT scans from ARDS patients due to direct lung injury have a prevalence of consolidation as opposed to more prevalent edema and alveolar collapse in ARDS patients with an indirect source (39). However, it is unclear whether the differentiation of direct and indirect lung injury is useful clinically. In an analysis of patients enrolled into one of the ARDSnet trials, the efficacy of low tidal volume ventilation was similar among patients with different clinical risk factors (41).

A. Comorbidity, Demographics, and Incidence of ARDS

As the previous studies have demonstrated, only a percentage of patients with an at-risk diagnosis will eventually develop ARDS. Therefore, other factors must play a role in determining which of these patients met the diagnostic criteria for ARDS. Alcohol is one of the most commonly used drugs in the world, and has been reported to alter susceptibility for the development of ARDS. In one cohort study of 351 critically ill patients, 43% of the patients with a prior history of alcohol abuse developed ARDS, compared to 22% in those patients without a history of alcohol abuse (42). This initial association between alcohol abuse and an increased susceptibility for ARDS has been validated in several other populations including patients with septic shock, critically ill patients requiring blood transfusions, surgical patients after lung resection, and in one epidemiological survey of ICUs in the Netherlands (43–46).

Diabetes mellitus is another chronic medical condition that theoretically alters susceptibility for ARDS. A multitude of studies supports the theory that proinflammatory cytokines, and more specifically the activation and recruitment of circulating neutrophils into the lung parenchyma, are an integral component of the pathogenesis of ARDS. The same alterations in the inflammatory cascade that predispose diabetic patients to develop serious infections were hypothesized to be protective for the development of ARDS. One study identified 113 patients with septic shock, of whom 28% had a history of diabetes (47). In both univariate and multivariable analyses, the incidence of ARDS was significantly greater in the nondiabetic patients when compared to those with a history of diabetes. These results have been validated in a subsequent study of 688 patients at risk for the development of ARDS, with an odds ratio for the development of ARDS of 0.58 in patients with a history of diabetes (48).

Older patients have also been reported to be at an increased risk of developing ARDS. Trauma patients over 70 were twice as likely to develop ARDS when compared to the patients between 18 and 29 years (13). Increasing age has also been reported to have positive association with the development of ARDS in burn patients (49).

Several recent studies have reported that a delay in the initiation of specific therapies during the initial resuscitation period can also alter susceptibility for the development of ARDS. In a study of 160 patients with septic shock, delayed initiation of early

goal-directed therapy and antibiotic treatment during the first six hours were both independently associated with an increased risk for the development of ARDS (50). The delayed
implementation of low tidal volume ventilation has also been reported to be associated
with the development of ARDS. Several single center studies and one secondary analysis
of a large international survey have reported that the early use of high tidal volume is
associated with the subsequent development of ARDS (51–53). Finally, an association
between the transfusion of blood products and the development of ARDS has been recognized for many years. This phenomenon called transfusion-associated acute lung injury
(TRALI) is discussed in more depth in chapter 10. These important studies identify potential therapeutic strategies that can be implemented to decrease the incidence of ARDS and
possibly improve outcome of critically ill patients who are at risk for the development
of ARDS.

VI. Clinical Risk Factors for Mortality from ARDS

The cause of death for patients with ARDS has been traditionally divided into early causes
(within 72 hours) and late causes (after three days) (54). Most early deaths are attributed
to the original presenting illness or injury. Sepsis, persistent respiratory failure, and the
development of multiple organ system dysfunction are the most common causes of death
in ARDS patients who survive at least three days. Several secondary factors have been
reported to influence mortality in ARDS. Patients with a primary at-risk diagnosis of
sepsis have a higher mortality rate when compared to trauma patients (55–57). Long-
term survival after ARDS also appears to be dependent on the primary at-risk diagnosis.
Trauma patients with ARDS who survive to hospital discharge have an excellent prognosis
over the following two years. However, survivors of sepsis-induced ARDS continue to be
at an increased risk of dying after hospital discharge (58). This difference in long-term
survival may be due to the presence of more significant and chronic comorbidities in
those patients with sepsis-induced ARDS. In addition, patients with a direct cause of lung
injury have been reported to have a higher mortality rate when compared to indirect at-risk
diagnoses (59).

Age is also associated with mortality from ARDS as older patients are more likely
to die from ARDS when compared to younger patients. Zilberberg and Epstein demonstrated that age greater than 65 years was an independent predictor of hospital mortality
in a cohort of 107 medical patients with ARDS (60). A study of 221 ARDS patients in
Scandinavia demonstrated similar effects of age on ARDS and reported a risk ratio for
mortality of nearly 2.0 when patients were stratified by age >65 (2). An analysis of
the 902 patients enrolled in ARDS network studies showed that patients over 70 years
old were twice as likely to die even after adjustments for covariates. Older survivors
recovered from respiratory failure at similar rates but had greater difficulty weaning from
the ventilator (61).

Pre-existing medical conditions appear to have a dramatic impact on the mortality
from ARDS. Although patients with cirrhosis of the liver are predisposed to several of
the at-risk diagnoses for ARDS, such as sepsis, only a few reports have examined a
possible association between cirrhosis and the mortality from ARDS (62). Matuschak
and colleagues retrospectively examined 29 patients with severe liver disease awaiting
transplantation and reported that their incidence of ARDS was higher than a random
control group of ICU patients (63). Doyle and colleagues reported that the mortality from

ALI was increased in 26 medical patients with chronic liver disease when compared to ALI patients without liver disease (64). Finally, cirrhosis was identified as the single most important predictive variable of mortality in a cohort of 259 patients with ARDS (59). Similarly, patients with a history of HIV disease, active malignancy, and organ transplantation appear to be at increased of dying from ARDS (60). Though obesity has been associated with an increased risk of complications and death in certain hospitalized patients, an effect of obesity on outcome has not been consistently observed in patients with ARDS (65,66). In a study of patients enrolled into the ARDS network low tidal volume ventilator trial, obesity was not associated with an increased mortality (67). However, patients with severe obesity defined as a BMI > 40 kg/m^2 were not enrolled into the study and therefore could not be analyzed. In a subsequent study that did not exclude ARDS patients based on their BMI, severe obesity was not associated with increased mortality but was associated with prolonged mechanical ventilation and hospital length of stay (68). In addition, severely obese patients were more likely to be discharged to a rehabilitation or skilled nursing facility.

No single pulmonary-specific variable, including the severity of hypoxemia, has been found to predict the risk of death independently when measured early in the course of the ARDS (69). The ARDSnet trial reported that the patients with improved survival due to low tidal volume ventilation actually had a worse Pao_2/Fio_2 ratio when compared to high tidal volume group (28). In addition, several studies have reported that the mortality rate among patients with ALI (Pao_2/Fio_2 ratio ≤ 300) is similar to those patients with ARDS (Pao_2/Fio_2 ratio ≤ 200) (13,60,64). However, a model that included oxygenation index defined as (mean airway pressure $\times Pao_2/Fio_2$) on day 3, the age of the patient, and the presence of cardiovascular failure on day 3 did accurately predict mortality in a cohort of ARDS patients (70). Abnormalities of pulmonary blood flow and injury to the microcirculation in ARDS result in compromised pulmonary blood flow to well-ventilated areas of the lung resulting in an increase in the physiological dead space. Pulmonary dead space is the component of ventilation that is wasted because it does not participate in gas exchange, and an increase in dead space represents an impaired ability to excrete carbon dioxide. One study of 179 patients with ARDS demonstrated that mean dead-space fraction, measured with a bedside metabolic monitor, was markedly elevated early in the course of ARDS and elevated values were associated with an increased risk of death (71).

There are racial and gender differences in ARDS mortality in the United States (72). Using multiple-cause mortality data compiled by the National Center for Health Statistics, annual ARDS mortality rates have been continuously higher for males when compared to females and for African-Americans when compared to white decedents and decedents of other racial backgrounds. When decedents were stratified by race and gender, black males had the highest ARDS mortality rates in comparison to all other subgroups (mean annual mortality rate of 12.8 deaths per 100,000 black males). In addition, a higher percentage of the black ARDS decedents were reported in the youngest age categories, as 27% of the decedents who were less than 35 were black. More recently, Erickson and colleagues examined the effect of race and ethnicity on outcome in 2362 patients who had been enrolled into previous ARDS network studies. The results of this study revealed that black and Hispanic patients with ALI had a significantly higher risk of death compared to white patients. This increased risk appeared to be mediated by increased severity of illness at presentation for blacks, but was unexplained among Hispanics (73).

Finally, differences in the ICU organizational model and structure have been reported to affect outcome of ARDS patients (74). Patients who were cared for in closed ICUs, defined as units that require patient transfer or mandatory patient comanagment by an intensivist, had reduced hospital mortality with an odds ratio of 0.68. Consultation by a pulmonologist for patients care in an open ICU model was not associated with an improved mortality. One possible explanation for this observation may be the higher physician and nurse availability that was reported to be present in the closed ICUs.

VII. Conclusions

Since 1967 the diagnostic criteria used to define ARDS have evolved. However, it remains difficult to answer the question, "Who has diffuse alveolar damage and ARDS?" (75). The ARDS definition is still based on classic physiological and radiographic alterations. These criteria are subject to variable interpretations that likely account for some of the discrepancy in the epidemiology of ARDS from different centers (76). Other questions still remain, such as, "Is ARDS a homogeneous syndrome or the combination of several different disorders loosely bound together by common physiological and radiographic abnormalities?" Schuster suggested the following general definition of ARDS: "It is a specific form of lung injury in which structural changes (characterized pathologically as diffuse alveolar damage) and functional abnormalities (principally a breakdown in the alveolar-capillary barrier function) leading first to proteinaceous alveolar edema, and then (as a consequence) to altered respiratory system mechanics and hypoxemia" (75). We would add that ARDS is an inflammatory disease and that inflammation begets lung injury and subsequent structural change. Presently, there is no clinically useful biochemical marker of alveolar-capillary injury or inflammation that can be used as part of the diagnostic criteria of ARDS (30). As the pathogenesis of ARDS is more completely understood, certain biochemical tests may become available that remove the inherent subjectivity in the AECC definition of this syndrome. The identification of such an inflammatory mediator that functions as an extremely sensitive and specific marker in diagnosing ARDS would constitute a major advance in this field. Future definitions, based on biochemical or even genetic predisposition to inflammation rather than on physiological and radiographic parameters, are likely to provide more homogeneous groups of patients within the overall population of what is now called ALI (77). This should allow investigators to target subgroups of patients based on their specific pattern of an inflammatory response, opening the door to individualized therapy for ARDS.

References

1. Rubenfeld GD, Caldwell E, Peabody E, et al. Incidence and outcomes of acute lung injury. N Engl J Med 2005; 353:1685–1693.
2. Luhr OR, Antonsen K, Karlsson M, et al. Incidence and mortality after acute respiratory failure and acute respiratory distress syndrome in Sweden, Denmark, and Iceland. The ARF Study Group. Am J Respir Crit Care Med 1999; 159:1849–1861.
3. Rubenfeld GD, Caldwell ES, Steinberg KP, et al. Persistent lung injury and ICU resource utilization. Am J Respir Crit Care Med 1998; 157:A498.
4. Ashbaugh DG, Bigelow DB, Petty TL, et al. Acute respiratory distress in adults. Lancet 1967; 2:319–323.

5. Fowler AA, Hamman RF, Good JT, et al. Adult respiratory distress syndrome: risk with common predispositions. Ann Intern Med 1983; 98:593–597.
6. Kraus PA, Lipman J, Lee CC, et al. Acute lung injury at Baragwanath ICU. An eight-month audit and call for consensus for other organ failure in the adult respiratory distress syndrome. Chest 1993; 103:1832–1836.
7. Murray JF, Matthay MA, Luce JM, et al. An expanded definition of the adult respiratory distress syndrome. Am Rev Respir Dis 1988; 138:720–723.
8. Parsons PE, Giclas PC. The terminal complement complex (sC5b-9) is not specifically associated with the development of the adult respiratory distress syndrome. Am Rev Respir Dis 1990; 141:98–103.
9. Pepe PE, Potkin RT, Reus DH, et al. Clinical predictors of the adult respiratory distress syndrome. Am J Surg 1982; 144:124–130.
10. Rinaldo JE. The prognosis of the adult respiratory distress syndrome. Inappropriate pessimism? Chest 1986; 90:470–471.
11. Moss M, Parsons PE. What is the acute respiratory distress syndrome? J Intensive Care Med 1998; 13:59–67.
12. Sloane PJ, Gee MH, Gottlieb JE, et al. A multicenter registry of patients with acute respiratory distress syndrome. Physiology and outcome. Am Rev Respir Dis 1992; 146:419–426.
13. Hudson LD, Milberg JA, Anardi D, et al. Clinical risks for development of the acute respiratory distress syndrome. Am J Respir Crit Care Med 1995; 151:293–301.
14. Wheeler AP, Bernard GR, Thompson BT, et al. Pulmonary-artery versus central venous catheter to guide treatment of acute lung injury. N Engl J Med 2006; 354:2213–2224.
15. Sandham JD, Hull RD, Brant RF, et al. A randomized, controlled trial of the use of pulmonary-artery catheters in high-risk surgical patients. N Engl J Med 2003; 348:5–14.
16. Moss M, Goodman PL, Heinig M, et al. Establishing the relative accuracy of three new definitions of the adult respiratory distress syndrome. Crit Care Med 1995; 23:1629–1637.
17. Bernard GR, Artigas A, Brigham KL, et al. The American-European Consensus Conference on ARDS. Definitions, mechanisms, relevant outcomes, and clinical trial coordination. Am J Respir Crit Care Med 1994; 149:818–824.
18. Ferguson ND, Davis AM, Slutsky AS, et al. Development of a clinical definition for acute respiratory distress syndrome using the Delphi technique. J Crit Care 2005; 20:147–154.
19. Esteban A, Fernandez-Segoviano P, Frutos-Vivar F, et al. Comparison of clinical criteria for the acute respiratory distress syndrome with autopsy findings. Ann Intern Med 2004; 141:440–445.
20. Pinheiro BV, Muraoka FS, Assis RV, et al. Accuracy of clinical diagnosis of acute respiratory distress syndrome in comparison with autopsy findings. J Bras Pneumol 2007; 33:423–428.
21. Ferguson ND, Frutos-Vivar F, Esteban A, et al. Acute respiratory distress syndrome: underrecognition by clinicians and diagnostic accuracy of three clinical definitions. Crit Care Med 2005; 33:2228–2234.
22. Rubenfeld GD, Caldwell E, Granton J, et al. Interobserver variability in applying a radiographic definition for ARDS. Chest 1999; 116:1347–1353.
23. Beards SC, Jackson A, Hunt L, et al. Interobserver variation in the chest radiograph component of the lung injury score. Anaesthesia 1995; 50:928–932.
24. Meade MO, Cook RJ, Guyatt GH, et al. Interobserver variation in interpreting chest radiographs for the diagnosis of acute respiratory distress syndrome. Am J Respir Crit Care Med 2000; 161:85–90.
25. Medoff BD, Harris RS, Kesselman H, et al. Use of recruitment maneuvers and high-positive end-expiratory pressure in a patient with acute respiratory distress syndrome. Crit Care Med 2000; 28:1210–1216.
26. Estenssoro E, Dubin A, Laffaire E, et al. Impact of positive end-expiratory pressure on the definition of acute respiratory distress syndrome. Intensive Care Med 2003; 29:1936–1942.

27. Neff MJ, Caldwell ES, Hudson LD, et al. The effect of definition of left atrial hypertension (LAH) on identification of patients with acute lung injury (ALI). Am J Respir Crit Care Med 2001; 144:124–130.

28. The Acute Respiratory Distress Syndrome Network. Ventilation with lower tidal volumes as compared with traditional tidal volumes for acute lung injury and the acute respiratory distress syndrome. N Engl J Med 2000; 342:1301–1308.

29. Wiedemann HP, Wheeler AP, Bernard GR, et al. Comparison of two fluid-management strategies in acute lung injury. N Engl J Med 2006; 354:2564–2575.

30. Pittet JF, Mackersie RC, Martin TR, et al. Biological markers of acute lung injury: prognostic and pathogenetic significance. Am J Respir Crit Care Med 1997; 155:1187–1205.

31. Calandrino FS Jr., Anderson DJ, Mintun MA, et al. Pulmonary vascular permeability during the adult respiratory distress syndrome: a positron emission tomographic study. Am Rev Respir Dis 1988; 138:421–428.

32. Kaplan JD, Calandrino FS, Schuster DP. A positron emission tomographic comparison of pulmonary vascular permeability during the adult respiratory distress syndrome and pneumonia. Am Rev Respir Dis 1991; 143:150–154.

33. Martin GS, Eaton S, Mealer M, et al. Extravascular lung water in patients with severe sepsis: a prospective cohort study. Crit Care 2005; 9:R74–R82.

34. Gattinoni L, Caironi P. Refining ventilatory treatment for acute lung injury and acute respiratory distress syndrome. JAMA 2008; 299:691–693.

35. Navarrete-Navarro P, Rivera-Fernandez R, Rincon-Ferrari MD, et al. Early markers of acute respiratory distress syndrome development in severe trauma patients. J Crit Care 2006; 21: 253–258.

36. White TO, Jenkins PJ, Smith RD, et al. The epidemiology of posttraumatic adult respiratory distress syndrome. J Bone Joint Surg Am 2004; 86-A:2366–2376.

37. Kutlu CA, Williams EA, Evans TW, et al. Acute lung injury and acute respiratory distress syndrome after pulmonary resection. Ann Thorac Surg 2000; 69:376–380.

38. Gattinoni L, Pelosi P, Suter PM, et al. Acute respiratory distress syndrome caused by pulmonary and extrapulmonary disease. Different syndromes? Am J Respir Crit Care Med 1998; 158:3–11.

39. Pelosi P, Gattinoni L. Acute respiratory distress syndrome of pulmonary and extra-pulmonary origin: fancy or reality? Intensive Care Med 2001; 27:457–460.

40. Pelosi P, Caironi P, Gattinoni L. Pulmonary and extrapulmonary forms of acute respiratory distress syndrome. Semin Respir Crit Care Med 2001; 22:259–268.

41. Eisner MD, Thompson T, Hudson LD, et al. Efficacy of low tidal volume ventilation in patients with different clinical risk factors for acute lung injury and the acute respiratory distress syndrome. Am J Respir Crit Care Med 2001; 164:231–236.

42. Moss M, Bucher B, Moore FA, et al. The role of chronic alcohol abuse in the development of acute respiratory distress syndrome in adults. JAMA 1996; 275:50–54.

43. Gajic O, Rana R, Winters JL, et al. Transfusion-related acute lung injury in the critically ill: prospective nested case-control study. Am J Respir Crit Care Med 2007; 176: 886–891.

44. Licker M, de PM, Spiliopoulos A, et al. Risk factors for acute lung injury after thoracic surgery for lung cancer. Anesth Analg 2003; 97:1558–1565.

45. Moss M, Parsons P, Steinberg K, et al. Chronic alcohol abuse is associated with an increased incidence of ARDS and severity of multiple organ dysfunction in patients with septic shock. Crit Care Med 2003; 31:869–877.

46. Wind J, Versteegt J, Twisk J, et al. Epidemiology of acute lung injury and acute respiratory distress syndrome in The Netherlands: a survey. Respir Med 2007; 101:2091–2098.

47. Moss M, Guidot DM, Steinberg KP, et al. Diabetic patients have a decreased incidence of acute respiratory distress syndrome. Crit Care Med 2000; 28:2187–2192.

48. Gong MN, Thompson BT, Williams P, et al. Clinical predictors of and mortality in acute respiratory distress syndrome: potential role of red cell transfusion. Crit Care Med 2005; 33:1191–1198.

49. Dancey DR, Hayes J, Gomez M, et al. ARDS in patients with thermal injury. Intensive Care Med 1999; 25:1231–1236.

50. Iscimen R, Cartin-Ceba R, Yilmaz M, et al. Risk factors for the development of acute lung injury in patients with septic shock: an observational cohort study. Crit Care Med 2008; 36:1518–1522.

51. Gajic O, Frutos-Vivar F, Esteban A, et al. Ventilator settings as a risk factor for acute respiratory distress syndrome in mechanically ventilated patients. Intensive Care Med 2005; 31:922–926.

52. Mascia L, Zavala E, Bosma K, et al. High tidal volume is associated with the development of acute lung injury after severe brain injury: an international observational study. Crit Care Med 2007; 35:1815–1820.

53. Gajic O, Dara SI, Mendez JL, et al. Ventilator-associated lung injury in patients without acute lung injury at the onset of mechanical ventilation. Crit Care Med 2004; 32:1817–1824.

54. Montgomery AB, Stager MA, Carrico CJ, et al. Causes of mortality in patients with the adult respiratory distress syndrome. Am Rev Respir Dis 1985; 132:485–489.

55. Knaus WA, Sun X, Hakim RB, et al. Evaluation of definitions for adult respiratory distress syndrome. Am J Respir Crit Care Med 1994; 150:311–317.

56. Ciesla DJ, Moore EE, Johnson JL, et al. Decreased progression of postinjury lung dysfunction to the acute respiratory distress syndrome and multiple organ failure. Surgery 2006; 140: 640–647.

57. Calfee CS, Eisner MD, Ware LB, et al. Trauma-associated lung injury differs clinically and biologically from acute lung injury due to other clinical disorders. Crit Care Med 2007; 35:2243–2250.

58. Davidson TA, Rubenfeld GD, Caldwell ES, et al. The effect of acute respiratory distress syndrome on long-term survival. Am J Respir Crit Care Med 1999; 160:1838–1842.

59. Monchi M, Bellenfant F, Cariou A, et al. Early predictive factors of survival in the acute respiratory distress syndrome. A multivariate analysis. Am J Respir Crit Care Med 1998; 158:1076–1081.

60. Zilberberg MD, Epstein SK. Acute lung injury in the medical ICU: comorbid conditions, age, etiology, and hospital outcome. Am J Respir Crit Care Med 1998; 157:1159–1164.

61. Ely EW, Wheeler AP, Thompson BT, et al. Recovery rate and prognosis in older persons who develop acute lung injury and the acute respiratory distress syndrome. Ann Intern Med 2002; 136:25–36.

62. Wyke RJ. Problems of bacterial infection in patients with liver disease. Gut 1987; 28:623–641.

63. Matuschak GM, Shaw BW Jr. Adult respiratory distress syndrome associated with acute liver allograft rejection: resolution following hepatic retransplantation. Crit Care Med 1987; 15:878–881.

64. Doyle RL, Szaflarski N, Modin GW, et al. Identification of patients with acute lung injury. Predictors of mortality. Am J Respir Crit Care Med 1995; 152:1818–1824.

65. Flegal KM, Graubard BI, Williamson DF, et al. Excess deaths associated with underweight, overweight, and obesity. JAMA 2005; 293:1861–1867.

66. Flegal KM. Estimating the impact of obesity. Soz Praventivmed 2005; 50:73–74.

67. O'Brien JM Jr., Welsh CH, Fish RH, et al. Excess body weight is not independently associated with outcome in mechanically ventilated patients with acute lung injury. Ann Intern Med 2004; 140:338–345.

68. Morris AE, Stapleton RD, Rubenfeld GD, et al. The association between body mass index and clinical outcomes in acute lung injury. Chest 2007; 131:342–348.

69. Ware LB, Matthay MA. The acute respiratory distress syndrome. N Engl J Med 2000; 342:1334–1349.

70. Gajic O, Afessa B, Thompson BT, et al. Prediction of death and prolonged mechanical ventilation in acute lung injury. Crit Care 2007; 11:R53.
71. Nuckton TJ, Alonso JA, Kallet RH, et al. Pulmonary dead-space fraction as a risk factor for death in the acute respiratory distress syndrome. N Engl J Med 2002; 346:1281–1286.
72. Moss M, Mannino DM. Race and gender differences in acute respiratory distress syndrome deaths in the United States: an analysis of multiple-cause mortality data (1979–1996). Crit Care Med 2002; 30:1679–1685.
73. Erickson SE, Shlipak MG, Martin GS, et al. Racial and ethnic disparities in mortality from acute lung injury. J Crit Care 2008; 37:1–6.
74. Treggiari MM, Martin DP, Yanez ND, et al. Effect of intensive care unit organizational model and structure on outcomes in patients with acute lung injury. Am J Respir Crit Care Med 2007; 176:685–690.
75. Schuster DP. What is acute lung injury? What is ARDS? Chest 1995; 107:1721–1726.
76. Garber BG, Hebert PC, Yelle JD, et al. Adult respiratory distress syndrome: a systemic overview of incidence and risk factors. Crit Care Med 1996; 24:687–695.
77. Abraham E. Toward new definitions of acute respiratory distress syndrome. Crit Care Med 1999; 27:237–238.

2
Epidemiology of Acute Lung Injury: A Public Health Perspective

GORDON D. RUBENFELD
Program in Trauma, Emergency, and Critical Care, Department of Critical Care, Sunnybrook Health Sciences Centre, University of Toronto, Toronto, Ontario, Canada

MARGARET J. NEFF
Division of Pulmonary and Critical Care, Harborview Medical Center, University of Washington, Seattle, Washington, U.S.A.

I. Introduction

Critical care clinicians are drawn to practice in the intensive care unit by the physiological nature of critical illness and the application of physiological principles to the care of critically ill patients. We frequently consider the physiological derangements of acute lung injury (ALI): the gas exchange abnormalities, the abnormal thoracic compliance, and the response to positive end-expiratory pressure (PEEP). We have come to appreciate the immunological and tissue repair abnormalities seen in patients with ALI. More recently, we have been able to link pathophysiology with cellular mechanisms in the concept of ventilator-induced lung injury and ventilator-induced organ failure. The clinical epidemiology of ALI in terms of its diagnostic criteria, risk factors, and prognostic factors has also evolved (1). However, it is unusual for critical care clinicians and investigators to consider the public health impact of critical illness syndromes in general and ALI, in particular.

Public health professionals are less interested in the exact pathophysiological mechanism of disease and focus more on the disease's impact on the health of the public and on mechanisms for reducing this impact. This is a particularly important perspective on disease, if an unusual one for critical care. Understanding the public health implications of ALI places it in relation to other common diseases and helps to prioritize research and clinical funding. Understanding changes in the burden and outcome of illness tells us whether we are doing a better job at what ultimately matters: improving the health of the public. To address these questions about ALI and critical illness syndromes, answers to some basic epidemiological questions are needed. What is the incidence of ALI? What are the attributable mortality and morbidity of ALI? Are effective treatments or preventive interventions being implemented in the community? Is the incidence, outcome, or use of effective therapies changing over time?

These data are available for a variety of diseases. There are a number of population-based studies on the incidence and outcome of cardiovascular, pulmonary, infectious, and neoplastic diseases. In the United States, the National Center for Health Statistics maintains data on the incidence and mortality of hundreds of diseases (2). Similarly, the

Surveillance, Epidemiology, and End Results (SEER) Program of the National Cancer Institute maintains high-quality data on cancer incidence and survival from selected areas across the United States (3). In contrast, similar data are not readily available for sepsis, ALI, or multiple organ failure.

Studying the epidemiology of ALI is not easy and may explain the lack of data. It is a syndrome that is operationally defined by laboratory, radiological, and physiological criteria that themselves have not been well defined in terms of reliability and validity (4–7) (see chap. 1). Even the terminology can be confusing. We will adopt the North American-European Consensus Conference (AECC) nomenclature and use ALI as a comprehensive term for the syndrome and acute respiratory distress syndrome (ARDS) to refer to a specific subset with more severe hypoxemia (8). There is no diagnostic test for ALI similar to troponin in myocardial infarction or serology in infectious diseases. Discharge diagnostic codes that are used to study the epidemiology of many diseases are extremely inaccurate in ALI. Compared to chronic diseases such as cancer or asthma, ALI has a short duration and high mortality rate, which makes the number of prevalent cases available for study at any given time small. Despite these challenges, a growing body of literature exists to allow us to estimate the public health implications of ALI.

II. Incidence

The incidence of a disease is defined as the number of new cases divided by the population at risk of developing the disease multiplied by the period of time they were at risk. Prevalence is the number of existing cases at any given time divided by the population at risk for developing the disease. Because ALI is a disease of relatively short duration, incidence and prevalence will approximate each other. It is important to distinguish which population constitutes the denominator in the incidence calculation. For population-based estimates of incidence, this will be the entire community from which patients are admitted to the hospital where ALI might be diagnosed. In epidemiological studies of ALI a more convenient denominator is often used, for example, the "incidence" of ALI in the intensive care unit (ICU) population, in the population with acute respiratory failure, or in the population of patients with a known risk factor for ALI. These numbers are not useful, however, for estimating the population burden of ALI.

Incidence figures for ALI are important because they establish the importance of the disease to justify research and health care funding, allow tracking to explore trends in the disease, and provide data to study the potential explanations of differences in the incidence of the disease. The earliest incidence figure for ARDS is an often quoted 1972 National Heart, Lung, and Blood Institute (NHLBI) report estimate of 150,000 cases per year in the United States or about 75 per 10^5 person-years (9). Relatively few empirical estimates of the incidence of ALI or ARDS exist (10–13). Available empirical studies place the incidence of ARDS at much lower rates than expected by the NHLBI report: approximately 2 to 12 per 10^5 person-years (Table 1). Only one of these studies used the AECC definition for ALI. The others used more restrictive criteria, including more severe hypoxemia, a risk factor for ALI, and reduced thoracic compliance. These studies were also limited by a variety of factors: relatively short observation periods, the potential for missed cases due to lack of a standardized definition, lack of a generalizable study population, and estimates of population incidence made from a small number of hospitals.

Table 1 Selected ALI and ARDS Incidence Studies

Study location (sample time of study)	Definition	Incidence	References
Grand Canaria (1983–1985)	1. Risk 2. $Pao_2 < 55$ or $Fio_2 > 0.5$ with PEEP 5 and no improvement in 24 hr and also $Pao_2/Fio_2 < 150$ 3. Bilateral infiltrates 4. No clinical left atrial hypertension	1.5 per 10^5 person-years for $Pao_2/Fio_2 < 110$ 3.5 per 10^5 person-years for $Pao_2/Fio_2 < 150$ 10.6 per 10^5 person-years for acute respiratory failure	(14)
Utah (12 mo, 1989–1990)	1. $Pao_2/PA_2 \leq 0.2$ 2. Bilateral infiltrates 3. No clinical evidence of left atrial hypertension 4. Static thoracic compliance < 50 mL/cm H_2O	4.8–8.3 per 10^5 person-years for ARDS	(15)
Berlin (8 wk in 1991)	Severe lung injury: Murray–Matthay score > 2.5	3.0 per 10^5 person-years for severe lung injury 88.6 per 10^5 person-years for acute respiratory failure	(16)
Maryland (1995)	ICD-9 codes	10.5–14.2 per 10^5 person-years	(17)
Sweden, Denmark, Iceland (8 wk in 1997)	AECC criteria	17.9 per 10^5 person-years for ALI 13.5 per 10^5 person-years for ARDS 77.6 per 10^5 person-years for acute respiratory failure	(18)
King County Washington, U.S.A. (12 mo 1999–2000)	AECC criteria	86.2 per 10^5 person-years for ALI 64 per 10^5 person-years for ARDS	(19)

Several lines of reasoning suggest these incidence estimates are, at least for the United States, as much as an order of magnitude too low. Analysis of the incidence of known associated risk conditions yields incidence rates for ALI that are higher than these published estimates. For example, in all epidemiological series and clinical trials, sepsis and pneumonia are the most common risk factors for ALI. Recent data suggest that the incidence of severe sepsis in patients in ICUs is 150 per 10^5 person-years (Table 2) (20). Epidemiological studies and clinical trials suggest that 30–43% of patients with

Table 2 ARDS Incidence Estimated from Associated Conditions

Associated condition	Incidence of associated condition	Patients without risk who develop ARDS	Calculated incidence of ARDS
Severe sepsis	150 per 10^5 person-years[a]	30–43%[b]	45–64 per 10^5 person-years
Severe trauma (ISS[g] > 15)	44 per 10^5 person-years[c]	25–40%[d]	11–18 per 10^5 person-years
Acute respiratory failure	137 per 10^5 person-years[e]	18%[f]	25 per 10^5 person-years

[a]*Source*: From Ref. 20.
[b]*Source*: From Refs. 21, 22.
[c]*Source*: From Ref. 23.
[d]*Source*: From Refs. 21, 24.
[e]*Source*: From Ref. 25.
[f]*Source*: From Ref. 26.
[g]Injury severity score.

severe sepsis develop ARDS (21,22). Combining these data yields incidence estimates for sepsis-associated ARDS of 45 to 64 cases per 10^5 person-years. A similar calculation for severe trauma (injury severity score >15) yields incidence rates for ARDS of 11 to 18 per 10^5 person-years associated with trauma alone. These estimates are conservative for the incidence of ALI because they do not include an estimate of the number of patients who meet the less strict hypoxemia criterion for ALI and do not include patients who develop lung injury from causes other than sepsis or trauma, for example, inhalation injuries, aspiration, and burns.

Several recent sources corroborate these higher incidence rates. Moss and coworkers analyzed national death data and, relying on ICD-9 coding, arrived at a figure of 19,460 deaths associated with ARDS in 1993 in the United States (1). Assuming a mortality rate for ARDS of approximately 40%, this yields a case incidence rate of 26 per 10^5 person-years. Goss and coworkers combined screening log data from the ARDS Network multicenter clinical trial with data on U.S. hospitals to arrive at ALI incidence rates of 45 to 65 per 10^5 person-years even assuming that ALI cases only occurred in hospitals with more than 20 ICU beds (27). Recently, epidemiologic data from a regional study in King County, Washington, using the AECC criteria for ALI have also validated these higher incidence rates for ALI, at least in the United States (19).

Finally, two recent studies have examined the incidence of ALI in Scandinavia and Berlin. Lewandowski and coworkers studied acute respiratory failure during a two-month period in Berlin in 1991 (16). They defined acute respiratory failure as intubation and mechanical ventilation of >24 hours. The incidence of acute respiratory failure was 88 per 10^5 person-years. The authors used a scoring system to categorize the severity of patients' lung injury, making direct comparison to the AECC criteria difficult. Patients with ALI by AECC criteria could have a score as low as 0.75 (1 point for $Pao_2/Fio_2 < 300$ and 2 points for two quadrants of radiographic opacity without receiving points for PEEP or compliance, which are not in the AECC definition). Using this cutoff and excluding 108 patients in the study with cardiogenic shock or cardiogenic edema leaves an incidence of 48 cases of ALI per 10^5 person-years. Luhr and coworkers (18) used similar methods to study the incidence of ALI and ARDS in 132 ICUs in Scandinavia over an eight-week period and found incidences of acute respiratory failure, ALI, and ARDS of 77.6, 17.9, and 13.5 per 10^5 person-years, respectively.

Despite the difficulties in comparing the incidence of ALI across these studies, two striking and consistent findings emerge. The incidence of ALI appears to be significantly higher than the 2 to 12 per 10^5 person-years rates previously estimated for ARDS. These studies indicate that all forms of acute respiratory failure have a high mortality rate. The overall mortality rate for acute respiratory failure was 43% in the Berlin study and 41% in the Scandinavian study. In both studies, patients with acute respiratory failure, regardless of etiology, had similar mortality to patients with ALI.

There is little support in the available data for a single incidence value for ALI. Variability in incidence rates between studies can reflect chance, true variability, or simply methodological differences. None of the existing studies on the population incidence of ALI use comparable methods or definitions: therefore, direct comparison of incidence rates is difficult. The studies used various observation periods, used different definitions for ALI and ARDS, and relied on varying degrees of quality control for case identification and data integrity. Given the evidence of interobserver variability in clinician radiographic interpretation and diagnosis of ALI (5,6), rigorous protocolized case identification is necessary in epidemiological studies of ALI. True variability in incidence is a potential explanation of the existing studies. No single number reflects the incidence rate for myocardial infarction, colon cancer, or motor vehicle collisions, and we should not expect a single incidence figure for ALI.

Potential explanations for this variability include differences in the incidence of risk factors, susceptibility (including genetic variation), and health care utilization. For example, differences in smoking, use of motor vehicles, population density, incidence of respiratory infections, and genetic factors might all influence geographic variability in the incidence of ALI. An interesting and unexplored source of variation is the effect of health care resource use on ALI incidence. Even within the United States there is wide variability in the number of hospital beds and ICU beds, emergency medical response time, and other medical resources. These may influence the observed incidence of ALI in two ways. To be diagnosed with ALI, patients must survive long enough to be admitted to an ICU, there must be an ICU bed to be admitted to, and they must have an arterial blood gas and a chest radiograph. Limited access to ICU care, implicit or explicit restriction of intensive care, or differences in emergency medical response time may reduce the number of observed cases of ALI. Similarly, the extent to which a region provides aggressive medical and surgical treatments may also affect the number of cases of ALI. For example, organ and bone marrow transplantation, coronary bypass grafting, and intensive chemotherapy all are associated with ALI, and countries that provide greater access to these treatments may have more cases of lung injury (28–30).

III. Attributable Mortality

Attributable mortality is relatively easy to define mathematically: it is the difference in mortality rates between patients with a disease or exposure and those without. Practically, it is much more difficult to attribute a given death to a specific disease. A 68-year-old man who is an alcoholic is severely injured in a motor vehicle crash and develops ALI. After 14 days of progressive organ failure, life-sustaining treatment is withdrawn at the request of the patient's family. Is the patient's death attributable to alcoholism? To motor vehicle trauma? To ARDS? To multiple organ failure? To the decision to withdraw medical therapy? To address these complexities, it is helpful to think of attributable mortality in two categories: as deaths associated with the disease and as deaths caused by the disease that could be prevented by some therapy or intervention. The former is much easier to calculate although the latter is more important for public health purposes.

A. Attributable Short-Term Mortality

Mortality rates attributed to various diseases and reported in cause-of-death tables are calculated based on death records and generally reflect deaths associated with the disease. Attributable mortality associated with ALI can be calculated by multiplying the incidence rate times the mortality rate from the disease. The U.S. adult population (over age 15) in 2000 was 215 million. While the above discussion indicates that the incidence of ALI in the United States has not been described, it is reasonable, based on the studies cited above, to estimate it at between 20 and 50 cases per 10^5 person-years, or 43,000 to 107,000 cases per year. Assuming the mortality rate of approximately 40% observed in the recent studies of acute respiratory failure, 17,000 to 43,000 deaths per year are associated with ALI. Although the figures are arrived at by different methods, it is important to place these numbers into context with other diseases with important public health impact (Table 3).

Many efforts have been undertaken to try to identify those at risk for death. A recent study of a population-based cohort of ALI patients revealed similar predictors of mortality in ALI patients as were seen in the overall ICU population (32). Another study exploring the influence of race and ethnicity on mortality found that black and Hispanic patients with ALI had a significantly higher risk of death compared to white patients (33). One of the surprising observations from recent epidemiological studies in ALI is the similar mortality, approximately 40%, that exists among the following different categories of respiratory failure: (1) patients with ARDS, (2) patients with ALI who meet other criteria for ARDS but with less severe hypoxemia ($200 < \mathrm{Pao_2/Fio_2} < 300$), and (3) patients with acute respiratory failure (intubation and mechanical ventilation >24 hours regardless of etiology, radiograph, or degree of hypoxemia) (26,34). This observation provides little

Table 3 Attributable Mortality for Acute Lung Injury, Acute Respiratory Failure, and Comparison Diseases

Disease	Attributable mortality
ALI[a]	17,000–43,000
Acute respiratory failure[b]	60,000–120,000
Acute myocardial infarction[c]	199,454
Breast cancer[c]	41,528
HIV disease[c]	14,802
Asthma[c]	4657

[a]Assumes incidence range of 20 to 50 per 10^5 person-years, mortality of 40%, and U.S. 2000 census population of 215 million > age 15.
[b]Assumes incidence range of 70 to 140 per 10^5 person-years, mortality of 40%, and U.S. 2000 census population of 215 million > age 15.
[c]Based on U.S. 1999 death certificate data (31).

insight into disease mechanisms in this heterogeneous population, but it has significant implications for public health. The incidence of acute respiratory failure is estimated at between 70 and 140 per 10^5 person-years. If 40% of these patients die, then up to 120,000 adult deaths per year are associated with mechanical ventilation. Even small reductions in the mortality or morbidity associated with mechanical ventilation would have significant implications for the public health.

Identifying the independent or causal contribution of ALI to mortality is much more difficult. Two options exist for identifying this figure. By examining observational epidemiological data, one can try to control for other factors associated with mortality and estimate the independent effect of ALI on mortality. This is an important analysis because it is possible that ALI is merely a marker of severity of illness and contributes little on its own to mortality. These are difficult studies to do because they require identifying a cohort of critically ill patients, only a minority of whom will develop lung injury, and following them to compare mortality. The study by Hudson and coworkers attempted to control for this by the epidemiological technique of restriction (21). By comparing patients with ARDS to those at similar risk who did not develop ARDS, they showed that ARDS increased the mortality rate in all risk conditions by an average of 3.3-fold. This ranged from a relative risk for death attributed to ARDS of 1.4 in sepsis to 4.3 in trauma to 8.6 in drug overdose. The authors further controlled for Acute Physiology and Chronic Health Evaluation (APACHE) in the septic patients and injury severity in the trauma patients without a significant effect on the attributable mortality. The evidence linking mortality to ALI is not uniform and may be risk factor dependent. After adjusting for age, severity of illness, and injury severity, ALI was not statistically significantly associated with mortality in patients sustaining severe trauma. The signal was particularly attenuated after excluding patients who died in the first 24 hours from their initial injury (35).

More compelling evidence of the attributable and preventable deaths in ALI would be reduction in mortality from an effective intervention to prevent ALI or to prevent death after ALI. No interventions have been shown to prevent ALI; however, recent data from two studies suggest that a ventilator strategy can reduce mortality in ALI by a risk difference of 8.8–33% (36,37). These data can be analyzed in light of the findings in Table 3 to estimate that 3800 to 35,000 deaths annually could be prevented in the United States by implementing lung-protective ventilation in ALI, depending on its incidence and the benefits of lung-protective ventilation beyond the clinical trial population (38,39).

A number of epidemiologic studies and meta-analyses of studies suggested that short-term mortality in ALI had been decreasing (40). These are challenging data, though, because no clear strategies for reducing mortality from ALI had been identified during the time period of those studies. A recent thorough meta-analysis that accounted for study type and year found that the mortality reduction being reported occurred before a consensus definition for the syndrome appeared (1994) and was limited to observational studies, suggesting that the "advances" in improved ALI outcome were more definitional than clinical (41).

B. Attributable Long-Term Mortality

There is growing interest in the effects of critical illness syndromes on long-term outcomes. The methodological challenges are similar to those encountered in establishing attributable short-term mortality rates. Trying to separate the independent and causal effect of ALI on long-term mortality from the effects of the risk factors that cause or are associated with ALI is a challenge. Two studies have documented an effect of sepsis on long-term survival. A study by Quartin and coworkers showed that, even after controlling for age and comorbidity using ICD-9 diagnostic codes, patients with sepsis have a higher mortality rate than control patients (42). Among patients who survive for a year, those who had an episode of sepsis have an approximately 1.5 times greater rate of death than similar patients without an episode of sepsis. Patients who survive for 30 days after sepsis still have a median survival that is reduced from 6.24 to 2.35 years. Concerns about this study relate to the quality of the ICD-9 coding of comorbidities and the possibility that patients who have been admitted to the hospital for a severe illness like sepsis have more comorbidities coded than controls.

A number of studies have followed ALI and ARDS patients beyond hospital discharge to explore the long-term survival in patients with lung injury. For example, a study of relatively young (mean age 48) and previously healthy ARDS patients enrolled in a clinical trial of inhaled nitric oxide showed that survivors of ARDS continued to accrue mortality from day 28 after ARDS until about day 180, where the mortality rate stabilized (43). However, these data cannot be used to assess attributable mortality of ARDS since it does not include control patients. Only one study has compared long-term survival in patients who survived to hospital discharge and compared it to controls matched on severity of sepsis or trauma (44). Patients with sepsis had reduced long-term survival compared to patients with trauma, regardless of the presence of ARDS; however, there was no independent effect of ARDS on long-term mortality when the analysis was restricted to patients who survived to hospital discharge. This study was limited by two factors. It was a relatively small study, so important effects of ARDS on long-term mortality may have been missed, and the authors could not completely exclude the possibility that the controls had some mild component of ALI. Nevertheless, the best current evidence suggests that ALI does not independently worsen long-term survival in patients who survive to hospital discharge. Importantly, this study found that 80% of all deaths occurred in the hospital, 77% of all deaths occurred by day 30 after the onset of ARDS, and 89% of all deaths occurred by day 100 after the onset of ARDS.

IV. Attributable Morbidity

If, as recent clinical evidence suggests, mortality after ALI is declining and, in some subgroups, may be as low as 20%, then the morbidity incurred by survivors of ALI becomes an increasingly significant clinical issue. We can estimate this burden by calculating the number of ALI five-year survivors in the U.S. health care system. Assuming that there are 107,500 cases of ALI per year (215 million adults × 50 cases/100,000 person-year) (Table 3), that 70% of patients with ALI survive their acute illness, and that all patients with trauma-associated ALI and 50% of sepsis associated-ALI survive for five years, then more than 280,000 ALI survivors are alive in the United States. This conservative estimate excludes all survivors whose ALI occurred more than 5 years ago. As we improve our acute care to critically ill patients, we must address the health care sequelae of the large group of ALI survivors we are creating. While information about the late outcomes of critical illness is growing, this is an evolving field with relatively few data particularly regarding mechanisms and treatments. The same methodological limitations apply to identifying the attributable effect of ALI on morbidity as was noted for its effect on mortality.

A. Attributable Effect of ALI on Functional Status

For the purposes of this discussion, functional status refers to objective and physiological measures of performances after an episode of ALI. This includes pulmonary function, gas exchange, exercise tolerance, and cognitive performance. A number of investigators have studied pulmonary function in survivors of ALI. Pulmonary function appears to be severely abnormal within one month of ALI onset. The abnormalities are primarily restrictive, although obstructive abnormalities have been reported (45). This is followed by a period of rapid improvement in pulmonary function of over three to six months. After approximately six months, most of the improvement that will occur has occurred. The majority of patients are left with little measurable pulmonary dysfunction except for a reduced diffusing capacity of the lung for carbon monoxide (DLCO). A small minority has a persistent severe restrictive defect. These physiological data are corroborated by similar changes in radiographic studies (46,47). Although it seems reasonable to assume that pulmonary function abnormalities are attributable to the parenchymal and vascular pathology of ALI, there are no studies comparing pulmonary function in ALI patients to a similar control group that tests this hypothesis. It is possible that diffusion abnormalities and restrictive disease in ALI survivors are due to the combination of a slowly resolving endothelial injury and critical illness polyneuropathy that are sequelae of systemic inflammation and have nothing to do with lung injury.

There is a growing body of literature demonstrating acute cognitive impairment in critically ill patients (48,49). However, the mechanism, persistence, and relationship to ALI, hypoxemia, or duration of mechanical ventilation are unclear. At one year, the majority of ALI survivors have impaired memory, attention, concentration, and/or decreased mental processing speed (50). The extent to which these cognitive abnormalities are attributable to ALI or to risk conditions is unknown, but they reflect significant morbidity in these patients.

B. Attributable Effect of ALI on Psychiatric Outcomes and Quality of Life

To an ALI survivor, quality of life is as important as any specific physical or functional parameter. Potential problems were initially appreciated only anecdotally as clinicians saw ALI survivors in follow-up and heard their patients describe depression or difficulty at work or with relationships. Subsequently, these outcomes have been more formally studied by means of standardized questionnaires and tools (45,51). Hopkins and coworkers confirmed results seen by other investigators who interviewed ALI survivors using the Medical Outcomes Study 36-item, short form health survey (SF-36) (50). ALI survivors showed continued poor scores when tested at one year in the categories of role emotional, mental health, bodily pain, and general health. Davidson and coworkers evaluated quality-of-life measures in ALI survivors as compared to matched critically ill controls who had not developed ALI and found worse results in the domains of physical functioning, general health, and vitality when measured on average two years after hospitalization (52). While the degree of impairment was not as profound as for patients with other severe lung diseases, many of these patients still found it difficult to function fully and to return to work.

In most studies and clinical reports, patients described feelings of fatigue, memory loss, depression, and fear of relapse. In fact, Weinert and coworkers found that over 75% of survivors had scores on a depression scale that qualified for a diagnosis of depression during the first 15 months after ALI (53). In addition, another study revealed that over 50% of a cohort of critically ill patients transferred to a long-term acute care facility were prescribed an antidepressant (54). While historically studied in people who have suffered from trauma or war experiences, post-traumatic stress disorder (PTSD) is a similarly important mental health assessment in critically ill patients. Many clinicians have questioned whether patients suffered from memories of their ICU experience, but except for anecdotes few data have been available. However, Schelling and coworkers have studied this issue using tools such as the SF-36 and the Post-Traumatic Stress Syndrome-10 (55). Of the 80 patients studied, there was evidence of PTSD in one-third of the patient population approximately four years posthospitalization. A higher prevalence of PTSD, anxiety, and depression was also seen in a systematic review of ALI patients (56). Patients with pneumonia as a risk factor for ALI tend to have worse health-related quality of life than patients with sepsis or trauma, although the patients spent similar time in the ICU and on mechanical ventilation (57). These remain important outcomes to be incorporated into the future clinical trials of ALI and to be studied among current survivors of ALI. Whether other aspects of the patient's hospitalization, for example, hypoxemia or level of sedation, may be associated with the development of depression or PTSD is unknown but is important to explore as we try to optimize the physical and mental well-being of ALI survivors.

V. Effect of Aging Population

Age is a complex "exposure" variable. Like gender or race, it is a surrogate marker for a variety of other social and biological exposures. Identifying an association between age and other variables sheds little light on the causal factors associated with age that may actually be driving the relationship. Because age is strongly associated with the decision to admit patients to the ICU and to withdraw life-sustaining treatments in the ICU, the relationships between age and other variables are confounded by these physician decisions. Similarly, associations between age and other variables may not reflect an effect of age, per se, but of other variables that are frequently associated with age. For example, while age is crudely associated with mortality in many studies of critical illness, the effect disappears or is mitigated when comorbidities are accounted for (58). Therefore, the effect of age alone is less than the effect of diabetes, heart failure, and malnutrition that occur more frequently in the elderly than in other populations.

These mechanistic issues are of less concern to the public health epidemiologist. Regardless of the mechanism, if older people are at greater risk of developing ALI or at greater risk of mortality and morbidity from ALI, then age is an important factor in the clinical epidemiology of the disease. It is particularly important given the realities of the aging population in the United States. By the year 2030, the proportion of people over the age of 65 will double to 20% of the population, with approximately 71 million people in this age group (59). There are relatively few data to model the effect of an aging population on the incidence and mortality from ALI. We know that the incidence of risk factors for ALI including sepsis and pneumonia increases with age (60). Older patients are also at greater risk of developing ALI after trauma, even after controlling for severity of injury (61). The effect of age on mortality in patients with ALI has recently been studied. Older patients with ALI are at significantly higher risk of death even after controlling for severity of illness and comorbidity (62,63). If the age-specific mortality and incidence rates of ALI in the United States remain stable, we can expect an additional

114,000 cases of ALI per year by 2030 with 59% of those cases occurring in patients over the age of 65 (calculations by authors using data from Ref. (19)).

VI. Pediatrics

ALI is not unique to the adult population. A similar clinical picture is seen among pediatric patients but is not well described. In talking about pediatric ALI, a distinction must first be made from neonatal respiratory distress syndrome (RDS) or hyaline membrane disease that is due to surfactant deficiency in neonates. This is in contrast to the mechanism in ALI where the surfactant may be present (or perhaps reduced) but is dysfunctional. ALI in children is felt to represent the same pathophysiological process as is seen in adults, but less is known about its risk factors, outcomes, and incidence. Most studies have represented single-site descriptions of their patient populations and outcomes (64–67). True incidence studies, where the total number of children at risk for the disease is truly known, have not been done. Most descriptions of pediatric ALI have defined a minimal age (e.g., one month), excluded congenital heart disease, and identified clinical criteria required to be diagnosed with ALI. These criteria have not been uniformly agreed upon but include some combination of radiographic abnormalities and hypoxemia.

Risk factors include those for ALI in adults but have not been rigorously studied. It is unknown if children with certain predisposing risks have better outcomes from ARDS. Also of interest to clinicians and investigators is identifying predictors of outcome. Airway pressures, degree of hypoxemia, and oxygen index have been used to try to predict who might benefit from extracorporeal membrane oxygenation and who might be at high risk of dying. Common among most published reports is a mortality rate of approximately 60%, considerably higher than the 30–40% currently quoted for adults with ALI. Unknown for children with ALI is whether their deaths are primarily due to respiratory failure, multiorgan failure, or central nervous system damage. While increasing interest is focused on functional and quality-of-life outcomes in adults, more work is needed to evaluate such outcomes as school performance, learning disabilities, or socialization problems in children. Much remains to be studied in this field, and a good understanding of the epidemiology of the disease including a standard definition will likely help. Particularly important will be risk factor identification in an attempt to impact the frequency of the disease in the same way that successful injury prevention programs (e.g., distribution of bike helmets and booster seats) have reduced unintentional injuries in children.

VII. Conclusions

ALI continues to challenge clinicians and investigators both in understanding the disease itself and in providing care destined to improve survival and long-term outcomes. While focusing on an individual patient's outcome is critically important, equally meaningful is the continued study of the epidemiology of this disease and, as a consequence, its impact on public health as a whole. Even if conservative estimates of the incidence of ALI in adults are used, this disease process is associated with up to 43,000 deaths per year in the United States. While research and clinical trials have led to new approaches to managing ALI patients that have positively impacted mortality, the study of long-term physical and emotional functioning has just begun. As clinicians see more and more survivors of ALI, issues such as pulmonary function, depression, and PTSD will become more prominent.

Finally, additional study is also needed to better understand the impact of ALI in special patient populations, such as in children and the elderly.

References

1. TenHoor T, Mannino DM, Moss M. Risk factors for ARDS in the United States: analysis of the 1993 National Mortality Followback Study. Chest 2001; 119:1179–1184.
2. National Vital Statistics Reports. http://www.cdc.gov/nchs/fastats (accessed September 2008).
3. National Cancer Institute. Surveillance, Epidemiology, and End Results Program. http://seer.cancer.gov (accessed September 2008).
4. American Educational Research Association, American Psychological Association, National Council on Measurement in Education, and Joint Committee on Standards for Educational and Psychological Testing (U.S.). Standards for educational and psychological testing. Washington, D.C.: American Educational Research Association, 1999: ix, 194.
5. Meade MO, Cook RJ, Guyatt GH, et al. Interobserver variation in interpreting chest radiographs for the diagnosis of acute respiratory distress syndrome. Am J Respir Crit Care Med 2000; 161:85–90.
6. Rubenfeld GD, Caldwell E, Granton J, et al. Interobserver variability in applying a radiographic definition for ARDS. Chest 1999; 116:1347–1353.
7. Moss M, Goodman PL, Heinig M, et al. Establishing the relative accuracy of three new definitions of the adult respiratory distress syndrome. Crit Care Med 1995; 23:1629–1637.
8. Bernard GR, Artigas A, Brigham KL, et al. The American-European Consensus Conference on acute respiratory distress syndrome. Definitions, mechanisms, relevant outcomes, and clinical trial coordination. Am J Respir Crit Care Med 1994; 149:818–824.
9. National Heart and Lung Institutes. Task Force Report on Problems, Research Approaches, Needs. Washington, D.C.: U.S. Government Printing Office, 1972:167–180.
10. Webster NR, Cohen AT, Nunn JF. Adult respiratory distress syndrome–how many cases in the UK? Anaesthesia 1988; 43:923–926.
11. Zaccardelli DS, Pattishall EN. Clinical diagnostic criteria of the adult respiratory distress syndrome in the intensive care unit. Crit Care Med 1996; 24:247–251.
12. Garber BG, H'Ebert PC, Yelle JD, et al. Adult respiratory distress syndrome: a systemic overview of incidence and risk factors. Crit Care Med 1996; 24:687–695.
13. Luce JM. Acute lung injury and the acute respiratory distress syndrome. Crit Care Med 1998; 26:369–376.
14. Villar J, Slutsky AS. The incidence of the adult respiratory distress syndrome. Am Rev Respir Dis 1989; 140:814–816.
15. Thomsen GE, Morris AH. Incidence of the adult respiratory distress syndrome in the state of Utah. Am J Respir Crit Care Med 1995; 152:965–971.
16. Lewandowski K, Metz J, Deutschmann C, et al. Incidence, severity, and mortality of acute respiratory failure in Berlin, Germany. Am J Respir Crit Care Med 1995; 151:1121–1125.
17. Reynolds HN, McCunn M, Borg U, et al. Acute respiratory distress syndrome: estimated incidence and mortality rate in a 5 million-person population base. Crit Care 1998; 2(1): 29–34.
18. Luhr OR, Antonsen K, Karlsson M, et al. Incidence and mortality after acute respiratory failure and acute respiratory distress syndrome in Sweden, Denmark, and Iceland. The ARF Study Group. Am J Respir Crit Care Med 1999; 159:1849–1861.
19. Rubenfeld GD, Caldwell E, Peabody E, et al. Incidence and outcomes of acute lung injury. N Engl J Med 2005; 353:1685–1693.
20. Angus DC, Linde-Zwirble WT, Lidicker J, et al. Epidemiology of severe sepsis in the United States: analysis of incidence, outcome, and associated costs of care. Crit Care Med 2001; 29:1303–1310.

21. Hudson LD, Milberg JA, Anardi D, et al. Clinical risks for development of the acute respiratory distress syndrome. Am J Respir Crit Care Med 1995; 151:293–301.

22. Bernard GR, Wheeler AP, Russell JA, et al. The effects of ibuprofen on the physiology and survival of patients with sepsis. The Ibuprofen in Sepsis Study Group. N Engl J Med 1997; 336:912–918.

23. National Center for Injury Prevention and Control. Scientific Data, Surveillance, and Injury Statistics. http://www.cdc.gov/injury (accessed February 2009).

24. Rainer TH, Lam PK, Wong EM, et al. Derivation of a prediction rule for post-traumatic acute lung injury. Resuscitation 1999; 42:187–196.

25. Behrendt CE. Acute respiratory failure in the United States: incidence and 31-day survival. Chest 2000; 118:1100–1105.

26. Roupie E, Lepage E, Wysocki M, et al. Prevalence, etiologies and outcome of the acute respiratory distress syndrome among hypoxemic ventilated patients. SRLF Collaborative Group on Mechanical Ventilation. Societe de Reanimation Langue Francaise. Intensive Care Med 1999; 25:920–929.

27. Goss CH, Brower RG, Hudson LD, et al. Incidence of acute lung injury in the United States. Crit Care Med 2003; 31:1607–1611.

28. Demertzis S, Haverich A. Adult respiratory distress syndrome and lung transplantation. J Heart Lung Transplant 1993; 12:878–879.

29. Kress JP, Christenson J, Pohlman AS, et al. Outcomes of critically ill cancer patients in a university hospital setting. Am J Respir Crit Care Med 1999; 160:1957–1961.

30. Winer-Muram HT, Gurney JW, Bozeman PM, et al. Pulmonary complications after bone marrow transplantation. Radiol Clin North Am 1996; 34:97–117.

31. Hoyert DL, Arias E, Smith BL, et al. Deaths: final data for 1999. Natl Vital Stat Rep 2001; 49:1–113.

32. Cook CR, Kahn JM, Caldwell E, et al. Predictors of hospital mortality in a population-based cohort of patients with acute lung injury. Crit Care Med 2008; 36:1412–1420.

33. Erickson SE, Shilpak MG, Martin GS, et al. Racial and ethnic disparities in mortality from acute lung injury. Crit Care Med 2009; 37:1–6.

34. Milberg JA, Davis DR, Steinberg KP, et al. Improved survival of patients with acute respiratory distress syndrome (ARDS): 1983–1993. JAMA 1995; 273:306–309.

35. Treggiari MM, Hudson LD, Martin DP, et al. Effect of acute lung injury and acute respiratory distress syndrome on outcome in critically ill trauma patients. Crit Care Med 2004; 32: 327–331.

36. Amato MB, Barbas CS, Medeiros DM, et al. Effect of a protective-ventilation strategy on mortality in the acute respiratory distress syndrome. N Engl J Med 1998; 338:347–354.

37. Acute Respiratory Distress Syndrome Network. Ventilation with lower tidal volumes as compared with traditional tidal volumes for acute lung injury and the acute respiratory distress syndrome. N Engl J Med 2000; 342(18):1301–1308.

38. Rothman KJ. Modern Epidemiology, 2nd ed. Philadelphia, PA: Lippincott-Raven, 1998.

39. Gordis L. Epidemiology. Philadelphia, PA: W.B. Saunders Company, 1996.

40. Zambon M, Vincent JL. Mortality rates for patients with acute lung injury/ARDS have decreased over time. Chest 2008; 133:1120–1127.

41. Phua J, Badia JR, Adhikari NK, et al. Has mortality from acute respiratory distress syndrome decreased over time? A systematic review. Am J Respir Crit Care Med 2009; 179:220–227.

42. Quartin AA, Schein RM, Kett DH, et al. Magnitude and duration of the effect of sepsis on survival. Department of Veterans Affairs Systemic Sepsis Cooperative Studies Group. JAMA 1997; 277:1058–1063.

43. Angus DC, Musthafa AA, Clermont G, et al. Quality-adjusted survival in the first year after the acute respiratory distress syndrome. Am J Respir Crit Care Med 2001; 163(6): 1389–1394.

44. Davidson TA, Rubenfeld GD, Caldwell ES, et al. The effect of acute respiratory distress syndrome on long-term survival. Am J Respir Crit Care Med 1999; 160:1838–1842.
45. McHugh LG, Milberg JA, Whitcomb ME, et al. Recovery of function in survivors of the acute respiratory distress syndrome. Am J Respir Crit Care Med 1994; 150:90–94.
46. Lakshminarayan S, Stanford RE, Petty TI. Prognosis after recovery from adult respiratory distress syndrome. Am Rev Respir Dis 1976; 113:7–16.
47. Desai SR, Wells AU, Rubens MB, et al. Acute respiratory distress syndrome: CT abnormalities at long-term follow-up. Radiology 1999; 210:29–35.
48. Ely EW, Inouye SK, Bernard GR, et al. Delirium in mechanically ventilated patients: validity and reliability of the confusion assessment method for the intensive care unit (CAM-ICU). JAMA 2001; 286:2703–2710.
49. Ely EW, Margolin R, Francis J, et al. Evaluation of delirium in critically ill patients: validation of the Confusion Assessment Method for the Intensive Care Unit (CAM-ICU). Crit Care Med 2001; 29:1370–1379.
50. Hopkins RO, Weaver LK, Pope D, et al. Neuropsychological sequelae and impaired health status in survivors of severe acute respiratory distress syndrome. Am J Respir Crit Care Med 1999; 160:50–56.
51. McSweeny AJ, Grant I, Heaton RK, et al. Life quality of patients with chronic obstructive pulmonary disease. Arch Intern Med 1982; 142:473–478.
52. Davidson TA, Caldwell ES, Curtis JR, et al. Reduced quality of life in survivors of acute respiratory distress syndrome compared with critically ill control patients. JAMA 1999; 281:354–360.
53. Weinert CR, Gross CR, Kangas JR, et al. Health-related quality of life after acute lung injury. Am J Respir Crit Care Med 1997; 156:1120–1128.
54. Weinert CR. Epidemiology of psychiatric medication use in patients recovering from critical illness at long-term acute-care facility. Chest 2001; 119:547–553.
55. Schelling G, Stoll C, Haller M, et al. Health-related quality of life and posttraumatic stress disorder in survivors of the acute respiratory distress syndrome. Crit Care Med 1998; 26:651–659.
56. Davydow D, Desai SV, Needham DM, et al. Psychiatric morbidity in survivors of the acute respiratory distress syndrome: a systematic review. Psychosom Med 2008; 70:512–519.
57. Parker CM, Heyland DK, Groll D, et al. Mechanism of injury influences quality of life in survivors of acute respiratory distress syndrome. Intensive Care Med 2006; 32:1895–1900.
58. Cohen IL, Lambrinos J. Investigating the impact of age on outcome of mechanical ventilation using a population of 41,848 patients from a statewide database. Chest 1995; 107:1673–1680.
59. Centers for Disease Control. National Center for Chronic Disease Prevention and Health Promotion. http://www.cdc.gov/aging (accessed September 2008).
60. Ely EW, Haponik EF. Pneumonia in the elderly. J Thorac Imaging 1991; 6:45–61.
61. Sprenkle MD, Caldwell ES, Rudenfeld GD, et al. Mortality following acute respiratory distress syndrome (ARDS) among the elderly. Am J Respir Crit Care Med 1999; 159:A717.
62. Suchyta MR, Clemmer TP, Elliott CG, et al. Increased mortality of older patients with acute respiratory distress syndrome. Chest 1997; 111:1334–1339.
63. Siner JM, Pisani MA. Mechanical ventilation and acute respiratory distress syndrome in older patients. Clin Chest Med 2007; 28:783–791.
64. Lyrene RK, Truog WE. Adult respiratory distress syndrome in a pediatric intensive care unit: predisposing conditions, clinical course, and outcome. Pediatrics 1981; 67:790–795.
65. Timmons OD, Dean JM, Vernon DD. Mortality rates and prognostic variables in children with adult respiratory distress syndrome. J Pediatr 1991; 119:896–899.
66. Davis SL, Furman DP, Costarino AT Jr. Adult respiratory distress syndrome in children: associated disease, clinical course, and predictors of death. J Pediatr 1993; 123:35–45.
67. Paret G, Ziv T, Barzilai A, et al. Ventilation index and outcome in children with acute respiratory distress syndrome. Pediatr Pulmonol 1998; 26:125–128.

3

Radiographic Findings of the Acute Respiratory Distress Syndrome

PHILIP C. GOODMAN
Radiology/Cardiac and Thoracic Imaging, Duke University Medical Center, Durham, North Carolina, U.S.A.

DESIRÉE M. QUIÑONES
Hospital del Maestro Avenida Domenech, Hato Rey, Puerto Rico

I. Introduction

In 1967, Ashbaugh and coworkers introduced the phrase *acute respiratory distress syndrome of adults,* now adult respiratory distress syndrome (ARDS), to describe an illness that resulted in severe respiratory failure in a group of 12 patients with different underlying etiologies (including pneumonia and trauma) (1). Ashbaugh and other investigators described the chest films of several of these patients; the radiographs demonstrated bilateral heterogeneous opacities that rapidly coalesced to become more homogeneous throughout both lungs. During the last three decades, many articles regarding ARDS have been published. The radiological features of the disease remain an integral part of its definition.

This chapter describes the imaging characteristics of ARDS as seen on chest radiographs and other imaging modalities such as computed tomography (CT), magnetic resonance imaging (MRI), and positron emission tomography (PET).

II. Definition and Causes of ARDS

Several definitions have been proposed for ARDS over the past decades. In 1994, the North American/European Consensus Conference Committee (NAECC) proposed the currently used criteria for the diagnosis of ARDS: (1) acute onset of lung injury, (2) diffuse bilateral infiltrates on chest radiography, (3) refractory hypoxemia, (4) no clinical evidence of congestive heart failure, and (5) decreased lung compliance (see chap. 2). Thus, imaging abnormalities are both a by-product of this disease and part of its definition.

Although the definition recommended by the NAECC includes simple criteria that are easy to apply in the clinical setting, some investigators believe that in a clinical trial setting its lack of specific criteria for radiological findings is a limitation. In a recent study by Rubenfeld and colleagues, the reliability of this consensus radiographic definition for ARDS was evaluated (2). Twenty-one experts, all pulmonologists or critical care physicians, including seven members of the National Institutes of Health ARDS Network, evaluated chest radiographs of critically ill patients with a Pao_2/Fio_2 ratio of <300 and were asked to decide whether the radiographs fulfilled the NAECC definition for acute lung injury (ALI)–ARDS. There was a high interobserver variability, which could affect the validity of investigators using results of their clinical trials on patients. Radiologists, the authors note, may have had less variability on interpreting the films but were specifically not involved because of the design and intent of the study.

Nevertheless, the NAECC 1994 definition has been helpful in understanding more about the disease and as a basis for defining members of a group who are being investigated regarding various treatment options. The NAECC 1998 recommendations revealed no formal changes but did emphasize the importance of recognizing etiological and epidemiological differences between patients when studying ALI–ARDS (3).

Major risk factors for ARDS are sepsis, aspiration of gastric contents, trauma (including long bone and pelvic fracture and pulmonary contusion), multiple blood transfusions, overwhelming pneumonia, and shock (4,5). Interventions directed at one of these etiologies may not be as effective if other etiologies are causative. Less commonly, near drowning, drug toxicity, major burns, and toxic inhalation may lead to ARDS. Often more than one etiology is responsible; thus, auxiliary-imaging findings in addition to those typically associated with ARDS may be present.

III. Pathophysiology

ARDS to some degree is a form of permeability defect with protein-rich pulmonary edema associated with diffuse alveolar damage. This explains the usual diffuse distribution of increased opacities seen on chest films.

The disease is characteristically described as having three overlapping phases: exudative, proliferative, and fibrotic (see chap. 5). The exudative phase, usually seen within hours of the instigating pulmonary insult, is associated with interstitial edema characterized by a high protein content and hemorrhage that rapidly fills the alveoli. Subsequently, hyaline membrane formation occurs. During the proliferative phase, organization of the fibrinous exudate and regeneration of the alveoli occur. These changes are seen 7 to 28 days after the onset of disease. Fibrosis, scarring, and formation of subpleural and intrapulmonary cysts characterize the third, fibrotic phase, which may begin within two or three weeks of the initial insult, and are recognized for weeks to months later.

IV. Chest Radiography

Frequently, the first chest film of a patient with ARDS demonstrates diffuse symmetrical bilateral heterogeneous or homogeneous opacities, the picture of pulmonary edema (Fig. 1). In a short time, within hours or days, the opacities become significantly more homogeneous while maintaining their symmetric bilateral distribution. This progression of interstitial edema to diffuse airspace disease corresponds to the rapid filling of alveolar spaces by edema and hemorrhage. Characteristically, the opacities on the initial chest radiograph have been described as being located predominantly in the lung periphery, but this should not dissuade one from suggesting the diagnosis when a more central or even involvement is observed (Fig. 2). On the other hand, in contrast to cardiogenic pulmonary edema, the heart size and vascular pedicle are generally normal in patients with ARDS. Kerley lines (e.g., interstitial edema or lymphatic engorgement) may or may not be seen; they are reported with various frequency. Pleural effusions, common with cardiogenic pulmonary edema, have been thought unusual with ARDS and in the past were assumed to occur late in the disease or suggest the development of acute pneumonia or pulmonary infarct. However, the use of CT in patients with ARDS has revealed an earlier, more common association of pleural fluid in this setting. Of course, this brings into question

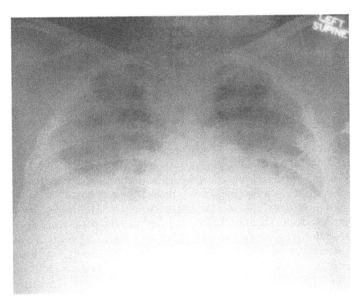

Figure 1   ARDS. A 27-year-old male developed respiratory failure after being hospitalized for a motor vehicle accident. Portable chest radiograph demonstrates low lung volumes with diffuse bilateral heterogeneous opacities. This is a typical picture of ARDS.

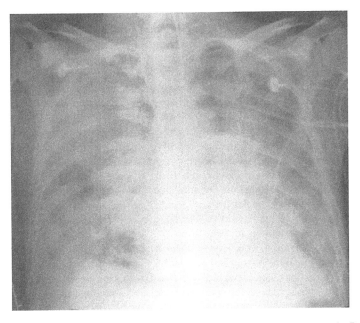

Figure 2   ARDS. A 44-year-old female with *Pseudomonas* pneumonia. Portable chest radiograph demonstrates bilateral homogeneous opacities with a central distribution. The radiographic abnormalities of ARDS may not be peripheral.

how often pleural fluid is really a marker of superimposed infection. As edema worsens, bilateral ill-defined opacities become more and more homogeneous, involving virtually all of the lungs with severe opacification with or without air bronchograms.

Some studies have shown, however, that distinguishing between cardiogenic and permeability pulmonary edema, as occurs in ARDS, is difficult (6). In a study by Aberle and coworkers, some features more typical of hydrostatic pulmonary edema such as widened vascular pedicle, pleural effusions, peribronchial cuffs, and septal lines were commonly found in patients with permeability pulmonary edema (7). Nevertheless, chest radiography remains a valuable tool in the evaluation of pulmonary edema.

In patients who survive the initial period, radiographs eventually improve slightly but continue to reveal diffuse bilateral homogeneous or heterogeneous opacities. As the disease enters the proliferative phase, characterized by an increasing fibroblast population and deposition of collagen, the chest film stabilizes as the radiographic pattern becomes more coarsely heterogeneous, linear, and reticular. In some patients, complete resolution of abnormalities ultimately occurs, but this may take several months. More commonly, patients develop chronic changes secondary to ARDS. The chest film demonstrates coarse linear, curvilinear, and reticular opacities representing fibrosis. Intrapulmonary air-filled cysts, which may form during the acute phase from abscesses or during the proliferative and fibrotic phases from barotrauma or cicatrization, frequently persist. Loculated pneumothoraces may also become common chronic abnormalities on the chest film of recovering patients.

V. Complications of ARDS
A. Support Lines

Most individuals with ARDS require days or weeks of endotracheal (ET) intubation with assisted mechanical ventilation. Chest films are frequently obtained to monitor the position of these tubes. The desired placement puts the tip 3–5 cm above the carina with the cervical spine in neutral position. If the patient's neck at the time the film is taken is flexed, this will drive the ET tube down toward the carina and spuriously misrepresent its position. In extension, the tip of the ET tube will appear higher than it is when the patient's neck is in the neutral position.

Because of the more vertical course of the right mainstem bronchus, most low malpositions place the ET tube in this bronchus, resulting in collapse of the left lung. If the misplaced tube is not adjusted, positive pressure ventilation delivered to one lung may result in more frequent episodes of barotrauma. If the ET tube is placed too high, adequate delivery of oxygen to the lungs may be inhibited, laryngeal injury may occur, and there is a great possibility that the patient may accidentally become extubated. Too high a placement, certainly above the level of the clavicles, may also lead to mistakes in establishing the proper pressure settings for ventilation.

Another important observation to make is the status of the ET tube balloon cuff. This structure, meant to partially seal the airway and prevent back flow of air, is situated near the tip of the ET tube. The balloon should not be overinflated, as this may lead to injury of the tracheal mucosa with subsequent edema and in some instances eventual stenosis. An overinflated ET tube balloon can be recognized as a round or oval lucency near the tip of the tube with expansion of the trachea at this site. In an analysis of 30 survivors of ARDS, Elliot and coworkers concluded that laryngotracheal stenosis is an important cause of exertional dyspnea following treatment of ARDS (8). Etiological factors in this group of patients included difficult orotracheal intubation and high tracheal cuff pressures.

Radiographs are usually obtained after placement of catheters within the thoracic deep venous system. The lines are frequently placed via a subclavian or internal jugular vein approach. Pneumothorax may occur in 5–6% of patients. It is also important to document catheter position. Ideally the tip of a central venous catheter should be placed within the central lumen of a large vein such that the tip does not abut the vein or heart wall end-on. Catheter tips can be safely located within the upper right atrium provided they do not abut the atrial wall or pass into the coronary sinus (9).

Pulmonary artery catheters are commonly used in critically ill patients for measurement of pulmonary capillary wedge pressure. These catheters are inserted via a subclavian or internal jugular vein and ideally terminate distal to the pulmonic valve with the tip in the right or left pulmonary artery or interlobar arteries. Complications include pulmonary infarction, knotting, and cardiac perforation.

B. Barotrauma

Mechanical ventilation is the mainstay of therapy in patients with ARDS. Different strategies of oxygen delivery have been tried since the disease was first described, but the most frequently used regimen remains positive pressure ventilation. Injury to the lungs has been a continuing problem with this therapy, and the incidence of barotrauma can be high. Gammon and colleagues investigated mediastinal emphysema and pneumothorax in a group of patients on mechanical ventilation for a variety of diseases (10). Of 29 patients with ARDS, 66% developed barotrauma, 62% developed mediastinal emphysema, and 60% developed pneumothorax. Recent studies, however, have not reported such a high incidence. A study by Schnapp and colleagues showed an incidence of barotrauma of 13% in 100 patients with ALI (11). In this study, mortality rates were not different in patients with and without barotrauma. Another study by Eisneggggr and colleagues demonstrated an incidence of barotrauma of 13% and that higher positive end-expiratory pressure (PEEP) is associated with an increased risk of barotrauma (12).

Patients with decreased lung compliance, one of the pathophysiological consequences of ARDS, are especially subject to this complication. The mechanism is associated with rupture of alveoli. Intense shearing forces develop in the alveolar walls as a result of the high pressures necessary to separate the collapsed walls of surfactant-deficient alveoli during inspiration. After rupture of alveoli, air is introduced into the interstitial space and from there spreads peripherally to the subpleural regions, either adjacent to fissures or along the lateral chest wall; another path takes air centrally into the mediastinum. At the lung periphery, rupture of the visceral pleura results in pneumothorax. Air that has dissected along bronchovascular bundles into the mediastinum (causing pneumomediastinum or pneumopericardium) may migrate into the soft tissues of the neck and chest, resulting in subcutaneous emphysema, or may break through the parietal pleura into the pleural space, resulting in pneumothorax.

The earliest radiographic finding of barotrauma is pulmonary interstitial emphysema (PIE). This arises when air first exits the alveoli into the interstitial space. Radiographically, PIE is recognized as linear or rounded lucencies radiating from the hilum, along bronchovascular pathways, and sometimes as a mottled or "salt and pepper" pattern throughout the lungs (Fig. 3). Larger collections of air may form radiolucencies

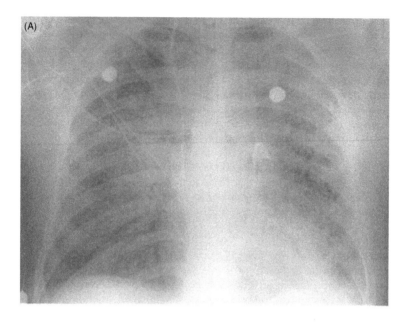

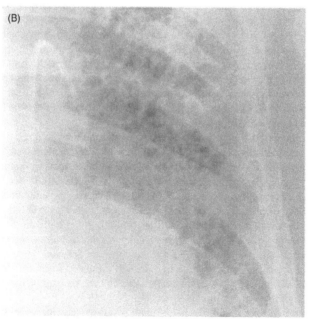

Figure 3 Pulmonary interstitial emphysema (PIE). A 24-year-old male with disseminated blastomycosis developed ARDS. A portable chest film (**A**) demonstrates a mottled heterogeneous opacification in the left lung. This is a typical appearance of PIE. A close-up of the left midlung (**B**) demonstrates PIE. *Source*: From Ref. 13.

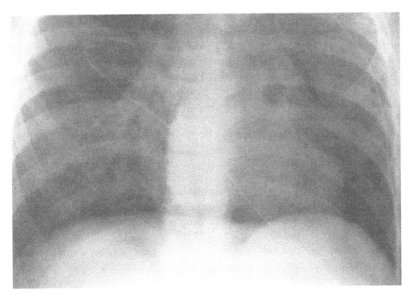

Figure 4   Pneumomediastinum. A close-up of the chest demonstrates sharp definition of the complete superior border of the diaphragm. This appearance of a continuous diaphragm is a classic example of pneumomediastinum. *Source*: From Ref. 13.

in the perihilar or subpleural regions and have been termed air cysts or pneumatoceles. Subpleural air collections have an increased risk of causing pneumothorax. The detection of PIE suggests that the patient has suffered barotrauma and may prompt an effort to lower airway pressures and the patient's tidal volume, if they are not already maximally reduced.

Pneumomediastinum is a sign of barotrauma in mechanically ventilated patients. Chest radiographs show a line or band of lucency outlining the contours of the heart or other mediastinal structures (Fig. 4). The continuous diaphragm sign, another indicator of pneumomediastinum, occurs when air overlying the central portion of the diaphragm under the heart allows the top of the diaphragm to be seen as a continuous structure (14). This sign should permit recognition of pneumomediastinum on supine or upright studies. Pneumopericardium or a medially placed pneumothorax may simulate pneumomediastinum. Decubitus views can help differentiate between these air collections as air in the mediastinal space rarely moves or moves slowly, whereas air in the pericardium or pleural space moves to nondependent locations within these compartments almost immediately with position changes.

Pneumothorax is the most feared form of barotrauma and the only one for which treatment is performed. Prolonged or high-pressure ventilation, especially in patients with decreased lung compliance, may lead to recurrent pneumothoraces or rapid enlargement of a small pneumothorax, occasionally producing tension physiology. A pneumothorax is typically thought of and identified as a thin white curved line (visceral pleura) above the lung apex with the absence of pulmonary vessels superiorly or laterally. But these abnormalities are typically seen in patients in upright position. In patients with ARDS, chest films are obtained in the intensive care unit with the patient usually in the supine position. In these cases, air in the pleura space may collect anteriorly in the most ventral, nondependent portion of the thorax, which is typically at the level of the diaphragm. The radiographic appearances caused by this location of pleural air include the deep sulcus sign, anterior sulcus sign, subpulmonic air collection, and occasionally epicardial fat sign (Fig. 5). The most common of these is the deep sulcus sign, which consists of a deep lateral costophrenic angle on the involved side (15).

Subpulmonic pneumothorax, like subpulmonic pleural fluid, is a collection within the pleural space above the diaphragm and can be recognized by a sharp thin curvilinear opacity representing the visceral pleura above and often parallel to the hemidiaphragm (16). Tocino and colleagues examined 88 critically ill patients with 112 pneumothoraces, and they found that the abnormal air collections were located in the anteromedial space in 38% and subpulmonic space in 26% of occurrences (17).

Tension physiology resulting from a pneumothorax may be suggested radiographically when complete collapse of the ipsilateral lung and mediastinal shift to the contralateral side are observed (18). However, in patients with ARDS and decreased lung compliance or "stiff lungs," tension pneumothorax can exist without complete lung collapse. Radiographic findings in these cases may include flattening of the ipsilateral diaphragm, enlarging loculated pneumothorax, and mediastinal shift accompanied by deterioration of clinical status.

C. Pneumonia

Nosocomial pneumonia is a common complication in patients who are intubated and occurs more often in patients with ARDS than in other ventilated patients. Chastre and colleagues reported a 55% incidence of nosocomial pneumonia in patients with ARDS, as compared to 28% incidence in those patients without ARDS (19). The same investigators found that the most frequently isolated organisms in these patients were methicillin-resistant *Staphylococcus aureus* (23%), nonfermenting gram-negative bacilli (*Pseudomonas aeruginosa*) (21%), and Enterobacteriaceae (21%).

The diagnosis of nosocomial pneumonia in ARDS is difficult as the patient's chest radiograph is already abnormal. An asymmetrical opacity or more homogeneous opacity than seen elsewhere in the lung may be a radiographic clue of superimposed pneumonia. However, this finding is not sensitive or specific for the diagnosis of pneumonia. Winer-Muram and coworkers studied the overall accuracy of chest radiography in diagnosing pneumonia in patients with ARDS and found it to be approximately 50% (20). They found that an increase in false-negative interpretations occurred because the diffuse opacities in ARDS obscure the radiographic findings of pneumonia. The same investigators also concluded that the presence of pleural effusion was not a helpful indicator in the diagnosis of superimposed pneumonia. This is supported by recent work with CT scanning of ARDS, which has revealed an unexpected higher incidence of pleural fluid in this setting even in patients not felt to be infected. Winer-Muram and colleagues also studied the ability of CT to detect pneumonia in patients with ARDS (21). They found that diagnostic accuracy was approximately 65–70% primarily because of a 70% true-negative result. Unfortunately, no individual CT findings were found to reliably differentiate pneumonia from ARDS.

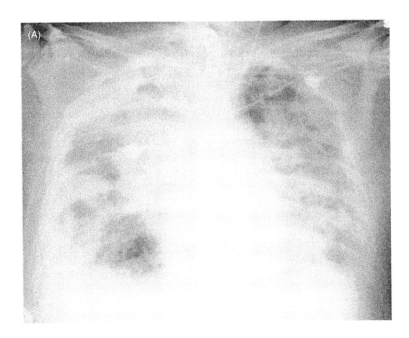

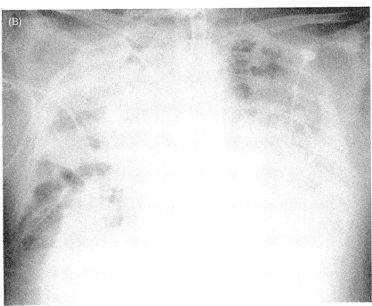

Figure 5 Pneumothorax. A 44-year-old male with aspiration pneumonia developed ARDS. Initial portable chest film (**A**) demonstrates bilateral heterogeneous opacities. The subsequent film (**B**) demonstrates lucency overlying the right costophrenic angle. Air collects in this location when patients are supine, creating a deep sulcus representing pneumothorax.

VI. CT and ARDS

For the last 20 years, CT has been used by some investigators to better understand the distribution of abnormalities in the lungs of patients with ARDS. Several studies using this modality have shown that ARDS does not affect the lungs homogeneously as frequently depicted on chest radiography (22–25).

During the early stages of disease, CT reveals: (1) normal or near normal lung frequently located in nondependent regions; (2) ground glass opacities in the anterior and middle portions; and (3) homogeneous opacities in the most dependent lung (Fig. 6). It is believed that the weight of adjacent pulmonary parenchyma causes compression of more dependent alveoli, resulting in this distribution of opacities. Furthermore, CT scanning has been used to demonstrate a reversal of lung opacification when patients with ARDS are placed in the prone position.

After approximately one week of initial lung injury, during the organizing phase of ARDS, there is a decrease in overall lung opacity and the pattern of disease becomes more linear or reticular. During this phase, the lung parenchyma undergoes extensive remodeling with development of some degree of pulmonary fibrosis. Desai and coworkers described the CT findings at long-term follow-up in 27 patients who survived ARDS (26). A coarse reticular pattern with distortion of lung parenchyma was the most frequent pattern in 23 patients (85%). This reticular pattern had an anterior distribution and was associated with CT signs of pulmonary fibrosis including architectural distortion and traction bronchiectasis. The extent of disease was related to the length of time that patients underwent pressure-controlled inverse ratio ventilation. Some feel that the anterior distribution of fibrosis occurs because alveolar overdistention is predominantly seen in this region, that the anterior ground glass opacities seen on CT acutely represent

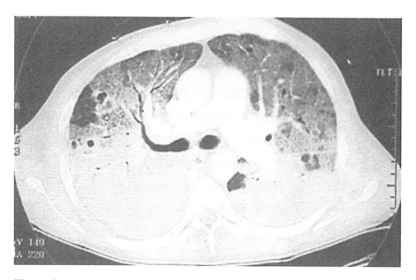

Figure 6   ARDS. This is the same patient as in Figure 4. CT study demonstrates ground glass opacities in the anterior and middle portions of the lungs and consolidation in the dependent regions. This is a typical distribution of abnormalities with ARDS.

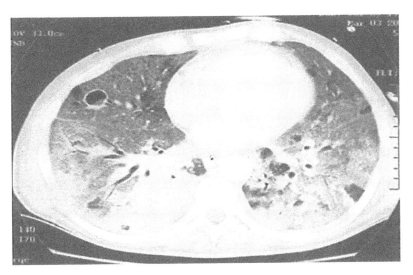

Figure 7 ARDS. This is the same patient as in Figures 4 and 5. Follow-up CT study demonstrates, in addition to ground glass and consolidative opacities, an intrapulmonary cyst in the right middle lobe likely secondary to barotrauma.

inter-alveolar septal inflammation from this overdistention, and that this ultimately results in fibrosis.

Complications of ARDS can also be detected using CT (Fig. 7). Some investigators have found that CT scans are more sensitive than chest radiographs in detecting PIE, the earliest sign of barotrauma (27). The CT findings of PIE in patients with ARDS include air within the interlobular septa, air around the pulmonary veins and bronchi, and variably sized subpleural, air-filled cysts. In regards to other evidence of barotrauma, Tagliabue and coworkers showed that 40% of pneumothoraces and 80% of pneumomediastinums seen on CT scan were not seen on chest radiographs (28). Pleural effusions and lung abscesses were also seen more frequently on CT than on plain chest films. On the other hand, the benefits of observing these abnormalities on patient outcome have not been proved, and some believe that CT for ARDS should be restricted to problem cases (29).

Finally, CT has been used as an investigative tool for studying the pathophysiology of ARDS and novel approaches to treatment of this disease. Pelosi and coworkers used CT to analyze the effects of prone positioning of patients with ARDS (30). They discovered that some otherwise atelectatic areas of lung near the diaphragm might be recruited while the patient was prone and that this could perhaps lead to improved oxygenation. Using dynamic CT, Helm and coworkers have investigated the degree of oxygenation in rabbits ventilated by negative pressure with an external device, "iron lung", versus rabbits ventilated with positive pressure and found a benefit with the former technique (31). Using a pig model, David and coworkers found that dynamic CT imaging permitted the quantification of the degree of inflation of the lungs, the discovery and quantification of recruitment and derecruitment in the lungs, and suggested that this technique may provide information that could alter therapy of early ARDS (32). A similar benefit for dynamic

CT in optimizing ventilator adjustments for pigs with early ARDS was observed by Markstarller and coworkers (33). Gattinoni has presented a number of revelations in regards to pathophysiology of ARDS, including the distribution of disease, differences in CT pattern based on etiology of ARDS, and the relationship of decreased lung compliance versus decreased lung size when volutrauma or barotrauma occurs (29). CT has been helpful in the management of complications due to barotrauma in some instances. Gattinoni also used whole-lung CT during breath-holding sessions to demonstrate what portion of lung might be recruitable with different airway pressures and found that anatomical and functional lung recruitment are not necessarily congruent (34). Caironi and coworkers discuss the use of CT and quantitative techniques to determine rational PEEP settings; and also predict that CT might become a tool with which to define ARDS as it can measure permeability pulmonary edema as distinct from atelectasis (35). Chon and coworkers used CT-guided percutaneous catheter drainage for loculated thoracic air collections (pneumothoraces, pneumatoceles, and tension pneumothorax) in nine patients mechanically ventilated for a clinical diagnosis of ARDS (36). Eight (89%) of the nine patients were successfully treated with CT-guided catheter placement, obviating the need for surgical intervention.

Miller and colleagues studied the value of CT scans in patients in the intensive care unit and concluded that, for the majority of patients, there was significant agreement between chest radiographs and CT (37). CT did demonstrate additional findings, but most of these were not clinically important. Those that were found useful were the identification of abscesses or postoperative mediastinal fluid collections and unsuspected pneumonia or pleural effusions. The conclusions of this investigation suggested that CT scanning may be beneficial in selected cases. In another study, Desai and Hansell concluded that CT is best reserved to detect occult complications in patients who are deteriorating or not responding to treatment at the expected rate (38). Moving patients from the ICU to the CT scanner is not a trivial matter as it puts the patient into a less optimal clinical environment and requires additional manpower. Thus, the widespread use of CT in ARDS patients cannot be advocated, but in selected cases CT should be considered. Some medical centers are considering the installation of CT scanners in their intensive care units to facilitate more expeditious and frequent use of this imaging modality.

VII. Other Imaging Modalities
A. Nuclear Medicine
Several investigators have studied the value of radioactive gallium studies in patients with ARDS. The primary mechanism of uptake of gallium is related to interstitial inflammation and repair of pulmonary tissue as occurs in ARDS (39). In one study, investigators used a dual-radionuclide method (gallium-67 transferrin and technetium-99 m red blood cells) to measure pulmonary microvascular permeability in patients with pulmonary edema due to ARDS and hydrostatic pulmonary edema (40). Radioactivity measurements over the lungs and blood were used to calculate the pulmonary leak index as a measure of pulmonary microvascular permeability. These investigators concluded that the gallium-67 pulmonary leak index is useful in differentiating ARDS and hydrostatic pulmonary edema. In a follow-up publication, the same investigative group discusses a modification of their work in which they show that a simple blood transcapillary escape rate of gallium-67 transferrin is comparable to the more complex method they previously describe. Thus

they postulate that the diagnosis of permeability edema of ARDS might be possible at the bedside (41).

Similarly, PET has been used as a tool in studying the physiology of ARDS. Mintun and colleagues quantified pulmonary vascular permeability with PET and gallium-68−labeled transferrin in normal volunteers, in six dogs after oleic acid-induced lung injury, and in patients with ARDS (42). These investigators measured the pulmonary transcapillary escape rate (PTCER) and demonstrated marked differences in PTCER between abnormal and normal lung tissue. In a recent case report, F-18 fluorodeoxyglucose PET/CT demonstrated diffuse hypermetabolic activity throughout the lungs in a patient with ARDS. This was presumed to be due to a high rate of glucose metabolism in inflammatory cells (43). In a series of eight patients with pulmonary contusion who underwent initial and repeat CT and fluorodeoxyglucose-PET scanning, another group of investigators found that diffuse FDG metabolic activity was seen one to three days prior to the development of ARDS in a subset of their patients (44).

B. MRI

There are several studies addressing the imaging of lung parenchyma and pulmonary edema using MRI. However, this imaging modality is not currently used in the evaluation of patients with ARDS. Caruthers and colleagues used three-dimensional MRI to measure pulmonary microvascular barrier permeability in animals after oleic acid-induced lung injury (45). They concluded that 3-D MRI imaging of pulmonary edema is sensitive for measuring small changes in lung water. In another study, contrast-enhanced MRI with a macromolecular agent was used to differentiate between hydrostatic pulmonary edema and edema caused by abnormal capillary permeability (46). However, widespread use of these methods has not yet occurred in critically ill patients.

VIII. Conclusions

Chest radiographs are essential for the diagnosis and monitoring of ARDS, although better methods are needed to standardize their interpretation. Although new imaging modalities have been developed since the first description of the disease, only CT has some clinical importance in complicated cases. CT and PET scanning have been useful modalities in better understanding the pathophysiology of the disease, particularly in recognizing the heterogeneity of intrapulmonary involvement. Imaging methods to measure lung vascular permeability or extravascular lung water have not been proven to be sufficiently reproducible or reliable for clinical use. In general, these imaging methods should be limited to clinical research endeavors. Perhaps new technological advances in radiology will lead to improved utilization of these modalities with subsequent better evaluation and treatment of ARDS patients.

References

1. Ashbaugh DG, Bigelow DB, Petty TL, et al. Acute respiratory distress in adults. Lancet 1967; 2:319–323.
2. Rubenfeld GD, Caldwell E, Granton J, et al. Interobserver variability in applying a radiographic definition for ARDS. Chest 1999; 116:1347–1353.

3. Ware LB, Matthay MA. The acute respiratory distress syndrome. N Engl J Med 2000; 342:1334–1349.
4. TenHoor T, Mannino DM, Moss M. Risk factors for ARDS in the United States: analysis of the 1993 National Mortality Followback Study. Chest 2001; 119:1179–1184.
5. Doyle RL, Szaflarski N, Modin GW, et al. Identification of patients with acute lung injury: predictors of mortality. Am J Respir Crit Care Med 1995; 152:1818–1824.
6. Thomason JW, Wesley Ely E, Chiles C, et al. Appraising pulmonary edema using supine chest roentgenograms in ventilated patients. Am J Respir Crit Care Med 1998; 157:1600–1608.
7. Aberle DR, Wiener-Kronish JP, Webb WR, et al. Hydrostatic vs. increased permeability pulmonary edema: diagnosis based on radiographic criteria in critically ill patients. Radiology 1988; 168:73–79.
8. Elliot CG, Rasmusson BY, Crapo RO. Upper airway obstruction following adult respiratory distress syndrome. An analysis of 30 survivors. Chest 1988; 94:526–530.
9. Fletcher SJ, Bodenham AR. Safe placement of central venous catheters: where should the tip of the catheter lie? Br J Anaesth 2000; 85:188–191.
10. Gammon RB, Shin MS, Buchalter SE. Pulmonary barotrauma and mechanical ventilation. Chest 1992; 102:568–572.
11. Schnapp LM, Chin DP, Szaflarski N, et al. Frequency and importance of barotrauma in 100 patients with acute lung injury. Crit Care Med 1995; 23:272–278.
12. Eisner MD, Thompson BT, Schoenfeld D, et al. Airway pressures and early barotrauma in patients with acute lung injury and acute respiratory distress syndrome. Am J Respir Crit Care Med 2002; 165:978–982.
13. Goodman PC. Radiographic findings in patients with acute respiratory distress syndrome. Clin Chest Med 2000; 21:419–433.
14. Bejvan SM, Godwin JD. Pneumomediastinum: old signs and new signs. AJR Am J Roentgenol 1996; 166:1041–1048.
15. Gordon R. The deep sulcus sign. Radiology 1980; 136:25–27.
16. Rhea JT, vanSonnenberg E, McLoud TC. Basilar pneumothorax in the supine adult. Radiology 1979; 133:593–595.
17. Tocino IM, Miller MH, Fairfax WR. Distribution of pneumothorax in the supine and semirecumbent critically ill adult. AJR Am J Roentgenol 1985; 144:901–905.
18. Gobien RP, Reiness, HD, Schabel SI. Localized tension pneumothorax: unrecognized form of barotrauma in adult respiratory distress syndrome. Radiology 1982; 142:15–19.
19. Chastre J, Trouillet JL, Vuagnat A, et al. Nosocomial pneumonia in patients with acute respiratory distress syndrome. Am J Respir Crit Care Med 1998; 157:1165–1172.
20. Winer-Muram HT, Rubin SA, Ellis JV, et al. Pneumonia and ARDS in patients receiving mechanical ventilation: diagnostic accuracy of chest radiography. Radiology 1993; 188: 479–485.
21. Winer-Muram HT, Steiner RM, Gurney JW, et al. Ventilator-associated pneumonia in patients with adult respiratory distress syndrome: CT evaluation. Radiology 1998; 208:193–199.
22. Gattinoni L, Bombino M, Pelosi P, et al. Lung structure and function in different stages of severe adult respiratory distress syndrome. JAMA 1994; 271:1772–1779.
23. Gattinoni L, Mascheroni D, Torresin A, et al. Morphological response to positive end expiratory pressure in acute respiratory failure: computerized tomography study. Intensive Care Med 1986; 12:137–142.
24. Gattinoni L, Presenti A, Bombino M, et al. Relationships between lung computed tomographic density, gas exchange, and PEEP in acute respiratory failure. Anesthesiology 1988; 69:824–832.
25. Gattinoni L, Presenti A, Torresin A, et al. Adult respiratory distress syndrome profiles by computed tomography. J Thorac Imaging 1986; 1(3):25–30.
26. Desai SR, Wells AU, Rubens MB, et al. Acute respiratory distress syndrome: CT abnormalities at long-term follow up. Radiology 1999; 210:29–35.

27. Kemper AC, Steinberg KP, Stern EJ. Pulmonary interstitial emphysema: CT findings. AJR Am J Roentgenol 1999; 172:1642.

28. Tagliabue M, Casella TC, Zincone GE, et al. CT and chest radiography in the evaluation of adult respiratory distress syndrome. Acta Radiol 1994; 35:230–234.

29. Gattinoni L, Caironi P, Pelosi P, et al. What has computed tomography taught us about the acute respiratory distress syndrome? Am J Respir Crit Care Med 2001; 164:1701–1711.

30. Pelosi P, Crotti S, Brazzi L, et al. Computed tomography in adult respiratory distress syndrome: what has it taught us? Eur Respir J 1996; 9:1055–1062.

31. Helm E, Talakoub O, Grasso, et al. Use of dynamic CT in acute respiratory distress syndrome (ARDS) with comparison of positive and negative pressure ventilation. Eur Radiol 2008; 19(1):50–57.

32. David M, Karmrodt J, Bletz C, et al. Analysis of atelectasis, ventilated, and hyperinflated lung during mechanical ventilation by dynamic CT. Chest 2005; 128(5):3757–3770.

33. Markstarller K, Kauczor HU, Weiler N, et al. Lung density distribution in dynamic CT correlates with oxygenation in ventilated pigs with lavage ARDS. Br J Anaesth 2003; 91(5):699–708.

34. Gattinoni L, Caironi P, Cressoni M, et al. Lung recruitment in patients with the acute respiratory distress syndrome. N Engl J Med 2006; 354(17):1775–1786.

35. Caironi P, Carlesso E, Gattinoni L. Radiological imaging in acute lung injury and acute respiratory distress syndrome. Semin Respir Crit Care Med 2006; 27(4):404–415.

36. Chon KS, vanSonnenberg E, D'Agostino HB, et al. CT-guided catheter drainage of loculated thoracic air collections in mechanically ventilated patients with acute respiratory distress syndrome. AJR Am J Roentgenol 1999; 173:1345–1350.

37. Miller WT Jr, Tino G, Friedburg JS. Thoracic CT in the intensive care unit: assessment of clinical usefulness. Radiology 1998; 209:491–498.

38. Desai SR, Hansell DM. Lung imaging in the adult respiratory distress syndrome: current practice and new insights. Intensive Care Med 1997; 23:7–15.

39. Passamonte PM, Martinez AJ, Singh A. Pulmonary gallium concentration in the adult respiratory distress syndrome. Chest 1984; 85:828–830.

40. Raijmakers PG, Groeneveld AB, Teule GJ, et al. Diagnostic value of the gallium-67 pulmonary leak index in pulmonary edema. J Nucl Med 1996; 37:1316–1322.

41. Verheij J, Raijmakers PG, Lingen A, et al. Simple vs. complex radionuclide methods of assessing capillary protein permeability for diagnosing acute respiratory distress syndrome. J Crit Care 2005; 20(2):162–171.

42. Mintun MA, Dennis DR, Welch MJ, et al. Measurements of pulmonary vascular permeability with PET and gallium-68 transferrin. J Nucl Med 1987; 28:1704–1716.

43. Jacene HA, Cohade C, Wahl RL. F-18FDG PET/CT in acute respiratory distress syndrome: a case report. Clin Nucl Med 2004; 29(12):786–788.

44. Rodrigues RS, Miller PR, Bozza FA, et al. FDG-PET in patients at risk for acute respiratory distress syndrome: a preliminary report. Intensive Care Med 2008; 34(12):2273–2278.

45. Caruthers SD, Pachal CB, Pou NA, et al. Regional measurements of pulmonary edema by using magnetic resonance imaging. J Appl Physiol 1998; 84:2143–2153.

46. Berthezene Y, Vexler V, Jerome H, et al. Differentiation of capillary leak and hydrostatic pulmonary edema with a macromolecular MR imaging contrast agent. Radiology 1991; 181:773–777.

4

Pulmonary Pathology of ARDS: Diffuse Alveolar Damage

LESTER KOBZIK
Department of Pathology, Brigham & Women's Hospital, Harvard Medical School and Harvard School of Public Health, Boston, Massachusetts, U.S.A.

LYNETTE SHOLL
Department of Pathology, Brigham and Women's Hospital, Harvard Medical School, Boston, Massachusetts, U.S.A.

I. Introduction

Diffuse alveolar damage (DAD) describes the pathology found in most patients with acute respiratory distress syndrome (ARDS). DAD represents a stereotypical response to one or more insults that injure the alveolocapillary unit (1). The injury may occur predominantly at the alveolar epithelium (as in inhalational exposures) or at the level of the capillary endothelium (such as in sepsis). Regardless of the site of initial injury, the tissue response is the same. Not surprisingly, it is typically difficult to determine the proximal cause based solely on finding DAD.

DAD follows a relatively predictable temporal course that has three phases, as summarized in Table 1: (1) an exudative phase occurring in the first week with a peak at 72 hours following the injury, (2) a proliferative phase that follows from approximately days 7 to 21, and (3) a later fibrotic phase that persists, in some cases, indefinitely (2). Each phase has characteristic histologic features that are readily recognized by light microscopy. This chapter will review the typical morphologic findings in each phase of DAD, will discuss elements of differential diagnosis that arise, and will also consider studies that have attempted to identify prognostic histologic features in open lung biopsies in patients with ARDS.

II. History and Overview

The first systematic descriptions of DAD in humans occurred in the 1960s in patients who had received oxygen therapy, at which time the findings were termed "respirator lung syndrome" (3). In retrospect, features of the exudative phase of DAD were described as early as 1947 in studies of atomic bomb victims who died in the first few weeks following the bombing in Hiroshima (4). Autopsy studies of Vietnam war casualties demonstrated the presence of "hyaline membranes" in a subset of patients suffering from traumatic war injuries (5). Early observers quickly noticed that the pathologic findings were similar to those seen in neonates with respiratory distress syndrome (6). In 1976, Katzenstein coined the term "diffuse alveolar damage" to describe the pathologic features of acute lung injury (7).

Table 1 Phases of Diffuse Alveolar Damage

	Exudative	Proliferative	Fibrosing
Synonym	Early, acute	Organizing	Late
Time following injury	1–7 days	1–3 wk	Weeks–months
Major features	Edema	Type II pneumocyte hyperplasia	Interstitial fibrosis
	Hemorrhage	Mononuclear cell predominance	Chronic inflammation
	Neutrophils	Organization of alveolar exudates	Type II pneumocyte
	Hyaline membranes		hyperplasia

DAD follows a predictable course, with characteristic histopathologic features present in three phases: exudative, proliferative, and fibrotic. The exudative and proliferative phases tend to overlap during the acute phase of DAD. The average in-hospital mortality during these phases is approximately 50% (2,8) but depends in part on the underlying disease process. Of the surviving patients, a subset has successful resolution of DAD at the proliferative phase (8). However, many cases progress to a fibrotic phase that is typically dominant by weeks three to four following injury (1).

III. Exudative Phase

Animal models of hyperoxic pulmonary injury show that pathologic changes precede the ARDS-like physiologic and radiologic changes seen later. In primate models of hyperoxic lung injury, endothelial cell swelling and vacuolation occur first and are detectable only by electron microscopy, followed by interstitial swelling and endothelial disruption visible by light microscopy (9). Both chest radiographs and fine section CT are relatively insensitive to these early changes (early exudative phase); the sensitivity of radiography increases with the onset of physiologic changes, including disordered gas exchange, at which time the histology demonstrates marked disruption of the endothelium and alveolar epithelium integrity, as well as interstitial swelling and leukocyte infiltration (9,10).

As noted in the patients with traumatic war injuries, patients with DAD have markedly heavy lungs, even more so than patients suffering from other processes such as hemorrhage or pneumonia (5). On average, the combined weight of lungs with DAD in the exudative phase is greater than 2000 g (1), over twice the normal combined weight, which averages 750 g in women and 850 g in men (11). Grossly, the lungs are firm and dusky, with a dense, hemorrhagic cut surface.

Microscopically, the lung shows "exudative" features with capillary congestion, intra-alveolar hemorrhage, and alveolar and interstitial edema. The earliest changes, manifesting as capillary congestion and intra-alveolar edema, have been seen as early as one to three days after injury in cases of hyperoxia (7). The pathognomic finding, however, is the presence of "hyaline membranes": acellular, eosinophilic membranes that adhere to the alveolar ducts and walls (Fig. 1). Hyaline membranes begin to form as the interstitial edema resolves, and are most prominent in the two to six days following injury (7) (Fig. 2). In the exudative phase of DAD, the hyaline material contains strands of fibrin and cellular debris, as well as high concentrations of immunoglobulins (particularly IgG) and

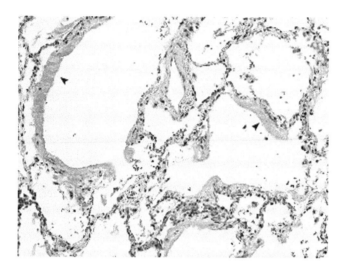

Figure 1   Hyaline membranes in early exudative phase DAD.

fibrinogen as demonstrated by immunofluorescence and immunohistochemical studies (12). Surfactant apoprotein can be found by immunohistochemistry in type II pneumocytes and in lesser amounts in the hyaline membranes (13). Several groups have contended that the composition of the hyaline membranes varies based on the underlying insult (14,15). Peres e Serra and coworkers found relatively more endothelial (Factor VIII) and less

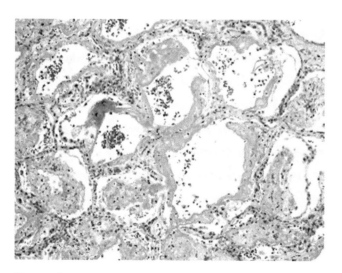

Figure 2   Hyaline membranes and type II pneumocyte hyperplasia in late exudative phase DAD.

epithelial cell components (keratin AE1/AE3) following idiopathic and extrapulmonary injuries (e.g., sepsis) as compared to primary pulmonary injuries (such as pneumonia). However, the expression of the component proteins has also been found to be variable within a single specimen (15), likely reflecting the temporal heterogeneity that can be seen in DAD when there are several physiologic or treatment-related insults.

Electron microscopic examination reveals that the type I pneumocytes comprising the alveolar epithelium are absent or markedly damaged and the underlying alveolar basement membrane is exposed. Hyaline membranes entrap conspicuous, hyperplastic type II pneumocytes (12). Temporal studies of exudative phase DAD in autopsy cases find that the hyaline membranes form along the alveolar septa and spread over time to cover the alveolar ducts (14). Immunohistochemical studies further suggest that more severe injury occurs along the ducts, which show loss of the epithelial cell-specific protein epithelial membrane antigen expression, contrasting to preserved expression in the alveolar walls (16). This finding provides a good example of the utility of immunohistochemistry in illuminating disease pathogenesis, as also discussed later. Following epithelial cell injury, alveolar ducts become dilated and the alveolar sacs that branch from the duct, collapse (12,17).

In another demonstration of potential insights from immunohistochemistry studies, Yamada and coworkers described a subset of patients with DAD and intracytoplasmic eosinophilic inclusion bodies within pneumocytes. They found that the presence of inclusion bodies, which contain ubiquitin and cytokeratin by immunohistochemistry, correlated with greater numbers of hyaline membranes and concluded that disordered ubiquitin-mediated proteolysis may play a role in the pathogenesis of DAD (18).

Endothelial injury is typically less prominent than epithelial injury by either microscopic or ultrastructural examination, and the degree of interstitial edema appears out of proportion to the degree of endothelial damage. However, endothelial cell swelling, widening of cell–cell junctions, and intravascular fibrin thrombi can be seen (1,7).

Inflammatory cells are a minor component of the histologic picture during this phase, often consisting of a mixed interstitial infiltrate comprising macrophages, lymphocytes and plasma cells (2). Neutrophils are most prominent in patients with ARDS secondary to pneumonia, sepsis, or trauma. In pneumonia, neutrophils are seen in the alveolar airspaces whereas in the latter two conditions they are more commonly seen as intracapillary aggregates (1).

In summary, the histologic manifestations of the acute, or exudative, phase of DAD reflect the underlying severe cellular injury within the alveolar walls and ducts. Although type II pneumocytes are retained and appear activated by cytologic criteria, they do not yet show the marked proliferation seen during attempts at repair, which are most evident in the next stage of DAD, the proliferative phase.

IV. Proliferative Phase

Grossly, the lungs remain heavy and solid in this phase of DAD. The red, hemorrhagic appearance of the exudative phase, however, is replaced by a diffuse gray and glistening cut surface, reflecting initial clearance of red cells by macrophages and an increase in new matrix produced by fibroblasts. Small, sub-millimeter cysts can often be appreciated grossly, corresponding to the alveolar duct dilatation that begins in the exudative phase (1).

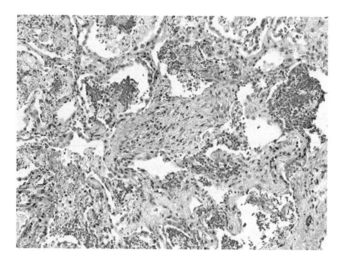

Figure 3   Proliferative phase DAD with interstitial and intra-alveolar fibroblast proliferation and type II pneumocyte hyperplasia.

The histologic changes characteristic of the proliferative phase of DAD, namely proliferation of type II pneumocytes and interstitial fibrosis, (Fig. 3) become readily apparent by day 6 following injury, but increased numbers of type II pneumocytes can be seen as early as day 3 (1,7). The cuboidal type II pneumocytes undergo differentiation to type I (or membranous) pneumocytes, and a combination of these two cells repopulate the alveolar ducts and septa by day 10 (7,19,20). The proliferating type II pneumocytes frequently display marked regenerative atypia, including nucleomegaly and prominent nucleoli, and frequent mitotic figures (21) (Fig. 4). Alveolar epithelium may also undergo squamous metaplasia, seen frequently in association with intra-alveolar fibrosis (12).

The underlying lung architecture becomes progressively distorted as DAD progresses through this stage, particularly in more clinically severe cases. Overall, the tissue becomes significantly more cellular, with the proliferation of epithelium and fibroblasts/myofibroblasts and influx of acute and chronic inflammatory cells into the interstitium and airspaces (2). Intra-alveolar fibrosis, including "alveolar duct fibrosis" and "alveolar bud" formation, leads to remodeling or obliteration of the normal underlying alveolar ducts or spaces, respectively (1). Hyaline membranes may be phagocytosed by intra-alveolar macrophages or may be covered by proliferating fibroblasts and ultimately incorporated into the interstitium (8,22,23). Epithelial cells can then migrate over this intra-alveolar fibrotic tissue and re-epithelialize the airspaces, and in these areas squamous metaplasia can appear prominent (22). Collapse of alveolar airspaces with re-epithelialization of apposed alveolar surfaces contributes to widening of the interstitium (2).

Changes at the hyaline membrane–alveolar septal interface appear to mediate the onset of fibrosis. During the late exudative and early proliferative phase, hyaline membranes acquire positivity for fibronectin (12) and reticulin fibers sprout from the alveolar

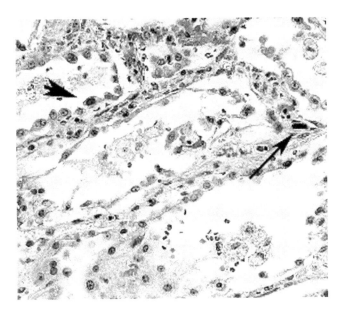

Figure 4 Proliferative phase DAD, high power magnification. Hyperplastic type II pneumo-cytes show marked atypia, including cellular pleomorphism, nucleomegaly, and hyperchroma-sia (short arrow). The airspaces containing foamy macrophages. An intravascular megakary-ocyte is seen (long arrow) (see also sec. VI "Pathologic Indicators of Outcome or Etiology").

septa into the overlying hyaline membranes (16). These events coincide with the migra-tion of fibroblasts/myofibroblasts from the interstitial compartment through gaps in the epithelial basement membrane and into the intra-alveolar spaces (12,22). Immunohisto-chemical studies using smooth muscle actin as a marker of myofibroblasts have shown that the cells are restricted to the septal compartment during the proliferative phase, but are found also in the hyaline membranes and comprising intra-alveolar fibroplasia in the proliferative phase (24). The infiltrating myofibroblasts in DAD, in contrast to uninjured lung, demonstrate intense expression of matrix metalloproteinases and tissue inhibitors of metalloproteinases, which likely permit rapid remodeling of the lung extracellular matrix during the proliferative phase (25).

The changes in the cellular content of the lung parenchyma, specifically the shift from epithelium- to fibroblast-predominance, and associated architectural remodeling, set the stage for the next phase of DAD, the fibrotic phase.

V.   Fibrotic Phase

Grossly, the lungs remain heavy, but now have a "cobblestone" appearance. The cut surface reveals alternating relatively preserved lung with microcystic change and patchy scarring. The proliferation of fibroblasts and myofibroblasts along with collapse and re-epithelialization of the pre-existing alveolar structures contribute to the prominent interstitial fibrosis characteristic of this stage of DAD (2).

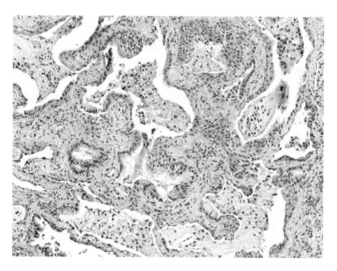

Figure 5 Fibrotic phase DAD with end-stage lung containing entrapped mucous and prominent squamous metaplasia of the residual airspaces.

Histologically, dilated alveolar ducts correlate with the microcystic change. Alveolar walls are irregularly thickened and elastic and trichrome stains (highlighting collagen deposition) demonstrate that the interstitium has undergone "fibroelastosis" (12,26). Dilated peripheral bronchi correspond to the radiologic appearance of traction bronchiectasis (1). In cases with progressive and fatal fibrosis, this ultimately leads to irreversible changes resembling those of "honeycomb" or end-stage lung (2) (Fig. 5). Rarely fibrotic DAD organizes into a pattern similar to bronchopulmonary dysplasia of infancy, with predominantly peripheral cyst formation apparently centered on the alveolar ducts. One report notes that clinically, patients with this outcome have been treated with higher than usual PEEP pressures and high concentrations for oxygen over a long period (27).

Marked changes are evident in the pulmonary vasculature, with capillary thrombi persisting early and large and small vessel remodeling occurring later in the fibrotic phase (2). Postmortem arteriography and venography studies have revealed vascular pruning, with abrupt narrowing of the peripheral third of the veins and intra-acinar narrowing of the arteries (28). Histologically, intra-acinar arteries and veins show intimal fibrosis and medial thickening and can be obliterated in areas of advanced fibrosis (28,29). Dilatation of veins can be seen in the pleura. Morphometric analysis demonstrates that the greatest arterial wall thickening occurs in the fibrotic phase of DAD (29). These changes undoubtedly contribute to the pathophysiology of this stage (e.g., V/Q mismatch), and the interested reader is referred to Tomashefski's excellent review of the vascular changes in DAD (1,29).

VI. Pathologic Indicators of Outcome or Etiology

The pathogenesis of DAD is under study using a variety of genomic, molecular and biochemical approaches, as detailed in other chapters in this volume. Here, we highlight two areas where pathologic evaluation of DAD is contributing to advances in our under-standing of ARDS.

First, tissue samples of DAD provide a critical testing ground for identifying and validating mediators of the injury or repair process. For example, a few groups have eval-uated the role of collagen subtypes and their mediators in fibrosis. Heat shock protein 47, a collagen-binding stress protein, appears to mediate intracellular procollagen processing. Immunohistochemical studies have demonstrated that Hsp47 is markedly upregulated in fibrotic lung in association with type III collagen deposition. This is not, however, unique to DAD as this relationship is found in other fibrosing diseases of the lung (30). In an lipopolysaccharide (LPS)-driven mouse model of ARDS, HSP47 and types I and III col-lagen mRNAs are upregulated in concert with fibrosis (31). Interestingly, the same group demonstrated that hyperthermic induction of another heat shock protein, Hsp70, could actually attenuate the fibrosis secondary to the LPS challenge (32).

Cell cycle regulators appear to be upregulated in DAD, as one might expect in response to tissue injury and repair. P53 and its effector CDKN1a (WAF1) are expressed in type II pneumocytes in association with apoptosis (33). Another downstream effector of apoptosis, BAX, is overexpressed in DAD as compared to normal lung, predominantly in alveolar pneumocytes and interstitial cells. A critical antiapoptotic protein and BAX homolog, BCL-2, is focally expressed in myofibroblasts in DAD, supporting a role for this protein in the proliferative activity of these cells (34).

The second area is the ongoing search for histopathologic features that may be predictive of resolution or progression, especially in the proliferative phase.

A subset of patients who survive ARDS have persistent lung function impair-ment, thought to be a function of degree of fibrosis and microvascular destruction (35). As in other fibrosing lung diseases (usual interstitial pneumonia/idiopathic pulmonary fibrosis, other interstitial pneumonias), the biological mediators of fibrosis in DAD are complex and currently not well defined, although defects in the surfactant biosynthe-sis pathway have been implicated in familial interstitial fibrosis (36) and the cytokine TGF-β appears to be an important mediator of both acute and chronic lung injury in ARDS (37).

Routine histopathologic evaluation is limited in its ability to predict the course of disease in terms of resolution versus progression versus stable fibrosis. This has sparked investigation of other morphologic approaches to identify possible predictive features.

Recent quantitative analyses of DAD histology have attempted to identify objective features that can predict clinical outcomes. Mandal and coworkers draw a distinction between a pure DAD pattern and DAD with organizing pneumonia (DAD-OP); the latter is defined as DAD with 20% or more of the examined tissue containing OP, which histologically appears as plugging of bronchioles and airspaces by fibroblast proliferations in a myxoid matrix. They also found that DAD-OP is associated with greater mean maximal lymphatic diameters as compared to DAD, a finding that suggests improved clearance of interstitial fluid in the former entity. Accordingly, patients with DAD-OP demonstrate improved survival over those with DAD alone (38).

The role of platelets in ARDS has also been studied. Thrombocytopenia with or without disseminated intravascular coagulation is associated with worse outcomes in patients with ARDS. In contrast, one retrospective study demonstrated improved survival in patients with ARDS and thrombocytosis (>350 th/cm^3). The same study quantitated megakaryocytes trapped in the pulmonary vasculature (Fig. 3) and found that they were significantly increased in DAD versus normal lung; however, this increase did not correspond with circulating platelet levels (39).

VII. The Role of Open Lung Biopsy in ARDS

Open lung biopsy plays an important role in guiding clinical management in a substantial percentage of patients with suspected ARDS. Although DAD is the underlying pathology in most cases of ARDS, there are some exceptions (40). According to the American European Consensus Conference, ARDS is defined as bilateral pulmonary infiltrates and a Pao_2/Fio_2 ratio of <200 mm Hg without evidence of left atrial hypertension (41). In one study of open lung biopsy specimens in patients fulfilling the AECC criteria, DAD represented the underlying pathology in 60% of cases and alternative diagnoses, including diffuse alveolar hemorrhage, bronchiolitis obliterans with organizing pneumonia (BOOP), pneumonia, neoplasia, and interstitial pneumonitides, comprised the remaining 40% of cases (42). Other studies also report that a significant minority of ARDS cases have other specific pathologic findings (43). A potential confounder in these analyses is that the process of DAD may be present, but not explicitly diagnosed, in ARDS biopsies that show other specific diagnostic patterns (e.g., infection, vasculitis, hemorrhage).

Conversely, in one study of patients diagnosed with DAD, approximately 90% fulfilled clinical criteria for ARDS (40). In this series, the authors examined 58 open lung biopsies performed on patients with diffuse lung infiltrates on radiology. Ten percent of the cases revealed a previously unrecognized causative or clinically important associated process, including viral or mycobacterial infections and underlying usual interstitial pneumonia (the pathologic correlate to idiopathic pulmonary fibrosis) (40). These findings clearly indicate the utility of open lung biopsy in treatment decisions: the current clinical criteria actually encompass a heterogeneous group of pathologic processes and in those cases with concordant ARDS and DAD, important causative factors can be detected by tissue examination.

VIII. Bronchoalveolar Lavage in DAD

Although tissue evaluation is the "gold standard" for diagnosis of DAD, several studies have evaluated the utility of bronchoalveolar lavage (BAL) samples. BAL fluid taken from patients with ARDS is typically moderate to highly cellular and contains a mixture of inflammatory cells and desquamated alveolar epithelial cells (44). Type II pneumocytes can be detected in the BAL fluid most readily in the first week from onset of symptoms and are uncommon or absent in the fibrotic stage (greater than 3–4 weeks from the onset of ARDS) (21). A spectrum of cytologic changes can be seen in the epithelial cells. Clumps of small cells with high nuclear: cytoplasmic ratios can resemble neoplastic cells and even be mistaken for adenocarcinoma. Other reactive pneumocytes appear large and highly atypical, changes reminiscent of radiation-induced atypia (21). Other features that can be seen in BAL fluids include squamous metaplasia and hyaline membranes. Neutrophils are a prominent feature in patients with sepsis-related ARDS, most notable at days 7 and 14 after the onset of symptoms, and their persistence at high concentrations in the BAL fluid is associated with higher mortality. Alveolar macrophages are another prominent component, but in contrast to neutrophils, high concentrations of alveolar macrophages are associated with improved survival (45). While these BAL features are satisfyingly concordant with biopsy findings, they are not diagnostic per se, since localized (nondiffuse) causes of pneumonitis can yield similar findings.

IX. DAD Superimposed on Other Interstitial Lung Diseases

DAD can complicate the course of other subacute or chronic lung diseases and in a minority of cases is the presenting feature of the disease. A leading example is the well-described acute exacerbation (AE) of idiopathic pulmonary fibrosis (IPF) (46,47). Clinically these patients present with one to a few weeks of worsening dyspnea; radiologically they show bilateral ground-glass opacities with or without consolidation combined with the peripheral honeycombing typical of usual interstitial pneumonia (UIP). Histologically, most cases demonstrate the features of DAD, with hyaline membranes as well as fibroblast/myofibroblast proliferation and intravascular fibrin thrombi superimposed on UIP, characterized by multifocal subpleural fibrosis and scarring with honeycomb change (47,48). One medical center's retrospective analysis of all patients diagnosed with IPF over a two-year period found an incidence of AE of IPF of 9%, a number that the authors suggest is likely an underestimate (48).

Some controversy surrounds predicting outcomes of AE in IPF patients, with some reports suggesting close to a 90% mortality rate (47) and others suggesting closer to 50% mortality rate (49). Churg and coworkers suggest that AE of interstitial lung disease be defined as the presence of new ground-glass opacities radiologically combined with evidence of acute injury on lung biopsy and expand the histologic definition of acute injury to include those specimens that demonstrate OP and/or numerous, large foci of fibroblast proliferation, essentially both features that can account for the ground glass appearance by CT scan (49). Similarly to the aforementioned study that demonstrated improved outcomes in patients with combined DAD and OP (38), these authors conclude that patients with interstitial lung disease (including UIP, nonspecific interstitial pneumonia, and hypersensitivity pneumonitis) and OP with or without large fibroblast foci have better outcomes than those with features of DAD (48).

X. Acute Interstitial Pneumonia

The main differential diagnosis for patients with idiopathic rapidly progressive respiratory failure is acute interstitial pneumonia (Hamman–Rich syndrome) (50). This is a rare disorder with high mortality. The histopathologic findings are identical to those of DAD, therefore this diagnosis can only be made clinically on the basis of excluding other factors that could trigger ARDS. However, open lung biopsy can serve an important role in excluding other processes including infection, underlying interstitial lung disease, or BOOP (also known as cryptogenic organizing pneumonia, or COP) and clinical correlation is necessary to exclude an underlying connective tissue disease or other systemic disorder (50,51).

XI. Summary

In summary, the pathology of DAD can be divided into three distinct but overlapping phases. (1) The exudative phase occurs within days following insult to the alveolocapillary unit. Epithelial and endothelial injuries lead to the characteristic edema, hemorrhage, and hyaline membrane formation. (2) The proliferative phase represents the early reparative stage of DAD, usually occurring by one week following the initial insult. Proliferating type II pneumocytes and fibroblasts dominate the histologic picture and drive remodeling of the alveolar architecture. (3) The fibrotic phase, for those patients who survive the acute stages of ARDS, is characterized by alveolar wall fibrosis and vascular wall thickening.

Although the histologic findings in DAD per se are nonspecific, other features seen on the open lung biopsy can uncover factors contributing to an individual case of ARDS. In particular, the open lung biopsy can aid in the identification of an infectious process or underlying pulmonary disease that may have significant implications for treatment or prognostication.

The pathology of DAD has been carefully examined by light microscopy and electron microscopy since its systematic description in the 1970s. Ancillary techniques, such as immunohistochemistry, have enhanced our understanding of the pathophysiology of DAD. We have limited ability, however, to predict the course of disease based on the histology alone, although recognition of certain features, such as OP or interstitial fibrosis, does permit some prognostic stratification. Future studies that bridge histology with advanced diagnostic techniques that examine protein expression and molecular genetic pathology may offer additional insight into an individual patient's predispositions and prognosis.

References

1. Tomashefski JF Jr. Pulmonary pathology of acute respiratory distress syndrome. Clin Chest Med 2000; 21(3):435–466.
2. Katzenstein AL. Katzenstein and Askin's surgical pathology of non-neoplastic lung disease. In: Livolsi VA, ed. Major Problems in Pathology, Vol. 13, 4 ed. Philadelphia, PA: Saunders Elsevier, 2006:17–49.
3. Nash G, Blennerhassett JB, Pontoppidan H. Pulmonary lesions associated with oxygen therapy and artificial ventilation. N Engl J Med 1967; 276(7):368–374.
4. Liebow AA, Warren S, De CE. Pathology of atomic bomb casualties. Am J Pathol 1949; 25(5):853–1027.
5. Martin AM Jr, Simmons RL, Heisterkamp CA III. Respiratory insufficiency in combat casualties. I. Pathologic changes in the lungs of patients dying of wounds. Ann Surg 1969; 170(1):30–38.
6. Claireaux AE. The effect of oxygen on the lung. J Clin Pathol Suppl (R Coll Pathol) 1975; 9:75–80.
7. Katzenstein AL, Bloor CM, Leibow AA. Diffuse alveolar damage—the role of oxygen, shock, and related factors. A review. Am J Pathol 1976; 85(1):209–228.
8. Wright JL. Adult respiratory distress syndrome. In: Churg AM, Myers JL, Tazelaar HD, et al. eds. Thurlbeck's Pathology of the Lung. New York: Thieme, 2005:355–370.
9. Fracica PJ, Knapp MJ, Piantadosis CA, et al. Responses of baboons to prolonged hyperoxia: Physiology and qualitative pathology. J Appl Physiol 1991; 71(6):2352–2362.
10. Ichikado K, Suga M, Gushima Y, et al. Hyperoxia-induced diffuse alveolar damage in pigs: correlation between thin-section CT and histopathologic findings. Radiology 2000; 216(2):531–538.
11. Whimster WF, Macfarlane AJ. Normal lung weights in a white population. Am Rev Respir Dis 1974; 110(4):478–483.

12. Fukuda Y, Ishizaki M, Masuda Y, et al. The role of intraalveolar fibrosis in the process of pulmonary structural remodeling in patients with diffuse alveolar damage. Am J Pathol 1987; 126(1):171–182.

13. Sugiyama K, Kawai T. Diffuse alveolar damage and acute interstitial pneumonitis: histochemical evaluation with lectins and monoclonal antibodies against surfactant apoprotein and collagen type IV. Mod Pathol 1993; 6(3):242–248.

14. Peres e Serra A, Parra ER, Eher E, et al. Nonhomogeneous immunostaining of hyaline membranes in different manifestations of diffuse alveolar damage. Clinics 2006; 61(6):497–502.

15. Sun AP, Ohtsuki Y, Fujita J, et al. Immunohistochemical characterisation of pulmonary hyaline membrane in various types of interstitial pneumonia. Pathology 2003; 35(2):120–124.

16. Kobashi Y, Manabe T. The fibrosing process in so-called organized diffuse alveolar damage. An immunohistochemical study of the change from hyaline membrane to membranous fibrosis. Virchows Arch A Pathol Anat Histopathol 1993; 422(1):47–52.

17. Katzenstein AL. Pathogenesis of "fibrosis" in interstitial pneumonia: an electron microscopic study. Hum Pathol 1985; 16(10):1015–1024.

18. Yamada T, Uehara K, Kawanishi R, et al. Immunohistochemical detection of ubiquitin-positive intracytoplasmic eosinophilic inclusion bodies in diffuse alveolar damage. Histopathology 2006; 48(7):846–854.

19. Evans MJ, Cabral LJ, Stephens RJ, et al. Transformation of alveolar type 2 cells to type 1 cells following exposure to NO2. Exp Mol Pathol 1975; 22(1):142–150.

20. Kawanami O, Ferrans VJ and Crystal RG. Structure of alveolar epithelial cells in patients with fibrotic lung disorders. Lab Invest 1982; 46(1):39–53.

21. Stanley MW, Henry-Stanley MJ, Gajl-Peczalska KJ, et al. Hyperplasia of type II pneumocytes in acute lung injury. Cytologic findings of sequential bronchoalveolar lavage. Am J Clin Pathol 1992; 97(5):669–677.

22. Fukuda Y, Ferrans VJ, Schoenberger CI, et al. Patterns of pulmonary structural remodeling after experimental paraquat toxicity. The morphogenesis of intraalveolar fibrosis. Am J Pathol 1985; 118(3):452–475.

23. Takahashi T, Takahashi Y and Nio M. Remodeling of the alveolar structure in the paraquat lung of humans: a morphometric study. Hum Pathol 1994; 25(7):702–708.

24. Pache JC, Christakos PG, Gannon DE, et al. Myofibroblasts in diffuse alveolar damage of the lung. Mod Pathol 1998; 11(11):1064–1070.

25. Hayashi T, Stetler-Stevenson WG, Fleming MV, et al. Immunohistochemical study of metalloproteinases and their tissue inhibitors in the lungs of patients with diffuse alveolar damage and idiopathic pulmonary fibrosis. Am J Pathol 1996; 149(4):1241–1256.

26. Rozin GF, Gomes MM, Parra ER, et al. Collagen and elastic system in the remodelling process of major types of idiopathic interstitial pneumonias (IIP). Histopathology 2005; 46(4):413–421.

27. Churg A, Golden J, Fligiel S, et al. Bronchopulmonary dysplasia in the adult. Am Rev Respir Dis 1983; 127(1):117–120.

28. Homma S, Jones R, Qvist J, et al. Pulmonary vascular lesions in the adult respiratory distress syndrome caused by inhalation of zinc chloride smoke: a morphometric study. Hum Pathol 1992; 23(1):45–50.

29. Tomashefski JF Jr, Davies P, Boggis C, et al. The pulmonary vascular lesions of the adult respiratory distress syndrome. Am J Pathol 1983; 112(1):112–126.

30. Razzaque MS, Nazneen A, Taguchi T. Immunolocalization of collagen and collagen-binding heat shock protein 47 in fibrotic lung diseases. Mod Pathol 1998; 11(12):1183–1188.

31. Hagiwara S, Iwasaka H, Matsumoto S, et al. Coexpression of HSP47 gene and type I and type III collagen genes in LPS-induced pulmonary fibrosis in rats. Lung 2007; 185(1):31–37.

32. Hagiwara S, Iwasaka H, Matsumoto S, et al. Association between heat stress protein 70 induction and decreased pulmonary fibrosis in an animal model of acute lung injury. Lung 2007; 185(5):287–293.

33. Guinee D Jr, Fleming M, Hayashi T, et al. Association of p53 and WAF1 expression with apoptosis in diffuse alveolar damage. Am J Pathol 1996; 149(2):531–538.

34. Guinee D Jr, Brambilla E, Fleming M, et al. The potential role of BAX and BCL-2 expression in diffuse alveolar damage. Am J Pathol 1997; 151(4):999–1007.

35. Neff TA, Stocker R, Frey HR, et al. Long-term assessment of lung function in survivors of severe ARDS. Chest 2003; 123(3):845–853.

36. Young LR, Nogee LM, Barnett B, et al. Usual interstitial pneumonia in an adolescent with ABCA3 mutations. Chest 2008; 134(1):192–195.

37. Dhainaut JF, Charpentier J, Chiche JD. Transforming growth factor-beta: a mediator of cell regulation in acute respiratory distress syndrome. Crit Care Med 2003; 31(Suppl. 4):S258–S264.

38. Mandal RV, Mark EJ, Kradin RL. Organizing pneumonia and pulmonary lymphatic architecture in diffuse alveolar damage. Hum Pathol 2008; 39(8):1234–1238.

39. Mandal RV, Mark EJ, Kradin RL. Megakaryocytes and platelet homeostasis in diffuse alveolar damage. Exp Mol Pathol 2007; 83(3):327–331.

40. Parambil JG, Myers JL, Aubry MC, et al. Causes and prognosis of diffuse alveolar damage diagnosed on surgical lung biopsy. Chest 2007; 132(1):50–57.

41. Bernard GR, Artigas A, Brigham KL, et al. The American-European Consensus Conference on ARDS. Definitions, mechanisms, relevant outcomes, and clinical trial coordination. Am J Respir Crit Care Med 1994; 149(3 Pt 1):818–824.

42. Patel SR, Karmpaliotis D, Ayas NT, et al. The role of open-lung biopsy in ARDS. Chest 2004; 125(1):197–202.

43. Esteban A, Fernández-Segoviano P, Frutos-Vivar F, et al. Comparison of clinical criteria for the acute respiratory distress syndrome with autopsy findings. Ann Intern Med 2004; 141(6):440–445.

44. Beskow CO, Drachenberg CB, Bourquin PM, et al. Diffuse alveolar damage. Morphologic features in bronchoalveolar lavage fluid. Acta Cytol 2000; 44(4):640–646.

45. Steinberg KP, Milberg JA, Martin TR, et al. Evolution of bronchoalveolar cell populations in the adult respiratory distress syndrome. Am J Respir Crit Care Med 1994; 150(1):113–122.

46. Kondoh Y, Taniguchi H, Kawabata Y, et al. Acute exacerbation in idiopathic pulmonary fibrosis. Analysis of clinical and pathologic findings in three cases. Chest 1993; 103(6):1808–1812.

47. Parambil JG, Myers JL, Ryu JH. Histopathologic features and outcome of patients with acute exacerbation of idiopathic pulmonary fibrosis undergoing surgical lung biopsy. Chest 2005; 128(5):3310–3315.

48. Kim DS, Park JH, Park BK, et al. Acute exacerbation of idiopathic pulmonary fibrosis: frequency and clinical features. Eur Respir J 2006; 27(1):143–150.

49. Churg A, Müller NL, Silva CI, et al. Acute exacerbation (acute lung injury of unknown cause) in UIP and other forms of fibrotic interstitial pneumonias. Am J Surg Pathol 2007; 31(2):277–284.

50. Katzenstein AL, Myers JL, Mazur MT. Acute interstitial pneumonia. A clinicopathologic, ultrastructural, and cell kinetic study. Am J Surg Pathol 1986; 10(4):256–267.

51. Bouros D, Nicholson AC, Polychronopoulos V, et al. Acute interstitial pneumonia. Eur Respir J 2000; 15(2):412–418.

5
Pathogenesis of Acute Lung Injury: Experimental Studies

REBECCA M. BARON
Department of Medicine, Division of Pulmonary and Critical Care, Brigham and Women's Hospital, Boston, Massachusetts, U.S.A.

MARK A. PERRELLA
Department of Medicine, Division of Pulmonary and Critical Care; and Newborn Medicine, Brigham and Women's Hospital, Boston, Massachusetts, U.S.A.

I. Introduction

Acute respiratory distress syndrome (ARDS) represents a devastating clinical condition for which there exist few treatment options. While great scientific strides have been made in the last decades in terms of defining molecular pathways, applicability of these discoveries to tangible treatments for human disease has been limited. A major challenge in generating effective therapeutics has been the ability to develop reliable animal models of critical illness that allow generation and testing of novel hypotheses and, ultimately, translatability of the findings to the human condition. While there exist larger animal models of critical illness, the expense and complexity of these studies have limited widespread use of these systems for basic experimentation. Murine models of ARDS are appealing for experimental design for many reasons, including the ability to rapidly breed large numbers of animals that can be carefully studied with appropriate controls and the capability of studying animals with complex genetic manipulations. However, disadvantages to the study of ARDS in mice include inherent differences in murine and human genetics and response to disease, as well as significant heterogeneity of the interaction of the human genome with a complex environment that is impossible to model. That being said, there exists a wealth of critical information that has yet to be gleaned from the study of mouse models of ARDS, and understanding of the methods of experimentation and their limitations are important for our ability to move forward with clinically relevant translational studies. The current understanding of ARDS pathophysiology and underlying mechanisms are reviewed elsewhere in detail in this book. We will therefore highlight how animal experimental studies have and can be applied toward discerning mechanisms of complex lung disease, through examining key pathophysiologic features of the development of ARDS.

II. The Lung Is Injured

ARDS represents a clinical syndrome that includes hypoxemia (in the presence of bilateral lung infiltrates not attributable to elevated left heart filling pressures) and is believed to be the end result of injury to the lung that arises through a variety of different possible mechanisms, including aspiration of gastric contents, pneumonia, sepsis, and trauma (1). Some studies have suggested that "direct" injury as a result of noxious inhalation (e.g., aspiration pneumonitis) may result in more severe damage than "indirect" injury incurred from infection or ischemia localized at a site distant from the lung (e.g., pancreatitis or peritonitis). Direct injury first affects the alveolar epithelium and results in alveolar inflammation, while indirect lung injury arises as a result of bloodstream mediators and dysregulation of the vascular endothelium, producing more pronounced lung interstitial inflammation. Hence, direct injury more classically results in alveolar consolidation, while indirect injury more typically produces diffuse ground glass opacification. It has been proposed that different mechanisms of injury result in distinct clinical ARDS syndromes, with indirect injury (also referred to as extrapulmonary ARDS) demonstrating more response to application of positive end-expiratory pressure as a result of less stiffness in the lung parenchyma, compared with direct injury (also referred to as pulmonary ARDS) (2,3). Irrespective of the mechanism of primary injury (or "1st-hit"), a downstream cascade of complex events is triggered that may be exacerbated by continued elaboration of inflammatory mediators from the primary injury and/or incursion of an additional injury (or "2nd-hit", e.g., pancreatitis followed by ventilator-induced lung injury) (Fig. 1). Pathologic hallmarks of human ARDS from any cause include (4,5):

(a) Neutrophilic alveolitis: presence of polymorphonuclear cells within the alveolar space;
(b) Hyaline membranes: reflecting serum protein transudation and precipitation in the airspaces;
(c) Microthrombi: reflecting endothelial injury and propagation of procoagulant mediators.

Each of these features will be discussed in more detail below. While it is not clear that outcomes are different from ARDS as a result of direct *versus* indirect injury (7), these paradigms represent an important framework for approaching mechanistic study using mouse models of ARDS.

There exist a variety of mouse models that have produced important biologic findings regarding mechanisms underlying propagation of lung injury, even though no model perfectly replicates the clinical and pathologic findings of ARDS. This has been borne out through failure of uniform translation of murine findings to human disease, as exemplified by the efficacy of inhibition of tumor necrosis factor alpha (TNF)-α in septic mice that was not reproducible in humans (8,9). It has become increasingly appreciated that different mouse models of ARDS represent varying aspects of human disease, and we have provided an overview of some of the more commonly used mouse models (Table 1) that have been reviewed recently in detail elsewhere (5).

III. Disruption of the Alveolar-Capillary Membrane
A. Increased Permeability

Irrespective of the mechanism of initial or propagating injury at the genesis of ARDS, disruption of the alveolar-capillary membrane (ACM) represents the hallmark of early physiologic derangement in lung injury (13,14). It has been suggested that the persistent

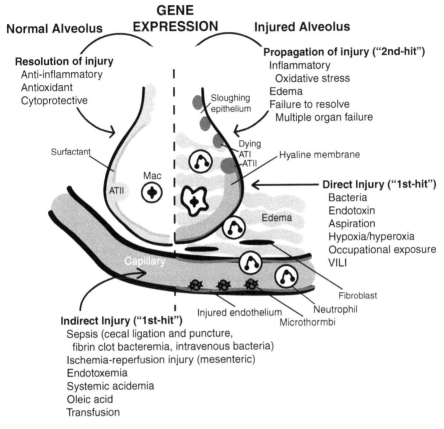

Figure 1   The lung is injured. ARDS is initiated with a variety of possible mechanisms of injury, including direct injury to the lung (e.g., aspiration pneumonia) or indirect injury at a distant site from the lung (e.g., bacterial peritonitis). These "1st-hit" injuries might be exacerbated with propagation of the injury process by a "2nd-hit" or by failure of the initial process to fully resolve. Alterations in gene expression underlie all of the processes that result in activation of distinct pathways. While a direct injury might first affect the pulmonary epithelium and an indirect injury might initially affect the endothelium, both types of injury result in disruption of the alveolar-capillary membrane, influx of protein-rich edema fluid, production of hyaline membranes, recruitment of neutrophils to the lung, and surfactant inactivation. Activated neutrophils can elaborate a variety of mediators, including proteases and oxidants. Activated macrophages can elaborate both pro and anti-inflammatory cytokines. Fibroblasts play an important role in production of extracellular matrix. *Abbreviations*: VILI, ventilator-induced lung injury; ATI and ATII, alveolar type I and II cells, respectively; Mac, macrophage. *Source*: From Ref. 6.

Table 1 Examples of Mouse Models of ARDS

Mechanism of injury	Model of injury	Features replicating human disease	Features not necessarily consistent with human disease
Direct lung injury	Intratracheal LPS	Produces significant alveolar neutrophil infiltration; heals without scarring or fibrosis; can produce some systemic hypotension	Injury can be patchy; may be mild effect on permeability
	Acid instillation	Intended to simulate aspiration pneumonitis (10); significant neutrophil infiltration and permeability (11)	Humans usually aspirate mixed gastric contents rather than pure hydrochloric acid
	Hyperoxia	Produces significant oxidative stress and hemorrhagic lung injury	Uncertain whether humans develop injury similar to mice in response to hyperoxia (12)
	VILI	Has direct clinical relevance; early phase results in interstitial edema and permeability with later phases producing interstitial and alveolar inflammation	Requires prolonged periods of ventilation to see alveolar inflammation, and therefore presents a challenge in studying large numbers of mice quickly with this model
Indirect lung injury	Systemic LPS (i.v. or i.p.)	Significant early hypotension (but not sustained)	Interstitial neutrophil infiltration with less pronounced alveolar injury and permeability
	CLP	Indwelling focus of ongoing source of systemic inflammation; interstitial and alveolar inflammation with epithelial permeability	Varying effect with use of fluid resuscitation, antibiotics, etc.; believed by many to be one of the best models of sepsis/organ injury, though with variable extent of lung injury
Combined direct and indirect injury	Intrapulmonary bacteria	Direct effect from localized delivery to the lung, with indirect effect from elaborated microbial products	Injury can be patchy
	Indirect injury (e.g., CLP) + VILI	Replicates sequential injury pattern of human ARDS	Time course of dual injury can be variable

Abbreviations: LPS, lipopolysaccharide; i.v., intravenous; i.p., intraperitoneal; CLP, cecal ligation and puncture; VILI, ventilator-induced lung injury.
Source: Adapted from Refs. 4,5.

impaired function of the ACM correlates with increased mortality (15). Mechanisms of more "direct" injury initially affect the alveolar epithelium, while "indirect" injuries attack the capillary endothelium primarily. Impairment of the protective ACM results in development of increased permeability edema, with transudation of serum proteins into the alveolar space. In contrast to hydrostatic pulmonary edema as a result of left heart dysfunction, analysis of bronchoalveolar lavage (BAL) fluid revealed an elevated ratio of protein in the edema fluid as compared with plasma in patients with ARDS (ratio >0.75 in ARDS *vs.* ratio <0.75 in congestive heart failure (CHF) or other forms of hydrostatic edema) (16). Animal models have been used extensively in deciphering the mechanisms of ACM dysregulation (17,18) and will be discussed in detail elsewhere in this book. Key techniques in evaluating the presence of increased permeability edema in animals are summarized in Table 2 and have been proven invaluable in assessing the reliability of various murine models of ARDS and in correlating findings from animal models with human disease.

B. Development of Lung Inflammation

Recruitment of inflammatory cells to the lung following injury has been observed in humans and in animal models of ARDS, and release of neutrophil contents has been implicated in propagating enhancement of ACM disruption (14; Fig. 1). While it is believed that alveolar inflammation is a hallmark of ARDS, treatment with anti-inflammatory agents in human ARDS has not been proven beneficial. Furthermore, animals and humans can develop ARDS in the setting of neutropenia (25–27). Thus, investigators are exploring therapeutic targets that extend beyond pure inhibition of the inflammatory response. For example, recent exciting work has demonstrated an important role for platelet-neutrophil aggregates in the development of acid-induced lung injury (28). Furthermore, increasingly, it is appreciated that there exists an important balance between pro and anti-inflammatory cytokines that are elaborated in ARDS, such that pure inhibition of proinflammatory cytokines might predispose the host toward an immune-deficient state (29). Relative immune deficiency may be particularly detrimental for the host when an infectious etiology (e.g., pneumonia, bacterial peritonitis) underlies the development of ARDS. Assessment of lung inflammation is a key component in evaluating murine models of ARDS, and some key techniques are outlined in Table 2. Mechanisms of lung inflammation have been investigated intensely in ARDS, and are discussed in detail in other chapters in this book.

C. Surfactant Dysfunction

Surfactant is a lipoprotein mixture that is secreted by type II pneumocytes and lines the alveolar surface. Surfactant plays important roles in host defense and in reduction of surface tension, thereby allowing for maintenance of alveolar patency. Loss of surfactant function has been implicated in causing significant physiologic lung dysfunction in ARDS that results in alveolar collapse (14). Dysregulated surfactant function arises from a variety of mechanisms, including injury to type II alveolar epithelial cells, influx of edema and proteins as a result of disruption of the ACM, and decreased transcription of key surfactant components in the setting of inflammation and oxidative stress (19,20,30). Although surfactant replacement has not shown benefit to date in adult ARDS, numerous unresolved issues remain, with timing of replacement, delivery to appropriate lung segments, and

Table 2 Examples of Laboratory-Based Techniques Commonly Used in Characterizing Lung Injury in Mouse Models

Parameter in ARDS	Common techniques for assessment in animal models	Variables in application of the technique
Permeability of the alveolar-capillary membrane (18)	Measurement of BAL protein content	Represents extent of serum protein transudation across the membrane; can be measured in humans and helps to distinguish CHF from ALI (13,16)
	Wet-to-dry weight	Lungs are removed from animal and weight obtained pre and postdesiccation to determine lung fluid content; technique is fairly insensitive but detection of differences are meaningful
	Evans blue dye	Dye is injected into the vascular system, and recovery of dye from the lung used to calculate extent of permeability; requires more technical skill than previous two techniques but is more sensitive
Surfactant disruption	Assessment of lung physiology	Mice are tracheotomized and assessed for physiologic parameters similar to those in humans (compliance and resistance) using a computerized mouse ventilator (e.g., Flexivent system); additionally, more complicated techniques for measuring surface tension to surface area of surfactant ex vivo have been applied (20,21)
Alteration of gene expression	Measurement of levels of RNA	Northern blots and real-time PCR allow for quantitative assessment of gene expression; reflect expression attributable in part to transcriptional regulation. Assessment of changes in gene expression of many genes can be performed using microarrays (genechips) (22,23). Western blots and immunohistochemistry allow for assessment of protein levels in cells and/or tissues, and changes in levels of a large number of proteins are increasingly being performed using proteomic techniques (24)
	Measurement of promoter activity	Regulatory regions of genes (promoter sequences) can be cloned into vectors and analyzed in transfections in cells (and in mice using transgenic techniques); such studies can help discern which sequence motifs within gene promoters are critical for regulating gene expression
	Assessment of transcription factor binding to DNA	Electrophoretic mobility shift assays (EMSA, in vitro) and chromatin immunoprecipitation assays (ChIP, in vivo) allow for examination of transcription factor binding to DNA motifs

Table 2 Examples of Laboratory-Based Techniques Commonly Used in Characterizing Lung Injury in Mouse Models (*Continued*)

Parameter in ARDS	Common techniques for assessment in animal models	Variables in application of the technique
Recruitment of inflammatory cells	Assessment of lung inflammation	Cell counts and differentials can be measured from BAL fluid to assess alveolar inflammation, and interstitial inflammation can be assessed by quantitation of immunohistochemical staining of lung sections; other methods include measurement of myeloperoxidase activity from cell or tissue lysates; further characterization of inflammatory cell populations from BAL fluid or digested lung tissue can be undertaken using flow cytometry analysis; levels of cytokines can be measured in plasma and in BAL fluid collected from mice

Abbreviations: BAL, bronchoalveolar lavage; CHF, congestive heart failure; ALI, acute lung injury; PCR, polymerase chain reaction.

optimal product constituents necessary for restoration of surfactant function. Moreover, with increasing sophistication of delivery mechanisms for targeting alveolar epithelial cells (e.g., inhalation technology and intratracheal administration (31)), there remains optimism for modulating surfactant properties beneficially in ARDS (32). Measurement of physiologic lung dysfunction and surfactant properties is feasible in mice and has contributed significantly toward modeling and studying lung dysfunction in translational models (Table 2). Further discussion of the role of surfactant dysfunction in ARDS will be discussed in more detail elsewhere in this book.

IV. Resolution of Lung Injury

Development of ARDS has traditionally been viewed as incurred injury with resultant dysregulation of gene expression and propagation of downstream events in the inflammatory cascade. It is increasingly appreciated that ARDS can also be viewed as syndrome in which lung injury "fails to resolve" (Fig. 1) and, moreover, that the process of resolution represents an "active" process that requires defined mechanistic stages of molecular events (33). The transition from the inflammatory/exudative phase of ARDS to the proliferative, followed by the fibrotic phase depends upon numerous biologic processes that are discussed in more detail elsewhere in this book. Optimal repair depends upon appropriate balances in cellular apoptosis, matrix metalloproteinase production, oxidative stress, fibrinolysis, the immune response, chemokines, growth factors, cytokines, and eicosanoid production. Thus, dysregulated repair can ensue for a variety of distinct biologic reasons, and persistent intra-alveolar fibrosis can result in obliteration of alveolar-capillary units and a phenotype similar to that studied in models of idiopathic pulmonary fibrosis. In fact, much of the information regarding later-stage ARDS has been inferred from murine models of intratracheal bleomycin that result in profound lung fibrosis.

Differential rates of repair have been invoked to account for the more rapid resolution of lung histologic changes in extrapulmonary-induced injury as compared with
direct pulmonary injury leading to ARDS (34,35). While it is not clear that there is a difference in overall outcomes based upon the mode of injury, these findings further suggest
that there might exist distinct possible therapeutic targets to enhance resolution of injury.
Much of therapeutics strategy has traditionally been aimed at preventing "upregulation"
of the injurious processes that result in ARDS. However, increasing recognition of key
factors in the resolution of lung injury suggests that enhancement of these pathways
might prove beneficial in disease (36). For example, recent years have produced exciting
studies that have suggested a role for bone marrow-derived progenitor cells in enhancing
the repair process following injury. Administration of intravenous and intratracheal bone
marrow-derived progenitor cells to mice subjected to acute lung injury through endotoxin
is feasible and has demonstrated ameliorated lung injury indices (37,38).

V. Alteration of Gene Expression
A. Changes in Expression of Single Genes
In Vivo: Genetically Engineered Mice

Despite the paucity of existing targeted treatment for ARDS, the last 100 years have
witnessed an explosion in molecular understanding of disease pathogenesis of critical
illness (39). While post-translational alterations to existing proteins are critical in disease
states, alteration in gene expression is also believed to play a key role in the multiple
dysregulated pathways in ARDS (touched upon in the sections above). Much of the
current scientific knowledge has arisen from study of the effects of a single gene on a
disease process, and the availability of genetically engineered mice for the last 20 years
has allowed further in vivo dissection of gene function using mouse models of ARDS
as described above. "Loss of function" studies have been facilitated by the development
of mice with targeted deletion of a candidate gene, and "gain of function" studies have
been possible with the development of transgenic mice capable of overexpressing a
candidate gene. Furthermore, the ability to conditionally express genes in mice during
different phases of development and/or disease and, in many cases, in specific cell types
using cell-specific promoters, has provided unprecedented ability to study the in vivo
effects of altered gene expression. For example, the surfactant protein C promoter has
been used to target candidate gene expression to the distal lung epithelium while the
Clara Cell Secretory Protein promoter has allowed for targeted proximal lung epithelial
cell expression (40). While development of genetically engineered mice has traditionally
been limited to a few number of laboratories with the funds and relevant expertise,
recent development of international consortia to catalog, generate, and freely distribute
genetically engineered mice will prevent reduplication of efforts and allow more uniform
access to these critical reagents (41).

B. Change in Expression of Individual Genes
In Vitro: Transcriptional Regulation

Alteration in gene expression can result from a variety of processes, including alteration in mRNA processing, mRNA stability, and recent increasing appreciation of the
importance of RNA-mediated gene silencing in gene regulation (42,43). To date, much

of our understanding of changes in gene expression has arisen from studies of alteration in gene promoter activity (Table 2). Transcriptional regulation involves binding of transcription factors to sequence-specific regulatory sequences (DNA-binding motifs) within the promoter (and/or enhancer) region of DNA that lies upstream from the transcription initiation start site (described in further detail in Fig. 2). RNA is transcribed, processed, then transported to the cytoplasm for translation of the functional protein. While

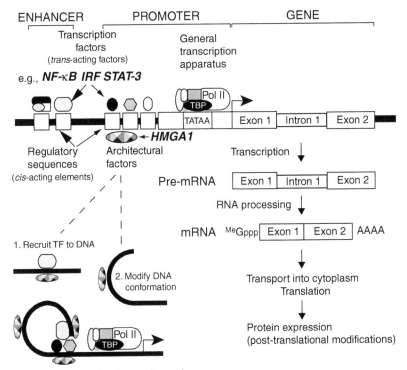

Figure 2 Overview of gene regulation. *Trans*-acting factors (transcription factors) bind to *cis*-acting elements (DNA regulatory sequences) in the 5′-flanking sequence of a gene (promoter and enhancer elements) to initiate and drive transcription. Key transcription factors in upregulation of genes in the inflammatory cascade are listed (NF-κB, IRF-1, Stat-3), and architectural transcription factors (e.g., HMGA1) play a role in recruiting multiple transcription factors to DNA to form an "enhanceosome" or regulatory complex. The general transcription apparatus contains RNA polymerase II (Pol II) and TATA-binding protein (TBP), as well as associated factors that form a transcriptional complex at the TATA box (TATAA) that is required for initiation of transcription (bent arrow represents the transcription initiation start site). mRNA is transcribed and is then processed (including splicing out of introns with joining of exons to generate the intact coding sequence, as well as addition of a 5′-methylated cap (^{Me}Gppp) and a poly(A) tail (AAAA)). The mature mRNA is transported to the cytoplasm for translation of the functional protein. *Source*: From Ref. 42.

activation of gene transcription depends upon numerous complex factors, including chromatin structure and modification of histone proteins, the binding of key transcription factors to their cognate promoter binding sites in a coordinated fashion plays a key role in changing gene expression in an orchestrated manner. The ability to study alteration in gene transcription and binding of transcription factors to specific promoter sequences have yielded important understanding of mechanisms underlying key pathophysiologic steps in ARDS. Common techniques used in laboratory studies of gene regulation are summarized in Table 2. Studies of multiple individual genes, as well as emerging data from microarray studies in ARDS (described below) have arrived at the same unifying concept that coordinated gene expression arises in large part from regulation of "families" of genes as a result of shared promoter motifs and binding of a few key transcription factors to produce pluripotent effects (44). For example, a large number of key mediators of the inflammatory cascade are regulated in part by a few common transcription factors, including NF-κB, Stat-3, and IRF-1 (45,46). Moreover, there exist a group of proteins termed architectural transcription factors that facilitate assembly of groups of transcription factors, termed "enhanceosomes" that drive gene transcription. For example, the High Mobility Group A1 (HMGA1) protein is an architectural transcription factor that has been shown to play an important role in transcriptional upregulation of a number of key target genes during inflammation, including E-selectin, VCAM-1, IFN-β, and NOS2 (47; Fig. 2). Thus, elucidation of key regulatory processes in ARDS presents increased availability of and understanding of targets for therapeutics development. The ability to control levels of expression of individual genes or "gene families" temporally under variable stimuli represents a powerful tool in improving outcomes from critical illness. The increasing understanding of molecular regulation of gene expression is making such "designer" drugs increasingly feasible.

C.   Changes in Expression of Many Genes: Microarray Technology

While significant biological progress has been made with the study of individual genes, many investigators have proposed that the failure to translate biological findings into therapeutic advances has arisen from the difficulty of analyzing large-scale expression of many genes simultaneously in a complex organism. The sequencing and mapping of the human genome, as well as that of the mouse and other organisms, coupled with technological advances allowing for complex gene expression analysis has led to use of microarray technology to assess expression of thousands of genes simultaneously (Table 2). Moreover, high-throughput genotyping has allowed for determination of sequence variants in the human genome on a larger scale than has ever been previously possible, thus further facilitating genetic association studies in critical illness that allow correlation of genetic variants with disease susceptibility and severity (22). Thus, investigators now have available capability of correlating large-scale gene expression patterns in human illness and in mice subjected to animal models of disease, such that relevant translational research can be carried out in the laboratory that ultimately will be clinically applicable (23). Increasing capability is emerging in assessing global changes in protein levels in critically ill patients that will allow further analysis of the complex biologic pathways that are activated during ARDS (24).

VI. Conclusion

Increasing understanding of molecular mechanisms underlying ARDS pathophysiology coupled with growing sophistication of murine models of lung injury provides a unique platform for translational research, with the ultimate goal of improved therapeutics for this devastating syndrome. Moreover, increasing ability to measure complex gene and protein expression patterns in human patients and in animals subjected to clinically relevant ARDS models will significantly enhance our ability to identify appropriate targets for drug development. Now represents an exciting time in which we can hope to apply our molecular understanding of biologic mechanisms toward improving outcomes from ARDS.

References

1. Hudson LD, Milberg JA, Anardi D, et al. Clinical risks for the development of the acute respiratory distress syndrome. Am J Respir Grit Care Med 1995; 151:293–301.
2. Gattinoni L, Pelosi P, Suter PM, et al. Acute respiratory distress syndrome caused by pulmonary and extrapulmonary disease. Different syndromes? Am J Respir Crit Care Med 1998; 158:3–11.
3. Pelosi P, D'Onofrio D, Chiumello D, et al. Pulmonary and extrapulmonary acute respiratory distress syndrome are different. Eur Respir J Suppl 2003; 42:48S–56S.
4. Adapted from Matute-Bello G, Matthay MA. "Animal Models of Acute Lung Injury". American Thoracic Society Website.
5. Matute-Bello G, Frevert CW, Martin TR. "Animal models of acute lung injury". Am J Physiol Lung Cell Mol Physiol 2008; 295:L379–L399.
6. Ware LW, Matthay MA. The acute respiratory distress syndrome. N Engl J Med 2000; 342:1334–1349.
7. Agarwal R, Srinivas R, Nath A, et al. Is the mortality higher in the pulmonary vs. the extrapulmonary ARDS? A meta analysis. Chest 2008; 133:1463–1473.
8. Rice TW, Bernard GR. Therapeutic intervention and targets for sepsis. Annu Rev Med 2005; 56:225–248.
9. Hite RD, Morris PE. Acute respiratory distress syndrome: pharmacological treatment options in development. Drugs 2001; 61:897–907.
10. Mendelson CL. The aspiration of stomach contents into the lungs during obstetric anesthesia. Am J Obstet Gynecol 1946; 52:191.
11. Wynne JW, Ramphal R, Hood Cl. Tracheal mucosal damage after aspiration: a scanning electron microscope study. Am Rev Respir Dis 1981; 124:728–732.
12. Barber RE, Hamilton WK. Oxygen toxicity in man. A prospective study in patients with irreversible brain damage. N Engl J Med 1970; 283:1478–1484.
13. Matthay MA, Zimmerman GA. Acute lung injury and the acute respiratory distress syndrome. Am J Respir Cell Mol Biol 2005; 33:319–327.
14. Suratt BT, Parsons PE. Mechanisms of acute lung injury/acute respiratory distress syndromes. Clin Chest Med 2006; 27:579–589.
15. Ware LB, Matthay MA. Alveolar fluid clearance is impaired in the majority of patients with acute lung injury and the acute respiratory distress syndrome. Am J Respir Crit Care Med 2001; 163:1376–1383.
16. Fein A, Grossman RF, Jones JG, et al. The value of edema fluid protein measurement in patients with pulmonary edema. Am J Med 1979; 67:32–38.
17. Matthay MA, Folkesson HG, Clerici C. Lung epithelial fluid transport and the resolution of pulmonary edema. Physiol Rev 2002; 82:569–600.

18. Parker JC, Townsley MI. Evaluation of lung injury in rats and mice. Am J Lung Cell Mol Physiol 2004; 286:L231–L246.
19. Sever-Chroneos Z, Bachurski CJ, Van C, et al. Regulation of mouse SP-B gene promoter by AP-1 family members. Am J Physiol 1999; 277:L79–L88.
20. Baron RM, Carvajal IM, Fredenburgh LE, et al. Nitric oxide synthase-2 down-regulates surfactant protein-B expression and enhances endotoxin-induced lung injury in mice. FASEB J 2004; 18:1276–1278.
21. Ingenito EP, Mora R, Cullivan M, et al. Decreased surfactant protein-B expression and surfactant expression in a murine model of acute lung injury. Am J Respir Cell Mol Biol 2001; 25:35–44.
22. Wurfel MM. Microarray-based analysis of ventilator-induced lung injury. Proc Am Thorac Soc 2007; 4:77–84.
23. Nonas SA, Finigan JH, Gao L, et al. Functional genomic insights into acute lung injury. Role of ventilators and mechanical stress. Proc Am Thorac Soc 2005; 2:188–194.
24. Chang DW, Hayashi S, Gharib SA, et al. Proteomic and computational analysis of bronchoalveolar proteins during the course of the acute respiratory distress syndrome. Am J Respir Crit Care Med 2008; 178:701–709.
25. Braude S, Krausz T, Apperley J, et al. Adult respiratory distress syndrome after allogeneic bone-marrow transplantation: evidence for a neutrophil-independent mechanism. Lancet 1985; 325:1239–1242.
26. Winn R, Maunder R, Chi E, et al. Neutrophil depletion does not prevent lung edema after endotoxin infusion in goats. J Appl Physiol 1987; 62:116–121.
27. Snapper JR, Hinson JM Jr, Hutchison AA, et al. Effects of platelet depletion on the unanesthetized sheep's pulmonary response to endotoxemia. J Clin Invest 1984; 74:1782–1791.
28. Zarbock A, Singbarti K, Ley K. Complete reversal of acid-induced acute lung injury by blocking of platelet-neutrophil aggregation. J Clin Invest 2006; 116:3211–3219.
29. Park WY, Goodman RB, Steinberg KP, et al. Cytokine balance in the lungs of patients with acute respiratory distress syndrome. Am J Respir Crit Care Med 2001; 164:1896–1903.
30. Salinas D, Sparkman L, Berhane K, et al. Nitric oxide inhibits surfactant protein B gene expression in lung epithelial cells. Am J Physiol Lung Cell Mol Physiol 2003; 285:L1153–L1165.
31. Weiss YG, Maloyan A, Tazelaar J, et al. Adenoviral transfer of HSP-70 into pulmonary epithelium ameliorates experimental acute respiratory distress syndrome. J Clin Invest 2002; 110:801–806.
32. Baudouin SV. Exogenous surfactant replacement in ARDS—one day, some day, or never? New Engl J Med 2004; 351:853–855.
33. Horowitz JC, Cui Z, Moore TA, et al. Constitutive activation of prosurvival signaling in alveolar mesenchymal cells isolated from patients with nonresolving acute respiratory distress syndrome. Am J Physiol 2006; 290:L415–L425.
34. Santos FB, Nagato LKS, Boechem NM, et al. Time course of lung parenchyma remodeling in pulmonary and extrapulmonary acute lung injury. J Appl Physiol 2006; 100:98–106.
35. Negri EM, Hoelz C, Barbas CS, et al. Acute remodeling of parenchyma in pulmonary and extrapulmonary ARDS. An autopsy study of collagen-elastic system fibers. Pathol Res Pract 2002; 198:355–361.
36. Dos Santos CC. Advances in mechanisms of repair and remodeling in acute lung injury. Intensive Care Med 2008; 34:619–630.
37. Yamada M, Kubo H, Kobayashi S, et al. Bone marrow-derived progenitor cells are important for lung repair after lipopolysaccharide-induced lung injury. J Immunol 2004; 172: 1266–1272.
38. Gupta N, Su X, Popov B, et al. Intrapulmonary delivery of bone marrow-derived mesenchymal stem cells improves survival and attenuates endotoxin-induced acute lung injury in mice. J Immunol 2007; 179:1855–1863.

39. Baron RM, Baron MJ, Perrella MA. Pathobiology of sepsis: are we still asking the same questions? Am J Respir Cell Mol Biol 2006; 34:129–134.
40. Glasser SW, Korfhagen TR, Wert SE, et al. Transgenic models for study of pulmonary development and disease. Am J Physiol 1994; 267:L489–L497.
41. Gondo Y. Trends in large-scale mouse mutagenesis: from genetics to functional genomics. Nat Rev Genet 2008; 9:803–810.
42. Perrella MA. Gene regulation. In: Laurent GJ, Shapiro SD, Editor(s)-in-Chief, Encyclopedia of Respiratory Medicine. Oxford: Academic Press, 2006:231–237.
43. Hawkins PG, Morris KV. RNA and transcriptional modulation of gene expression. Cell Cycle 2008; 7:602–607.
44. Gharib SA, Liles WC, Matute-Bello G, et al. Computational identification of key biological modules and transcription factors in acute lung injury. Am J Respir Crit Care Med 2006; 173:653–658.
45. Mizgerd JP. Acute lower respiratory tract infection. N Engl J Med 2008; 358:716–727.
46. Sunil VR, Connor AJ, Guo Y, et al. Activation of type II alveolar epithelial cells during acute endotoxemia. Am J Physiol Lung Cell Mol Physiol 2002; 282:L872–L880.
47. Carvajal IM, Baron RM, Perrella MA. High mobility group-I/Y proteins: potential role in the pathophysiology of critical illnesses. Crit Care Med 2002; 30:S36–S42.

6

Pathogenesis of Acute Lung Injury: Clinical Studies

Benedict C. Creagh-Brown and Timothy W. Evans
Department of Critical Care Medicine, Imperial College School of Medicine, Royal Brompton
Hospital, London, U.K.

I. Introduction

Over the past three decades, experimental studies have contributed substantially to an increased understanding of the pathogenesis of acute lung injury (ALI) and its extreme manifestation, the acute respiratory distress syndrome (ARDS). However, many investigators have employed animal models that fail to accurately reproduce the heterogeneity of human ALI/ARDS, and which are difficult to sustain for the protracted periods needed to permit an assessment of the effects of mechanical ventilation and other supportive measures upon the evolution of the syndrome. Clinical studies are therefore critical to expanding our understanding of ALI/ARDS, and those that have contributed significantly to progress in this area are summarized herein. Trials of putative treatment strategies for ALI/ARDS are discussed elsewhere. For brevity, the abbreviation ALI is employed throughout, unless studies were performed specifically in patients with ARDS.

II. Methodologies Used

The methodology employed in clinical studies of the pathogenesis of ALI is limited compared to that which can be applied in animals. Nevertheless, a variety of useful and innovative techniques have been developed (Table 1). A major focus of clinical studies has been the measurement of biological markers of lung inflammation and injury in blood, edema, and bronchoalveolar lavage (BAL) fluids (1), which has improved understanding of the pathophysiology of ALI. Measurement of biological markers may have prognostic utility both in patients with established lung injury and in "at-risk" patient populations.

A. Bronchoalveolar Lavage

Bronchoalveolar lavage has been widely used to characterize the cellular content and fluid composition of the alveolar space and affords several advantages over other techniques. First, it can be performed at any time point and does not require that pulmonary edema be present for sampling. Thus, BAL has been carried out in patient populations at risk for ALI in the hope of identifying soluble factors that might predict the development of lung injury. Second, a large volume of lavage is returned, allowing measurement of multiple mediators in one patient. Third, BAL is probably the most reliable technique for sampling the cell population present in alveolar lining fluid. By contrast, BAL is invasive (2) and introduces sample dilution that is variable and difficult to quantify accurately.

Table 1 Methodologies Used in Clinical Studies of Acute Lung Injury and the Acute Respiratory Distress Syndrome

Methodology	Advantages	Disadvantages
Bronchoalveolar lavage	• Can be done at any time during the course of ALI • Can be done in at-risk patients • Can be done serially in same patient • Can sample the alveolar cell population	• Variable dilution factor • Invasive • Not feasible if severe hypoxemia is present
Pulmonary edema fluid sampling	• No dilutional factor • Simultaneous edema fluid and plasma levels of mediators can be compared • Relatively noninvasive • Can be used to calculate rate of alveolar fluid clearance	• Only feasible when alveolar flooding is present • Not all patients will have aspirable edema fluid
Blood sampling	• Relatively noninvasive • Can be done at any time during the course of ALI	• Samples only the intravascular compartment
Exhaled breath condensate	• Completely noninvasive • Can be done at any time during the course of ALI	• Source of exhaled molecules unclear (nasopharynx, airway, alveolus) • Evaporation may affect concentrations • Relationship to alveolar lining fluid unclear
Exhaled gas analysis	• Completely noninvasive	• Only useful for volatile compounds • May be technically difficult
Imaging	• Provides information about distribution of disease • Completely noninvasive	• Descriptive • Patient transport may be required • Radiation exposure
Extravascular lung water measurements	• Provides better quantification of degree of pulmonary edema than chest radiograph • Can be used to guide fluid management	• Does not distinguish between hydrostatic and increased permeability pulmonary edema • Relatively invasive
Lung microvascular permeability	• Can quantify protein permeability of the alveolar-capillary barrier • Relatively noninvasive	• May require patient transport • Findings differ depending on tracer used
Wasted ventilation	• Completely noninvasive • Quantifies degree of lung microvascular destruction/obstruction	• Does not differentiate cause of lung microvascular destruction/obstruction

(Continued)

Table 1   Methodologies Used in Clinical Studies of Acute Lung Injury and the Acute
Respiratory Distress Syndrome (*Continued*)

Methodology	Advantages	Disadvantages
Genetic studies	• Has the potential to identify genetic predispositions for the development of ALI	• Given the large number of factors that probably determine whether someone develops ALI, it may be difficult to pinpoint specific mutations that increase risk
Lung biopsy	• Allows histological and ultrastructural analysis at various time points during ALI	• Very invasive • Rarely done for diagnosis
Autopsy	• Allows histological and ultrastructural analysis of entire lung	• Samples only sickest patients who die from their illness • Not done routinely

The degree of dilution may render undetectable some factors that are present in very low
concentrations.

B.   Pulmonary Edema Fluid and Pulmonary Epithelial Lining Fluid

ALI is characterized by the presence of high-permeability pulmonary edema. Alveolar
fluid can be sampled using a standard tracheal suction catheter wedged into a distal airway.
The application of gentle suction yields a few milliliters of undiluted alveolar edema
that can be collected in a suction trap (3,4). This technique is less invasive than BAL
and obviates the problems associated with sample dilution. Concentrations of relevant
mediators can be compared directly to those in plasma sampled simultaneously. If serial
samples of edema fluid are obtained, their protein content can be used to calculate the
rate of alveolar fluid clearance, an indicator of alveolar epithelial fluid transport function
(3). Patients with hydrostatic pulmonary edema can serve as appropriate controls (5).
However, the technique is usually only successful when alveolar flooding is present; the
optimal time to sample pulmonary edema fluid being 15−30 minutes after endotracheal
intubation. From this point, serial samples can frequently be obtained for up to 12 hours,
but thereafter only in patients with severe and unremitting alveolar edema. Further, the
technique cannot be used in patients at risk for ALI or in those in whom overt pulmonary
edema has given way to fibroproliferation.

A newer technique, bronchoscopic microsampling involves the passage of a sampling probe down the working channel of a flexible bronchoscope that is wedged in a
distal airway. The probe has a protected cotton bud that is gently introduced into the distal
airway and absorbs fluid. This allows measurement of epithelial lining fluid of the small
airways without dilution (6) and in patients without alveolar edema.

C.   Exhaled Gas and Breath Condensate

Exhaled breath condensate (EBC) is a noninvasive, safe technique with which to obtain
direct samples from the lower respiratory tract. The technique is based on the hypothesis
that particles exhaled in breath reflect the composition of the alveolar lining fluid. A variety

of molecules have been measured in this fashion, including H_2O_2 (7–9), markers of lipid peroxidation (10), eicosanoids (11), and cytokines (12,13). This technique has several potential advantages. First, it is noninvasive and can be performed easily on ventilated patients or healthy controls. Second, repeated measures can be made over time. Third, it is very sensitive; for example, it can detect evidence of subclinical lung injury in patients after lung resection (14). Disadvantages include the lack of evidence for the origin of the aerosolized molecules (e.g., airway vs. alveoli), the susceptibility to concentration artifact due to evaporation, and the extent to which derived values depend upon variations in pulmonary or bronchial blood flow (15). The lack of standardization and variability in methods may have improved since the publication of ATS/ERS guidelines (16). Direct analysis of a variety of exhaled gases in patients with ALI has also been reported, including nitric oxide (NO) measured by chemiluminescence (17) and gas chromatographic analysis of exhaled gas after charcoal absorption (18).

D. Urine

A novel medium for the investigation of ALI is analysis of urinary markers. The clear advantage is that sampling urine is noninvasive and is available in all patients passing urine. Higher urinary NO is associated with survival and urinary desmosine with mortality (discussed below), and higher urine H_2O_2 levels are associated with worse clinical outcomes (19).

E. Imaging

A variety of imaging techniques have been used in patients with ALI to enhance the understanding of the clinical syndrome. These include chest radiography, computed tomographic (CT) scanning, and positron emission tomography (PET). Electrical impedance tomography is gaining attention as it is radiation free, is applicable at the bedside, and allows a direct estimate of regional lung ventilation during breathing (20). Lung ultrasound is excellent at visualizing both pleural effusions and parenchymal consolidation, and early reports suggest utility in assessing reaeration as an aid to monitoring treatment (21).

New techniques are under development to quantify lung water by CT imaging (22). A variety of radionuclide compounds have been used to make noninvasive measurements of lung microvascular permeability (23). Quantification of lung microvascular permeability to proteins can be achieved using an intravenously injected labeled tracer protein such as [67]gallium-transferrin, but immobile detection systems such as PET or gamma camera are required. Portable techniques more suited to mechanically ventilated patients have been employed, including mobile gamma cameras and microscintillation counter probes (23).

F. Physiological Measurements

Historically, measurements of extravascular lung water (EVLW) using the thermal-dye double indicator technique have been used to quantify the severity of pulmonary edema formation (24). A device using the transpulmonary thermodilution technique (PiCCO[TM], PULSION Medical Systems, Germany) has been shown to correlate well with the double indicator technique (25). Measures of EVLW in humans with ARDS correlated well with measures of lung weight assessed by CT scan (26). In human septic shock, EVLW correlates moderately well with markers of ALI (27). A decrease in EVLW as ALI evolves clinically is associated with better outcome (28) and in a recent large, retrospective study of 373 critically ill patients, EVLW was significantly higher in nonsurvivors (29). The use of the pulmonary artery catheter in ALI is diminishing, in part due to studies failing to show benefit (30).

Finally, simple lung function studies are possible in patients with ALI (31,32). Indeed, measurements of wasted ventilation have been used to quantify physiological dead space that represents a simple, noninvasive quantification of the extent of pulmonary vascular injury. Dead-space ventilation was elevated in patients with ALI and was an independent predictor of mortality by multivariate analysis (33).

G. Genetic Analysis

Determination of genetic factors that influence susceptibility to, and outcome from, ALI is a promising new area of research that is still in its infancy. Preliminary reports suggest that polymorphisms in the surfactant protein-B gene may affect the risk of developing ALI (34). Polymorphisms in the promoter region of the IL-6 gene have been shown to be associated with reduced gene promoter activity and lower circulating IL-6 concentrations. However, assessing polymorphisms in patients with ALI there was no difference in genotype or allele frequencies for IL-6 between the ARDS and controls. By contrast, the frequency of the DD ACE genotype (associated with higher tissue and circulating ACE) was increased in the ARDS group and was strongly associated with adverse outcome, suggesting a role for renin-angiotensin system in the development and progression of ALI (35). Others have shown that the ferritin light-chain gene genotype may confer susceptibility to ARDS, whilst the heme oxygenase-2 haplotype is protective against the onset of the syndrome. Such data support further previous findings that suggest abnormalities in iron handling resulting in redox imbalance are implicated in the pathogenesis of ARDS (36).

H. Autopsy and Lung Biopsy

Classic reports by Bachofen and Weibel defined the histopathological and ultrastructural changes typical in ALI (37,38). However, autopsy studies have the inherent limitation that only the most advanced and severe disease can be studied. Further, autopsies are obtained less frequently today than previously. Lung biopsy may be undertaken for diagnosis in patients with unexplained acute respiratory failure and although is generally considered too invasive to be used routinely there are reports of its utility and safety (39,40).

III. The Alveolar-Capillary Membrane
A. The Alveolar Unit

The concept of ventilator-associated lung injury (41) and the role of protective ventilation strategy in managing patients with established ALI are now accepted (42). By contrast, the role of ventilation in the pathogenesis of ALI remains underappreciated, although a strong association between higher initial tidal volumes and the incidence of subsequent ALI has been demonstrated (43).

B. Endothelium

Injury and activation of the lung microvascular endothelium is a critical component of ALI and was defined in early ultrastructural studies (37,38). Subsequently, simultaneous measurements of the protein concentration of pulmonary edema fluid and plasma confirmed that increased endothelial permeability, with an edema fluid-to-plasma protein ratio of >0.75, is present in early ALI (3,4,44,45). By contrast, patients with hydrostatic pulmonary edema have an edema fluid-to-plasma protein ratio of <0.65 (5). Studies using radiolabeled tracer proteins confirmed that lung microvascular permeability is increased in patients with ALI compared to those with hydrostatic pulmonary edema (46). Focal, reversible gap formation between endothelial cells is thought to occur (47).

Endothelin-1 (ET-1) is a vasoconstrictor peptide released by the injured endothelium (48). Patients with ALI have marked early increases in circulating plasma ET-1 levels, associated with abnormal pulmonary ET-1 metabolism (49). Several studies have measured increased plasma levels of ET-1 in patients with ALI, due both to increased production and decreased metabolism by the pulmonary vasculature (49–51). In autopsy studies of lungs taken from patients who died with ARDS, ET-1 immunostaining was diffusely increased in the vascular endothelium, alveolar macrophages, smooth muscle, and airway epithelium (52). Whether ET-1 is a marker of endothelial injury, has a proinflammatory action (51), or contributes to increased pulmonary vascular resistance in ALI is unclear. Specific endothelin receptor antagonists (used therapeutically in patients with pulmonary arterial hypertension) have not yet been used in clinical studies.

Von Willebrand factor (VWF) is a marker of endothelial activation and injury. It is a high molecular weight antigen produced by endothelial cells and to a lesser extent by platelets. In the setting of endothelial injury or activation, VWF is released from preformed stores into the circulation. Measuring plasma levels of VWF in patients with ALI at enrolment to a randomized trial of different ventilatory strategies revealed several findings: baseline VWF levels were similar in patients with and without sepsis, and were significantly higher in nonsurvivors versus survivors, even when controlling for severity of illness, sepsis, and ventilator strategy (53). These findings are in agreement with previous studies (54–56).

C. Epithelium

Increasingly, the critical role of injury to the alveolar epithelium in the pathogenesis of ALI has been recognized (57), although ultrastructural studies as early as 1977 showed evidence of substantial alveolar epithelial injury and necrosis (37). The alveolar epithelium has multiple functions that can be impaired in ALI.

First, the alveolar epithelium is responsible for the active transport of fluid and solute out of the alveolar space. Removal of fluid is driven by the active transport of sodium from the alveolar space to the interstitium by alveolar epithelial type II cells. In early ALI, clearance of fluid from the alveolar space is impaired in the majority of patients, a finding with adverse prognostic significance (3,4). By contrast, the majority of patients with hydrostatic pulmonary edema have intact alveolar fluid clearance, and many have very rapid rates of clearance (5). Under conditions of microvascular injury, lung water accumulates to a greater degree compared with normal lung at the same microvascular pressures (58) and clinically there is a greater increase in extravascular water for a given rise in pulmonary capillary wedge pressure compared to patients with cardiogenic pulmonary edema (24). In order to reduce the passage of intravascular fluid into the alveolar space, the pulmonary venous pressure should be restricted and excessive exogenous fluid administration represents a threat to this precarious balance. In the multicenter Fluid and Catheter Treatment Trial, patients with established ALI were randomized to either a liberal or conservative fluid management strategy. Patients randomized to the latter regimen displayed improved lung function and shortened duration of mechanical ventilation and intensive care length of stay without increasing nonpulmonary organ failures (59). β-agonists are believed to enhance alveolar fluid clearance through the upregulation of sodium transport mechanisms located on the alveolar epithelial cells. A trial assessing the effects of intravenous salbutamol (beta-agonist lung injury trial, BALTI) demonstrated a reduction in EVLW (assessed by a transpulmonary thermodilution system) (57). The primary mechanism through which β-agonists are believed to enhance alveolar fluid clearance is through the upregulation of sodium transport mechanisms located on the alveolar epithelial cells. Salbutamol does not affect neutrophil function or recruitment but does stimulate wound repair in alveolar epithelial cells (60,61).

Second, the alveolar epithelium acts as a barrier to the influx of bacteria from the alveolar space into the circulation. In experimental pneumonia, breakdown of the alveolar epithelial barrier leads to bacteremia and sepsis (62). Third, alveolar epithelial type II cells produce both the protein and lipid components of surfactant. Surfactant function is inhibited in patients with ALI (63–66) and its components may be inactivated by proteolysis (67) or through the flooding of the alveolar space with serum proteins (63). Plasma levels of surfactant protein A and surfactant protein D (SP-A and SP-D) rise early in the course of ALI and may reflect epithelial injury with the consequent increase in permeability. Consistent with this, BAL (65) and pulmonary edema (66) fluid levels of SP-D are lower in patients with ALI and are associated with higher mortality. Analysis of plasma levels of SP-A and SP-D from patients in the ARDSNet trial of lower tidal volumes (68) demonstrated that higher baselines levels of SP-D are associated with increased mortality and morbidity. Moreover, patients with a low tidal volume ventilation strategy showed attenuation of the rise in SP-D (69).

Further potential explanations for the decline in alveolar levels of SP-D include either decreased production of SP-D by alveolar type 2 cells in response to injury, inflammatory cytokines or bacterial products; or increased degradation of SP-D (66). Whether decreased SP-D has pathogenetic consequences or is merely a marker of lung injury is unclear. Decreased SP-D levels might have more of an impact on host defense than on alveolar surface tension (70).

A phase I/II human trial of recombinant surfactant protein C did not show a significant treatment benefit (71). Using proteomics to study the pattern of air space proteins in ALI patients revealed further evidence of damage to the selectivity of the alveolar-capillary barrier—high-molecular mass proteins such as albumin, immunoglobulin, and transferrin were pathologically increased, diminished SP-A, and abnormal truncated proteins with novel evidence of subtle post-translational modifications (72).

There are several potential biomarkers of alveolar epithelial damage. Levels of the epithelial cell marker Krebs van den Lungen 6 antigen (KL-6) reflect the severity of lung injury in patients with ALI. Increased levels are strongly associated with adverse outcome (73). Two cell surface receptors that mediate TNF-α inflammatory effects are TNF receptor 1 and 2 (TNFRI and TNFRII) and of these, alveolar epithelial cells express TNFRI. In ALI, TNF-α was undetectable in the majority of patients but soluble TNFRI and TNFRII are independently related to mortality. Analysis of plasma levels of soluble TNFRI in patients in the ARDSNet trial of lower tidal volumes demonstrated attenuation of plasma levels that could reflect an attenuation of alveolar epithelial injury (74). HTI56, an integral apical plasma membrane protein of human alveolar epithelial type I cells (75), is increased in both plasma and pulmonary edema fluid in patients with ALI compared to those with hydrostatic edema (76).

Epithelial cell-lining fluid changes are thought to be reflected in EBC, and acidification of EBC has been suggested as marker of inflammation in airway disease. EBC-pH was significantly decreased in patients with ALI, correlating with markers of local inflammation and indices of severity of lung injury but not markers of systemic inflammation (77). Interestingly, in a small study of patients with ALI the administration of inhaled salbutamol attenuated the EBC-pH and was associated with a trend toward decreased markers of nitrosative and oxidative stress (78).

D. Extracellular Matrix

The extracellular matrix (ECM) provides structural support to the lungs and comprises of the region of the lung between the alveolar epithelium and the vascular endothelium. Elevations of ECM proteins have been reported in the BAL, pulmonary edema fluid, and serum from patients with ALI implicating damage to the ECM. In the absence of pathological process, the elastin content of the pulmonary ECM remains stable for the lifetime of the individual. Desmosine is a stable breakdown product of elastin that can be reliably measured in urine samples. In a large group of ALI patients, urinary desmosine levels at enrolment to (a low tidal volume ventilation in ARDS study) were positively correlated to mortality. The intervention group had lower urinary desmosine levels and lower mortality, although this was only weakly correlated with markers of disease severity (79).

IV. Specific Inflammatory Cells, Pathways, and Mediators
A. Neutrophils

The accumulation of activated neutrophils in the lungs is an early step in the pulmonary inflammatory process that leads to ALI (80,81) and is a histological hallmark (37,38). Pulmonary edema and BAL fluids from ALI patients also have a predominance of neutrophils (82,83), the resolution of which is a good prognostic indicator (84). Labeled autologous neutrophils localize to the lung when reinfused into patients with ALI (85).

However, ARDS can occur in patients with neutropenia (86). In a large case series of oncology patients with neutropenia, 58% developed ARDS either during recovery from neutropenia, during a neutropenic episode or after neutropenia recovery (87). In contrast to other reports of ALI in neutropenia, there was no association with administration of granulocyte-colony-stimulating factor (G-CSF). Neutrophils mediate lung injury by a number of mechanisms, including the release of reactive oxygen and nitrogen species (ROS, RNS), the production of cytokines and growth factors that can amplify the inflammatory response, and the release of proteolytic enzymes. Proteolytic enzymes are potentially injurious to the lung, predominant among which is neutrophil elastase. Plasma levels of neutrophil elastase are elevated in patients at risk for ARDS after trauma (88) and in those with established ARDS after trauma (89). In samples of BAL fluid from patients with ALI, variable levels of functional neutrophil elastase have been measured (90–94), and most of that recovered is complexed to endogenous inhibitors such as α_2-macroglobulin or α_1-antitrypsin. The presence of endogenous inhibitors of elastase activity suggests that the overall degree of proteolytic activity caused by neutrophil activation and degranulation may be attenuated to a great extent by endogenous inhibitors. Other proteases that are elevated in BAL fluid from patients with ALI include collagenase (95) and gelatinases A and B (96,97). High levels of endogenous metalloproteinase inhibitors such as tissue inhibitor of metalloproteinases (TIMP) have also been identified (98), indicating that it is the overall protease/antiprotease balance that determines neutrophil-induced proteolytic damage.

Multiple mechanisms contribute to pulmonary neutrophil influx. A number of cytokines and chemokines commonly implicated in ALI can render neutrophils stiffer and less able to deform experimentally, hindering their passage through the pulmonary capillary bed (99–101). A study of neutrophil deformability in critical illnesses, including ARDS, confirmed diminished active and passive deformability compared to healthy controls (102). The diminished deformability was associated with higher circulating levels of proinflammatory cytokines such as TNF-α.

Nuclear factor κB (NFκB) is a transcription regulation factor with proinflammatory roles, is implicated in the development of ALI (103–106). Specifically, it regulates the transcription of interleukin-1β (IL-1β), interleukin-8 (IL-8), and TNF-α. Assessment of the activation of NFκB within peripheral neutrophils in patients with early ALI (i.e., within 24 hours of invasive ventilation) revealed increased NFκB activation compared to controls, but no correlation between this and clinical outcome (ventilator-free days). However, a failure of neutrophils to increase their NFκB activation to in vitro stimulation with lipopolysaccharide correlated with improved clinical outcome. These findings suggest that early alterations in neutrophil function have profound clinical implications (107).

Dysregulation of neutrophil turnover is thought to play a major role in the resolution of the inflammatory response. Neutrophil apoptosis (programmed cell death) with subsequent phagocytosis by macrophages provides a way of removing neutrophils without damage to surrounding tissue. BAL fluid from patients with ARDS has been shown to have an antiapoptotic effect on normal human neutrophils, an effect mediated predominantly by G-CSF and granulocyte-macrophage colony-stimulating factor (GM-CSF), cytokines with antiapoptotic activity. Further, neutrophil apoptosis is markedly reduced in patients with ARDS (108,109). A variety of natural inhibitors of neutrophil function have also been identified in BAL from ARDS patients (110), including CC16, an inhibitor of neutrophil chemotaxis, levels of which correlate inversely with levels of neutrophil elastase (111).

B. Cytokines

Levels of a wide variety of cytokines are increased in biological fluids from patients with ALI (1). In early studies focused on identifying proinflammatory cytokines in biological fluids from patients with ALI, levels of most mediators were not clearly prognostic. Interleukin (IL)-6 is a pleiotropic cytokine that is both a marker and a mediator of sepsis. IL-8 is a prototypical chemotactic cytokine that induces chemotaxis of inflammatory cells and in particular, recruitment of neutrophils. Elevated IL-6 and IL-8 levels at enrolment to the ARDSNet trial (68) were associated with increased mortality and morbidity. Moreover, lower tidal volume ventilation was associated with more rapid attenuation of the inflammatory response (112). Levels of IL-6 and IL-8 were significantly higher in patients with sepsis as the cause of their ALI.

Anti-inflammatory strategies targeted at specific cytokines such as IL-1β and TNF-α have been unsuccessful clinically (111). It is now clear that the cytokine response in ALI/ARDS is complex and involves both pro and anti-inflammatory cytokines as well as endogenous inhibitors of proinflammatory cytokines. A variety of endogenous inhibitors have been identified, including the IL-1 receptor antagonist, soluble IL-1 receptor, soluble TNF receptors I and II, and autoantibodies to IL-8. Although individual cytokines such as TNF-α and IL1-β increased before and after the onset of lung injury, greater increases in the levels of relevant endogenous inhibitors such as IL1-β receptor antagonist and soluble TNF-α receptors were measured (113). This study provides convincing evidence of a significant anti-inflammatory response early in the course of ALI that counteracts the proinflammatory response. Measuring levels of proinflammatory and anti-inflammatory molecules using immunological methods provide insufficient information concerning the complex cytokine milieu that characterizes ALI. For example, relative molar concentrations of pro and anti-inflammatory cytokines do not necessarily predict biological activity of a given cytokine (111). In a second study, levels of IL-8/anti-IL-8 autoantibody complexes correlated better with ARDS outcome than levels of IL-8 alone (114), even though complexing of anti-IL-8 antibody with IL-8 is thought to neutralize its chemotactic activity for neutrophils (115). A better way to assess the net pro or anti-inflammatory activity of a given cytokine in human samples may be through assays of biological activity. Using cell surface expression of ICAM-1 on alveolar epithelial cell monolayers as a measure of proinflammatory activity, both pulmonary edema fluid (97) and BAL fluid (116) from patients with ALI were shown to have potent proinflammatory activity, due predominantly to biologically active IL-1. Moreover, pulmonary edema fluid from ALI patients has been shown to stimulate repair in cultured alveolar epithelial monolayers, an effect mediated, in part, by biologically active IL-1 (117).

C. Pro-Oxidant/Antioxidant Balance

There is a severe imbalance between pro-oxidant and antioxidant activity in the lung in patients with ALI (118). Under normal conditions, the generation of ROS or RNS is counteracted by a complex network of antioxidant defense systems (119) including several low molecular weight compounds, such as reduced glutathione (GSH), ascorbic (vitamin C), and uric acids; lipophilic antioxidants, such as α-tocopherol (vitamin E), retinol (vitamin A), and plasmalogens (1-alkenyl-phospholipids); and antioxidant enzymes including superoxide dismutases, catalase, and the glutathione peroxidizes. There are also mechanisms to remove or repair oxidatively damaged molecules, including DNA and proteins (118). There is no consensus on the amount of antioxidants in the alveolar space. In a study of BAL fluid in 40 patients with ALI, a significant increase was found in the concentrations of antioxidants, particularly vitamins A, C, and E and uric acid compared to healthy controls. Consistent with previous investigations, there are also elevations in markers of oxidant stress (oxidized glutathione and F2 isoprostanes) (120). However, in a study of pulmonary edema fluid in 29 patients with ALI there were lower concentrations of vitamin C and uric acid and additionally, lower levels of glutathione compared to healthy controls (121). Alterations in the levels of endogenous antioxidants may also affect the risk of developing ALI. Chronic alcohol abuse is associated with an increased incidence and severity of ALI (122). This has been linked with depletion of pulmonary glutathione and chronic oxidant stress (123), via a significant shift in lung redox potential toward a more oxidized state. This shift is not accurately predicted by changes in redox potential in the blood (124).

Despite the growing body of evidence that supports a role for altered pro-oxidant/ antioxidant imbalance in clinical ALI, the results of clinical trials of antioxidants have been disappointing (125).

Important markers of oxidative injury in the lung include nitrogen oxide species (NOx), particularly NO, nitrite (NO_2^-), and nitrate (NO_3^-). Pulmonary NO production is stimulated by mechanical forces and inflammatory processes within the lung. Higher urine NO levels in a subgroup of 566 of the 861 patients included in the ARDSNet study (68) were independently predictive of lower mortality (126). NO may confer improved outcome through free radical scavenging, pulmonary vasodilatation, protection of type II alveolar cells from stretch injury, protection of systemic endothelial function, or higher levels may reflect a greater percentage of intact lung endothelium and epithelium (i.e., a less severe insult). Nitrite and nitrate are also found both in the plasma and edema fluid in patients with ALI and the levels in the edema fluid are greater than the levels in plasma suggesting that local NO exists (127). Nitrate and nitrite are also elevated in BAL from patients at risk of developing ALI (128), but levels are not individually predictive. A strong correlation has been demonstrated between EBC NO_2^- and tidal volume (V_t) unrelated to parameters of pulmonary or systemic inflammation. Moreover, the ratio of EBC NO_2^- and V_t correlated closely with the extent of lung injury, suggesting that levels of nitrite could reflect extent of alveolar injury due to pulmonary distension (129).

Iron is a fundamental biological catalyst for oxygen utilization that can also induce formation of ROS. Aberrant iron regulation may contribute to susceptibility to, and progression of ALI (36). Inducible heme oxygenase (HO)-1 catalyzes the catabolism of heme and is upregulated by a diverse array of stimuli, in what is considered to be a protective response to oxidative stress. The products of heme catabolism biliverdin, bilirubin, and carbon monoxide have anti-inflammatory and antioxidant properties. However, another product of heme catabolism, low molecular mass redox active iron, is a pro-oxidant with potentially adverse effects. In patients with ALI, there are significantly raised amounts of HO-1 protein in lung biopsies and BAL fluid compared with controls and these levels correlate significantly with indexes of iron mobilization (130). As carbon monoxide is a product of HO-1 activity, and accounts for 85% of endogenous CO production, measuring carboxy-hemoglobin (CO-Hb) is considered a surrogate for HO-1 activity. In mixed critically ill cardiothoracic patients, there is an association between both low and high levels of CO-Hb and mortality. This suggests that activity of the HO system is protective and that either a dampened or excessive response to proinflammatory stress is deleterious (131).

D. Coagulation Pathway

Platelet activation and aggregation, microthrombi, and intra-alveolar deposition are major components of the histologic appearance of ALI (37,38,132) and alterations in coagulation and fibrinolysis are of major pathogenic importance in ALI (133,134). Fibrin deposition in the alveolar space results from an imbalance between coagulation, fibrinolytic proteases (plasmin and urokinase type plasminogen activators or u-PA) and antiproteases (plasminogen activator inhibitor-1 (PAI-1) and α_2-antiplasmin), and the availability of plasma-derived fibrinogen.

An increase in procoagulant activity is seen both in patients at risk of ALI (135) and those with established ALI (136) and is related to an increase in expression of procoagulant (tissue factor) and antifibrinolytic (PAI-1) proteins (137,138). The increase in plasma and edema levels of PAI-1 is discriminative for ALI (as opposed to hydrostatic pulmonary edema) and predicts increased mortality (139). PAI-1 is thought to be released locally by the epithelial cells, endothelial cells, and fibroblasts. Tissue factor (TF) is a highly thrombogenic mediator in the extrinsic coagulation pathway leading to fibrin formation. In ALI, the alveolar compartment contains high levels of TF (140,141) and this may be due partly to alveolar epithelium reacting to proinflammatory stimuli (142). The endogenous inhibitor to TF is tissue factor pathway inhibitor (TFPI), and levels are elevated in edema fluid from patients with ARDS compared to levels in patients with hydrostatic pulmonary edema. However, levels of intra-alveolar TFPI in ARDS are insufficient to counteract intra-alveolar TF procoagulant activity, due to truncation and inactivation of intra-alveolar TFPI. This may be partly explained through a failure to increase TFPI gene transcription or protein production (143).

Protein C is an endogenous circulating plasma anticoagulant that promotes fibrinolysis and inhibits thrombosis and inflammation. Lower levels of plasma protein C are associated with worse clinical outcomes in ALI (144). Activation of protein C requires binding to the endothelial protein C receptor and the thrombomodulin–thrombin complex. In patients with sepsis, increased circulating thrombomodulin results from cleavage from the cell surface of the endothelium, resulting in reduced availability for activation of protein C on the endothelial surface. Levels of plasma thrombomodulin are increased in plasma from ALI patients compared with controls, hold prognostic significance, and are higher in edema fluid, suggesting local release (144).

A common genetic polymorphism, factor V Leiden (FVL) mutation results in partial resistance to inactivation by activated protein C and creates a mildly prothrombotic state. A heterozygous FVL genotype is associated with improved 30-day survival in patients with ARDS, although severity and ICU length of stay were unchanged. The underlying mechanisms may relate to augmentation of endogenous protein C activation (145). Instillation of endotoxin into bronchopulmonary segments of normal volunteers induced local activation of coagulation, inhibited by prior administration of recombinant human activated protein C (rhAPC). Fibrinolysis was suppressed and protein C concentrations were reduced (146), suggesting that rhAPC exerts an anticoagulant effect in these circumstances.

Restoration of procoagulant/anticoagulant balance may have an important therapeutic role in ALI. Despite these and other results in patients with severe sepsis (147), a recent placebo control, efficacy study of rhAPC in patients with ALI was terminated prematurely by the Data and Safety Monitoring Board after 75 patients were enrolled and a planned interim analysis showed no difference in the primary outcome variable of ventilator-free days (148).

E. Damage-Associated Molecular Pattern (DAMP) Recognition

Stressed, injured, and dead cells release signals, termed alarmins or DAMPs, that are recognized by the innate immune system and cause an inflammatory response (149).

These include the high-mobility group box 1 protein (HMGB1), serum amyloid A protein (SAAP), and the S100 proteins. The receptor for advanced glycated end-products (RAGE) was initially identified as a receptor for advanced glycated proteins, but is also a pattern-recognition receptor that also ligates with DAMPS including HMGB1, SAAP, and the S100 proteins. RAGE activity is proinflammatory via NFkB and its expression is upregulated in the presence of its ligands--therefore it is thought to potentiate and perpetuate inflammation. RAGE has been detected in many tissues but is particularly densely expressed in the lung, specifically in alveolar type 1 cells and as such, is also considered to be a marker of alveolar injury.

Soluble RAGE levels in pulmonary edema and plasma are significantly higher than in patients with ALI than those with hydrostatic pulmonary edema (150). Plasma levels of RAGE were measured at enrolment and at day 3 in a subset of patients from the ARDSNet trial (68). Higher baseline levels of plasma RAGE were significantly associated with more severe ALI and with adverse clinical outcomes in the higher V_t group. With both ventilatory strategies, the levels decreased by day 3 but there was a greater decline in the lower tidal ventilation group (151). These studies indicate that severity of alveolar epithelial injury is associated with susceptibility to ventilator associated lung injury (VALI). An alternative hypothesis is that higher levels of plasma RAGE reflect a proinflammatory milieu that predisposes to VALI and is exacerbated by injurious ventilation. In those without pre-existent lung pathology undergoing prolonged mechanical ventilation, increased BAL levels of HMGB1 were shown (152) implicating the interaction of HMGB1 with RAGE as a contributory mechanism of VALI.

F. Glycemia and Glycated Proteins

Diabetes has been found to be a negative predictor for ARDS (153). There is evidence from a murine model of leptin-resistant mice exposed to hyperoxic lung injury that leptin resistance (as a model for type II diabetes and/or obesity) might provide protection against the development of ALI. There are no supportive data from human studies and humans exposed to experimental endotoxinemia do not have a rise in circulating leptin (154).

G. Uncharacterized Mechanisms

The risk of transfusion-related lung injury is higher when plasma-rich blood products (fresh frozen plasma and platelets) are used compared to red cells (155). The hypothesized mechanisms include the passive transfer of antileukocyte antibodies in plasma-rich blood products and the accumulation of inflammatory mediators and bioactive lipids in stored platelets. Antileukocyte antibodies are only found in 15–17% of female donors and 25% of multiparous donors but are rare in male donors; their presence resulting from alloimmunization. Evidence supporting the pathogenic role of these antibodies is provided by the significant reduction in incidence of ALI in recipients of blood products after the exclusion of donations from female donors (156). Figure 1 diagrammatically represents the changes in the alveolus during ALI.

V. Future Directions

Clinical studies will continue to contribute to our understanding of the pathogenesis of ALI. The advent of genomics and proteomics has the potential to greatly expand the

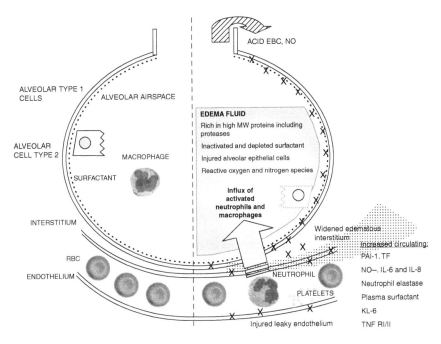

Figure 1 The alveolus in health and in acute lung injury.

amount of information that can be gained from patient-based studies. The formation of large multicenter clinical trials groups such as the NIH ARDS Network also provides the impetus and potential to study pathophysiological mechanisms in large numbers of patients as an adjunct to clinical trials.

References

1. Pittet JF, Mackersie RC, Martin TR, et al. Biological markers of acute lung injury: prognostic and pathogenetic significance. Am J Respir Crit Care Med 1997; 155(4):1187–1205.
2. Steinberg KP, Mitchell DR, Maunder RJ, et al. Safety of bronchoalveolar lavage in patients with adult respiratory distress syndrome. Am Rev Respir Dis 1993; 148(3):556–561.
3. Ware LB, Matthay MA. Alveolar fluid clearance is impaired in the majority of patients with acute lung injury and the acute respiratory distress syndrome. Am J Respir Crit Care Med 2001; 163(6):1376–1383.
4. Matthay MA, Wiener-Kronish JP. Intact epithelial barrier function is critical for the resolution of alveolar edema in humans. Am Rev Respir Dis 1990; 142(6, pt 1):1250–1257.
5. Verghese GM, Ware LB, Matthay BA, et al. Alveolar epithelial fluid transport and the resolution of clinically severe hydrostatic pulmonary edema. J Appl Physiol 1999; 87(4):1301–1312.
6. Ishizaka A, Watanabe M, Yamashita T. et al. New bronchoscopic microsample probe to measure the biochemical constituents in epithelial lining fluid of patients with acute respiratory distress syndrome. Crit Care Med 2001; 29(4):896–898.
7. Heard SO, Longtine K, Toth I, et al. The influence of liposome-encapsulated prostaglandin E1 on hydrogen peroxide concentrations in the exhaled breath of patients with the acute respiratory distress syndrome. Anesth Analg 1999; 89(2):353–357.

8. Baldwin SR, Simon RH, Grum CM, et al. Oxidant activity in expired breath of patients with adult respiratory distress syndrome. Lancet 1986; 1(8471):11–14.

9. Sznajder JI, Fraiman A, Hall JB, et al. Increased hydrogen peroxide in the expired breath of patients with acute hypoxemic respiratory failure. Chest 1989; 96(3):606–612.

10. Carpenter CT, Price PV, Christman BW. Exhaled breath condensate isoprostanes are elevated in patients with acute lung injury or ARDS. Chest 1998; 114(6):1653–1659.

11. Tufvesson E, Bjermer L. Methodological improvements for measuring eicosanoids and cytokines in exhaled breath condensate. Respir Med 2006; 100(1):34–38.

12. Scheideler L, Manke HG, Schwulera U, et al. Detection of nonvolatile macromolecules in breath. A possible diagnostic tool? Am Rev Respir Dis 1993; 148(3):778–784.

13. Sack U, Scheibe R, Wotzel M, et al. Multiplex analysis of cytokines in exhaled breath condensate. Cytometry A 2006; 69(3):169–172.

14. Moloney ED, Mumby SE, Gajdocsi R, et al. Exhaled breath condensate detects markers of pulmonary inflammation after cardiothoracic surgery. Am J Respir Crit Care Med 2004; 169(1):64–69.

15. Mutlu GM, Garey KW, Robbins RA, et al. Collection and analysis of exhaled breath condensate in humans. Am J Respir Crit Care Med 2001; 164(5):731–737.

16. Horvath I, Hunt J, Barnes PJ, et al. Exhaled breath condensate: methodological recommendations and unresolved questions. Eur Respir J 2005; 26(3):523–548.

17. Brett SJ, Evans TW. Measurement of endogenous nitric oxide in the lungs of patients with the acute respiratory distress syndrome. Am J Respir Crit Care Med 1998; 157(3, pt 1): 993–997.

18. Schubert JK, Muller WP, Benzing A, et al. Application of a new method for analysis of exhaled gas in critically ill patients. Intensive Care Med 1998; 24(5):415–421.

19. Mathru M, Rooney MW, Dries DJ, et al. Urine hydrogen peroxide during adult respiratory distress syndrome in patients with and without sepsis. Chest 1994; 105(1):232–236.

20. Caironi P, Langer T, Gattinoni L. Acute lung injury/acute respiratory distress syndrome pathophysiology: what we have learned from computed tomography scanning. Curr Opin Crit Care 2008; 14(1):64–69.

21. Bouhemad B, Zhang M, Lu Q, et al. Clinical review: bedside lung ultrasound in critical care practice. Crit Care 2007; 11(1):205.

22. Malbouisson LM, Preteux F, Puybasset L, et al. Validation of a software designed for computed tomographic (CT) measurement of lung water. Intensive Care Med 2001; 27(3):602–608.

23. Groeneveld AB, Raijmakers PG. The 67gallium-transferrin pulmonary leak index in pneumonia and associated adult respiratory distress syndrome. Clin Sci (Lond) 1997; 93(5):463–470.

24. Sibbald WJ, Short AK, Warshawski FJ, et al. Thermal dye measurements of extravascular lung water in critically ill patients. Intravascular starling forces and extravascular lung water in the adult respiratory distress syndrome. Chest 1985; 87(5):585–592.

25. Sakka SG, Ruhl CC, Pfeiffer UJ, et al. Assessment of cardiac preload and extravascular lung water by single transpulmonary thermodilution. Intensive Care Med 2000; 26(2):180–187.

26. Patroniti N, Bellani G, Maggioni E, et al. Measurement of pulmonary edema in patients with acute respiratory distress syndrome. Crit Care Med 2005; 33(11):2547–2554.

27. Kuzkov VV, Kirov MY, Sovershaev MA, et al. Extravascular lung water determined with single transpulmonary thermodilution correlates with the severity of sepsis-induced acute lung injury. Crit Care Med 2006; 34(6):1647–1653.

28. Mitchell JP, Schuller D, Calandrino FS, et al. Improved outcome based on fluid management in critically ill patients requiring pulmonary artery catheterization. Am Rev Respir Dis 1992; 145(5):990–998.

29. Sakka SG, Klein M, Reinhart K, et al. Prognostic value of extravascular lung water in critically ill patients. Chest 2002; 122(6):2080–2086.

30. Wheeler AP, Bernard GR, Thompson BT, et al. Pulmonary-artery versus central venous catheter to guide treatment of acute lung injury. N Engl J Med 2006; 354(21):2213–2224.
31. Macnaughton PD, Morgan CJ, Denison DM, et al. Measurement of carbon monoxide transfer and lung volume in ventilated subjects. Eur Respir J 1993; 6(2):231–236.
32. Macnaughton PD, Evans TW. Measurement of lung volume and DLCO in acute respiratory failure. Am J Respir Crit Care Med 1994; 150(3):770–775.
33. Nuckton TJ, Alonso JA, Kallet RH, et al. Pulmonary dead-space fraction as a risk factor for death in the acute respiratory distress syndrome. N Engl J Med 2002; 346(17):1281–1286.
34. Lin Z, Pearson C, Chinchilli V, et al. Polymorphisms of human SP-A, SP-B, and SP-D genes: association of SP-B Thr131Ile with ARDS. Clin Genet 2000; 58(3):181–191.
35. Marshall RP, Webb S, Hill MR, et al. Genetic polymorphisms associated with susceptibility and outcome in ARDS. Chest 2002; 121(Suppl. 3):68S–69S.
36. Lagan AL, Quinlan GJ, Mumby S, et al. Variation in iron homeostasis genes between patients with ARDS and healthy control subjects. Chest 2008; 133(6):1302–1311.
37. Bachofen M, Weibel ER. Alterations of the gas exchange apparatus in adult respiratory insufficiency associated with septicemia. Am Rev Respir Dis 1977; 116(4):589–615.
38. Bachofen M, Weibel ER. Structural alterations of lung parenchyma in the adult respiratory distress syndrome. Clin Chest Med 1982; 3(1):35–56.
39. Patel SR, Karmpaliotis D, Ayas NT, et al. The role of open-lung biopsy in ARDS. Chest 2004; 125(1):197–202.
40. Baumann HJ, Kluge S, Balke L, et al. Yield and safety of bedside open lung biopsy in mechanically ventilated patients with acute lung injury or acute respiratory distress syndrome. Surgery 2008; 143(3):426–433.
41. Pinhu L, Whitehead T, Evans T, et al. Ventilator-associated lung injury. Lancet 2003; 361(9354):332–340.
42. Leaver SK, Evans TW. Acute respiratory distress syndrome. BMJ 2007; 335(7616):389–394.
43. Gajic O, Dara SI, Mendez JL, et al. Ventilator-associated lung injury in patients without acute lung injury at the onset of mechanical ventilation. Crit Care Med 2004; 32(9):1817–1824.
44. Fein A, Grossman RF, Jones JG, et al. The value of edema fluid protein measurement in patients with pulmonary edema. Am J Med 1979; 67(1):32–38.
45. Sprung CL, Rackow EC, Fein IA, et al. The spectrum of pulmonary edema: differentiation of cardiogenic, intermediate, and noncardiogenic forms of pulmonary edema. Am Rev Respir Dis 1981; 124(6):718–722.
46. Raijmakers PG, Groeneveld AB, Teule GJ, et al. Diagnostic value of the gallium-67 pulmonary leak index in pulmonary edema. J Nucl Med 1996; 37(8):1316–1322.
47. Hurley JV. Types of pulmonary microvascular injury. Ann N Y Acad Sci 1982; 384:269–286.
48. Pittet JF, Morel DR, Hemsen A, et al. Elevated plasma endothelin-1 concentrations are associated with the severity of illness in patients with sepsis. Ann Surg 1991; 213(3):261–264.
49. Langleben D, DeMarchie M, Laporta D, et al. Endothelin-1 in acute lung injury and the adult respiratory distress syndrome. Am Rev Respir Dis 1993; 148(6, pt 1):1646–1650.
50. Druml W, Steltzer H, Waldhausl W, et al. Endothelin-1 in adult respiratory distress syndrome. Am Rev Respir Dis 1993; 148(5):1169–1173.
51. Sanai L, Haynes WG, MacKenzie A, et al. Endothelin production in sepsis and the adult respiratory distress syndrome. Intensive Care Med 1996; 22(1):52–56.
52. Albertine KH, Wang ZM, Michael JR. Expression of endothelial nitric oxide synthase, inducible nitric oxide synthase, and endothelin-1 in lungs of subjects who died with ARDS. Chest 1999; 116(Suppl. 1):101S–102S.
53. Ware LB, Eisner MD, Thompson BT, et al. Significance of von Willebrand factor in septic and nonseptic patients with acute lung injury. Am J Respir Crit Care Med 2004; 170(7):766–772.

54. Ware LB, Conner ER, Matthay MA. von Willebrand factor antigen is an independent marker of poor outcome in patients with early acute lung injury. Crit Care Med 2001; 29(12):2325–2331.

55. Carvalho AC, Bellman SM, Saullo VJ, et al. Altered factor VIII in acute respiratory failure. N Engl J Med 1982; 307(18):1113–1119.

56. Kayal S, Jais JP, Aguini N, et al. Elevated circulating E-selectin, intercellular adhesion molecule 1, and von Willebrand factor in patients with severe infection. Am J Respir Crit Care Med 1998; 157(3, pt 1):776–784.

57. Berthiaume Y, Lesur O, Dagenais A. Treatment of adult respiratory distress syndrome: plea for rescue therapy of the alveolar epithelium. Thorax 1999; 54(2):150–160.

58. Bernard GR. Acute respiratory distress syndrome: a historical perspective. Am J Respir Crit Care Med 2005; 172(7):798–806.

59. Wiedemann HP, Wheeler AP, Bernard GR, et al. Comparison of two fluid-management strategies in acute lung injury. N Engl J Med 2006; 354(24):2564–2575.

60. Perkins GD, Gao F, Thickett DR. In vivo and in vitro effects of salbutamol on alveolar epithelial repair in acute lung injury. Thorax 2008; 63(3):215–220.

61. Perkins GD, Nathani N, McAuley DF, et al. In vitro and in vivo effects of salbutamol on neutrophil function in acute lung injury. Thorax 2007; 62(1):36–42.

62. Kurahashi K, Kajikawa O, Sawa T, et al. Pathogenesis of septic shock in Pseudomonas aeruginosa pneumonia. J Clin Invest 1999; 104(6):743–750.

63. Lewis JF, Jobe AH. Surfactant and the adult respiratory distress syndrome. Am Rev Respir Dis 1993; 147(1):218–233.

64. Gregory, TJ, Steinberg KP, Spragg R, et al. Bovine surfactant therapy for patients with acute respiratory distress syndrome. Am J Respir Crit Care Med 1997; 155(4):1309–1315.

65. Greene KE, Wright JR, Steinberg KP, et al. Serial changes in surfactant-associated proteins in lung and serum before and after onset of ARDS. Am J Respir Crit Care Med 1999; 160(6):1843–1850.

66. Cheng IW, Ware LB, Greene KE, et al. Prognostic value of surfactant proteins A and D in patients with acute lung injury. Crit Care Med 2003; 31(1):20–27.

67. Baker CS, Evans TW, Randle BJ, et al. Damage to surfactant-specific protein in acute respiratory distress syndrome. Lancet 1999; 353(9160):1232–1237.

68. Brower RG, Matthay MA, Morris A, et al. Ventilation with lower tidal volumes as compared with traditional tidal volumes for acute lung injury and the acute respiratory distress syndrome. The Acute Respiratory Distress Syndrome Network. N Engl J Med 2000; 342(18):1301–1308.

69. Eisner MD, Parsons P, Matthay MA, et al. Plasma surfactant protein levels and clinical outcomes in patients with acute lung injury. Thorax 2003; 58(11):983–988.

70. Wright JR. Immunomodulatory functions of surfactant. Physiol Rev 1997; 77(4):931–962.

71. Spragg RG, Lewis JF, Wurst W, et al. Treatment of acute respiratory distress syndrome with recombinant surfactant protein C surfactant. Am J Respir Crit Care Med 2003; 167(11):1562–1566.

72. Bowler, RP, Duda B, Chan ED, et al. Proteomic analysis of pulmonary edema fluid and plasma in patients with acute lung injury. Am J Physiol Lung Cell Mol Physiol 2004; 286(6):L1095–L1104.

73. Ishizaka A, Matsuda T, Albertine KH, et al. Elevation of KL-6, a lung epithelial cell marker, in plasma and epithelial lining fluid in acute respiratory distress syndrome. Am J Physiol Lung Cell Mol Physiol 2004; 286(6):L1088–L1094.

74. Parsons PE, Matthay MA, Ware LB, et al. Elevated plasma levels of soluble TNF receptors are associated with morbidity and mortality in patients with acute lung injury. Am J Physiol Lung Cell Mol Physiol 2005; 288(3):L426–L431.

75. Dobbs LG, Gonzalez RF, Allen L, et al. HTI56, an integral membrane protein specific to human alveolar type I cells. J Histochem Cytochem 1999; 47(2):129–137.

76. Newman, V, Gonzalez RF, Matthay MA, et al. A novel alveolar type I cell-specific biochemical marker of human acute lung injury. Am J Respir Crit Care Med 2000; 161(3, pt 1):990–995.
77. Gessner C, Hammerschmidt S, Kuhn H, et al. Exhaled breath condensate acidification in acute lung injury. Respir Med 2003; 97(11):1188–1194.
78. Roca O, Gomez-Olles S, Cruz MJ, et al. Effects of salbutamol on exhaled breath condensate biomarkers in acute lung injury: prospective analysis. Crit Care 2008; 12(3):R72.
79. McClintock DE, Starcher B, Eisner MD, et al. Higher urine desmosine levels are associated with mortality in patients with acute lung injury. Am J Physiol Lung Cell Mol Physiol 2006; 291(4):L566–L571.
80. Lee WL, Downey GP. Neutrophil activation and acute lung injury. Curr Opin Crit Care 2001; 7(1):1–7.
81. Abraham E. Neutrophils and acute lung injury. Crit Care Med 2003; 31(Suppl. 4):S195–S199.
82. Steinberg KP, Milberg JA, Martin TR, et al. Evolution of bronchoalveolar cell populations in the adult respiratory distress syndrome. Am J Respir Crit Care Med 1994; 150(1):113–122.
83. Parsons PE, Fowler AA, Hyers TM, et al. Chemotactic activity in bronchoalveolar lavage fluid from patients with adult respiratory distress syndrome. Am Rev Respir Dis 1985; 132(3):490–493.
84. Baughman RP, Gunther KL, Rashkin MC, et al. Changes in the inflammatory response of the lung during acute respiratory distress syndrome: prognostic indicators. Am J Respir Crit Care Med 1996; 154(1):76–81.
85. Warshawski FJ, Sibbald WJ, Driedger AA, et al. Abnormal neutrophil-pulmonary interaction in the adult respiratory distress syndrome. Qualitative and quantitative assessment of pulmonary neutrophil kinetics in humans with in vivo 111indium neutrophil scintigraphy. Am Rev Respir Dis 1986; 133(5):797–804.
86. Laufe MD, Simon RH, Flint A, et al. Adult respiratory distress syndrome in neutropenic patients. Am J Med 1986; 80(6):1022–1026.
87. Azoulay E, Darmon M, Delclaux C, et al. Deterioration of previous acute lung injury during neutropenia recovery. Crit Care Med 2002; 30(4):781–786.
88. Donnelly SC, MacGregor I, Zamani A, et al. Plasma elastase levels and the development of the adult respiratory distress syndrome. Am J Respir Crit Care Med 1995; 151(5):1428–1433.
89. Gando S, Kameue T, Nanzaki S, et al. Increased neutrophil elastase, persistent intravascular coagulation, and decreased fibrinolytic activity in patients with posttraumatic acute respiratory distress syndrome. J Trauma 1997; 42(6):1068–1072.
90. Weiland JE, Davis WB, Holter JF, et al. Lung neutrophils in the adult respiratory distress syndrome. Clinical and pathophysiologic significance. Am Rev Respir Dis 1986; 133(2):218–225.
91. Lee CT, Fein AM, Lippmann M, et al. Elastolytic activity in pulmonary lavage fluid from patients with adult respiratory-distress syndrome. N Engl J Med 1981; 304(4):192–196.
92. McGuire WW, Spragg RG, Cohen AB, et al. Studies on the pathogenesis of the adult respiratory distress syndrome. J Clin Invest 1982; 69(3):543–553.
93. Suter PM, Suter S, Girardin E, et al. High bronchoalveolar levels of tumor necrosis factor and its inhibitors, interleukin-1, interferon, and elastase, in patients with adult respiratory distress syndrome after trauma, shock, or sepsis. Am Rev Respir Dis 1992; 145(5):1016–1022.
94. Idell S, Kucich U, Fein A, et al. Neutrophil elastase-releasing factors in bronchoalveolar lavage from patients with adult respiratory distress syndrome. Am Rev Respir Dis 1985; 132(5):1098–1105.
95. Christner P, Fein A, Goldberg S, et al. Collagenase in the lower respiratory tract of patients with adult respiratory distress syndrome. Am Rev Respir Dis 1985; 131(5):690–695.
96. Delclaux C, d'Ortho MP, Delacourt C, et al. Gelatinases in epithelial lining fluid of patients with adult respiratory distress syndrome. Am J Physiol 1997; 272(3, pt 1):L442–L451.

97. Pugin J, Verghese G, Widmer MC, et al. The alveolar space is the site of intense inflammatory and profibrotic reactions in the early phase of acute respiratory distress syndrome. Crit Care Med 1999; 27(2):304–312.

98. Ricou B, Nicod L, Lacraz S, et al. Matrix metalloproteinases and TIMP in acute respiratory distress syndrome. Am J Respir Crit Care Med 1996; 154(2, pt 1):346–352.

99. Worthen GS, Schwab B III, Elson EL, et al. Mechanics of stimulated neutrophils: cell stiffening induces retention in capillaries. Science 1989; 245(4914):183–186.

100. Lavkan AH, Astiz ME, Rackow EC. Effects of proinflammatory cytokines and bacterial toxins on neutrophil rheologic properties. Crit Care Med 1998; 26(10):1677–1682.

101. Erzurum SC, Downey GP, Doherty DE, et al. Mechanisms of lipopolysaccharide-induced neutrophil retention. Relative contributions of adhesive and cellular mechanical properties. J Immunol 1992; 149(1):154–162.

102. Skoutelis AT, Kaleridis V, Athanassiou GM, et al. Neutrophil deformability in patients with sepsis, septic shock, and adult respiratory distress syndrome. Crit Care Med 2000; 28(7):2355–2359.

103. Everhart MB, Han W, Sherrill TP, et al. Duration and intensity of NF-kappaB activity determine the severity of endotoxin-induced acute lung injury. J Immunol 2006; 176(8):4995–5005.

104. Blackwell TS, Blackwell TR, Holden EP, et al. In vivo antioxidant treatment suppresses nuclear factor-kappa B activation and neutrophilic lung inflammation. J Immunol 1996; 157(4):1630–1637.

105. Christman JW, Sadikot RT, Blackwell TS. The role of nuclear factor-kappa B in pulmonary diseases. Chest 2000; 117(5):1482–1487.

106. Fan J, Ye RD, Malik AB. Transcriptional mechanisms of acute lung injury. Am J Physiol Lung Cell Mol Physiol 2001; 281(5):L1037–L1050.

107. Yang KY, Arcaroli JJ, Abraham E. Early alterations in neutrophil activation are associated with outcome in acute lung injury. Am J Respir Crit Care Med 2003; 167(11):1567–1574.

108. Lesur O, Kokis A, Hermans C, et al. Interleukin-2 involvement in early acute respiratory distress syndrome: relationship with polymorphonuclear neutrophil apoptosis and patient survival. Crit Care Med 2000; 28(12):3814–3822.

109. Matute-Bello G, Liles WC, Radella F II, et al. Neutrophil apoptosis in the acute respiratory distress syndrome. Am J Respir Crit Care Med 1997; 156(6):1969–1977.

110. Geerts L, Jorens PG, Willems J, et al. Natural inhibitors of neutrophil function in acute respiratory distress syndrome. Crit Care Med 2001; 29(10):1920–1924.

111. Opal, SM, Cross AS. Clinical trials for severe sepsis. Past failures, and future hopes. Infect Dis Clin North Am 1999; 13(2):285–297, vii.

112. Parsons PE, Eisner MD, Thompson BT, et al. Lower tidal volume ventilation and plasma cytokine markers of inflammation in patients with acute lung injury. Crit Care Med 2005; 33(1):1–6; discussion 230–232.

113. Park WY, Goodman RB, Steinberg KP, et al. Cytokine balance in the lungs of patients with acute respiratory distress syndrome. Am J Respir Crit Care Med 2001; 164(10, pt 1):1896–1903.

114. Kurdowska A, Noble JM, Steinberg KP, et al. Anti-interleukin 8 autoantibody: interleukin 8 complexes in the acute respiratory distress syndrome. Relationship between the complexes and clinical disease activity. Am J Respir Crit Care Med 2001; 163(2):463–468.

115. Kurdowska A, Miller EJ, Noble JM, et al. Anti-IL-8 autoantibodies in alveolar fluid from patients with the adult respiratory distress syndrome. J Immunol 1996; 157(6):2699–2706.

116. Pugin J, Ricou B, Steinberg KP, et al. Proinflammatory activity in bronchoalveolar lavage fluids from patients with ARDS, a prominent role for interleukin-1. Am J Respir Crit Care Med 1996; 153(6 pt 1):1850–1856.

117. Geiser T, Atabai K, Jarreau PH, et al. Pulmonary edema fluid from patients with acute lung injury augments in vitro alveolar epithelial repair by an IL-1beta-dependent mechanism. Am J Respir Crit Care Med 2001; 163(6):1384–1388.

118. Chabot F, Mitchell JA, Gutteridge JM, et al. Reactive oxygen species in acute lung injury. Eur Respir J 1998; 11(3):745–757.

119. Gutteridge J, Halliwell, B. Antioxidants in Nutrition, Health and Disease. Oxford: Oxford University Press, 1994.

120. Schmidt R, Luboeinski T, Markart P, et al. Alveolar antioxidant status in patients with acute respiratory distress syndrome. Eur Respir J 2004; 24(6):994–999.

121. Bowler RP, Velsor LW, Duda B, et al. Pulmonary edema fluid antioxidants are depressed in acute lung injury. Crit Care Med 2003; 31(9):2309–2315.

122. Moss M, Bucher B, Moore FA, et al. The role of chronic alcohol abuse in the development of acute respiratory distress syndrome in adults. JAMA 1996; 275(1):50–54.

123. Moss M, Guidot DM, Wong-Lambertina M, et al. The effects of chronic alcohol abuse on pulmonary glutathione homeostasis. Am J Respir Crit Care Med 2000; 161(2, pt 1): 414–419.

124. Yeh MY, Burnham EL, Moss M, et al. Chronic alcoholism alters systemic and pulmonary glutathione redox status. Am J Respir Crit Care Med 2007; 176(3):270–276.

125. Conner BD, Bernard GR. Acute respiratory distress syndrome. Potential pharmacologic interventions. Clin Chest Med 2000; 21(3):563–587.

126. McClintock DE, Ware LB, Eisner MD, et al. Higher urine nitric oxide is associated with improved outcomes in patients with acute lung injury. Am J Respir Crit Care Med 2007; 175(3):256–262.

127. Zhu S, Ware LB, Geiser T, et al. Increased levels of nitrate and surfactant protein a nitration in the pulmonary edema fluid of patients with acute lung injury. Am J Respir Crit Care Med 2001; 163(1):166–172.

128. Sittipunt C, Steinberg KP, Ruzinski JT, et al. Nitric oxide and nitrotyrosine in the lungs of patients with acute respiratory distress syndrome. Am J Respir Crit Care Med 2001; 163(2):503–510.

129. Gessner C, Hammerschmidt S, Kuhn H, et al. Exhaled breath condensate nitrite and its relation to tidal volume in acute lung injury. Chest 2003; 124(3):1046–1052.

130. Mumby S, Upton RL, Chen Y, et al. Lung heme oxygenase-1 is elevated in acute respiratory distress syndrome. Crit Care Med 2004; 32(5):1130–1135.

131. Melley DD, Finney SJ, Elia A, et al. Arterial carboxyhemoglobin level and outcome in critically ill patients. Crit Care Med 2007; 35(8):1882–1887.

132. Rinaldo JE, Rogers RM. Adult respiratory-distress syndrome: changing concepts of lung injury and repair. N Engl J Med 1982; 306(15):900–909.

133. Ware LB, Camerer E, Welty-Wolf K, et al. Bench to bedside: targeting coagulation and fibrinolysis in acute lung injury. Am J Physiol Lung Cell Mol Physiol 2006; 291(3):L307–L311.

134. Abraham E. Coagulation abnormalities in acute lung injury and sepsis. Am J Respir Cell Mol Biol 2000; 22(4):401–404.

135. Seeger W, Hubel J, Klapettek K, et al. Procoagulant activity in bronchoalveolar lavage of severely traumatized patients—relation to the development of acute respiratory distress. Thromb Res 1991; 61(1):53–64.

136. Fuchs-Buder T, de Moerloose P, Ricou B, et al. Time course of procoagulant activity and D dimer in bronchoalveolar fluid of patients at risk for or with acute respiratory distress syndrome. Am J Respir Crit Care Med 1996; 153(1):163–167.

137. Gunther A, Mosavi P, Heinemann S, et al. Alveolar fibrin formation caused by enhanced procoagulant and depressed fibrinolytic capacities in severe pneumonia. Comparison with the acute respiratory distress syndrome. Am J Respir Crit Care Med 2000; 161(2, pt 1):454–462.

138. Idell S. Coagulation, fibrinolysis, and fibrin deposition in acute lung injury. Crit Care Med 2003; 31(Suppl. 4):S213–S220.
139. Prabhakaran P, Ware LB, White KE, et al. Elevated levels of plasminogen activator inhibitor-1 in pulmonary edema fluid are associated with mortality in acute lung injury. Am J Physiol Lung Cell Mol Physiol 2003; 285(1):L20–L28.
140. Idell S, Gonzalez K, Bradford H, et al. Procoagulant activity in bronchoalveolar lavage in the adult respiratory distress syndrome. Contribution of tissue factor associated with factor VII. Am Rev Respir Dis 1987; 136(6):1466–1474.
141. Idell S, Peters J, James KK, et al. Local abnormalities of coagulation and fibrinolytic pathways that promote alveolar fibrin deposition in the lungs of baboons with diffuse alveolar damage. J Clin Invest 1989; 84(1):181–193.
142. Bastarache JA, Wang L, Geiser T, et al. The alveolar epithelium can initiate the extrinsic coagulation cascade through expression of tissue factor. Thorax 2007; 62(7):608–616.
143. Bastarache JA, Wang L, Wang Z, et al. Intra-alveolar tissue factor pathway inhibitor is not sufficient to block tissue factor procoagulant activity. Am J Physiol Lung Cell Mol Physiol 2008; 294(5):L874–L881.
144. Ware LB, Fang X, Matthay MA. Protein C and thrombomodulin in human acute lung injury. Am J Physiol Lung Cell Mol Physiol 2003; 285(3):L514–L521.
145. Adamzik M, Frey UH, Riemann K, et al. Factor V Leiden mutation is associated with improved 30-day survival in patients with acute respiratory distress syndrome. Crit Care Med 2008; 36(6):1776–1779.
146. van der Poll T, Levi M, Nick JA, et al. Activated protein C inhibits local coagulation after intra-pulmonary delivery of endotoxin in humans. Am J Respir Crit Care Med 2005; 171(10):1125–1128.
147. Bernard GR, Vincent JL, Laterre PF, et al. Efficacy and safety of recombinant human activated protein C for severe sepsis. N Engl J Med 2001; 344(10):699–709.
148. Liu KD, Levitt J, Zhuo H, et al. Randomized clinical trial of activated protein C for the treatment of acute lung injury. Am J Respir Crit Care Med 2008; 178(6):618–623.
149. Bianchi ME. DAMPs, PAMPs and alarmins: all we need to know about danger. J Leukoc Biol 2007; 81(1):1–5.
150. Uchida T, Shirasawa M, Ware LB, et al. Receptor for advanced glycation end-products is a marker of type I cell injury in acute lung injury. Am J Respir Crit Care Med 2006; 173(9):1008–1015.
151. Calfee CS, Ware LB, Eisner MD, et al. Plasma receptor for advanced glycation end-products and clinical outcomes in acute lung injury. Thorax 2008; 63:1083–1089.
152. van Zoelen MA, Ishizaka A, Wolthuis EK, et al. Pulmonary levels of high-mobility group box 1 during mechanical ventilation and ventilator-associated pneumonia. Shock 2008; 29(4):441–445.
153. Gong MN, Thompson BT, Williams P, et al. Clinical predictors of and mortality in acute respiratory distress syndrome: potential role of red cell transfusion. Crit Care Med 2005; 33(6):1191–1198.
154. Bornstein SR, Preas HL, Chrousos GP, et al. Circulating leptin levels during acute experimental endotoxemia and antiinflammatory therapy in humans. J Infect Dis 1998; 178(3):887–890.
155. Khan H, Belsher J, Yilmaz M, et al. Fresh-frozen plasma and platelet transfusions are associated with development of acute lung injury in critically ill medical patients. Chest 2007; 131(5):1308–1314.
156. Wright, SE, Snowden CP, Athey SC, et al. Acute lung injury after ruptured abdominal aortic aneurysm repair: the effect of excluding donations from females from the production of fresh frozen plasma. Crit Care Med 2008; 36(6):1796–1802.

7

Apoptosis in the Pathogenesis and Resolution of Acute Lung Injury

GUSTAVO MATUTE-BELLO
Division of Pulmonary and Critical Care Medicine, Department of Medicine,
University of Washington School of Medicine, Seattle, Washington, U.S.A.

THOMAS R. MARTIN
Veteran's Affairs Puget Sound Health Care System, and Division of Pulmonary
and Critical Care Medicine, Department of Medicine, University of Washington
School of Medicine, Seattle, Washington, U.S.A.

I. Introduction

Apoptosis is a controlled process of cell death, which is triggered by specific stimuli and is carried out by intracellular pathways. The outcome of this process is a decrease in cell size, fragmentation of the DNA, and ultimately uptake of the apoptotic cell by a phagocyte. In contrast, in necrosis the homeostatic mechanisms of a cell are disrupted, leading to swelling and eventually bursting of the necrotic cell with spillage of its contents into the surrounding microenvironment. A key aspect of apoptosis (as opposed to necrosis) is that it is a process controlled at several different levels, some of which are susceptible to therapeutic intervention designed to induce or inhibit the occurrence of cell death. Thus, knowledge of the role of apoptosis in the pathogenesis and/or resolution of a disease may lead to novel therapeutic strategies aimed at modifying the course of that disease by manipulating the apoptotic process.

Theoretically, apoptosis could be involved in disease processes by at least three separate mechanisms: inappropriate induction of apoptosis resulting in loss of "desired" cells; inappropriate inhibition of apoptosis allowing persistence of "nondesired" cells; and disruption of the apoptotic clearance process leading to secondary necrosis of apoptotic cells and spillage of their cellular contents. All three of these processes have been implicated in the pathogenesis of acute lung injury (ALI) and its more severe form, the acute respiratory distress syndrome (ARDS), as well as in the repair process that follows lung injury. ALI/ARDS is characterized pathologically by neutrophilic alveolitis, microthrombi, interstitial edema, destruction of the alveolar epithelial layer with exposure of the basement membrane, and proteinaceous exudates in the airspaces (1,2). The cells involved in this area are neutrophils (polymorphonuclear leukocytes, PMN), alveolar macrophages, alveolar epithelial cells, and capillary endothelial cells. We will review the evidence suggesting that alterations in the apoptotic process of each of these cells might be involved in the pathogenesis and resolution of ALI/ARDS.

II. Apoptosis in the Pathogenesis of Lung Injury
A. Neutrophil Apoptosis

Apoptosis of PMN has been proposed as a key mechanism of resolution of inflammation (3–5). After migrating from a blood vessel into tissues, PMN cannot return to the circulation, and thus their fate is either to necrose and disintegrate or to become apoptotic and be phagocytized by macrophages and other phagocytic cells. Clearance of inflammation would occur primarily by induction of PMN apoptosis and subsequent uptake of apoptotic PMN by phagocytes. Thus, inhibition of PMN apoptosis and/or impaired phagocytosis of apoptotic PMN would result in persistence of inflammation and, potentially, increased necrosis, with PMN disintegration and spillage of toxic PMN contents into the surrounding microenvironment. This hypothesis predicts that PMN apoptosis should be inhibited during early ALI/ARDS, then increase as inflammation resolves. Presumably, inhibition of PMN apoptosis or impaired clearance of apoptotic neutrophils would be associated with persistence of inflammation and a worse outcome. Several studies in animals support the hypothesis that neutrophil apoptosis is important for clearance of inflammation in the lungs. Mice lacking caspase-1 have delayed neutrophil apoptosis and show prolonged neutrophilic inflammation when challenged with intratracheal lipopolysaccharide (LPS) (6). Thus, in experimental models of ALI, impairment of neutrophil apoptosis results in a prolonged inflammatory response.

Studies performed in patients with ARDS showed that the percentage of apoptotic PMN in bronchoalveolar lavage (BAL) fluid from patients with early ARDS is relatively low (7) (Fig. 1). However, this was true throughout ARDS, and the percentage of apoptotic PMN did not increase as inflammation resolved. Thus, it would appear that the proportion of PMN that are apoptotic at any given time in the airspaces of patients with ARDS is relatively constant. However, this does not necessarily mean that apoptosis of PMN is unchanged during ARDS. If phagocytosis of apoptotic cells is very rapid there could be major changes in the *number* of PMN that develop apoptosis, even *if the proportion* of PMN that are apoptotic remains constant. Additional studies demonstrated that soluble mediators present in BAL fluid and plasma from patients with early ARDS inhibit PMN apoptosis (8–10). This inhibition was mediated primarily by the cytokine granulocyte-macrophage colony-stimulating factor (GM-CSF) and, to a lesser extent, by the cytokines granulocyte-stimulating factor (G-CSF) and interleukin-2 (IL-2) (Fig. 2). Lung fluids from patients at later stages of ARDS or at risk for ARDS had lower concentrations of GM-CSF (Fig. 3). These BAL fluids did not inhibit PMN apoptosis (Fig. 4). These studies suggest that high concentrations of GM-CSF in BAL fluid and plasma inhibit PMN apoptosis during acute inflammation and that as inflammation resolves and GM-CSF concentrations return to normal, PMN apoptosis also returns to baseline levels. However, it is not clear whether GM-CSF-mediated inhibition of PMN apoptosis is involved in the pathogenesis of the disease. Although there are anecdotal reports of patients developing ARDS after receiving recombinant GM-CSF (11), in more recent series, higher concentrations of GM-CSF in BAL fluid from patients with early ARDS are associated with increased survival (8). In summary, studies in humans with ARDS have confirmed that PMN apoptosis is modulated throughout the course of the disease, but a clear link between PMN apoptosis and pathogenesis has not been established.

In addition to G-CSF and GM-CSF, a number of other mediators have been shown to inhibit neutrophil apoptosis; these include the complement component C5a, cytokines

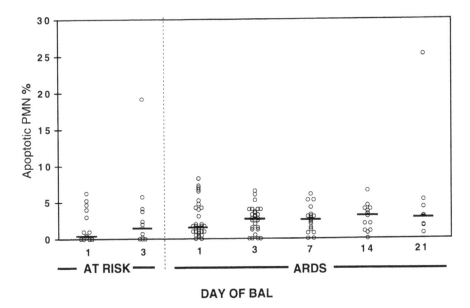

Figure 1 Percentage of apoptotic PMN on cytospin preparations of BAL fluid from patients at risk for ARDS and patients with ARDS, measured by morphologic criteria. Each point represents data from one patient. Bars represent medians. The horizontal axis shows the day of illness on which the BAL procedure was performed. *Source*: From Ref. 7.

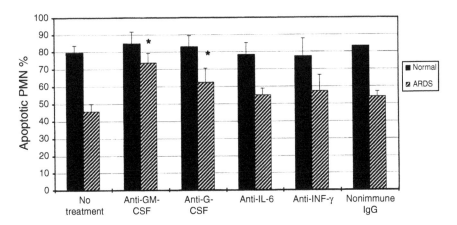

Figure 2 Effect of immunodepleting BAL of GM-CSF, G-CSF, IL-6, and IFN-γ on PMN apoptosis. BAL fluid from patients with ARDS was immunodepleted of GM-CSF, G-CSF, IL-6, and IFN-γ using blocking monoclonal antibodies. Then normal PMNs were incubated in either untreated or depleted BAL for 18 hours, and apoptosis was measured by Annexin-V binding. The asterisks show statistical significance ($p < 0.05$) compared to the "no treatment" group. *Source*: From Ref. 7.

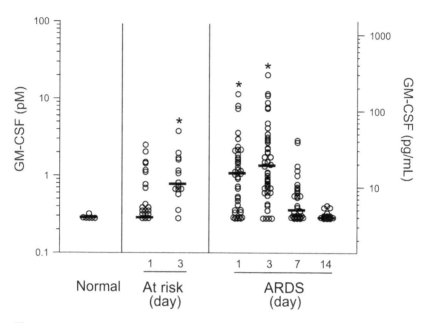

Figure 3 Concentration of GM-CSF in BALF from normal volunteers, BALF from patients on days 1 and 3 of being identified as being at risk for ARDS, and BALF from patients on days 1, 3, 7, and 14 of established ARDS. Each dot represents a single individual, and the bars show median values. $* = p < 0.05$, compared to BALF from normal volunteers (ANOVA with Fischer's posthoc analysis performed using $\log_{10}$ transformed data). *Source*: From Ref. 8.

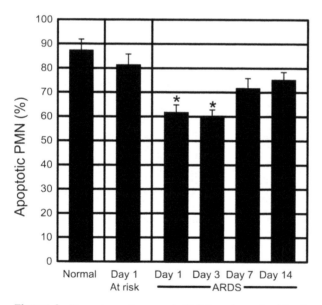

Figure 4 Percentage of apoptotic PMN, as determined by flow cytometry and Annexin-V binding, after incubation of normal PMN for 18 hours in either BALF from normal volunteers, or BALF from patients on days 1,3,7, and 14 of ARDS. $* = p < 0.05$ compared to normal BALF (ANOVA with Scheffe's posthoc analysis). *Source*: From Ref. 8.

such as IL-2, IL-6, and IL-10; bacterial products such as LPS, components of the coagulation cascade such as plasminogen and fibrinogen, and immune complexes (12–18).
However, the role of these mediators in neutrophil apoptosis during human ALI/ARDS
remains unclear.

The role of PMN apoptosis in lung injury has also been investigated in animal
studies. Parsey and coworkers (19) isolated parenchymal PMN from mice subject to
either hemorrhage or endotoxemia and measured the percent of apoptotic PMN over
48 hours using Annexin-V. At baseline, 18.5 ± 1.9% of the PMN in the lungs were
apoptotic (Fig. 5). The percentage of apoptotic PMN decreased significantly after one
hour of either hemorrhage or endotoxemia, remained low for 24 hours, and returned to
baseline levels at 48 hours. This study is important because it measured apoptosis in
lung PMN, thus providing direct information about the apoptotic process in lung PMN,

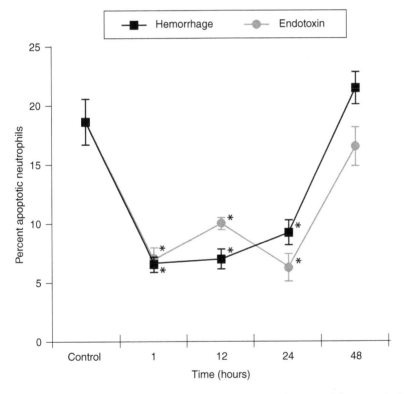

Figure 5 Hemorrhage or endotoxemia causes changes in neutrophil apoptosis. Mice were
either sham-hemorrhaged, hemorrhaged 30% blood volume, or injected i.p. with 5 mg/kg LPS.
At the times indicated, lung intraparenchymal pulmonary neutrophils and mononuclear cells
were isolated and Annexin-V assays performed while gating on the neutrophil population. The
rate of neutrophil apoptosis in sham-hemorrhaged controls was the same as in unmanipulated
control mice. Results are presented as the mean percentage of apoptotic cells ± SEM. * = p
< 0.01 compared to baseline (control). *Source*: From Ref. 19.

as opposed to measuring the effects of lung fluids on PMN apoptosis. Parsey's study confirms the human observations suggesting that PMN apoptosis is inhibited during acute inflammation, but does not clarify the importance of modulation of PMN apoptosis in the pathogenesis of lung injury.

The question of biological relevance was addressed in a study by Sookhai and coworkers (20), who investigated the consequences of inhibiting PMN apoptosis on the development of lung injury following ischemia/reperfusion (I/R) in mice. They found that PMN apoptosis was enhanced by the administration of aerosolized dead opsonized *Escherichia coli* to the animals. The improvement in PMN apoptosis was associated with enhanced survival and decreased severity of lung injury following I/R (measured by BAL protein concentrations and myeloperoxidase (MPO) activity in lung homogenates). Thus, enhancement of PMN apoptosis was beneficial and resulted in less lung injury and improved survival after ischemia reperfusion.

In summary, the role of PMN apoptosis in the pathogenesis of ALI remains unclear. Studies in animals and humans support the hypothesis that PMN apoptosis is inhibited during acute inflammation and suggest that this inhibition is mediated by soluble mediators, in particular GM-CSF. However, in humans with early ARDS, higher concentrations of GM-CSF are associated with improved survival, suggesting that inhibition of PMN apoptosis may be beneficial. In contrast to the human studies, in one animal study, enhancement rather than inhibition of PMN apoptosis was beneficial to the host. Additional studies are required to determine the biological importance of changes in PMN apoptosis in the pathogenesis of ALI.

B. Epithelial Cell Apoptosis

The death of epithelial cells during ARDS is likely to result from both necrosis and apoptosis, but the relative contribution of each of these processes to epithelial injury remains unknown. Bardales and coworkers (21) identified features consistent with apoptosis in the alveolar epithelium of patients who died with lung injury. Guinee and coworkers (22) found that *bax*, a *bcl-2* analog that promotes apoptosis, is upregulated in alveolar pneumocytes of humans with diffuse alveolar damage but not in control lungs. Fujita and coworkers (23) found that the administration of LPS to the lungs of mice is followed 6 hours later by endothelial and alveolar epithelial apoptosis. Perl confirmed that extensive alveolar epithelial cell apoptosis occurs in mice following the combination of hemorrhagic shock and cecal ligation and puncture (24). Alveolar epithelial cell apoptosis has also been identified in other lung diseases, such as pulmonary fibrosis (25). Several mechanisms have been implicated in the development of epithelial cell apoptosis, including activation of the proteinase-activated receptor (PAR)-1 by elastase, but accumulating evidence suggests that the Fas/FasL system plays a central role in alveolar cell apoptosis during human and experimental ALI (26–28).

The Fas/FasL system has an important role in the regulation of cell life and death. This system comprises the cell membrane surface receptor Fas (CD95) and its natural ligand (FasL) (29). Fas is a 45 kD type I membrane protein member of the TNF family of surface receptors (30). The natural ligand of Fas is Fas-ligand (FasL), a 37 kD type II protein (31). FasL exists as membrane-bound and soluble forms (sFasL) (32). Binding of Fas to FasL induces apoptosis of susceptible cells, by a mechanism involving activation of the interleukin-1 converting enzyme (ICE)-related proteases, caspase-8 and caspase-3 (33).

Membrane-bound FasL mediates lymphocyte-dependent cytotoxicity, clonal deletion of alloreactive T-cells, and activation-induced suicide of T-cells (34–36). The soluble form of FasL can induce apoptosis of human and rabbit lung epithelial cells but the murine form of soluble FasL has little bioactivity (28,37).

Subsets of alveolar epithelial cells express Fas on their surface and undergo apoptosis in response to sFasL ligation (38,39). Pulmonary alveolar and airway epithelial cells express Fas and FasL on their surface (39–42), and expression of mRNA for Fas and FasL in whole lungs increases following the administration of LPS (43). Fas-mediated apoptosis of alveolar epithelial cells is modulated by at least two important mediators: surfactant protein A (SP-A) and angiotensin II (AII). SP-A, the primary protein present in pulmonary surfactant, inhibits type II cell apoptosis in vivo (44,45). This is important because the concentration of SP-A is decreased in BAL fluid from patients with ARDS, which would favor apoptosis of type II cells (46). Interaction of AII with its ATi receptor on epithelial cells is required for Fas-mediated apoptosis of alveolar epithelial cells in vitro (47). This might be relevant for ARDS because the concentration of angiotensin-converting enzyme (ACE), which catabolizes the conversion of angiotensin I to AII is increased in BAL fluid from patients with ARDS (48).

In humans with ARDS, the soluble form of FasL (sFasL) can be detected in BAL fluid (28,49) (Fig. 6) and patients who die have higher concentrations of sFasL in BAL fluid than patients who survive. The sFasL present in lung fluids from patients with ARDS is biologically active and can induce apoptosis of distal lung epithelial cells (28) (Fig. 7). Thus, the alveolar microenvironment of patients with ARDS appears to favor alveolar epithelial cell apoptosis.

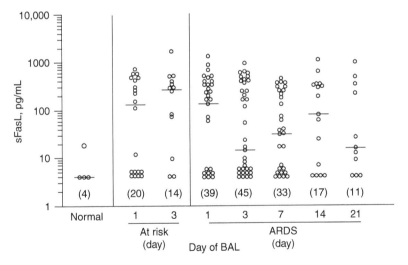

Figure 6 Soluble FasL concentrations measured by immunoassay in BALF from four normal volunteers, 20 patients at risk for ARDS, and 45 patients with ARDS. The bars represent median values. The numbers in parenthesis indicate the number of patients studied on each day. *Source*: From Ref. 28.

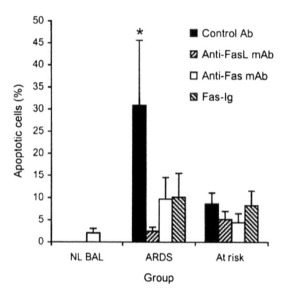

Figure 7 Effect of ARDS BAL fluid on primary distal lung epithelial cells (DLECs). DLECs were incubated in a medium supplemented at a 50% concentration with either BAL fluid from four normal volunteers (NL), BAL fluid from five patients studied on day 1 of ARDS, or BAL fluid from four patients studied on day 1 of becoming at risk for ARDS. The cells were incubated for 18 hours at 37°C, 5% CO_2, then stained with acridine orange and examined by fluorescence microscopy. The total number of cells and total number of apoptotic cells were counted on a low power field (160×), and the percent of apoptotic cells was calculated. * = $p < 0.05$ by ANOVA with Fischer's posthoc analysis, as compared with normal BALF. *Source*: From Ref. 28.

Animal studies support the hypothesis that activation of the Fas/FasL system is involved in the pathogenesis of acute and chronic lung injury. The administration of the Fas-activating mAb Jo2 to the lungs of mice results in alveolar epithelial cell apoptosis, permeability changes, and lung inflammation (36,50); and instillation of recombinant human sFasL into the lungs of rabbits causes acute alveolar injury with hemorrhage (37). Studies with chimeric mice expressing Fas in either myeloid or nonmyeloid cells demonstrated that Fas-mediated lung injury requires expression of Fas in lung nonmyeloid cells, and studies using intratracheal clodronate to deplete alveolar macrophages suggested that macrophage depletion does not prevent, and may worsen, Fas-mediated lung injury (51,52). Among the nonmyeloid cells of the lungs, distal epithelial cells are particularly susceptible to Fas-mediated apoptosis, as compared with large airway epithelial cells (53). Thus, distal lung epithelial cells, and in particular alveolar epithelial cells, appear to be the primary target for FasL in the lungs, at least in the development of ALI.

The role of the Fas/FasL system in ALI has been confirmed in several models of experimental lung injury. Mice deficient in Fas or FasL are protected in a model of hemorrhagic shock followed by cecal ligation and puncture, and this protection has been reproduced with the use of siRNA technology in vivo (24,27). Fas may also have a role in LPS-induced lung injury. In mice, the administration of LPS either intravenously or by intratracheal instillation is followed by increased alveolar epithelial permeability and apoptosis of both alveolar epithelial and endothelial cells and also bronchial epithelial cells (23,43,54). Interestingly, very early after LPS instillation, significant numbers of alveolar wall cells show DNA fragmentation by in situ nick-end labeling (TUNEL), suggesting that cell death can occur very rapidly after an injurious stimulus. Blockade of apoptosis by the broad caspase inhibitor ZVAD-fmk improves the histological picture and decreases alveolar epithelial apoptosis (55), whereas blockade of the Fas/FasL system with the anti-Fas antibody P2 inhibits apoptosis, and attenuates increases in albumin leak and alveolar neutrophilia following intratracheal LPS administration in mice (43). Thus, recent evidence suggests that the Fas/FasL pathway is important in the pathogenesis of epithelial injury in ALI in animals and humans.

These considerations lead to a Fas-centered hypothesis for the pathogenesis of septic lung injury, according to which soluble FasL released by monocytes, macrophages, and epithelial cells induces apoptosis of the alveolar epithelium (and endothelium), leading to disruption of the alveolar-epithelial barrier and increased permeability. This hypothesis has certain limitations, however. First, it has not been shown that in vivo, macrophages or epithelial cells in the lung release sFasL in response to activation. Second, while apoptotic epithelial cells can be identified in animal models of lung injury, they seem to be sparse, although this apparent paucity could be a result of the techniques used to measure apoptosis. Third, other mediators such as NO have been implicated in the development of apoptosis in epithelial cells (56,57). Finally, activation of the Fas/FasL system can result in activation of inflammatory pathways in macrophages, further complicating the model.

In addition to triggering apoptotic pathways, and independently of its proapoptotic function, activation of Fas can also lead to NFκB translocation and cytokine production (58). Evidence suggests that the Fas/FasL system can modulate host defenses. First, in addition to apoptosis, Fas activation also induces cytokine release in alveolar epithelial cells (24,52). Second, alveolar macrophages, which express Fas on their surface, do not become apoptotic in response to Fas ligation, but instead release inflammatory cytokines such as IL-8 (59,60). Third, mice deficient in Fas (*lpr*) show impaired PMN recruitment in response to intratracheal bacteria, although bacterial clearance is not affected (61). Fourth, animals deficient in Fas (*lpr*) are prone to systemic dissemination of *Pseudomonas aeruginosa* pneumonia, suggesting that the Fas/FasL system is involved in host defenses against bacteria (62). And finally, activation of the Fas/FasL system also leads to additional nonapoptotic consequences such as upregulation of metalloproteinases, in particular metalloproteinase-12 (MMP-12) (63). Thus, the associations between sFasL and ALI noted above could be due to the proinflammatory effects of the Fas/FasL system. In other words, it is unclear whether the changes in alveolar permeability and the alveolar epithelial injury seen in response to Fas ligation in the lungs result primarily from the proapoptotic effect of Fas ligation on the alveolar epithelium or instead are secondary to the proinflammatory effects of the Fas/FasL system on macrophages and on PMN recruitment.

C. Endothelial Cell Apoptosis

There is less information about apoptosis of endothelial cells as a possible pathogenic mechanism of endothelial dysfunction in ARDS. Assaly and coworkers have shown that serum from patients with systemic capillary leak syndrome and shock induces apoptosis of dermal microvascular endothelial cells, and this is associated with increases in intracellular ROS and in the bax/bc12 expression ratio (64). However, such a study has not been done in a systematic way using serum or plasma from patients with ARDS. In mice, the systemic administration of LPS is associated with endothelial cell apoptosis in several tissues, including the lung (23,65,66). Endothelial cell apoptosis can be detected as early as six hours after LPS administration (23) and appears to involve primarily the mitochondrial pathway by a mechanism involving intracellular ceramide generation (65,67,68). The administration of ceramide induces apoptosis in the lungs, but this is associated with emphysema rather than ALI (69). In addition, targeted apoptosis of lung endothelial cells by means of a lung endothelial cell-binding peptide fused to a proapoptotic motif resulted in development of emphysema, rather than ALI (70). Thus, endothelial cell apoptosis is present in ALI induced by LPS, but it appears to be primarily important in the development of emphysema, rather than ALI. Although the evidence supporting a pathogenic role of endothelial apoptosis is limited, the available studies suggest that circulating mediators, in particular TNF-α, may induce apoptosis of alveolar capillary endothelial cells.

III. Apoptosis in the Resolution of ALI/ARDS

Apoptosis occurs in alveolar airspaces during the repair phase of ALI. Polunovsky and coworkers suggested that apoptosis of fibroblasts and endothelial cells is an important method of elimination of granulation tissue during the repair phase of ALI (71). They showed that (1) BAL fluids from patients during lung repair induce apoptosis of fibroblasts and endothelial cells, and (2) lung tissue from patients recovering from lung injury shows evidence of apoptosis (71). Madden and Henke have shown that fibronectin peptides induce lung fibroblast death in vitro by anoikis (detachment), by blocking adhesion of fibroblasts to the extracellular matrix (72).

Fibroblasts themselves may contribute to apoptosis of lung epithelial cells and disruption of the repair process (73). Foci of apoptotic alveolar epithelium are present near areas of fibroblast proliferation in patients with pulmonary fibrosis (25). This appears to be mediated by release of angiotensinogen by myofibroblasts, subsequent conversion into AII, and angiotensin-mediated apoptosis of epithelial cells (47,74,75).

Studies by Teder and coworkers suggest that failure to clear apoptotic PMN may lead to persistence of inflammation and increased death (76). In a mouse model of bleomycin-induced lung injury, they found that mice deficient in the transmembrane adhesion receptor CD44 failed to clear inflammation, as compared to wild-type mice (Fig. 8). This was associated with increased numbers of apoptotic cells in the lungs and a significant failure to clear apoptotic PMN. The effect was reversed by adoptive transfer of normal marrow cells. This is important, because CD44 increases phagocytosis of apoptotic neutrophils by macrophages in vitro (77). However, CD44 has other functions such as clearance of the glycosaminoglycan hyaluronan, which in turn can increase the synthesis of chemokines such as IL-8 (78). A drawback of this study is that it does not show whether the findings were primarily due to the effects of CD44 on the clearance of apoptotic PMN or on clearance of hyaluronan and decreased production of chemokines.

In another study using a rat model of oleic acid-induced lung injury, Hussain and coworkers demonstrated that the resolution phase of lung injury is associated with generalized apoptosis of PMN and uptake of apoptotic PMN by macrophages (79). Thus, the studies of Teder and Hussain support the hypothesis that PMN apoptosis is an important mechanism of resolution of inflammation, but these studies do not clarify whether this

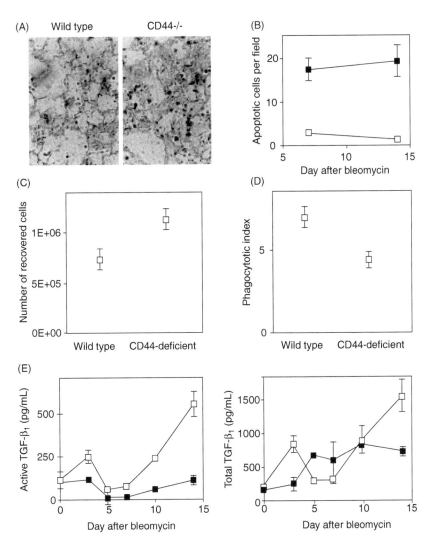

Figure 8 Clearance of apoptotic cells during lung inflammation. (**A**) Apoptotic cells (dark black) in lungs of wild type and CD44-deficient mice at day 7 after bleomycin. Magnification ×100. (**B**) Quantitation of apoptotic cells after bleomycin treatment. Fifty fields were counted at a magnification of ×400 from four experiments. Results are mean + SE, $n = 4$. CD44-deficient (black boxes) and wild-type (white boxes) mice, $n = 3$. (**C**) Human apoptotic PMNs were instilled into the lungs of LPS-treated mice; the numbers of recovered cells by BAL were counted ($p = 0.0096$) and (**D**) phagocytotic index was calculated ($p = 0.0029$). Values reported are the mean + SE from 12 animals in each group. (**E**) CD44-deficient mice generate decreased concentrations of active TGF-β1. TGF-β1 was measured in 10-fold concentrated BAL fluids, combined from four different wild type (white boxes) and CD44-deficient mice (black boxes) at each time point, $n = 3$. Results are mean + SE from three experiments. Active TGF-β1 is shown in the left panel and total TGF-β1 in the right panel. *Source*: From Ref. 76.

is the most important mechanism, or whether the key mechanism is downregulation of chemokine production pathways.

Neutrophil apoptosis may also indirectly contribute to resolution of inflammation by modulating the production of proinflammatory cytokines by alveolar macrophages. Macrophage phagocytosis of apoptotic PMN inhibits macrophage production of the proinflammatory cytokines IL-1β, IL-8, IL-10, GM-CSF, TNF-α, and increases TGF-β1, PGE2, and platelet-activating factor, all of which have anti-inflammatory properties (77). Thus, an increase in PMN apoptosis leading to increases in phagocytosis of apoptotic PMN could "turndown" the inflammatory phenotype in activated alveolar macrophages, favoring resolution of inflammation, while at the same time increasing fibroblast proliferation mediated by TGF-β1.

IV. Summary and Conclusions

An important difficulty regarding the interpretation of available studies on apoptosis and ARDS is that the current methods available to study the apoptotic process are limited. The apoptotic process is a dynamic process, involving not only the development or inhibition of apoptosis in a specific cell, but also its removal by nearby phagocytes. An increase in the number of apoptotic cells in tissue could be due to impairment of the clearance process or to an increase in apoptosis. Yet the majority of studies available rely on measurements of apoptotic cells, and no effective method is available to evaluate apoptotic cell clearance in vivo.

Another problem is that some of the methods available to detect apoptosis are controversial. This controversy stems from two facts: first, some of these methods, like the end-nick labeling assay (TUNEL) and also Annexin-V labeling, sometimes become positive in necrotic cells. Second, in the absence of effective clearance mechanisms, apoptotic cells will undergo secondary necrosis. No method exists at the present time that can reliably differentiate necrotic cells that have died from primary necrosis from cells that are apoptotic and undergoing secondary necrosis.

Another limitation of available studies is that most of our knowledge is derived from either animal studies or in vitro studies, rather than human studies, and extrapolating the results from animal studies to human ARDS is difficult because none of the animal models of lung injury currently available accurately reproduces clinical ARDS (80).

Despite these limitations, some conclusions can be drawn from the literature about the role of apoptosis in lung injury. It is likely that PMN apoptosis is inhibited during the early phase of ARDS, compared to normal lungs, and that this inhibition is mediated primarily by GM-CSF. However, the biological consequences of inhibiting PMN apoptosis are unclear, and may actually be beneficial. Despite the prevalent paradigm that PMN apoptosis is an important mechanism of resolution of inflammation, this hypothesis has not been proven true in human ARDS. Additional studies are required to clarify these issues.

The evidence suggesting a possible role for apoptosis of alveolar epithelial cells in the pathogenesis of the epithelial injury seen in ARDS is stronger, particularly because Fas activation can induce in mice a form of lung injury characterized by PMN infiltration and permeability increases, whereas inhibition of the Fas/FasL system protects against LPS-induced lung injury. However, the exact role of alveolar epithelial cell apoptosis (whether mediated by the Fas/FasL system or other mediators) in ARDS is also unclear at this time.

Finally, the evidence regarding a role for apoptosis in the repair process and resolution of inflammation is very exciting. An interesting hypothesis can be derived from the available data suggesting that release of angiotensinogen by fibroblasts and FasL by macrophages could result in apoptosis of the alveolar epithelium. Phagocytosis of these apoptotic cells by macrophages would induce release of TGF-β1, and this TGF-β1 would then promote further proliferation of fibroblasts, resulting in fibrosis.

In conclusion, the current evidence suggests that apoptosis has a role in the pathogenesis and repair of acute lung injury, but the evidence remains inconclusive and further studies are needed to determine its true biological relevance.

References

1. Katzenstein AL, Bloor CM, Leibow AA. Diffuse alveolar damage—the role of oxygen, shock, and related factors. A review. Am J Pathol 1976; 85:210–222.
2. Bachofen M, Weibel ER. Structural alterations of lung parenchyma in the adult respiratory distress syndrome. Clin Chest Med 1982; 3:35–56.
3. Cox G, Gauldie J, Jordana M. Bronchial epithelial-cell derived cytokines (G-CSF and GM-CSF) promote the survival of peripheral blood neutrophils in vitro. Am J Respir Cell Mol Biol 1992; 7:507–513.
4. Grigg JM, Savill, JS, Sarraf C, et al. Neutrophil apoptosis and clearance from neonatal lungs. Lancet 1991; 338:720–722.
5. Tang PS, Mura M, Seth R, et al. Acute lung injury and cell death: how many ways can cells die? Am J Physiol Lung Cell Mol Physiol 2008; 294:L632–L641.
6. Rowe SJ, Allen L, Ridger VC, et al. Caspase-1-deficient mice have delayed neutrophil apoptosis and a prolonged inflammatory response to lipopolysaccharide-induced acute lung injury. J Immunol 2002; 169:6401–6407.
7. Matute-Bello G, Liles WC, Radella F, et al. Neutrophil apoptosis in the acute respiratory distress syndrome. Am J Respir Crit Care Med 1997; 156:1969–1977.
8. Matute-Bello G, Liles WC, Radella II F, et al. Modulation of neutrophil apoptosis by G-CSF and GM-CSF during the course of the acute respiratory distress syndrome (ARDS). Crit Care Med 2000; 28:1–7.
9. Lesur O, Kokis A, Hermans C, et al. Interleukin-2 involvement in early acute respiratory distress syndrome: relationship with polymorphonuclear neutrophil apoptosis and patient survival. Crit Care Med 2000; 28:3814–3822.
10. Goodman ER, Strieker P, Velavicius M, et al. Role of granulocyte-macrophage colony-stimulating factor and its receptor in the genesis of acute respiratory distress syndrome through an effect on neutrophil apoptosis. Arch Surg 1999; 134:1049–1054.
11. Verhoef G, Boogaerts M. Treatment with granulocyte-macrophage colony stimulating factor and the adult respiratory distress syndrome. Am J Hematol 1991; 36:285–287.
12. Guo RF, Sun L, Gao H, et al. In vivo regulation of neutrophil apoptosis by C5a during sepsis. J Leukoc Biol 2006; 80:1575–1583.
13. Lee A, Whyte MK, Haslett C. Inhibition of apoptosis and prolongation of neutrophil functional longevity by inflammatory mediators. J Leukoc Biol 1993; 54:283–288.
14. Pericle F, Liu JH, Diaz JI, et al. Interleukin-2 prevention of apoptosis in human neutrophils. Eur J Immunol 1994; 24:440–444.
15. Biffl WL, Moore EE, Moore FA, et al. Interleukin-6 suppression of neutrophil apoptosis is neutrophil concentration dependent. J Leukoc Biol 1995; 58:582–584.
16. Cox G. IL-10 enhances resolution of pulmonary inflammation in vivo by promoting apoptosis of neutrophils. Am J Physiol Lung Cell Mol Physiol 1996; 271 (4, pt 1):L566–L571.
17. Pluskota E, Soloviev DA, Szpak D, et al. Neutrophil apoptosis: selective regulation by different ligands of integrin alphaMbeta2. J Immunol 2008; 181:3609–3619.

18. Fudala R, Krupa A, Matthay MA, et al. Anti-IL-8 autoantibody: IL-8 immune complexes suppress spontaneous apoptosis of neutrophils. Am J Physiol Lung Cell Mol Physiol 2007; 293:L364–L374.

19. Parsey MV, Kaneko D, Shenkar R, et al. Neutrophil apoptosis in the lung after hemorrhage or endotoxemia: apoptosis and migration are independent of IL-lbeta. Clin Immunol 1999; 91:219–225.

20. Sookhai S, Wang JJ, McCourt M, et al. A novel therapeutic strategy for attenuating neutrophil-mediated lung injury in vivo. Ann Surg 2002; 235:285–291.

21. Bardales RH, Xie SS, Schaefer RF, et al. Apoptosis is a major pathway responsible for the resolution of type II pneumocytes in acute lung injury. Am J Pathol 1996; 149:845–852.

22. Guinee DJ, Brambilla E, Fleming M, et al. The potential role of BAX and BCL-2 expression in diffuse alveolar damage. Am J Pathol 1997, 151:999–1007.

23. Fujita M, Kuwano K, Kunitake R, et al. Endothelial cell apoptosis in lipopolysaccharide-induced lung injury in mice. Int Arch Allergy Immunol 1998; 117:202–208.

24. Perl M, Chung CS, Perl U, et al. Fas-induced pulmonary apoptosis and inflammation during indirect acute lung injury. Am J Respir Crit Care Med 2007; 176:591–601.

25. Uhal BD, Gidea C, Bargout R, et al. Captopril inhibits apoptosis in human lung epithelial cells: a potential antifibrotic mechanism. Am J Physiol Lung Cell Mol Physiol 1998; 275:L1013–L1017.

26. Suzuki T, Moraes TJ, Vachon E, et al. Proteinase-activated receptor-1 mediates elastase-induced apoptosis of human lung epithelial cells. Am J Respir Cell Mol Biol 2005; 33: 231–247.

27. Perl M, Chung CS, Lomas-Neira J, et al. Silencing of Fas, but not caspase-8, in lung epithelial cells ameliorates pulmonary apoptosis, inflammation, and neutrophil influx after hemorrhagic shock and sepsis. Am J Pathol 2005; 167:1545–1559.

28. Matute-Bello G, Liles WC, Steinberg KP, et al. Soluble Fas ligand induces epithelial cell apoptosis in humans with acute lung injury (ARDS). J Immunol 1999; 163:2217–2225.

29. Nagata S, Golstein P. The Fas death factor. Science 1995; 267:1449–1456.

30. Itoh N, Yonehara S, Ishii A, et al. The polypeptide encoded by the cDNA for human cell surface antigen Fas can mediate apoptosis. Cell 1991; 66:233–243.

31. Suda T, Takahashi T, Golstein P, et al. Molecular cloning and expression of the Fas ligand, a novel member of the tumor necrosis factor family. Cell 1993; 75:1169–1178.

32. Tanaka M, Suda T, Takahashi T, et al. Expression of the functional soluble form of human Fas ligand in activated lymphocytes. EMBO J 1995; 14:1129–1135.

33. Takahashi A, Hirata H, Yonehara S, et al. Affinity labeling displays the stepwise activation of ICE-related proteases by Fas, staurosporine, and CrmA-sensitive caspase-8. Oncogene 1997; 14:2741–2752.

34. Kagi D, Vignaux F, Ledermann B, et al. Fas and perforin pathways as major mechanisms of T-cell mediated cytotoxicity. Science 1994; 265: 528–530.

35. Dhein J, Walczak H, Baumler C, et al. Autocrine T-cell suicide mediated by APO-1/(Fas/CD95). Nature 1995; 373:438–441.

36. Matute-Bello G, Winn RK, Jonas M, et al. Fas (CD95) induces alveolar epithelial cell apoptosis in vivo: implications for acute pulmonary inflammation. Am J Pathol 2001; 158: 153–161.

37. Matute-Bello G, Liles WC, Frevert CW, et al. Recombinant human Fas-ligand induces alveolar epithelial cell apoptosis and lung injury in rabbits. Am J Physiol Lung Cell Mol Physiol 2001; 281:L328–L335.

38. Wen L, Madani K, Fahrni JA, et al. Dexamethasone inhibits lung epithelial cell apoptosis induced by IFN-γ and Fas. Am J Physiol Lung Cell Mol Physiol 1997; 273:L921–L929.

39. Fine A, Anderson NL, Rothstein TL, et al. Fas expression in pulmonary alveolar type II cells. Am J Physiol Lung Cell Mol Physiol 1997; 273:L64–L71.

40. Hamann KJ, Dorscheid DR, Ko FD, et al. Expression of Fas (CD95) and FasL (CD95L) in human airway epithelium. Am J Respir Cell Mol Biol 1998; 19:537–542.
41. Druilhe A, Wallaert B, Tsicopoulos A, et al. Apoptosis, proliferation, and expression of Bcl-2, Fas, and Fas ligand in bronchial biopsies from asthmatics. Am J Respir Cell Mol Biol 1998; 19:747–757.
42. Gochuico BR, Miranda KM, Hessel EM, et al. Airway epithelial Fas ligand expression: potential role in modulating bronchial inflammation. Am J Physiol Lung Cell Mol Physiol 1998; 274:L444–L449.
43. Kitamura Y, Hashimoto S, Mizuta N, et al. Fas/FasL-dependent apoptosis of alveolar cells after lipopolysaccharide-induced lung injury in mice. Am J Respir Crit Care Med 2001; 163:762–779.
44. Vazquez de Lara L, Becerril C, Montano M, et al. Surfactant components modulate fibroblast apoptosis and type I collagen and collagenase-1 expression. Am J Physiol Lung Cell Mol Physiol 2000; 279: L950–L957.
45. White MK, Baireddy V, Strayer DS. Natural protection from apoptosis by surfactant protein A in type II pneumocytes. Exp Cell Res 2001; 263:183–192.
46. Greene KE, Wright JR, Steinberg KP, et al. Serial changes in surfactant-associated proteins in lung and serum before and after the onset of ARDS. Am J Respir Crit Care Med 1999; 160:1843–1850.
47. Wang R, Zagariya A, Ang E, et al. Fas-induced apoptosis of alveolar epithelial cells requires ANG II generation and receptor interaction. Am J Physiol Lung Cell Mol Physiol 1999; 277:L1245–L1250.
48. Idell S, Kueppers F, Lippmann M, et al. Angiotensin converting enzyme in bronchoalveolar lavage in ARDS. Chest 1987; 91:52–56.
49. Hashimoto S, Kobayashi A, Kooguchi K, et al. Upregulation of two death pathways of perforin/granzyme and FasL/Fas in septic acute respiratory distress syndrome. Am J Respir Crit Care Med 2000; 161:237–243.
50. Kuwano K, Miyazaki H, Hagimoto N, et al. The involvement of Fas-Fas ligand pathway in fibrosing lung diseases. Am J Respir Cell Mol Biol 1999; 20:53–60.
51. Matute-Bello G, Lee JS, Liles WC, et al. Fas-mediated acute lung injury requires fas expression on nonmyeloid cells of the lung. J Immunol 2005; 175:4069–4075.
52. Bern RA, Farnand AW, Wong V, et al. Depletion of resident alveolar macrophages does not prevent Fas-mediated lung injury in mice. Am J Physiol Lung Cell Mol Physiol 2008; 295:L314–L325.
53. Nakamura M, Matute-Bello G, Liles WC, et al. Differential response of human lung epithelial cells to Fas-induced apoptosis. Am J Pathol 2004; 164:1949–1958.
54. Vernooy JHJ, Dentener MA, van Suylen RJ, et al. Intratracheal instillation of lipopolysaccharide in mice induces apoptosis in bronchial epithelial cells. No role for tumor necrosis factor-{alpha} and infiltrating neutrophils. Am J Respir Cell Mol Biol 2001; 24:569–576.
55. Kuwano K, Kunitake R, Maeyama T, et al. Attenuation of bleomycin-induced pneumopathy in mice by a caspase inhibitor. Am J Physiol Lung Cell Mol Physiol 2001; 280:L316–L325.
56. Janssen YM, Matalon S, Mossman BT. Differential induction of c-fos, c-jun, and apoptosis in lung epithelial cells exposed to ROS or RNS. Am J Physiol Lung Cell Mol Physiol 1997; 273:L789–L796.
57. Smith JD, McLean SD, Nakayama DK. Nitric oxide causes apoptosis in pulmonary vascular smooth muscle cells. J Surg Res 1998; 79:121–127.
58. Rensing-Ehl A, Hess S, Ziegler-Heitbrock HW, et al. Fas/Apo-1 activates nuclear factor kB and induces interleukin-6 production. J Inflamm 1995; 45:161–174.
59. Park DR, Thomsen AR, Frevert CW, et al. Fas (CD95) induces proinflammatory cytokine responses by human monocytes and monocyte-derived macrophages. J Immunol 2003; 12:6209–6216.

60. Altemeier WA, Zhu X, Berrington WR, et al. Fas (CD95) induces macrophage proinflammatory chemokine production via a MyD88-dependent, caspase-independent pathway. J Leukoc Biol 2007; 82:721–728.

61. Matute-Bello G, Frevert CW, Liles WC, et al. The Fas/FasL system mediates epithelial injury, but not pulmonary host defenses, in response to inhaled bacteria. Infect Immun 2001; 69:5768–5776.

62. Grassme H, Kirschnek S, Riethmueller J, et al. CD95/CD95 ligand interactions on epithelial cells in host defense to pseudomonas aeruginosa. Science 2000; 290:527–530.

63. Matute-Bello G, Wurfel MM, Lee JS, et al. Essential role of MMP-12 in Fas-induced fibrosisis. Am J Respir Cell Mol Biol 2007; 37:210–221.

64. Assaly R, Olson D, Hammersley J, et al. Initial evidence of endothelial cell apoptosis as a mechanism of systemic capillary leak syndrome. Chest 2001; 120:1301–1308.

65. Haimovitz-Friedman A, Cordon-Cardo C, Bayoumy S, et al. Lipopolysaccharide induces disseminated endothelial apoptosis requiring ceramide generation. J Exp Med 1997; 186:1831–1841.

66. Kawasaki M, Kuwano K, Hagimoto N, et al. Protection from lethal apoptosis in lipopolysaccharide-induced acute lung injury in mice by a caspase inhibitor. Am J Pathol 2000; 157:597–603.

67. Polunovsky VA, Wendt CH, Ingbar DH, et al. Induction of endothelial cell apoptosis by TNF alpha: modulation by inhibitors of protein synthesis. Exp Cell Res 1994; 214:584–594.

68. Wang HL, Akinci IO, Baker CM, et al. The intrinsic apoptotic pathway is required for lipopolysaccharide-induced lung endothelial cell death. J Immunol 2007; 179:1834–1841.

69. Petrache I, Natarajan V, Zhen L, et al. Ceramide upregulation causes pulmonary cell apoptosis and emphysema-like disease in mice. Nat Med 2005; 11:491–498.

70. Giordano RJ, Lahdenranta J, Zhen L, et al. Targeted induction of lung endothelial cell apoptosis causes emphysema-like changes in the mouse. J Biol Chem 2008; 283:29447–29460.

71. Polunovsky VA, Chen B, Henke C, et al. Role of mesenchymal cell death in lung remodeling after injury. J Clin Invest 1993; 92:388–397.

72. Madden HL, Henke CA. Induction of lung fibroblast apoptosis by soluble fibronectin peptides. Am J Respir Crit Care Med 2000; 162:1553–1560.

73. Uhal B, Joshi I, True A, et al. Fibroblasts isolated after fibrotic lung injury induce apoptosis of alveolar epithelial cells in vitro. Am J Physiol Lung Cell Mol Physiol 1995; 269:L819–L828.

74. Wang R, Zagariya A, Ibarra-Sunga O, et al. Angiotensin II induces apoptosis in human and rat alveolar epithelial cells. Am J Physiol Lung Cell Mol Physiol 1999; 276:L885–L889.

75. Wang R, Ramos C, Joshi I, et al. Human lung myofibroblast-derived inducers of alveolar epithelial apoptosis identified as angiotensin peptides. Am J Physiol Lung Cell Mol Physiol 1999; 277:L1158–L1164.

76. Teder P, Vandivier RW, Jiang D, et al. Resolution of lung inflammation by CD44. Science 2002; 296:155–158.

77. Fadok VA, Bratton DL, Konowal A, et al. Macrophages that have ingested apoptotic cells in vitro inhibit proinflammatory cytokine production through autocrine/paracrine mechanisms involving TGF-beta, PGE2, and PAF. J Clin Invest 1998; 101:890–898.

78. Haslinger B, Mandl-Weber S, Sellmayer A, et al. Hyaluronan fragments induce the synthesis of MCP-1 and IL-8 in cultured human peritoneal mesothelial cells. Cell Tissue Res 2001; 305:79–86.

79. Hussain N, Wu F, Zhu L, et al. Neutrophil apoptosis during the development and resolution of oleic acid-induced acute lung injury in the rat. Am J Respir Cell Mol Biol 1998; 19:867–874.

80. Matute-Bello G, Frevert CW, Martin TR. Animal models of acute lung injury. Am J Physiol Lung Cell Mol Physiol 2008; 295:L379–L399.

8
Pathogenesis of Ventilator-Induced Lung Injury

FRANCO VALENZA
Dipartimento di Anestesiologia, Rianimazione e Scienze Dermatologiche, Fondazione
Ospedale Maggiore Policlinico, Mangiagalli e Regina Elena – IRCSS, Università degli Studi di
Milano, Milan, Italy

JAMES A. FRANK
University of California, San Francisco VA Medical Center, San Francisco, California, U.S.A.

YUMIKO IMAI
Department of Physiology and Pharmacology, Akita University School of Medicine, Akita,
Japan

ARTHUR S. SLUTSKY
Keenan Research Center at the Li Ka Shing Knowledge Institute of St. Michael's Hospital and
the University of Toronto, Toronto, Ontario, Canada

I. Introduction

From the time of its inception, the role of mechanical ventilation in acute respiratory failure has been duplicitous—life saving on one hand, while injury promoting on the other. Before the use of positive pressure ventilation became widespread, mortality from acute hypoxemic respiratory failure was nearly 100%. In 1971, when Petty and Ashbaugh (1) first reported on the use of positive pressure ventilation for the treatment of ARDS mortality was still nearly 60%. At that time, clinicians had already raised concerns about the potential harmful effects of mechanical ventilation. For example, in 1968 Sladen and coworkers (2) reported that prolonged mechanical ventilation resulted in worsening oxygenation, increased lung water, and decreased compliance in patients with ventilatory failure. Similar findings had been reported in animal models as early as the 1940s (3–5).

The active role of mechanical ventilation in determining patient outcome was convincingly demonstrated by the National Institute of Health (NIH)-sponsored ARDS Network study of 861 patients, which compared low tidal volume ventilation to conventional ventilation. Tidal volume reduction to 6 mL/kg (predicted body weight) from the conventional 12 mL/kg at similar levels of positive end-expiratory pressure (PEEP) resulted in an absolute 9% reduction in mortality (6). This is the only intervention that in a large study has convincingly demonstrated a reduction in mortality from ARDS since the initial description of the syndrome; however, the mechanisms of this protective effect are largely unknown.

The spectrum of ventilator-induced lung injury extends from macroscopic air leaks to ultrastructural changes and molecular/cellular responses. In this chapter, we will review the proposed mechanisms for ventilator-induced lung injury, focusing primarily on pathophysiological and molecular/cellular principles.

II. Adverse Effects of Mechanical Ventilation

Two general terms are used to describe the injury that is thought to be caused by mechanical ventilation. Ventilator-induced lung injury (VILI) is usually used in the context of animal studies, where the direct effect of mechanical ventilation on lung injury can be definitively ascertained since it is possible to perform appropriate controls. In clinical studies, it is often difficult to determine whether the lung injury is due to de novo injury directly attributable to the ventilatory strategy or due to amplification of pre-existing injury or simply due to worsening of the underlying disease process that precipitated the acute respiratory failure. Thus, in the clinical context the term that is often used is ventilator-associated lung injury (VALI). For this chapter, we will use the term VILI in a general sense to refer to investigations in this area of research and also in the specific context of animal models of injurious ventilation in previously normal lungs. The term VALI will be used to refer to clinical studies and animal models where the direct role of mechanical ventilation on producing the injury is less clear, as is often the case when injurious ventilation is applied to previously injured lungs.

Although the focus of this chapter is the cellular and molecular basis of VILI, it is important to acknowledge the other unintended adverse events associated with mechanical ventilation (Table 1). These include large air leaks, which result in the extravasation of air into the pleural space, mediastinum, peritoneum, or subcutaneous tissue. Although such leaks occur in approximately 10% of patients with ARDS, the development of an air leak is not a major factor contributing to increased mortality in the vast majority of these

Table 1 Complications of Mechanical Ventilation

Complication	Clinical results
Air leaks	Pneumothorax
	Pneumomediastinum
	Pneumoperitoneum
	Subcutaneous emphysema
Ventilator-induced alveolar epithelial and endothelial injury	Increased permeability/pulmonary edema formation
	Increased plasma and edema fluid levels of inflammatory cytokines
	Impaired alveolar fluid transport
	Impaired gas exchange
	Loss of compartmentalization
	Multisystem organ failure
Infectious	Ventilator-associated pneumonia
	Sinusitis
Traumatic	Tracheal stenosis
	Unplanned extubation
	Dental
	Nasopharyngeal/oral trauma
Other	Hemodynamic compromise
	Aspiration
	Respiratory alkalosis/acidosis
	Oxygen toxicity

patients (7,8). Endotracheal intubation and mechanical ventilation also increase the risk of aspiration, nosocomial pneumonia, and sinusitis.

How does mechanical ventilation injure the lung? Clearly, mechanical stresses can lead to gross cell death by disruption of the cytoskeleton or plasma membrane. However, at the cellular level, mechanical stresses induce changes in intra- and intercellular signaling cascades. This conversion of a physical stimulus into chemical signals inside the cell is termed mechanotransduction. The extent to which these more subtle changes in cell function influence permeability, ion transport, structural and functional protein expression, inflammation, and cell death in VILI is the focus of ongoing research.

III. Mechanical Forces During Positive-Pressure Ventilation

During tidal breathing, the lung is exposed to a variety of mechanical forces. On the most basic level, these include tensile strain, stress, and shear stress (9–11). Strain, commonly referred to as stretch, is defined as a change in length relative to the original length. Stress is the force per unit area as in compression. Shear stress is the force per unit area in the direction of flow.

A. Nature of Mechanical Forces During Ventilation

Figure 1 schematically illustrates the forces that have been postulated to act on the pulmonary airways, alveoli, and capillaries. Alveolar inflation results from an increased pressure gradient across the alveolar wall. Alveolar wall tension increases according to Laplace's law: $T = P \times r/2$, where T is wall tension, P is the pressure gradient across the alveolar wall, and r is the radius of the alveolus. Intrinsic elasticity of the lung and surface tension at the air/liquid interface in the alveolus oppose expansion, whereas the forces due to adjacent expanded alveoli and elasticity of the chest wall oppose collapse. Surface tension also serves to support the capillary endothelium by opposing endothelial cell bowing into the alveolus induced by vascular hydrostatic pressure (10,12).

The blood vessels of the lung are exposed to additional forces. As lung volume increases, blood vessels are exposed to longitudinal tension. Extra-alveolar blood vessels are potentially exposed to greater wall tension as lung volume increases because perivascular pressure decreases with lung expansion resulting in increased transmural pressure. It is also important to note that gravitational forces affect distribution of blood flow and therefore may affect regional transmural vascular pressure.

In addition, shear forces due to blood, pulmonary edema fluid, and air flow affect the luminal cells of both the capillary and airspaces. Commonly, shear stress refers to the mechanical stress experienced by endothelial cells during blood flow, but in the injured lung, airway and alveolar epithelial cells may also experience shear stress as edema fluid moves through the airways and as collapsed lung units are reinflated (13).

Therefore, changes in lung inflation affect both the endothelium and epithelium. This conclusion is supported by the studies of Costello and coworkers (14) in which pulmonary capillary hypertension (33–39 cm H_2O) induced both endothelial and alveolar epithelial cell breaks, especially at high lung volumes. VILI is thus the result of a complex interplay among various mechanical forces acting on lung structures during mechanical ventilation. Because of the complexity of the lung, the variety of cell types,

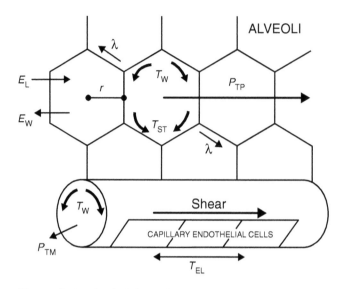

Figure 1 Mechanical forces in the lung during ventilation. Alveolar wall tension (T_w) increases with transpulmonary pressure (P_{TP}) and alveolar size (r = radius) according to the law of Laplace ($T_w = P_{TP} \times r/2$). Force from the inflation of adjacent alveoli (λ) also favors alveolar expansion (interdependence). Elastic recoil of the chest wall (E_w) also favors alveolar expansion when lung volume is low. Surface tension (T_{ST}) at the air/liquid interface in the alveolus favors alveolar collapse, as does the elastic recoil of the lung (E_L). Lung capillaries are also exposed to increasing wall tension as transmural vascular pressure (P_{TM}) increases with lung inflation. Vessels are also exposed to tensile elongation (T_{EL}) during lung inflation. Capillary endothelial cells are exposed to shear stress in the direction of blood flow. Airway and alveolar epithelial cells are also exposed to shear stress as air and edema fluid are displaced during reinflation of collapsed lung (not shown).

and the variety of mechanical forces to which cells are exposed, possible mechanisms of cellular/molecular responses caused by mechanical ventilation may vary widely.

B. Mechanical Forces and Injury

In experimental studies of positive-pressure ventilation, lung injury primarily results from excessive lung volume, particularly at end inspiration, and from insufficient functional residual capacity (FRC) where repetitive opening and collapse of atelectatic lung regions could generate strain and shear forces. Under this paradigm, the mechanical forces that precipitate VILI are amplified in the heterogeneously injured lung (Fig. 2). This results in large part from airspace edema formation as edema fills airspaces and inactivates surfactant, resulting in increased surface tension and alveolar and small airway collapse (15,16). Accordingly, heterogeneous lung injury can be modeled as having three different compartments: (1) regions of airway and alveolar flooding, in which minimal lung volume can be recruited during tidal breathing; (2) regions with normal compliance and aeration, appearing to be uninvolved with disease; (3) intermediate regions in which alveolar

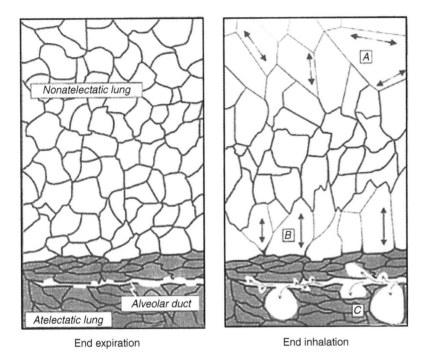

Nonatelectatic lung

Alveolar duct

Atelectatic lung

End expiration   End inhalation

Figure 2 Mechanisms of ventilator-associated lung injury. Left panel shows lung regions at end expiration. Right panel shows the same lung regions at end inspiration. (A) Patent alveoli are exposed to increased strain during tidal ventilation due to the uneven distribution of the inflated volume. (B) Some alveoli are damaged by excessive stress caused by the uneven expansion of surrounding lung regions at the margins between atelectatic and aerated alveoli. (C) Small bronchioles and alveoli may be injured by mechanical forces resulting from repeated opening and closing. *Source*: From Ref. 213.

collapse and flooding are apparent but where aeration can be restored. At the frequencies associated with conventional ventilation, a positive pressure tidal breath will distribute preferentially to the normally aerated areas (17). As a result, these regions are vulnerable to alveolar overdistension.

ARDS is characterized by the formation of protein-rich pulmonary edema, diffuse alveolar damage, and impaired airspace edema clearance in most patients (18). The result is a heterogeneous distribution of injury and edema in the lung. Interdependence refers to the regional traction forces exerted by adjacent lung segments that favor uniform expansion of the lung. These forces arise within the lung because the wall of each alveolar space is also the wall of the neighboring alveolus. In fully recruited normal lung, the alveolar-distending force can be thought of as the transpulmonary pressure (alveolar pressure–pleural pressure). However, once heterogeneity is introduced, the local distending forces will differ in a manner so as to oppose the heterogeneity and restore lung expansion. As a result, these regions are vulnerable to alveolar overdistension.

Mead and coworkers (5) postulated that at a transpulmonary pressure of 30 cm H_2O, "the pressure tending to expand an atelectatic region surrounded by a fully expanded lung would be approximately 140 cm H_2O." Therefore, in the heterogeneously injured lung, strain may be greater at areas where inflated lung is adjacent to atelectatic or fluid-filled lung due to interdependence. This may also explain in part why traditional tidal volumes (10–15 mL/kg) can result in alveolar overdistension and subsequent VILI in patients with ARDS and, in part, why ventilatory strategies aimed at maintaining uniform lung recruitment are less injurious than those strategies that permit development of marked regional disparities in lung volumes (11).

At the cellular and molecular levels, the distribution of forces across the fused cytoskeleton-extracellular matrix scaffold of the alveolar-capillary barrier is complex; however, it is reasonable to assume that some of the force applied to one side of the barrier is transmitted to neighboring cells, the extracellular matrix (ECM), and the cytoskeletal structure of the cells on the opposite side of the barrier. As proposed by Ingber and coworkers (19,20), the cytoskeleton behaves as a tensegrity structure referring to the architectural principle whereby continuous tension is coupled with compression-resistant supports yielding an efficient structure that yields without breaking. External force applied to this type of structure disrupts the tensional equilibrium and is distributed throughout the entire structure regardless of where the force is applied. In this way, mechanical strain may be focused to specific regions of the cytoskeleton—for example, at focal adhesion complexes (FACs). FACs are formed by integrin clusters bound to the ECM and the cytoskeleton that create a physical link between the ECM and the cytoskeleton. Multiple other intracellular signaling proteins are associated with the FAC, including focal adhesion kinases (FAKs), p60src, actin filament-associated proteins, among other proteins (see sec. VI). Alternatively, mechanical force may act on cells in a more local fashion. For example, plasma membrane disruption resulting from strain or shear stress and independent of changes in the cytoskeleton may predominate.

IV. Lung Injury from Overdistension

Although all of the forces listed above occur in the lung during the respiratory cycle, it stands to reason that alveolar epithelial cell tensile strain is greatest at end inspiration. Therefore, the larger the lung volume/transpulmonary pressure at end inspiration, the greater the strain; however, in normal rat lungs, alveolar strain as estimated by the change in basement membrane surface area is not linearly related to lung volume (21). Tschumperlin and Margulies (21) and Bachofen and coworkers (22) found that, following volume history standardization, epithelial basement membrane surface area increased only 12% as lung volume increased from 24% to 82% of total lung capacity (TLC). When lung volume was increased from 82% to 100% of TLC, the epithelial basement membrane surface area sharply increased an additional 20% (for a total increase of 40% from surface area at 24% TLC). This finding is best explained by an initial unfolding of the alveolar epithelial basement membrane during lung inflation at low lung volumes, followed by stretching at higher lung volumes. The simplified model of lung fiber system based on elastin/collagen unit proposed by Gattinoni and coworkers support this view: since collagen is inelastic, it works as a stop-length fiber, preventing further strain of the elastin/collagen unit. However, this leads to abrupt increases of stress for small volume (hence strain) changes (11).

A. Excessive Lung Volume in Clinical Studies

The most convincing evidence that excessive end-inspiratory lung volume is injurious to patients came from the ARDS Network study, which compared low tidal volume ventilation (6 mL/kg ideal body weight) and an inspiratory plateau pressure limit of 30 cm H_2O to conventional mechanical ventilation with a tidal volume of 12 mL/kg and a similar level of PEEP (6). In this study of 861 patients with ARDS or ALI, low tidal volume ventilation reduced mortality from 40% to 31% compared with conventional tidal volume ventilation. The protective effect persisted regardless of the underlying etiology of ARDS or the respiratory system compliance (23). As with other studies of ARDS, the most common causes of death were withdrawal of care, sepsis, and multiple organ dysfunction syndrome (MODS), not hypoxemia. In fact, oxygenation was not different between the groups (6). Other studies of protective ventilation incorporating low tidal volumes have yielded conflicting results (24–28). Part of the discrepancies may be due to the fact that plateau pressure and tidal volumes, used to titrate ventilator settings, are inadequate surrogates of stress and strain (29). Transpulmonary pressure is a potential candidate: in fact, it is more reliable as an indicator of lung stress than airway pressure alone since it takes into account chest wall elastance that is often affected during the course of ARDS (30,31). Talmor and coworkers clearly showed the discrepancy between airway pressure and transpulmonary pressure as assessed by means of esophageal pressure (32). A potential rational guide for setting PEEP and tidal volume in mechanically ventilated patients may also be the direct measurement of lung volumes to assess lung strain (tidal volume/end-expiratory lung volume). Unfortunately, these measurements are difficult to obtain clinically.

B. Experimental Models of Lung Overdistension

In the years following the first clinical reports of the adverse effects of positive-pressure ventilation, researchers investigated the effects of high-volume ventilation strategies on normal animal lungs. The lung injury induced by mechanical ventilation in these experimental models is characterized by high-protein pulmonary edema, diffuse alveolar damage, and infiltration by inflammatory cells. These findings were also reported in ex vivo and in vivo animal models of ARDS (injured animal lungs). The pathological lesion of VILI in these studies is not specific and closely resembles lung injury resulting from clinical ARDS (33–35). These experimental studies serve as the foundation of our understanding of the potential mechanisms of VILI in ARDS patients who have underlying lung disease.

Pulmonary Edema and High Tidal Volume Ventilation

The first comprehensive report of the harmful effects of high-pressure/high-volume ventilation in normal lungs was that of Webb and Tierney (35). In this classic study, the investigators ventilated rats for up to one hour with one of three tidal volumes (12.5 ± 0.1, 30 ± 0.2, or 43 ± 0.7 mL/kg) without PEEP, or with 10 cm H_2O of PEEP and a tidal volume of either 11.6 ± 0.4 or 15.6 ± 0.48 mL/kg (Fig. 3). These volumes were the result of matching peak inspiratory pressures in the two highest tidal volume groups. High tidal volume, zero PEEP ventilation resulted in the development of severe, protein-rich interstitial and airspace edema. Ventilation with a tidal volume of 30 mL/kg compared to 43 mL/kg resulted in a significant reduction in the severity of edema as measured by wet lung weight and a histological edema score. Further reducing tidal volume to 12.5 mL/kg

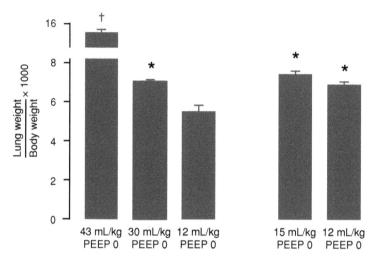

Figure 3   Ventilator-induced pulmonary edema in a rat model. Pulmonary edema, measured as lung weight/body weight, increased within one hour of high tidal volume ventilation without positive end-expiratory pressure (PEEP). A tidal volume of 43 mL/kg [peak inspiratory pressure (PIP) 40 cm H_2O] induced alveolar flooding, resulting in mortality in less than one hour. A tidal volume of 30 mL/kg and no PEEP (PIP 30 cm H_2O) induced significantly less edema. Ventilation with 12 mL/kg did not increase lung weight compared with unventilated controls. When a PEEP of 10 cm H_2O was applied and tidal volume was reduced such that peak inspiratory pressure was matched to 40 cm H_2O (tidal volume 15 mL/kg), lung water was significantly lower than with zero PEEP ventilation. When PIP was matched to 30 cm H_2O with a PEEP of 10 cm H_2O (tidal volume 12 mL/kg), lung water was not significantly different compared with a tidal volume of 30 mL/kg and no PEEP, but was significantly higher compared with the same tidal volume without PEEP. *Source*: From Ref. 35.

prevented the development of edema in their model. Combining PEEP with reduced tidal volume ventilation also reduced the severity of pulmonary edema. The rats ventilated with a tidal volume of 11.6 or 15.6 mL/kg and a PEEP level of 10 cm H_2O developed significantly less pulmonary edema compared with the rats ventilated with similar peak inspiratory pressures but with large tidal volumes (43 or 30 mL/ kg) and no PEEP. An additional important finding was that ventilation with a tidal volume of approximately 12 mL/kg without PEEP did not induce edema, but the same tidal volume with a PEEP of 10 cm H_2O induced mild edema (Fig. 3). These data demonstrate that ventilator-induced pulmonary edema develops when end-inspiratory lung volume is excessive whether the increase in lung volume results from a change in tidal volume alone or from a combination of PEEP and tidal volume (note that end-inspiratory lung volumes were not measured per se in this study). However, the combination of high tidal volume and no PEEP resulted in more severe edema (35).

Subsequent studies by others (36–38) have confirmed the findings of Webb and Tierney (35) and have found that the change in lung volume rather than airway pressure may be the critical factor in lung edema formation. In one such study, rats were ventilated with a similar high tidal volume (40 mL/kg), but with either positive-pressure or negative-pressure ventilation. A comparison group was ventilated with the same peak inspiratory pressure as the group ventilated with the positive pressure, but with approximately half the tidal volume. This was achieved by applying rubber bands to the abdomen and chest. High tidal volumes resulting from either positive or negative pressure ventilation induced severe edema and similar changes in endothelial permeability to albumin. High-pressure, low-volume ventilation did not induce edema or any change in albumin permeability (38). The role of tidal volume and hyperventilation on VILI was also confirmed in a long-term experiment conducted on sheep by Mascheroni and coworkers (39).

In another study, isolated perfused dog lungs injured by acid instillation were ventilated with a constant tidal volume of 15 mL/kg and increasing levels of PEEP. Although oxygenation initially increased with higher PEEP, the severity of lung edema increased with lung volume. This effect on edema formation was modest when PEEP was raised from 0 to 10 cm H_2O, but when PEEP was increased to 15 cm H_2O, lung water increased over 400% (40). Others have found that ventilation with increasing PEEP, but a constant end-inspiratory volume, reduces the rate of edema formation but affects endothelial protein permeability to a smaller degree (38). Therefore, increasing end-inspiratory lung volume increases edema formation and endothelial permeability. Adding PEEP attenuates edema formation. Similarly, PEEP may delay the progression of lung injury during ventilator strategies involving high airway pressure and lung overdistension (41).

However, part of this effect is explained by the changes in hemodynamics. When tidal volume, inspiratory time, and especially PEEP are increased in vivo, intrathoracic and mean alveolar pressures increase. In general, this has negative consequences on cardiac output and pulmonary blood flow in healthy animals. This partly explains the protective effect of PEEP on edema formation in in vivo models (37,38). For example, Dreyfuss and Saumon (37) have shown that rats submitted to high peak airway pressure ventilation with 10 cm H_2O PEEP had more severe edema when the hemodynamic alterations produced by PEEP were corrected with dopamine. Taken together with other studies, the reason why PEEP reduces the amount of edema may be a combination of such hemodynamic alterations, preservation of lung volume, and preservation of surfactant properties (see sec. V). In contrast, excessive lung volume, even when the result of high PEEP, can promote edema formation by increasing transmural vascular pressures for extra-alveolar vessels (42,43) and alveolar vessels (44,45). This partly explains the lack of a protective effect of PEEP on edema formation when the levels of PEEP are above a threshold point.

In previously injured lungs, the effects of high tidal volume ventilation on edema formation are more pronounced. Ventilation with high tidal volumes that do not induce injury in normal lungs can result in more severe edema formation during acute lung injury compared with lower tidal volumes (38,46–49). The increase in edema is largely due to differences in endothelial permeability and injury as assessed by histological and ultrastructural analysis (38,49).

Airspace Edema Clearance in VILI

The presence of edema fluid in the airspaces is both an effect of lung injury and a potential mechanism by which VILI is amplified. Edema fluid fills alveoli and promotes airspace collapse by inactivating surfactant and filling airways. This loss of lung volume leads to heterogeneity of the lung, resulting in even greater overdistension of the remaining lung units (21). Therefore, if the active sodium transport-dependent clearance of edema fluid from the distal airspaces is reduced, a vicious cycle of airspace edema leading to greater lung overdistension and shear stress will ensue. For example, flooding distal lung units of rats with saline was found to act synergistically with high tidal volume ventilation to increase endothelial permeability to albumin (50). In this study, the authors also found that as respiratory system compliance decreased, permeability to albumin increased, suggesting that as edema worsened, a smaller lung volume was ventilated and greater injury resulted (50).

The mechanical strain-induced reduction in energy-dependent sodium transport described by Lecuona and coworkers (51) may further impair airspace edema clearance promoting VILI. Using alveolar type II cells isolated from rats ventilated with a tidal volume of either 30 or 40 mL/kg, these authors reported that sodium–potassium ATPase activity was reduced, but mRNA for the α-1 subunit of this transporter was not reduced compared with rats ventilated with lower tidal volume (10 mL/kg). In another study, airspace edema clearance in lungs isolated from rats ventilated for 40 minutes with a tidal volume of 40 mL/kg was reduced by approximately 50%. Instilling the airspaces of the isolated lungs with the β-adrenergic agonists restored the rate of airspace edema clearance by increasing the activity and quantity of sodium–potassium ATPase in the basolateral membrane. This effect was blocked by disrupting microtubule assembly with colchicine, suggesting that it is the translocation of sodium–potassium ATPase from intracellular pools to the plasma membrane that accounts for much of the effect (52). In a rat model of acute lung injury, tidal volume reduction from 12 to 3 mL/kg resulted in greater preservation of airspace fluid transport. This effect persisted when either end-inspiratory lung volume or end-expiratory lung volume was constant (49).

Increased Endothelial Permeability with High Tidal Volume Ventilation

Ventilator-induced pulmonary edema is characterized by a high protein concentration indicating increased microvascular permeability. Dreyfuss and coworkers (36) demonstrated this increase in microvascular permeability using a rat model. They found that endothelial permeability to radiolabeled albumin increased as soon as five minutes after initiating ventilation with a peak airway pressure of 45 cm H_2O (tidal volume 40 mL/kg). This has also been demonstrated in larger animals, including lambs and dogs; however, a longer duration of ventilation was required (34,53,54). Although filtration pressure, or the transmural vascular pressure, also increases with high-volume ventilation, it is the increase in permeability resulting in part from increased wall tension that is the most important determinant of edema formation in intact animals (34,55,56). As discussed above, changes in cardiac output and blood flow will also influence the rate of edema formation.

There are at least two potential mechanisms for the rapid increase in capillary endothelial permeability that occurs during high-volume mechanical ventilation. First, high lung volume increases capillary wall strain (Fig. 2). This potentially results in the opening of stretch pores in the endothelium and eventually breaks in endothelial cells and the basement membrane, termed capillary stress failure (44,54,57). This mechanism is consistent with experimental studies demonstrating edema formation resulting from lung overinflation achieved by either high tidal volume or by the combination of tidal volume and PEEP (37,40). Recent in vitro data provide evidence that excessive cell stretch increases paracellular transport of micromolecules across the alveolar epithelium in association with increases of pore radii (58,59), even if the extent to which stretch pore formation contributes to edema formation has been questioned (60).

A second potential mechanism is strain-induced changes in the cytoskeleton and adhesion junctions of endothelial cells that result in a more permeable endothelial barrier. Such changes in endothelial barrier integrity have been well described in vascular endothelial cells in response to shear stress (44). This same process may occur in response to the mechanical forces associated with positive-pressure ventilation. Evidence supporting this hypothesis has been reported by Parker and coworkers. These investigators found that the increase in endothelial permeability associated with high-volume ventilation could be prevented by increasing intracellular cAMP or by inhibiting calcium/calmodulin-dependent myosin light chain kinase. Administration of β-adrenergic agonists (61), or inhibitors of phosphodiesterase (62), which increase intracellular cAMP, was found to prevent edema formation in isolated lungs exposed to high-volume ventilation. Gadolinium (an inhibitor of strain-gated calcium channels) also prevented edema formation in this model (63). In addition, the inhibition of tyrosine kinase with either genistein or phenylarsine oxide or the inhibition of myosin light chain kinase (MLCK) and protein kinase C (PKC) activity also attenuated the increase in endothelial permeability in rat lungs (62,64). Taken together, these data indicate that the calcium/calmodulin-MLCK pathway augments edema formation during high tidal volume ventilation (Fig. 4). This effect is attenuated by increasing intracellular cAMP, inhibiting MLCK and PKC, or the nonspecific inhibition of tyrosine kinases. Accordingly, the increased endothelial permeability in VILI may be regulated by a variety of signaling pathways and not only the result of breaks in endothelial cells and basement membrane. Czarny and Schnitzer have shown that after the distention of endothelium there is activation of caveolar neutral sphingomyelinase as well as downstream tyrosine and mitogen-activated protein kinases by generation of the lipid second messenger ceramide which is able to activate the Akt/endothelial nitric oxide synthase pathway (65).

Increased Epithelial Permeability with High Tidal Volume Ventilation

As with endothelial permeability, alveolar epithelial permeability increases with increasing lung volume. For example, increasing FRC by the application of PEEP during mechanical ventilation results in increased clearance of inhaled ^{99m}Tc-DPTA (MW 393 daltons) in excess of what would be predicted from a change in surface area alone (66,67). Alveolar epithelial permeability to albumin also increases with increasing lung volume (57,68). Egan (68) distended isolated rabbit and sheep lung lobes with fluid to a pressure of 40 cm H_2O and found that the equivalent pore radius increased from approximately 1 to 5 nm. This translated into mildly increased epithelial permeability; however, large irreversible leaks developed in some lobes. It is important to note that the distending pressure used in these studies resulted in a lung volume in excess of TLC. When entire lungs rather than isolated lobes were tested, the effect was less pronounced in that permeability to small molecules increased, but permeability to albumin was not altered (57). Similar findings were described in a report by Kim and Crandall (69) in which alveolar epithelial permeability in bullfrog lungs was not altered by ventilation within a physiological range. Therefore, lung distention near or exceeding the limits of normal physiology results in increased epithelial permeability in uninjured lungs.

Ventilation of injured lungs with tidal volumes within a physiological range can also exacerbate epithelial permeability changes. In a rat model of acid-induced acute lung injury, ventilation with 6 mL/kg resulted in less alveolar flooding and less alveolar epithelial injury as measured by plasma levels of a type I cell-specific marker of injury (RTI40)

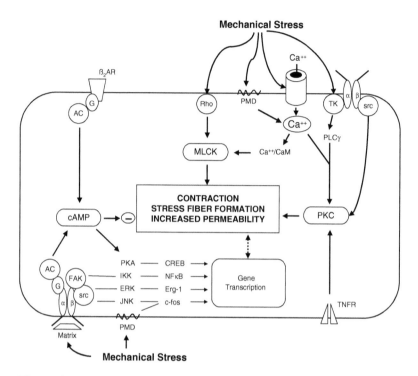

Figure 4 Effect of mechanical stresses on endothelial permeability in VILI. Mechanical forces associated with high tidal volume ventilation and shear stress activate strain-gated cation channels, resulting in increased intracellular calcium concentration. This activates calcium/calmodulin (Ca/CaM), which phosphorylates myosin light chain kinase (MLCK), resulting in stress fiber formation, cell contraction, and increased paracellular permeability to fluid and leukocytes. Stress-induced plasma membrane disruption (PMD) also increases intracellular calcium and increases expression of the transcription factor c-fos. Shear stress also induces phosphorylation and activation of focal adhesion complex tyrosine kinases (TK), including src, and the small GTPase Rho. Rho acts indirectly to inhibit myosin light chain phosphatase, thereby increasing MLCK activity. TK and src activate protein kinase C (PKC) directly and through phospholipase C-γ (PLCγ). PKC induces stress fiber formation and increased permeability by an MLCK-independent mechanism. Tumor necrosis factor receptor (TNFR) also activates PKC, in response to ligand binding, via phosphorylation of the 27 kDa heat shock protein (HSP-27). Increased endothelial permeability is inhibited by cAMP. Intracellular cAMP increases in response to ligand binding to the β_2-adrenergic receptor (β_2-AR) via G-protein-mediated activation of adenylate cyclase (AC). Mechanical stress is also transduced into chemical signals in the cell by extracellular matrix-bound integrins. Integrins bind the extracellular matrix. Bound integrins exposed to mechanical stress initiate a variety of signals from the focal adhesion complex. These signals include activation of AC, which increases cAMP, thereby activating protein kinase A (PKA). PKA affects gene transcription through CREB in the nucleus. Focal adhesion kinase (FAK) phosphorylates IKK, which in turn phosphorylates IκB to activate NFκB. Activation of src at the focal adhesion complex also results in the phosphorylation and activation of the mitogen-activated protein kinases (MAPK) ERK and JNK. These act in part to increase expression of the transcription factors Erg-1 and c-fos to modulate gene transcription.

compared with 12 mL/kg and a similar level of PEEP. This finding correlated with histological and ultrastructural differences in airspace edema and epithelial cell injury. When tidal volume was further reduced to 3 mL/kg, epithelial injury and airspace edema improved even more. Reducing PEEP during ventilation with a tidal volume of 12 mL/kg such that end-inspiratory lung volume and mean airway pressures were similar to the 6 mL/kg group did not prevent epithelial injury or edema (49). Similar findings have also been reported following surfactant depletion. In this model, tidal volume reduction prevented airspace edema formation and preserved oxygenation, suggesting preserved epithelial barrier function. Interestingly, when animals were ventilated with high-frequency oscillatory ventilation, edema and histological injury were further reduced (70,71).

ECM Constituents and High Tidal Volume Ventilation
In a study by Berg and coworkers, open-chested rabbits were ventilated for four hours with one lung at a PEEP of 9 cm H_2O and the other at a PEEP of 2 cm H_2O. Compared with rabbits ventilated with a PEEP of 2 cm H_2O on both lungs, the higher lung volume ventilation resulted in increased expression of mRNA for type III and type IV procollagen, fibronectin, basic fibroblast growth factor, and transforming growth factor-β1. Expression of mRNA for type I procollagen and vascular endothelial growth factor was not different between the groups (72). Interestingly, elevated edema fluid levels of procollagen III predict poor outcome in patients with ARDS (73).

Other investigators have found that high airway pressure ventilation increases expression of type IV and type I procollagen in isolated rat lungs (74) and in vitro (75). ECM proteoglycans and expression of enzymes active in matrix remodeling, including matrix metalloproteinases (MMPs) and the extracellular matrix metalloproteinase inducer (EMMPRIN), are also increased following high tidal volume ventilation in rats (76,77). Pretreatment with a nonspecific inhibitor of MMPs reduced the severity of lung injury following high-volume ventilation (77). The role of EMMPRIN and MMPs and of cyclic mechanical strain-induced proliferation and migration of human airway smooth muscle cells has also been recently shown. (78). These data suggest that alveolar overdistension may initiate an ECM remodeling process that potentially exacerbates lung injury or impairs healing.

C. Effects of Mechanical Strain In Vitro
An improved understanding of the effects of mechanical ventilation at the cellular level has come from in vitro studies using cell stretch devices, applied to a variety of cells including alveolar epithelial cells, fibroblasts, airway epithelial and smooth muscle cells, pulmonary vascular endothelial and smooth muscle cells. This section will review the effects of stretch on the cytoskeleton, plasma membrane, and ECM constituent expression.

Disruption of the Cytoskeleton and Plasma Membrane In Vitro
Studies of alveolar epithelial type II cells grown on flexible membranes have provided insight into the mechanical properties of these cells. In one study, increasing the duration, amplitude, or frequency of cyclic strain increased cellular uptake of ethidium homodimer-1 (ED-1), a marker of plasma membrane injury and cell death. Most cell injury occurred within five minutes of initiating the cyclic strain. If small amplitude deformation was superimposed on basal tonic strain, there was less membrane disruption and cell death compared with large amplitude stain to same peak level. The rate of

cellular deformation during a single strain did not affect ED-1 uptake (79). These finding are not surprising if one assumes that mechanical disruption of the cytoskeleton and plasma membrane is the etiology of the injury in this model and that the cytoskeletal structure of cultured cells behaves as most other solids. In a more recent study, plasma membrane disruption (PMD) induced by mechanical strain in vitro was primarily dependent on the rate of plasma membrane trafficking to the cell surface. Inhibition of cytoskeletal remodeling had little impact on the cell injury as measured by propidium iodide (PI) uptake. Although these data do not exclude strain-induced signaling through the cytoskeleton as an important mechanism of VILI, they support the hypothesis that PMD and lipid trafficking may be a major mechanism (80,81).

Effect of Mechanical Strain on Cell Adhesion In Vitro

Cyclic strain also affects cell–cell and cell–ECM attachment. Cavanaugh and coworkers (82) showed that cyclic stretch of alveolar epithelial cells corresponding to lung inflation to TLC (37% increase in surface area) resulted in decreased intercellular attachment and decreased expression of occludin, a major constituent of tight junctions. Lesser degrees of cyclic stretch did not have these effects. Interestingly, cyclic stretch to near-total lung capacity also resulted in a decrease in intracellular adenosine triphosphate (ATP); pharmacological inhibition of glycolytic metabolism also reduced cell–cell attachment and resulted in an abnormal cytoplasmic accumulation of occludin. Although these investigators did not measure permeability, the loss of cell–cell adhesion and disruption of tight junctions potentially contribute to increased alveolar epithelial permeability, as has been shown in endothelial cells (83).

V.   Injury from Low Lung Volume Ventilation

Although the forces described above occur to some extent at all volumes, additional sources of mechanical force at low lung volume may be important in VILI. The main additional force is that which resulted from the repeated opening and closing of small airways, alveolar ducts, and possibly individual alveoli during tidal ventilation. This cyclic recruitment of lung units may be partially or completely prevented by the application of PEEP, which likely accounts for some of the protective effect of PEEP in experimental models.

Airway closure has been observed to occur by one of the two mechanisms: development of a fluid meniscus, which occludes a patent bronchiole, or "compliant collapse" of small airways in which opposing walls buckle and become apposed owing to the "adhesive" forces of the airway lining fluid and peribronchiolar pressure. Reopening of the airways requires sufficient force either to rupture the meniscus or to peel the opposing wall and push the fluid interface toward the alveolus. During this process, shear stress sufficient to cause epithelial disruption may be generated. Surface tension forces of airway lining fluid in collapsed or occluded airway create a capillary pressure that must be exceeded for airway opening to occur. In conditions of increased surface tension, the tendency for airways to collapse significantly increases, as do the pressures required to reopen and keep open the airways.

Using surfactant-depleted isolated rat lungs, Muscedere and coworkers (84) reported that ventilation with low tidal volume of 7 mL/kg and low or no PEEP resulted in poorer lung compliance and more severe lung injury versus ventilation with the same tidal volume and a PEEP level higher than the lower inflection point on the respiratory system pressure volume curve. Histological injury such as epithelial necrosis, sloughing, and development of hyaline membranes was observed in alveolar ducts as well as respiratory and membranous bronchioles. This may explain, in part, the protective effects of ventilatory strategies that maintain lung volume with PEEP.

Repetitive airway opening and collapse may also explain the distribution of dependent lesions, especially in larger species. As pleural pressure is higher in the dependent than in the nondependent lung zones, the airspaces in the dependent zone would be more likely to collapse. In patients with ARDS, the regional cyclic recruitment of lung units can be demonstrated with computed tomographic imaging. When PEEP is applied at increasing levels, the proportion of lung undergoing cyclic recruitment decreases. This is associated with improved oxygenation and improved quasi-static lung compliance (17). Gattinoni and coworkers (17,85,86) demonstrated that the volume of the injured lung exposed to a tidal breath was markedly reduced when low levels of PEEP were used. When PEEP was increased, the proportion of the tidal volume delivered to the nonaerated lung regions gradually increased, becoming more evenly distributed (17). Similar results may be obtained by using the prone position with a benefit on ventilator-induced injury progression (87). In contrast, Martynowicz and coworkers (15) documented that regional tidal expansion of dependent regions was significantly reduced after oleic acid injury and was restored by application of PEEP. However, oleic acid injury did not lead to the collapse of dependent lung units at FRC, suggesting an alternative mechanism for topographic variability in regional impedance and lung expansion after injury in a model characterized by marked alveolar flooding (15).

A.   Clinical Studies of Protective Ventilation

In prospective studies, ventilation strategies that incorporate relatively high levels of PEEP and low tidal volumes reduce mortality from ARDS and acute lung injury (6,24,88).

As described above, PEEP could be responsible for minimizing VILI by reducing shear forces created by opening and collapse of alveoli.

The best method to select the ideal level of PEEP for a given patient with ARDS is yet to be determined. Although some studies have used the pressure volume curve of the respiratory system to set PEEP above the lower inflection point (P_{inf}), others have used arbitrary scales of PEEP. Both strategies, when combined with low tidal volume ventilation, reduce mortality from ARDS. Amato and coworkers (24) used a lung protective strategy based on (1) a PEEP level greater than the inflection point (14.7 ± 3.9 cm H_2O at baseline), (2) recruitment maneuver at start of study, and (3) peak airway pressure <40 cm H_2. In this study of 53 patients, there was a reduction in mortality from 71% to 38% using this strategy. Whether the marked decrease in mortality in this study was due to the lung protection due to an excessive mortality in the control group is uncertain. In the ARDS Network study, PEEP was set according to a predetermined scale and not the P_{inf}. A predetermined PEEP/F_{IO_2} table was used because the relationship between the shape of the pressure–volume curve and events at the alveolar level is affected by numerous factors and is the subject of ongoing research and debate (89–92). Interestingly, in a subsequent study by the ARDS Network combining low tidal volume with a scale incorporating high PEEP levels, no additional mortality benefit was observed (93). Similar results were found in the two recent large-scale trials on the use of PEEP in ARDS patients: the Lung Open Ventilation (LOV) (94) and the Expiratory pressure (Express) (95) trials. The level of PEEP in the LOV study was selected according to an oxygenation scale conceptually similar to that of the ALVEOLI study, while the Express study used a more physiological approach. Despite the differences, the PEEP levels were similar in the two studies (15.8 cm H_2O and 15.6 in the LOV and Express trials, respectively). However, in both trials mortality was not significantly different from the control groups. There is still debate on the use of PEEP in ARDS. It is possible that high PEEP levels may be beneficial in patients who have "recruitable" lungs, and may be detrimental in patients whose lungs are not recruitable, since in the latter group increases in PEEP may simply result in greater overdistension at end inspiration with no beneficial effect at low lung volumes (96). The approach seems rationale and in line with most of the knowledge derived from experimental data; however, no clinical outcome data, at the present, support the view.

Currently, there is renewed interest in high-frequency oscillatory ventilation (HFOV) combined with strategies of lung volume maintenance for adults with ARDS. This strategy would potentially prevent excessive end-inspiratory lung volume and maintain sufficient end-expiratory lung volume to a greater degree than conventional ventilation. Two randomized trials have shown HFO to be effective and safe in ARDS patients (97,98). HFO also may be useful when combined with other interventions such as recruitment maneuvers, prone positioning, or nitric oxide (99).

B. Experimental Studies of Low Lung Volume Ventilation

The strongest evidence that low end-expiratory lung volume ventilation promotes VALI comes from experimental studies. Following lung injury, low-volume ventilation inactivates surfactant and promotes edema formation in vivo and in isolated lungs (92,100,101). In surfactant-depleted isolated rat lungs, ventilation with low tidal volume of 7 mL/kg and a PEEP level below the lower inflection point of the lung pressure volume curve resulted in poorer lung compliance and more severe lung injury. The greatest increase in injury was found to be to the epithelium of membranous bronchioles (84). Although the injured lung is predisposed to cyclic recruitment of lung units with tidal ventilation due to the inactivation of surfactant and the resultant increase in surface tension, D'Angelo and coworkers (102) found that zero PEEP ventilation can induce small airway injury in normal rabbit lungs. Rabbits were ventilated open-chested for four hours with a tidal volume of approximately 10 mL/kg, with or without a PEEP level of 2 cm H_2O. Ventilation without PEEP resulted in injury to small (<1 mm diameter) airways as assessed by histological analysis. Airway resistance and elastance increased during zero PEEP ventilation. When PEEP was restored, elastance but not airway resistance returned to normal values. These data indicate that ventilation of normal lungs with an end-expiratory lung volume less than FRC induces small airway injury presumably due to the repetitive opening and closing of these airways.

In animal models of surfactant-deficient lungs, the preservation of lung volume with PEEP and periodic recruitment maneuvers improves oxygenation, compliance, and reduces histological lung injury (103). Combining HFOV with a strategy to recruit and maintain lung volume has also been found to prevent lung injury in premature baboons and in surfactant-depleted rabbits (104–106). In acid-injured rats, ventilation with low tidal volume and no PEEP resulted in 100% mortality by two hours, while rats ventilated with a higher tidal volume or with PEEP survived beyond four hours (46,38).

VI. Mechanotransduction in VILI

In the context of VILI, mechanotransduction refers to the mechanism(s) by which mechanical stimuli are converted into chemical signals within the cell. Although our understanding of the precise mechanisms and importance of mechanotransduction in VILI is far from complete, there is increasing evidence that these signaling mechanisms play an important role. Examples of mechanotransduction potentially important in VILI include impaired endothelial barrier function in response to shear stress, integrin-mediated signal transduction, mechanosensitive ion channels, and PMD-mediated signaling.

A. Endothelial Cells

The vascular endothelium forms the primary barrier between the vessel lumen and the interstitial space of the lung. As discussed earlier, increased permeability of the endothelium to fluid and proteins is a hallmark of VILI and ARDS. Although VILI can induce breaks in the endothelial barrier that contribute to the observed increase in permeability, modifications to the endothelial cytoskeleton in response to physical or inflammatory stimuli also increase permeability. Endothelial cell contraction and stress fiber formation are associated with increased paracellular movement of fluid and leukocytes from the bloodstream into the interstitial compartment and airspaces. In addition, ligand binding and endothelial cell activation result in the disruption of cell–cell adherens and tight junctions (107–109).

A well-described mechanism of increased permeability in endothelial cells is MLCK-dependent cell contraction. Phosphorylation of calcium/calmodulin-dependent MLCK results in contraction of the actin cytoskeleton, stress fiber formation, and the formation of paracellular gaps (110,111). MLCK phosphorylation is regulated by intracellular calcium via calcium/calmodulin as well as by tyrosine kinases, including p60src, tyrosine phosphatase activity of the SH2 domain of MLCK, and by the small GTPase Rho, which indirectly inhibits myosin light chain phosphatase (PPI), resulting in increased MLCK phosphorylation (112–114). As discussed above, Parker and coworkers have demonstrated that increased intracellular cAMP or inhibition of the MLCK activation pathway prevents ventilator-induced increases in permeability in isolated lungs (61–64).

Endothelial cell contraction can also be initiated by MLCK-independent pathways. For example, PKC, TNF-α, lipopolysaccharide (LPS), and p38MAPK all induce stress fiber formation and impair endothelial barrier function by mechanisms independent of MLCK (83,115–119). Taken together, these data indicate that increased endothelial permeability in VILI is regulated by a variety of signaling pathways, including MLCK-dependent cytoskeletal contraction and ligand-dependent disruption of adherens junctions, and is not only the result of breaks in endothelial cells and the basement membrane.

B. Signaling Pathways

Mechanical stresses also influence gene expression through a variety of signaling pathways in both endothelial and epithelial cells. In bovine endothelial cells, shear stress is transduced into increased cAMP via integrin-dependent, G-protein-mediated activation of adenylate cyclase. This increase in cAMP activates protein kinase A (PKA), which in turn phosphorylates cAMP-response element-binding protein (CREB) to mediate gene transcription. This signaling pathway is dependent on integrin binding to the tripeptide sequence Arg-Gly-Asp (RGD), abundant on ECM proteins. Integrin distortion in the absence of binding does not increase intracellular cAMP (120). Shear stress also activates NFκB in endothelial cells by an integrin binding-dependent mechanism (121). Activation and translocation of NFκB to the nucleus is important in signal transduction of various inflammatory stimuli and apoptosis.

Integrin-mediated signaling in response to fluid shear stress also activates the mitogen-activated protein kinases (MAPKs)/extracellular signal-regulated kinase (ERK) and c-Jun NH2-terminal kinase (JNK), in a process dependent on FAK activation (122). ERK has been shown to increase expression of the early response transcription factor Egr-1, which transactivates genes involved in inflammation and injury in response to fluid shear stress (123). Integrin binding to ECM also mediates the rapid translation of existing mRNAs and translocation of mRNA and ribosomes to FACs, thereby exerting local control over protein translation at the FAC (124). Although the role of this regulatory mechanism in VILI is not known, cytoskeletal stiffness, measured by magnetic twisting cytometry, increases during static conditions, but decreases in response to cyclic stress in cultured alveolar epithelial cells (125). Using this model, Berrios and coworkers found that stiffness correlated with integrin binding-mediated FAC formation (125). The precise mechanisms of the decrease in stiffness with shear stress are not clear, but changes in protein expression are one potential mechanism. Another potential mechanism for the decrease in cytoskeletal stiffness is the change in phosphorylation state of cytoskeletal scaffolding protein (126). In experimental VILI, high-volume ventilation has been shown to increase endothelial cell tyrosine kinase-mediated phosphorylation of focal adhesion proteins, including focal adhesion kinase (FAK), paxillin, JNK, and p38MAPK. In fetal lung cells, Liu and coworkers (127) demonstrated that mechanical strain in a three-dimensional culture system induced activation of p60src and its localization to the cytoskeleton. They identified several substrates for src, including the 110 kDa actin filament-associated protein (AFAP) and PLCgamma. Activation of this pathway affects gene transcription and cell proliferation, but the precise effect on cytoskeletal mechanics and cell adhesion is not known (128). Cytoskeleton fluidizes in response to stretch, thereby implicating mechanisms mediated not only by specific signaling intermediates but also by nonspecific physical forces (129).

Much of the knowledge on lung epithelial cell signaling comes from studies on cytokine production. Oudin and Pugin subjected bronchial epithelial cells to cyclic stretch and reported that IL-8 mRNA and protein production increased in a strain-amplitude manner (130). This deformation response could be inhibited by a MAPK inhibitor as well as with specific inhibitors of p38 and ERK kinases. Correa-Meyer and coworkers recently described a new mechanism of mechanotransduction: they reported that cyclic stretch of primary alveolar type II epithelial cells results in phosphorylation of ERK1 and ERK2 via G proteins end epidermal growth factor receptor signaling (131). Of note, this pathway was not related to ion channels, suggesting diversification of signaling pathways after cell deformation.

An interesting concept recently shown by microarray analysis is that there are regional responses to local mechanical stress in acute lung injury (132). Major functional grouping of differentially regulated genes, including inflammation and immune response, cell proliferation, adhesion, signaling, and apoptosis has been shown to be markedly different between nondependent compared to dependent lung regions, further underlying the importance of lung in-homogeneity in ARDS.

C. Indirect Mechanical Signaling

Recent studies have demonstrated that signals initiated by mechanical stimuli can be transmitted between cell types. For example, mechanical stress sensed by airway epithelial cells can be transmitted to unstressed adjacent endothelial cells in the absence of any physical connection. In these experiments, cultured bronchial epithelial cells exposed to a tonic pressure for four hours exhibited increased expression of Egr-1, fibronectin, and MMP-9, which degrades type IV collagen. In cocultured fibroblasts at atmospheric pressure, stress applied to the epithelial cells induced increased expression of type III collagen (133). Moreover, Tschumperlin and coworkers found that compressive stress shrinks the lateral intercellular space surrounding epithelial cells, and triggers cellular signaling via autocrine binding of epidermal growth factor family ligands to the epidermal growth factor receptor. This is a novel mechanism that is independent of force-dependent biochemical processes within the cell or cell membrane (134).

Another important indirect signaling mechanism proposed by Torday and Rehan (135): using primary fetal rat alveolar cells and lipofibroblasts they provide evidence for paracrine epithelial-mesenchymal signaling coordinated by mechanical stretch that ultimately leads to surfactant secretion.

VII. Alterations in Surfactant Secretion and Function

Surfactant lipid and protein turnover is rapid, and surfactant synthesis and secretion are affected by mechanical factors (136–138). Accordingly, impairment in surfactant metabolism is a potential mechanism of VILI. Data from even the earliest studies of VILI have supported the conclusion that large lung volume ventilation impairs surfactant function, resulting in increased surface tension and reduced lung compliance (35,139–141). The reduction in lung compliance and associated lung volume loss resulting from injurious ventilation potentially exacerbates the detrimental forces acting on the lung.

In an isolated, nonperfused lung model of injurious ventilation, Veldhuizen and coworkers (142) found that ventilation with a tidal volume of 40 mL/kg and without PEEP for two hours resulted in a decrease in surfactant proteins B and C mRNA, but surfactant protein A mRNA was not different from controls. Surfactant proteins B and C are the major surface active proteins, but surfactant protein A acts in part to prevent the inactivation of other surfactant proteins by plasma proteins (143–145). A subsequent study using a similar model found that the surface activity of large aggregate surfactant from lungs ventilated with an injurious tidal volume was reduced, but the amount of large aggregate surfactant was not changed (146). These authors concluded that the presence of protein-rich edema fluid in the airway combined with reduced synthesis of surfactant proteins B and C contributed to the observed decrease in surface activity.

Using models of preterm delivery and acute lung injury, others have found that mechanical ventilation with lung volumes in excess of TLC or without PEEP results in the loss of surfactant function (147–149). In one study, rabbits given *N*-nitroso-*N*-methylurethane (NNMU) to induce lung injury were ventilated with a tidal volume of either 5 or 10 mL/kg. Ventilation with the higher tidal volume resulted in more rapid inactivation of large aggregate surfactant compared with the lower tidal volume (149). Altering the level of PEEP from 3.5 to 12 cm H_2O with a tidal volume of 5 mL/kg did not alter the rate of surfactant inactivation. These authors concluded that large tidal excursions in lung volume, and therefore large changes in alveolar surface area, were important in surfactant inactivation (i.e., changes in PEEP affected lung volume much less than changes in tidal volume). Others have found that low lung volume also inactivates surfactant (100,101,150,151). For example, in experimental lung injury due to sepsis, the use of PEEP is associated with greater preservation of large aggregate surfactant pools when compared with a similar tidal volume and no PEEP (147).

In the injured lung, there are several potential mechanisms for the observed loss of surface active properties. First, because surfactant lipid has little surface activity alone, the loss of surfactant proteins results in a less active surfactant (152). Accordingly, decreased synthesis or secretion of these proteins would result in reduced surfactant function. Second, because plasma proteins bind and inactivate surfactant proteins B and C, the presence of protein-rich edema fluid in the airways reduces lung compliance in part by inactivating surfactant (153). Furthermore, airspace edema can act to wash away surfactant from the alveoli (16,139). Therefore, mechanical ventilation with high tidal volume and frequency or without PEEP can reduce surfactant function directly by affecting surfactant protein synthesis and secretion and indirectly by inducing airspace edema formation.

VIII. Effects of Hypercapnia

Another potential mechanism for the protective effect of low tidal volume ventilation is the hypercapnia that may occur with low tidal volume ventilation. Experimental models of ischemia-reperfusion injury have demonstrated reduced tissue injury in association with hypercapnia and acidosis. The presumed mechanisms, possibly mediated by pH changes, include a reduction in reactive oxygen and nitrogen species and an adaptive alteration in oxygen supply and demand kinetics (154,155). At least one experimental study of VILI demonstrated a similar protective effect of hypercapnia in isolated rabbit lungs (156). Any potential protective effect of hypercapnia in patients has not been clearly demonstrated. However, there is evidence that stretch and CO_2 modulate the inflammatory response of alveolar macrophages through independent changes in metabolic activity (157).

IX. Ventilator-Induced Pulmonary and Systemic Inflammation

One of the primary mechanisms of lung injury propagation in models of VALI is increased inflammation as measured by increases in edema fluid and plasma markers, and by an increase in neutrophil infiltration and macrophage activation. This section will review data from clinical, experimental, and in vitro studies supporting the role of increased inflammation in the pathogenesis of VILI.

A. Biomarkers of Inflammation in Clinical Studies

Elevated levels of proinflammatory mediators have been measured in airspace lavage fluid and in the plasma of patients with ARDS. Ranieri and coworkers (158) measured bronchoalveolar lavage (BAL) and plasma levels of several proinflammatory cytokines in 44 patients with ARDS. At study entry, patients were randomized to receive mechanical ventilation with a conventional strategy (mean tidal volume of 11.1 mL/kg, mean plateau airway pressure 31 $cm\,H_2O$, and mean PEEP of 6.5 $cm\,H_2O$), or a reduced tidal volume

(7.6 mL/kg) and higher PEEP (14.8 cm H_2O) with a mean plateau airway pressure of 24.6 cm H_2O. PEEP in the latter group was set above the lower inflection point of the respiratory system pressure volume curve. Baseline measurements of cytokines were made at the time of admission (study entry) and were then measured serially for two days. By 36 hours, BAL fluid from patients in the protective ventilation group had significantly fewer polymorphonuclear cells and lower concentrations of TNF-α, IL-1β, IL-6, and IL-8. Plasma levels of IL-6 were also significantly lower in the patients receiving protective ventilation (158).

The NIH ARDS Network study found a similar difference in plasma IL-6 levels at three days among patients ventilated with low tidal volume compared with conventional tidal volume (6) and in subsequent studies performed on subset of patients taken from that investigation (159–161). In another study of 27 consecutive patients with ARDS, Meduri and coworkers (162) found that persistent elevation of plasma IL-6 or IL-1β was associated with decreased survival although all patients were ventilated with the same strategy. Others have also found that persistent elevation of IL-1β is associated with increased mortality in patients with ARDS (163). Although plasma and BAL levels of cytokines are elevated early in the course of ARDS, the molar ratios of individual cytokines to anti-inflammatory soluble receptors and receptor antagonists may be more important in determining the pulmonary and systemic proinflammatory effects of these mediators (164). In another study of 39 patients with normal lungs, ventilation for one hour with a high tidal volume (15 mL/kg) and zero PEEP did not affect plasma levels of either IL-6, TNF-α, IL-1 receptor antagonist, or IL-10 (165).

In summary, these and other data (166) indicate that in ARDS patients, higher tidal volume ventilation is associated with poor outcome and higher BAL and plasma levels of proinflammatory mediators, especially IL-6. Higher plasma levels of IL-6 are associated with poor outcome independent of the ventilation strategy used. Interestingly, biological markers are also released from patients without ARDS ventilated with high tidal volumes (165,167,168).

B. Mediators of Inflammation in Experimental Studies

Under experimental conditions, high tidal volume, low PEEP ventilation induces increased release of proinflammatory cytokines into the airspaces and bloodstream, increased neutrophil infiltration into the lung, and activation of alveolar macrophages (169). Although there is some debate about the potential importance of proinflammatory cytokines in the development of VILI (170), there is considerable evidence supporting a role for the release of inflammatory mediators in VILI.

Tremblay and coworkers (171) found that ventilation of isolated, nonperfused rat lungs with a tidal volume of 40 mL/kg without PEEP for two hours resulted in large increases in lavage concentrations of TNF-α, IL-1β, IL-6, and MIP-2 (Fig. 5). Reducing tidal volume to 15 or 7 mL/kg reduced the lavage concentrations of these mediators even if end-inspiratory lung volume was similar. The increase in these cytokines was greater if rats were pretreated with LPS, but the differences among the groups persisted. Northern blot analysis of whole lung homogenates revealed increased expression of c-fos mRNA, a transcription factor important in the early stress response, with both high and moderate tidal volume, zero PEEP ventilation. The increase in c-fos was greater in saline-treated control rats than in LPS-pretreated rats (172). Early response genes, such as c-fos, as

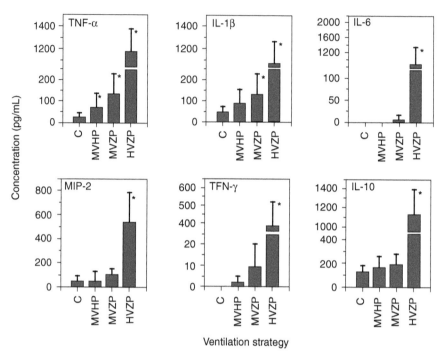

Figure 5 Effect of ventilation strategy on absolute lung lavage cytokine concentrations in isolated, nonperfused rat lungs. Two hours of high tidal volume ventilation in association with zero PEEP increased lavage levels of each of these cytokines. The lowest levels were found in the unventilated controls (C). MVHP: moderate volume (15 mL/kg), high PEEP (10 cm H$_2$O). MVZP: moderate tidal volume, zero PEEP. HVZP: high tidal volume (40 mL/kg), zero PEEP. *Source*: From Ref. 171.

well as NFκB contain *cis*-acting shear stress response elements in their promoter regions (171,173). Similar results were confirmed later by Veldhuizen and coworkers in a model of isolated mouse lung ventilated with 20 mL/kg of tidal volume without PEEP (146).

Chiumello and coworkers (46) demonstrated that injurious ventilatory strategies increased release of proinflammatory cytokines [TNF-α and macrophage inflammatory protein-2 (MIP-2)] in the lung as well as systemic circulation in an acid aspiration model in rats. Others have found that in a rat model of cecal ligation-induced sepsis, injurious ventilation with a tidal volume of 20 mL/kg, without PEEP, resulted in higher BAL levels of TNF-α, IL-1β, and IL-6 compared with unventilated controls and rats ventilated with a tidal volume of 10 mL/kg and PEEP level of 3 cm H$_2$O. Whole lung mRNA levels for each of these cytokines were also elevated after one hour of injurious ventilation in this study (174). Others reported similar results (70,172,175) suggesting a pathogenetic role for TNF-α and IL-1 in VALI (176).

Further evidence of the importance of these inflammatory mediators in the development of VILI comes from experimental studies of the effects of anti-TNF antibody and IL-1 receptor antagonist on lung injury following surfactant depletion. Administration of anti-TNF antibody to surfactant-depleted rabbits prior to the initiation of conventional mechanical ventilation resulted in less severe histological lung injury and preserved oxygenation (172). In a similar model, IL-1 receptor antagonist reduced endothelial albumin permeability and neutrophil infiltration at eight hours (177). The prominent role of neutrophils in VILI was subsequently shown by Belperio and coworkers (178).

The signaling pathway by which mechanical distention mediates the release of inflammatory cytokines involves translocation of NFκB to the nucleus. However, initiation of NFκB activation with VILI is independent of TRL-4/LPS receptor and is inhibited by corticosteroids (179). Moreover, a role of G-protein coupled receptors has been shown (180).

These data raise the possibility that pharmacological inhibition of VILI-mediated NFκB activation could be achieved without the complete inhibition of the potentially adaptive innate immune response.

Proinflammatory signals can also be transmitted across the ECM from alveolar epithelial cells to endothelial cells. Kuebler and coworkers (181) found that intra-alveolar TNF-α increased intracellular calcium in alveolar epithelial cells and activated phospholipase A_2. This in turn induced an increase in intracellular calcium in adjacent endothelial cells that was not dependent on gap junctions. The increase in intracellular calcium in the endothelial cells resulted in increased expression of P-selectin, a neutrophil adhesion molecule. Therefore, intra-alveolar TNF-α induces a proinflammatory response in adjacent endothelial cells in the absence of direct TNF-endothelial interaction.

C. Strain-Induced Inflammatory Response

Mechanical stimulation of epithelial cells, macrophages, endothelial cells, fibroblasts, and smooth muscle cells induces a change in protein phosphorylation and alterations in cytoskeleton proteins. In VILI, it is the alveolar epithelial cells and lung macrophages that are perhaps most responsible for the transcription and secretion of inflammatory mediators. Vlahakis and coworkers (182) found that in cultured A549 cells, mRNA for IL-8 increased fourfold after four hours of cyclic strain sufficient to change the cell surface area by 30%. Continued strain for up to 48 hours resulted in a nearly 50% increase in IL-8 secretion compared with nonstrained controls. A lesser degree of strain did not affect IL-8 secretion. Interestingly, the frequency of stretch does not interfere with IL-8 mRNA and protein in normal cells (183), but has a synergistic effect with LPS (184). Quinn and coworkers (185), who also found that the increase in IL-8 secretion was associated with activation of the JNK family MAPKs. Cyclic strain of 15% for two hours induced a 237% increase in phosphorylation of JNK in A549 cells. Phosphorylation of p38MAPK increased by 468%, but phosphorylation of ERK1/2 was not changed. A role for NFκB stretch-induced transcriptional regulation of IL-8 mRNA and IL-8 production was also shown by Li and coworkers (186).

IL-1β signaling activates ERK, JNK, and p38MAPK by different mechanisms. MacGillivray and coworkers have found that in fibroblasts, the IL-1β-dependent ERK activation depends on the localization of IL-1 receptor-associated kinase (IRAK) to the FAC (187). FACs are comprised of cell surface integrins that connect the cytoskeleton to the ECM. In addition, FACs contain a variety of other signaling proteins, including FAK and src tyrosine kinases as discussed above. Interestingly, FACs also colocalize with the IL-1 receptor-1 (187).

To identify the source of inflammatory cytokines in VILI, Dunn and Pugin (188) cultured human alveolar macrophages on flexible silastic membranes and exposed the cells to cyclic stretch for up to 32 hours. These authors found that cyclic strain increased secretion of IL-8 and MMP-9 (gelatinase b—a type IV collagenase), but not TNF-α or IL-6. When the macrophages were pretreated with LPS, TNF-α and IL-6 secretion increased to greater extent in strained cells compared with static cultures. Mechanical strain also activated NFκB in macrophages after 30 minutes.

In another study, a variety of cell types including macrophages, A549 cells, a bronchial epithelial cell line, two endothelial cell lines, and primary lung fibroblasts were exposed to the same cyclic strain. Of these cell types, only macrophages and A549 cells secreted IL-8 in response to mechanical distention. The relative amount of IL-8 secreted from macrophages was much greater than the amount secreted from A549 cells. In the absence of LPS stimulation, cytokines were not secreted in appreciable amounts from the other cell types (188). Importantly, IL-8 is present in high levels in the edema fluid of ventilated patients with ARDS (189,190). Furthermore, the activation of NFκB in response to intratracheal instillation of immune complexes is dependent on the presence of alveolar macrophages (191). Taken together, these data implicate the alveolar macrophage as the initial stretch-responsive cell in the initiation of the inflammatory response observed in VILI.

This does not negate a possible role for other cell types in the propagation of early proinflammatory signaling in VILI. For example, Grembowicz and coworkers (192) reported that sublethal PMD results in increased expression of c-fos, a transcription factor important in cytokine expression and activation of NFκB in vascular endothelial cells and smooth muscle cells. NFκB activation via IkappaB kinase (IKK) upregulates the expression of a variety of proinflammatory mediators, including IL-6, IL-8, IL-1β, and TNF-α (191,193,194). Tracheal epithelial cells exposed to either magnetic twisting cytometry or to static compressive stress were found to upregulate expression of Egr-1, another early response gene that encodes a transcription factor with binding sites in the promoter regions of genes such as TNF-α, PDGF, TGF-β, and PAI-1 (195–197).

Other in vivo studies underline the relationship between mechanical stretch and neutrophils. It is known from 1987 that neutrophils play a crucial role in VILI (198). Choudhury and coworkers showed that mechanical stress initiates pulmonary sequestration of polymorphonuclear cells (PMN) early during the course of VILI (199) and Belperio demonstrated that PMN accumulation causes microvascular permeability changes (178). However, recently Steinberg and coworkers showed that mechanical injury initiates an inflammatory response independently of neutrophils resulting in a secondary neutrhophil-mediated injury.

X. Biotrauma: Mechanical Ventilation and MODS

An interesting observation in most clinical studies of ARDS is that most patients die from MODS rather than respiratory failure. As confirmed in the clinical studies discussed above, injurious mechanical ventilation results in an increase in proinflammatory cytokines in the systemic circulation as well as in the airspaces of the lung (6,46,200,201).

A. Can Lung Injury/Inflammation Lead to Systemic Inflammation?

The lungs are uniquely poised anatomically to affect distant organs. The pulmonary vasculature not only receives the entire cardiac output, but also harbors a large reservoir of macrophages and marginated neutrophils. Thus, significant potential exists for the lungs to interact with, and contribute to, the circulating pool of inflammatory cells. In addition, inflammation in the lung caused by mechanical ventilation or injury to the alveolar-capillary interface may cause release or allow efflux of inflammatory mediators from the alveolar space into the circulation. Several investigators have also shown that increased permeability of the alveolar/capillary interface as a result of lung injury leads to the release of mediators into circulation. Von Bethmann and coworkers (201) reported that in an isolated perfused murine lung model, ventilation with higher transpulmonary pressure (25 cm H_2O) compared with a normal pressure (10 cm H_2O) leads to a significant increase in concentration of both TNF-α and IL-6 in the perfusate. In patients with ARDS, concentrations of TNF-α, IL-1β, and IL-6 were higher in the arterial blood (obtained via a wedged pulmonary artery catheter) as compared with mixed venous blood, suggesting that the lungs in these patients were contributing cytokines to the systemic circulation (202).

Another mechanism whereby mechanical ventilation may contribute to the development of a systemic inflammatory response is by promoting bacterial translocation from the airspaces into the circulation—analogous to the gut bacterial translocation hypothesis of multiple organ failure (203). Two studies evaluated the influence of mechanical ventilation strategy on the translocation of bacteria from the lung into the bloodstream in dogs (204) and rats (205). After intratracheal instillation of bacteria, these animals were ventilated with a high transpulmonary pressure ($\sim$30 cm H_2O) and minimal (0–3 cm H_2O) or 10 cm H_2O PEEP. Bacteremia seldom occurred in control animals ventilated with low airway pressure, whereas it was found in nearly all animals ventilated with high tidal volume and a low PEEP. In contrast, ventilation with the same transpulmonary pressure but with 10 cm H_2O PEEP resulted in rates of bacteremia as low as in controls. Subsequent studies added evidence to the hypothesis (201,206). Interestingly, alveolar collapse (207) or low PEEP levels (208) contribute to the translocation of bacteria suggesting that an individually tailored ventilator settings would be ideal (209).

B. Is There Evidence of MODS Secondary to Mechanical Ventilation?

The NIH ARDS Network has recently reported the results of a randomized, controlled multicenter study in 861 patients comparing a tidal volume of 12 mL/kg (predicted by body weight) with 6 mL/kg (6). The main finding was a 9% reduction in absolute mortality; plasma levels of IL-6 in the 6 mL/kg tidal volume group were also significantly lower than in the conventional tidal volume group. This was associated with a greater number of organ failure–free days, although this outcome variable may not be independent of mortality. However, it appears plausible that VILI in humans may affect the outcome of ARDS by affecting the systemic inflammatory response leading to MODS. It is important to emphasize that MODS is a complex syndrome, often precipitated and intensified by a series of events rather than a single event. A likely scenario is that there is an ongoing inflammatory response as a result of the persistence of the factors that either initiated or exacerbated the response and/or failure of intrinsic regulatory mechanisms. In an experimental study of acid aspiration, eight hours of mechanical ventilation with an injurious strategy led to an increase in pulmonary and systemic production of cytokines, as well as to elevations of biochemical markers indicating organ dysfunction (e.g., creatinine). Mechanical ventilation may also affect distal organ function via effects on cardiac output, as well as on the levels of oxygenation and the distribution of blood to the various organ systems (e.g., mesenteric, renal, and hepatic perfusion). For example, although fluid resuscitation of rats ventilated with PEEP returned cardiac output to normal values, mesenteric

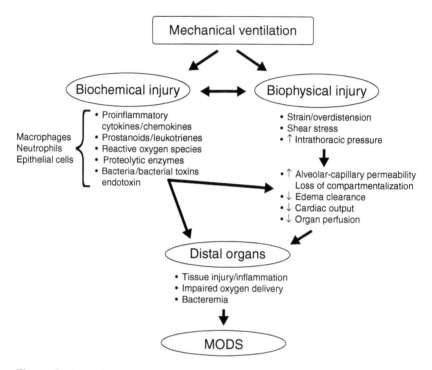

Figure 6 Potential mechanisms by which mechanical ventilation may contribute to multiple organ dysfunction syndrome (MODS). *Source*: From Ref. 214.

blood flow remained significantly reduced (210). An increase in distal ileal permeability has also been reported in rats ventilated with larger (20 mL/kg) versus smaller (10 mL/kg) tidal volumes (211).

An interesting concept that has recently been suggested links injurious mechanical ventilation, apoptosis and organ dysfunction. Imai and coworkers showed that low levels of lung stretch caused high levels of apoptosis while high stretch was associated with decreased apoptosis and increased necrosis (212). The stretch-induced activation of Akt-ERK1/2 via a G-protein-dependent pathway plays a key role. Oudin and Pugin reported that cyclic stretch of bronchial epithelial cells in culture led to IL-1 mRNA and protein production that could be inhibited by protein kinase inhibitors (130), while Correa-Meyer and coworkers showed that mechanical stretch of primary alveolar type II epithelial cells results in phosphorylation of ERK1/2 via G proteins (131). These observations suggest the hypothesis that mechanical deformation may trigger G-protein-mediated pathways that activate Akt/ERK1/2 thus inhibiting apoptosis and enhancing necrosis.

The potential effects of VILI on systemic inflammation and MODS are summarized in Figure 6.

XI. Summary

Recent clinical studies of protective ventilation have confirmed that VALI contributes to patient mortality. However, the mechanisms by which low tidal volume ventilation reduces mortality are poorly understood. On the most basic level, our current understanding is that tidal volume reduction prevents excessive end-inspiratory lung volume in the heterogeneously injured and edema-filled lung. This prevents the mechanical disruption of the alveolar-capillary barrier and potentially attenuates strain-induced functional changes in alveolar macrophages, epithelial cells, and endothelial cells. These cellular responses to mechanical stimuli include changes in the secretion of proinflammatory mediators, alterations in surfactant secretion and function, increased permeability, edema formation, and the loss of lung compartmentalization. Substantial experimental evidence also suggests that excessively low FRC results in surfactant inactivation, promotes lung inflammation, and results in the loss of compartmentalization.

Injurious mechanical ventilation may contribute to patient mortality by exacerbating existing lung injury and thereby prolonging the need for mechanical ventilation and exposing the patient to greater risk of other complications of intensive care. Injurious ventilation may also directly mediate MODS by affecting the release of inflammatory mediators into the systemic blood stream resulting in the dysfunction of other organs. Furthermore, it is likely that low tidal volume strategies of ventilation currently in clinical use do not entirely prevent VALI. An improved understanding of the cellular mechanisms of VALI may further guide the development of ventilation strategies and other therapies for patients with ARDS.

References

1. Petty TL, Ashbaugh DG. The adult respiratory distress syndrome. Clinical features, factors influencing prognosis and principles of management. Chest 1971; 60(3):233–239.
2. Sladen A, Laver MB, Pontoppidan H. Pulmonary complications and water retention in prolonged mechanical ventilation. N Engl J Med 1968; 279(9):448–453.
3. Greenfield LJ, Ebert PA, Benson DW. Effects of positive pressure ventilation on surface tension properties of lung extracts. Anesthesiology 1964; 25:312–316.
4. Mackline M, Mackline C. Malignant interstitial emphysema of the lungs and mediastinum as an important occult complication in many respiratory diseases and other conditions: an interpretation of the clinical literature in light of laboratory experiments. Medicine 1944; 23:281–352.
5. Mead J, Takishima T, Leith D. Stress distribution in lungs: a model of pulmonary elasticity. J Appl Physiol 1970; 28(5):596–608.
6. The Acute Respiratory Distress Syndrome Network. Ventilation with lower tidal volumes as compared to traditional tidal volumes for acute lung injury and the acute respiratory distress syndrome. N Engl J Med 2000; 342:1301–1308.
7. Schnapp LM, Chin DP, Szaflarski N, et al. Frequency and importance of barotrauma in 100 patients with acute lung injury. Crit Care Med 1995; 23(2):272–278.
8. Weg JG, Anzueto A, Balk RA, et al. The relation of pneumothorax and other air leaks to mortality in the acute respiratory distress syndrome. N Engl J Med 1998; 338(6):341–346.
9. Wirtz HR, Dobbs LG. The effects of mechanical forces on lung functions. Respir Physiol 2000; 119(1):1–17.
10. Bachofen H, Schurch S. Alveolar surface forces and lung architecture. Comp Biochem Physiol A Mol Integr Physiol 2001; 129(1):183–193.
11. Gattinoni L, Carlesso E, Cadringher P, et al. Physical and biological triggers of ventilator-induced lung injury and its prevention. Eur Respir J Suppl 2003; 47:15s–25s.
12. West JB. Invited review: pulmonary capillary stress failure. J Appl Physiol 2000; 89(6):2483–2489.
13. Martynowicz MA, Walters BJ, Hubmayr RD. Mechanisms of recruitment in oleic acid-injured lungs. J Appl Physiol 2001; 90(5):1744–1753.

14. Costello ML, Mathieu-Costello O, West JB. Stress failure of alveolar epithelial cells studied by scanning electron microscopy. Am Rev Respir Dis 1992; 145(6):1446–1455.

15. Martynowicz MA, Minor TA, Walters BJ, et al. Regional expansion of oleic acid-injured lungs. Am J Respir Crit Care Med 1999; 160(1):250–258.

16. Wyszogrodski I, Kyei-Aboagye K, Taeusch HW Jr, et al. Surfactant inactivation by hyperventilation: conservation by end-expiratory pressure. J Appl Physiol 1975; 38(3): 461–466.

17. Gattinoni L, Pelosi P, Crotti S, et al. Effects of positive end-expiratory pressure on regional distribution of tidal volume and recruitment in adult respiratory distress syndrome. Am J Respir Crit Care Med 1995; 151(6):1807–1814.

18. Ware LB, Matthay MA. Alveolar fluid clearance is impaired in the majority of patients with acute lung injury and the acute respiratory distress syndrome. Am J Respir Crit Care Med 2001; 163(6):1376–1383.

19. Ingber DE. Tensegrity: the architectural basis of cellular mechanotransduction. Annu Rev Physiol 1997; 59:575–599.

20. Wang N, Naruse K, Stamenovic D, et al. Mechanical behavior in living cells consistent with the tensegrity model. Proc Natl Acad Sci U S A 2001; 98(14):7765–7770.

21. Tschumperlin DJ, Margulies SS. Alveolar epithelial surface area-volume relationship in isolated rat lungs. J Appl Physiol 1999; 86(6):2026–2033.

22. Bachofen H, Schurch S, Urbinelli M, et al. Relations among alveolar surface tension, surface area, volume, and recoil pressure. J Appl Physiol 1987; 62(5):1878–1887.

23. Eisner MD, Thompson T, Hudson LD, et al. Efficacy of low tidal volume ventilation in patients with different clinical risk factors for acute lung injury and the acute respiratory distress syndrome. Am J Respir Crit Care Med 2001; 164(2):231–236.

24. Amato MB, Barbas CS, Medeiros DM, et al. Effect of a protective-ventilation strategy on mortality in the acute respiratory distress syndrome. N Engl J Med 1998; 338(6): 347–354.

25. Brochard L, Roudot-Thoraval F, Roupie E, et al. Tidal volume reduction for prevention of ventilator-induced lung injury in acute respiratory distress syndrome. The Multicenter Trail Group on Tidal Volume reduction in ARDS. Am J Respir Crit Care Med 1998; 158(6):1831–1838.

26. Brower RG, Shanholtz CB, Fessler HE, et al. Prospective, randomized, controlled clinical trial comparing traditional versus reduced tidal volume ventilation in acute respiratory distress syndrome patients. Crit Care Med 1999; 27(8):1492–1498.

27. Stewart TE, Meade MO, Cook DJ, et al. Evaluation of a ventilation strategy to prevent barotrauma in patients at high risk for acute respiratory distress syndrome. Pressure- and Volume-Limited Ventilation Strategy Group. N Engl J Med 1998; 338(6):355–361.

28. Ware LB, Matthay MA. The acute respiratory distress syndrome. N Engl J Med 2000; 342(18):1334–1349.

29. Chiumello D, Carlesso E, Cadringher P, et al. Lung stress and strain during mechanical ventilation for acute respiratory distress syndrome. Am J Respir Crit Care Med 2008; 178(4): 346–355.

30. Pelosi P, Caironi P, Gattinoni L. Pulmonary and extrapulmonary forms of acute respiratory distress syndrome. Semin Respir Crit Care Med 2001; 22(3):259–268.

31. Ranieri VM, Brienza N, Santostasi S, et al. Impairment of lung and chest wall mechanics in patients with acute respiratory distress syndrome: role of abdominal distension. Am J Respir Crit Care Med 1997; 156(4, pt 1):1082–1091.

32. Talmor D, Sarge T, O'Donnell CR, et al. Esophageal and transpulmonary pressures in acute respiratory failure. Crit Care Med 2006; 34(5):1389–1394.

33. Bachofen M, Weibel ER. Structural alterations of lung parenchyma in the adult respiratory distress syndrome. Clin Chest Med 1982; 3(1):35–56.

34. Dreyfuss D, Saumon G. Ventilator-induced lung injury: lessons from experimental studies. Am J Respir Crit Care Med 1998; 157(1):294–323.
35. Webb HH, Tierney DF. Experimental pulmonary edema due to intermittent positive pressure ventilation with high inflation pressures. Protection by positive end-expiratory pressure. Am Rev Respir Dis 1974; 110(5):556–565.
36. Dreyfuss D, Basset G, Soler P, et al. Intermittent positive-pressure hyperventilation with high inflation pressures produces pulmonary microvascular injury in rats. Am Rev Respir Dis 1985; 132(4):880–884.
37. Dreyfuss D, Saumon G. Role of tidal volume, FRC, and end-inspiratory volume in the development of pulmonary edema following mechanical ventilation. Am Rev Respir Dis 1993; 148(5):1194–1203.
38. Dreyfuss D, Soler P, Basset G, et al. High inflation pressure pulmonary edema. Respective effects of high airway pressure, high tidal volume, and positive end-expiratory pressure. Am Rev Respir Dis 1988; 137(5):1159–1164.
39. Mascheroni D, Kolobow T, Fumagalli R, et al. Acute respiratory failure following pharmacologically induced hyperventilation: an experimental animal study. Intensive Care Med 1988; 15(1):8–14.
40. Toung T, Saharia P, Permutt S, et al. Aspiration pneumonia: beneficial and harmful effects of positive end-expiratory pressure. Surgery 1977; 82(2):279–283.
41. Valenza F, Guglielmi M, Irace M, et al. Positive end-expiratory pressure delays the progression of lung injury during ventilator strategies involving high airway pressure and lung overdistention. Crit Care Med 2003; 31(7):1993–1998.
42. Albert RK, Lakshminarayan S, Charan NB, et al. Extra-alveolar vessel contribution to hydrostatic pulmonary edema in in situ dog lungs. J Appl Physiol 1983; 54(4):1010–1017.
43. Hotchkiss JR Jr, Blanch L, Naveira A, et al. Relative roles of vascular and airspace pressures in ventilator-induced lung injury. Crit Care Med 2001; 29(8):1593–1598.
44. West JB, Tsukimoto K, Mathieu-Costello O, et al. Stress failure in pulmonary capillaries. J Appl Physiol 1991; 70(4):1731–1742.
45. Clements JA. Pulmonary edema and permeability of alveolar membranes. Arch Environ Health 1961; 2:280–283.
46. Chiumello D, Pristine G, Slutsky AS. Mechanical ventilation affects local and systemic cytokines in an animal model of acute respiratory distress syndrome. Am J Respir Crit Care Med 1999; 160(1):109–116.
47. Colmenero-Ruiz M, Fernandez-Mondejar E, Fernandez-Sacristan MA, et al. PEEP and low tidal volume ventilation reduce lung water in porcine pulmonary edema. Am J Respir Crit Care Med 1997; 155(3):964–970.
48. Corbridge TC, Wood LD, Crawford GP, et al. Adverse effects of large tidal volume and low PEEP in canine acid aspiration. Am Rev Respir Dis 1990; 142(2):311–315.
49. Frank JA, Gutierrez JA, Jones KD, et al. Low tidal volume reduces epithelial and endothelial injury in acid-injured rat lungs. Am J Respir Crit Care Med 2002; 165(2):242–249.
50. Dreyfuss D, Martin-Lefevre L, Saumon G. Hyperinflation-induced lung injury during alveolar flooding in rats: effect of perfluorocarbon instillation. Am J Respir Crit Care Med 1999; 159(6):1752–1757.
51. Lecuona E, Saldias F, Comellas A, et al. Ventilator-associated lung injury decreases lung ability to clear edema and downregulates alveolar epithelial cell Na,K-adenosine triphosphatase function. Chest 1999; 116(Suppl 1):29S–30S.
52. Saldias FJ, Lecuona E, Comellas AP, et al. Beta-adrenergic stimulation restores rat lung ability to clear edema in ventilator-associated lung injury. Am J Respir Crit Care Med 2000; 162(1):282–287.
53. Carlton DP, Cummings JJ, Scheerer RG, et al. Lung overexpansion increases pulmonary microvascular protein permeability in young lambs. J Appl Physiol 1990; 69(2):577–583.

54. Parker JC, Hernandez LA, Longenecker GL, et al. Lung edema caused by high peak inspiratory pressures in dogs. Role of increased microvascular filtration pressure and permeability. Am Rev Respir Dis 1990; 142(2):321–328.

55. Hopewell PC. Failure of positive end-expiratory pressure to decrease lung water content in alloxan-induced pulmonary edema. Am Rev Respir Dis 1979; 120(4):813–819.

56. Hopewell PC, Murray JF. Effects of continuous positive-pressure ventilation in experimental pulmonary edema. J Appl Physiol 1976; 40(4):568–574.

57. Egan EA. Lung inflation, lung solute permeability, and alveolar edema. J Appl Physiol 1982; 53(1):121–125.

58. Cavanaugh KJ, Cohen TS, Margulies SS. Stretch increases alveolar epithelial permeability to uncharged micromolecules. Am J Physiol Cell Physiol 2006; 290(4):C1179–C1188.

59. Cohen TS, Cavanaugh KJ, Margulies SS. Frequency and peak stretch magnitude affect alveolar epithelial permeability. Eur Respir J 2008; 32(4):854–861.

60. Nicolaysen G, Waaler BA, Aarseth P. On the existence of stretchable pores in the exchange vessels of the isolated rabbit lung preparation. Lymphology 1979; 12(3):201–207.

61. Parker JC, Ivey CL. Isoproterenol attenuates high vascular pressure-induced permeability increases in isolated rat lungs. J Appl Physiol 1997; 83:1962–1967.

62. Parker JC. Inhibitors of myosin light chain kinase and phosphodiesterase reduce ventilator-induced lung injury. J Appl Physiol 2000; 89(6):2241–2248.

63. Parker JC, Ivey CL, Tucker JA. Gadolinium prevents high airway pressure-induced permeability increases in isolated rat lungs. J Appl Physiol 1998; 84(4):1113–1118.

64. Parker JC, Ivey CL, Tucker A. Phosphotyrosine phosphatase and tyrosine kinase inhibition modulate airway pressure-induced lung injury. J Appl Physiol 1998; 85(5):1753–1761.

65. Czarny M, Schnitzer JE. Neutral sphingomyelinase inhibitor scyphostatin prevents and ceramide mimics mechanotransduction in vascular endothelium. Am J Physiol Heart Circ Physiol 2004; 287(3):H1344–H1352.

66. Cooper JA, Van Der ZH, Line BR, et al. Relationship of end-expiratory pressure, lung volume, and 99mTc-DTPA clearance. J Appl Physiol 1987; 63(4):1586–1590.

67. Marks JD, Luce JM, Lazar NM, et al. Effect of increases in lung volume on clearance of aerosolized solute from human lungs. J Appl Physiol 1985; 59(4):1242–1248.

68. Egan EA. Response of alveolar epithelial solute permeability to changes in lung inflation. J Appl Physiol 1980; 49(6):1032–1036.

69. Kim KJ, Crandall ED. Effects of exposure to acid on alveolar epithelial water and solute transport. J Appl Physiol 1982; 52(4):902–909.

70. Imai Y, Nakagawa S, Ito Y, et al. Comparison of lung protection strategies using conventional and high-frequency oscillatory ventilation. J Appl Physiol 2001; 91(4):1836–1844.

71. Simma B, Luz G, Trawoger R, et al. Comparison of different modes of high-frequency ventilation in surfactant-deficient rabbits. Pediatr Pulmonol 1996; 22(4):263–270.

72. Berg JT, Fu Z, Breen EC, et al. High lung inflation increases mRNA levels of ECM components and growth factors in lung parenchyma. J Appl Physiol 1997; 83(1):120–128.

73. Chesnutt AN, Matthay MA, Tibayan FA, et al. Early detection of type III procollagen peptide in acute lung injury. Pathogenetic and prognostic significance. Am J Respir Crit Care Med 1997; 156(3, pt 1):840–845.

74. Parker JC, Breen EC, West JB. High vascular and airway pressures increase interstitial protein mRNA expression in isolated rat lungs. J Appl Physiol 1997; 83:1697–1705.

75. Breen EC. Mechanical strain increases type I collagen expression in pulmonary fibroblasts in vitro. J Appl Physiol 2000; 88(1):203–209.

76. Al Jamal R, Ludwig MS. Changes in proteoglycans and lung tissue mechanics during excessive mechanical ventilation in rats. Am J Physiol Lung Cell Mol Physiol 2001; 281(5):L1078–L1087.

77. Foda HD, Rollo EE, Drews M, et al. Ventilator-induced lung injury upregulates and activates gelatinases and EMMPRIN: attenuation by the synthetic matrix metalloproteinase inhibitor, prinomastat (AG3340). Am J Respir Cell Mol Biol 2001; 25(6):717–724.

78. Hasaneen NA, Zucker S, Cao J, et al. Cyclic mechanical strain-induced proliferation and migration of human airway smooth muscle cells: role of EMMPRIN and MMPs. FASEB J 2005; 19(11):1507–1509.

79. Tschumperlin DJ, Oswari J, Margulies AS. Deformation-induced injury of alveolar epithelial cells. Effect of frequency, duration, and amplitude. Am J Respir Crit Care Med 2000; 162(2, pt 1):357–362.

80. Vlahakis NE, Schroeder MA, Pagano RE, et al. Deformation-induced lipid trafficking in alveolar epithelial cells. Am J Physiol Lung Cell Mol Physiol 2001; 280(5):L938–L946.

81. Vlahakis NE, Schroeder MA, Pagano RE, et al. The role of the cytoskeleton in deformation induced alveolar epithelial wounding and repair. Am J Respir Crit Care Med 2002; 165: A379.

82. Cavanaugh KJ Jr, Oswari J, Margulies SS. Role of stretch on tight junction structure in alveolar epithelial cells. Am J Respir Cell Mol Biol 2001; 25(5):584–591.

83. Dudek SM, Garcia JG. Cytoskeletal regulation of pulmonary vascular permeability. J Appl Physiol 2001; 91(4):1487–1500.

84. Muscedere JG, Mullen JB, Gan K, et al. Tidal ventilation at low airway pressures can augment lung injury. Am J Respir Crit Care Med 1994; 149(5):1327–1334.

85. Gattinoni L, D'Andrea L, Pelosi P, et al. Regional effects and mechanism of positive end-expiratory pressure in early adult respiratory distress syndrome. JAMA 1993; 269(16):2122–2127.

86. Crotti S, Mascheroni D, Caironi P, et al. Recruitment and derecruitment during acute respiratory failure: a clinical study. Am J Respir Crit Care Med 2001; 164(1):131–140.

87. Valenza F, Guglielmi M, Maffioletti M, et al. Prone position delays the progression of ventilator-induced lung injury in rats: does lung strain distribution play a role? Crit Care Med 2005; 33(2):361–367.

88. Hickling KG, Walsh J, Henderson S, et al. Low mortality rate in adult respiratory distress syndrome using low-volume, pressure-limited ventilation with permissive hypercapnia: a prospective study. Crit Care Med 1994; 22(10):1568–1578.

89. Adams AB, Cakar N, Marini JJ. Static and dynamic pressure-volume curves reflect different aspects of respiratory system mechanics in experimental acute respiratory distress syndrome. Respir Care 2001; 46(7):686–693.

90. Hickling KG. The pressure-volume curve is greatly modified by recruitment. A mathematical model of ARDS lungs. Am J Respir Crit Care Med 1998; 158(1):194–202.

91. Jonson B, Richard JC, Straus C, et al. Pressure-volume curves and compliance in acute lung injury: evidence of recruitment above the lower inflection point. Am J Respir Crit Care Med 1999; 159(4, pt 1):1172–1178.

92. Karason S, Sondergaard S, Lundin S, et al. Evaluation of pressure/volume loops based on intratracheal pressure measurements during dynamic conditions. Acta Anaesthesiol Scand 2000; 44(5):571–577.

93. Brower RG, Lanken PN, MacIntyre N, et al. Higher versus lower positive end-expiratory pressures in patients with the acute respiratory distress syndrome. N Engl J Med 2004; 351(4):327–336.

94. Meade MO, Cook DJ, Guyatt GH, et al. Ventilation strategy using low tidal volumes, recruitment maneuvers, and high positive end-expiratory pressure for acute lung injury and acute respiratory distress syndrome: a randomized controlled trial. JAMA 2008; 299(6):637–645.

95. Mercat A, Richard JC, Vielle B, et al. Positive end-expiratory pressure setting in adults with acute lung injury and acute respiratory distress syndrome: a randomized controlled trial. JAMA 2008; 299(6):646–655.

96. Gattinoni L, Caironi P, Cressoni M, et al. Lung recruitment in patients with the acute respiratory distress syndrome. N Engl J Med 2006; 354(17):1775–1786.
97. Derdak S, Mehta S, Stewart TE, et al. High-frequency oscillatory ventilation for acute respiratory distress syndrome in adults: a randomized, controlled trial. Am J Respir Crit Care Med 2002; 166(6):801–808.
98. Bollen CW, van Well GT, Sherry T, et al. High frequency oscillatory ventilation compared with conventional mechanical ventilation in adult respiratory distress syndrome: a randomized controlled trial [ISRCTN24242669]. Crit Care 2005; 9(4):R430–R439.
99. Chan KP, Stewart TE, Mehta S. High-frequency oscillatory ventilation for adult patients with ARDS. Chest 2007; 131(6):1907–1916.
100. Oyarzun MJ, Stevens P, Clements JA. Effect of lung collapse on alveolar surfactant in rabbits subjected to unilateral pneumothorax. Exp Lung Res 1989; 15(6):909–924.
101. Albert RK, Lakshminarayan S, Hildebrandt J, et al. Increased surface tension favors pulmonary edema formation in anesthetized dogs' lungs. J Clin Invest 1979; 63(5):1015–1018.
102. D'Angelo E, Pecchiari M, Baraggia P, et al. Low-volume ventilation causes peripheral airway injury and increased airway resistance in normal rabbits. J Appl Physiol 2002; 92(3):949–956.
103. Rimensberger PC, Cox PN, Frndova H, et al. The open lung during small tidal volume ventilation: concepts of recruitment and "optimal" positive end-expiratory pressure. Crit Care Med 1999; 27(9):1946–1952.
104. Yoder BA, Siler-Khodr T, Winter VT, et al. High-frequency oscillatory ventilation: effects on lung function, mechanics, and airway cytokines in the immature baboon model for neonatal chronic lung disease. Am J Respir Crit Care Med 2000; 162(5):1867–1876.
105. Sugiura M, McCulloch PR, Wren S, et al. Ventilator pattern influences neutrophil influx and activation in atelectasis-prone rabbit lung. J Appl Physiol 1994; 77(3):1355–1365.
106. McCulloch PR, Forkert PG, Froese AB. Lung volume maintenance prevents lung injury during high frequency oscillatory ventilation in surfactant-deficient rabbits. Am Rev Respir Dis 1988; 137(5):1185–1192.
107. Del Maschio A, Zanetti A, Corada M, et al. Polymorphonuclear leukocyte adhesion triggers the disorganization of endothelial cell-to-cell adherens junctions. J Cell Biol 1996; 135(2):497–510.
108. Ukropec JA, Hollinger MK, Salva SM, et al. SHP2 association with VE-cadherin complexes in human endothelial cells is regulated by thrombin. J Biol Chem 2000; 275(8):5983–5986.
109. Hirata A, Baluk P, Fujiwara T, et al. Location of focal silver staining at endothelial gaps in inflamed venules examined by scanning electron microscopy. Am J Physiol 1995; 269(3, pt 1):L403–L418.
110. Tinsley JH, De Lanerolle P, Wilson E, et al. Myosin light chain kinase transference induces myosin light chain activation and endothelial hyperpermeability. Am J Physiol Cell Physiol 2000; 279(4):C1285–C1289.
111. Wysolmerski RB, Lagunoff D. Regulation of permeabilized endothelial cell retraction by myosin phosphorylation. Am J Physiol 1991; 261(1, pt 1):C32–C40.
112. Garcia JG, Verin AD, Herenyiova M, et al. Adherent neutrophils activate endothelial myosin light chain kinase: role in transendothelial migration. J Appl Physiol 1998; 84(5):1817–1821.
113. Shi S, Garcia JG, Roy S, et al. Involvement of c-Src in diperoxovanadate-induced endothelial cell barrier dysfunction. Am J Physiol Lung Cell Mol Physiol 2000; 279(3):L441–L451.
114. Ridley AJ, Hall A. The small GTP-binding protein rho regulates the assembly of focal adhesions and actin stress fibers in response to growth factors. Cell 1992; 70(3):389–399.
115. Petrache I, Verin AD, Crow MT, et al. Differential effect of MLC kinase in TNF-alpha-induced endothelial cell apoptosis and barrier dysfunction. Am J Physiol Lung Cell Mol Physiol 2001; 280(6):L1168–L1178.
116. Rousseau S, Houle F, Kotanides H, et al. Vascular endothelial growth factor (VEGF)-driven actin-based motility is mediated by VEGFR2 and requires concerted activation of

stress-activated protein kinase 2 (SAPK2/p38) and geldanamycin-sensitive phosphorylation of focal adhesion kinase. J Biol Chem 2000; 275(14):10661–10672.

117. Zhao Y, Davis HW. Endotoxin causes phosphorylation of MARCKS in pulmonary vascular endothelial cells. J Cell Biochem 2000; 79(3):496–505.

118. Schneider GB, Hamano H, Cooper LF. In vivo evaluation of hsp27 as an inhibitor of actin polymerization: hsp27 limits actin stress fiber and focal adhesion formation after heat shock. J Cell Physiol 1998; 177:575–584.

119. Borbiev T, Birukova A, Liu F, et al. p38 MAP kinase-dependent regulation of endothelial cell permeability. Am J Physiol Lung Cell Mol Physiol 2004; 287(5):L911–L918.

120. Meyer CJ, Alenghat FJ, Rim P, et al. Mechanical control of cyclic AMP signalling and gene transcription through integrins. Nat Cell Biol 2000; 2(9):666–668.

121. Bhullar IS, Li YS, Miao H, et al. Fluid shear stress activation of IkappaB kinase is integrin-dependent. J Biol Chem 1998; 273(46):30544–30549.

122. Li S, Kim M, Hu YL, et al. Fluid shear stress activation of focal adhesion kinase. Linking to mitogen-activated protein kinases. J Biol Chem 1997; 272(48):30455–30462.

123. Schwachtgen JL, Houston P, Campbell C, et al. Fluid shear stress activation of egr-1 transcription in cultured human endothelial and epithelial cells is mediated via the extracellular signal-related kinase 1/2 mitogen-activated protein kinase pathway. J Clin Invest 1998; 101(11):2540–2549.

124. Chicurel ME, Singer RH, Meyer CJ, et al. Integrin binding and mechanical tension induce movement of mRNA and ribosomes to focal adhesions. Nature 1998; 392(6677):730–733.

125. Berrios JC, Schroeder MA, Hubmayr RD. Mechanical properties of alveolar epithelial cells in culture. J Appl Physiol 2001; 91(1):65–73.

126. Cai S, Pestic-Dragovich L, O'Donnell ME, et al. Regulation of cytoskeletal mechanics and cell growth by myosin light chain phosphorylation. Am J Physiol 1998; 275(5, pt 1):C1349–C1356.

127. Liu M, Qin Y, Liu J, et al. Mechanical strain induces pp60src activation and translocation to cytoskeleton in fetal rat lung cells. J Biol Chem 1996; 271(12):7066–7071.

128. Liu M, Xu J, Liu J, et al. Mechanical strain-enhanced fetal lung cell proliferation is mediated by phospholipase C and D and protein kinase C. Am J Physiol 1995; 268(5, pt 1):L729–L738.

129. Trepat X, Deng L, An SS, et al. Universal physical responses to stretch in the living cell. Nature 2007; 447(7144):592–595.

130. Oudin S, Pugin J. Role of MAP kinase activation in interleukin-8 production by human BEAS-2B bronchial epithelial cells submitted to cyclic stretch. Am J Respir Cell Mol Biol 2002; 27(1):107–114.

131. Correa-Meyer E, Pesce L, Guerrero C, et al. Cyclic stretch activates ERK1/2 via G proteins and EGFR in alveolar epithelial cells. Am J Physiol Lung Cell Mol Physiol 2002; 282(5):L883–L891.

132. Simon BA, Easley RB, Grigoryev DN, et al. Microarray analysis of regional cellular responses to local mechanical stress in acute lung injury. Am J Physiol Lung Cell Mol Physiol 2006; 291(5):L851–L861.

133. Swartz MA, Tschumperlin DJ, Kamm RD, et al. Mechanical stress is communicated between different cell types to elicit matrix remodeling. Proc Natl Acad Sci U S A 2001; 98(11):6180–6185.

134. Tschumperlin DJ, Dai G, Maly IV, et al. Mechanotransduction through growth-factor shedding into the extracellular space. Nature 2004; 429(6987):83–86.

135. Torday JS, Rehan VK. Stretch-stimulated surfactant synthesis is coordinated by the paracrine actions of PTHrP and leptin. Am J Physiol Lung Cell Mol Physiol 2002; 283(1):L130–L135.

136. Gutierrez JA, Ertsey R, Scavo LM, et al. Mechanical distention modulates alveolar epithelial cell phenotypic expression by transcriptional regulation. Am J Respir Cell Mol Biol 1999; 21(2):223–229.

137. Nakamura T, Liu M, Mourgeon E, et al. Mechanical strain and dexamethasone selectively increase surfactant protein C and tropoelastin gene expression. Am J Physiol Lung Cell Mol Physiol 2000; 278(5):L974–L980.
138. Wirtz HR, Dobbs LG. Calcium mobilization and exocytosis after one mechanical stretch of lung epithelial cells. Science 1990; 250(4985):1266–1269.
139. Faridy EE. Effect of ventilation on movement of surfactant in airways. Respir Physiol 1976; 27(3):323–334.
140. Faridy EE, Permutt S, Riley RL. Effect of ventilation on surface forces in excised dogs' lungs. J Appl Physiol 1966; 21(5):1453–1462.
141. McClenahan JB, Urtnowski A. Effect of ventilation on surfactant, and its turnover rate. J Appl Physiol 1967; 23(2):215–220.
142. Veldhuizen RA, Tremblay LN, Govindarajan A, et al. Pulmonary surfactant is altered during mechanical ventilation of isolated rat lung. Crit Care Med 2000; 28(7):2545–2551.
143. Yukitake K, Brown CL, Schlueter MA, et al. Surfactant apoprotein A modifies the inhibitory effect of plasma proteins on surfactant activity in vivo. Pediatr Res 1995; 37(1):21–25.
144. Veldhuizen RA, Welk B, Harbottle R, et al. Mechanical ventilation of isolated rat lungs changes the structure and biophysical properties of surfactant. J Appl Physiol 2002; 92(3):1169–1175.
145. Cockshutt AM, Weitz J, Possmayer F. Pulmonary surfactant-associated protein A enhances the surface activity of lipid extract surfactant and reverses inhibition by blood proteins in vitro. Biochemistry 1990; 29(36):8424–8429.
146. Veldhuizen RA, Slutsky AS, Joseph M, et al. Effects of mechanical ventilation of isolated mouse lungs on surfactant and inflammatory cytokines. Eur Respir J 2001; 17(3):488–494.
147. Malloy JL, Veldhuizen RA, Lewis JF. Effects of ventilation on the surfactant system in sepsis-induced lung injury. J Appl Physiol 2000; 88(2):401–408.
148. Ogawa A, Brown CL, Schlueter MA, et al. Lung function, surfactant apoprotein content, and level of PEEP in prematurely delivered rabbits. J Appl Physiol 1994; 77(4):1840–1849.
149. Ito Y, Veldhuizen RA, Yao LJ, et al. Ventilation strategies affect surfactant aggregate conversion in acute lung injury. Am J Respir Crit Care Med 1997; 155(2):493–499.
150. Krause M, Olsson T, Law AB, et al. Effect of volume recruitment on response to surfactant treatment in rabbits with lung injury. Am J Respir Crit Care Med 1997; 156(3, pt 1):862–866.
151. Krause MF, Jakel C, Haberstroh J, et al. Alveolar recruitment promotes homogeneous surfactant distribution in a piglet model of lung injury. Pediatr Res 2001; 50(1):34–43.
152. Clements JA. Lung surfactant: a personal perspective. Annu Rev Physiol 1997; 59:1–21.
153. Baker CS, Evans TW, Randle BJ, et al. Damage to surfactant-specific protein in acute respiratory distress syndrome. Lancet 1999; 353(9160):1232–1237.
154. Laffey JG, Engelberts D, Kavanagh BP. Buffering hypercapnic acidosis worsens acute lung injury. Am J Respir Crit Care Med 2000; 161(1):141–146.
155. Laffey JG, Tanaka M, Engelberts D, et al. Therapeutic hypercapnia reduces pulmonary and systemic injury following in vivo lung reperfusion. Am J Respir Crit Care Med 2000; 162(6):2287–2294.
156. Broccard AF, Hotchkiss JR, Vannay C, et al. Protective effects of hypercapnic acidosis on ventilator-induced lung injury. Am J Respir Crit Care Med 2001; 164(5):802–806.
157. Pugin J, Dunn-Siegrist I, Dufour J, et al. Cyclic stretch of human lung cells induces an acidification and promotes bacterial growth. Am J Respir Cell Mol Biol 2008; 38(3):362–370.
158. Ranieri VM, Suter PM, Tortorella C, et al. Effect of mechanical ventilation on inflammatory mediators in patients with acute respiratory distress syndrome: a randomized controlled trial. JAMA 1999; 282(1):54–61.
159. Ware LB, Eisner MD, Thompson BT, et al. Significance of von Willebrand factor in septic and nonseptic patients with acute lung injury. Am J Respir Crit Care Med 2004; 170(7):766–772.

160. Eisner MD, Parsons P, Matthay MA, et al. Plasma surfactant protein levels and clinical outcomes in patients with acute lung injury. Thorax 2003; 58(11):983–988.

161. Parsons PE, Matthay MA, Ware LB, et al. Elevated plasma levels of soluble TNF receptors are associated with morbidity and mortality in patients with acute lung injury. Am J Physiol Lung Cell Mol Physiol 2005; 288(3):L426–L431.

162. Meduri GU, Headley S, Kohler G, et al. Persistent elevation of inflammatory cytokines predicts a poor outcome in ARDS. Plasma IL-1 beta and IL-6 levels are consistent and efficient predictors of outcome over time. Chest 1995; 107(4):1062–1073.

163. Goodman RB, Strieter RM, Martin DP, et al. Inflammatory cytokines in patients with persistence of the acute respiratory distress syndrome. Am J Respir Crit Care Med 1996; 154(3, pt 1):602–611.

164. Park WY, Goodman RB, Steinberg KP, et al. Cytokine balance in the lungs of patients with acute respiratory distress syndrome. Am J Respir Crit Care Med 2001; 164(10, pt 1):1896–1903.

165. Wrigge H, Zinserling J, Stuber F. Effects of mechanical ventilation on release of cytokines into systemic circulation in patients with normal pulmonary function. Anesthesiology 2000; 93:1413–1417.

166. Frank JA, Parsons PE, Matthay MA. Pathogenetic significance of biological markers of ventilator-associated lung injury in experimental and clinical studies. Chest 2006; 130(6):1906–1914.

167. Wrigge H, Uhlig U, Zinserling J, et al. The effects of different ventilatory settings on pulmonary and systemic inflammatory responses during major surgery. Anesth Analg 2004; 98(3):775–781, table.

168. Tsangaris I, Lekka ME, Kitsiouli E, et al. Bronchoalveolar lavage alterations during prolonged ventilation of patients without acute lung injury. Eur Respir J 2003; 21(3):495–501.

169. Imanaka H, Shimaoka M, Matsuura N, et al. Ventilator-induced lung injury is associated with neutrophil infiltration, macrophage activation, and TGF-beta 1 mRNA upregulation in rat lungs. Anesth Analg 2001; 92(2):428–436.

170. Ricard JD, Dreyfuss D, Saumon G. Production of inflammatory cytokines in ventilator-induced lung injury: a reappraisal. Am J Respir Crit Care Med 2001; 163(5):1176–1180.

171. Tremblay L, Valenza F, Ribeiro SP, et al. Injurious ventilatory strategies increase cytokines and c-fos m-RNA expression in an isolated rat lung model. J Clin Invest 1997; 99(5):944–952.

172. Imai Y, Kawano T, Iwamoto S, et al. Intratracheal anti-tumor necrosis factor-alpha antibody attenuates ventilator-induced lung injury in rabbits. J Appl Physiol 1999; 87(2):510–515.

173. Blackwell TS, Christman JW. The role of nuclear factor-kappa B in cytokine gene regulation. Am J Respir Cell Mol Biol 1997; 17(1):3–9.

174. Nakamura T, Malloy J, McCaig L, et al. Mechanical ventilation of isolated septic rat lungs: effects on surfactant and inflammatory cytokines. J Appl Physiol 2001; 91(2):811–820.

175. Steinberg JM, Schiller HJ, Halter JM, et al. Alveolar instability causes early ventilator-induced lung injury independent of neutrophils. Am J Respir Crit Care Med 2004; 169(1):57–63.

176. Frank JA, Matthay MA. Science review: mechanisms of ventilator-induced injury. Crit Care 2003; 7(3):233–241.

177. Narimanbekov IO, Rozycki HJ. Effect of IL-1 blockade on inflammatory manifestations of acute ventilator-induced lung injury in a rabbit model. Exp Lung Res 1995; 21(2):239–254.

178. Belperio JA, Keane MP, Burdick MD, et al. Critical role for CXCR2 and CXCR2 ligands during the pathogenesis of ventilator-induced lung injury. J Clin Invest 2002; 110(11):1703–1716.

179. Held HD, Boettcher S, Hamann L, et al. Ventilation-induced chemokine and cytokine release is associated with activation of nuclear factor-kappaB and is blocked by steroids. Am J Respir Crit Care Med 2001; 163(3, pt 1):711–716.

180. Lionetti V, Lisi A, Patrucco E, et al. Lack of phosphoinositide 3-kinase-gamma attenuates ventilator-induced lung injury. Crit Care Med 2006; 34(1):134–141.
181. Kuebler WM, Parthasarathi K, Wang PM, et al. A novel signaling mechanism between gas and blood compartments of the lung. J Clin Invest 2000; 105(7):905–913.
182. Vlahakis NE, Schroeder MA, Limper AH, et al. Stretch induces cytokine release by alveolar epithelial cells in vitro. Am J Physiol 1999; 277(1, pt 1):L167–L173.
183. Ning Q, Wang X. Role of Rel A and IkappaB of nuclear factor kappaB in the release of interleukin-8 by cyclic mechanical strain in human alveolar type II epithelial cells A549. Respirology 2007; 12(6):792–798.
184. Ning QM, Wang XR. Response of alveolar type II epithelial cells to mechanical stretch and lipopolysaccharide. Respiration 2007; 74(5):579–585.
185. Quinn D, Tager A, Joseph PM, et al. Stretch-induced mitogen-activated protein kinase activation and interleukin-8 production in type II alveolar cells. Chest 1999; 116(Suppl. 1): 89S–90S.
186. Li LF, Ouyang B, Choukroun G, et al. Stretch-induced IL-8 depends on c-Jun NH2-terminal and nuclear factor-kappaB-inducing kinases. Am J Physiol Lung Cell Mol Physiol 2003; 285(2):L464–L475.
187. MacGillivray MK, Cruz TF, McCulloch CA. The recruitment of the interleukin-1 (IL-1) receptor-associated kinase (IRAK) into focal adhesion complexes is required for IL-1beta-induced ERK activation. J Biol Chem 2000; 275(31):23509–23515.
188. Dunn I, Pugin J. Mechanical ventilation of various human lung cells in vitro: identification of the macrophage as the main producer of inflammatory mediators. Chest 1999; 116(Suppl. 1):95S–97S.
189. Kurdowska A, Miller EJ, Noble JM, et al. Anti-IL-8 autoantibodies in alveolar fluid from patients with the adult respiratory distress syndrome. J Immunol 1996; 157(6):2699–2706.
190. Miller EJ, Cohen AB, Matthay MA. Increased interleukin-8 concentrations in the pulmonary edema fluid of patients with acute respiratory distress syndrome from sepsis. Crit Care Med 1996; 24(9):1448–1454.
191. Lentsch AB, Czermak BJ, Bless NM, et al. Essential role of alveolar macrophages in intrapulmonary activation of NF-kappaB. Am J Respir Cell Mol Biol 1999; 20(4):692–698.
192. Grembowicz KP, Sprague D, McNeil PL. Temporary disruption of the plasma membrane is required for c-fos expression in response to mechanical stress. Mol Biol Cell 1999; 10(4):1247–1257.
193. McRitchie DI, Isowa N, Edelson JD, et al. Production of tumour necrosis factor alpha by primary cultured rat alveolar epithelial cells. Cytokine 2000; 12(6):644–654.
194. Schwartz MD, Moore EE, Moore FA, et al. Nuclear factor-kappa B is activated in alveolar macrophages from patients with acute respiratory distress syndrome. Crit Care Med 1996; 24(8):1285–1292.
195. Liu C, Yao J, de Belle I, et al. The transcription factor EGR-1 suppresses transformation of human fibrosarcoma HT1080 cells by coordinated induction of transforming growth factor-beta1, fibronectin, and plasminogen activator inhibitor-1. J Biol Chem 1999; 274(7):4400–4411.
196. Ressler B, Lee RT, Randell SH, et al. Molecular responses of rat tracheal epithelial cells to transmembrane pressure. Am J Physiol Lung Cell Mol Physiol 2000; 278(6):L1264–L1272.
197. Silverman ES, Collins T. Pathways of Egr-1-mediated gene transcription in vascular biology. Am J Pathol 1999; 154(3):665–670.
198. Kawano T, Mori S, Cybulsky M, et al. Effect of granulocyte depletion in a ventilated surfactant-depleted lung. J Appl Physiol 1987; 62(1):27–33.
199. Choudhury S, Wilson MR, Goddard ME, et al. Mechanisms of early pulmonary neutrophil sequestration in ventilator-induced lung injury in mice. Am J Physiol Lung Cell Mol Physiol 2004; 287(5):L902–L910.

200. Murphy DB, Cregg N, Tremblay L, et al. Adverse ventilatory strategy causes pulmonary-to-systemic translocation of endotoxin. Am J Respir Crit Care Med 2000; 162(1):27–33.
201. von Bethmann AN, Brasch F, Nusing R, et al. Hyperventilation induces release of cytokines from perfused mouse lung. Am J Respir Crit Care Med 1998; 157(1):263–272.
202. Douzinas EE, Tsidemiadou PD, Pitaridis MT, et al. The regional production of cytokines and lactate in sepsis-related multiple organ failure. Am J Respir Crit Care Med 1997; 155(1): 53–59.
203. Marshall JC, Cook DJ, Christou NV, et al. Multiple organ dysfunction score: a reliable descriptor of a complex clinical outcome. Crit Care Med 1995; 23(10):1638–1652.
204. Nahum A, Hoyt J, Schmitz L, et al. Effect of mechanical ventilation strategy on dissemination of intratracheally instilled Escherichia coli in dogs. Crit Care Med 1997; 25(10):1733–1743.
205. Verbrugge SJ, Sorm V, van 't Veen A, et al. Lung overinflation without positive end-expiratory pressure promotes bacteremia after experimental Klebsiella pneumoniae inoculation. Intensive Care Med 1998; 24(2):172–177.
206. Ozcan PE, Cakar N, Tugrul S, et al. The effects of airway pressure and inspiratory time on bacterial translocation. Anesth Analg 2007; 104(2):391–396.
207. van Kaam AH, Lachmann RA, Herting E, et al. Reducing atelectasis attenuates bacterial growth and translocation in experimental pneumonia. Am J Respir Crit Care Med 2004; 169(9):1046–1053.
208. Schortgen F, Bouadma L, Joly-Guillou ML, et al. Infectious and inflammatory dissemination are affected by ventilation strategy in rats with unilateral pneumonia. Intensive Care Med 2004; 30(4):693–701.
209. Lachmann RA, van Kaam AH, Haitsma JJ, et al. High positive end-expiratory pressure levels promote bacterial translocation in experimental pneumonia. Intensive Care Med 2007; 33(10):1800–1804.
210. Love R, Choe E, Lippton H, et al. Positive end-expiratory pressure decreases mesenteric blood flow despite normalization of cardiac output. J Trauma 1995; 39(2):195–199.
211. Guery B, Neviere R, Fialdes P. Mechanical ventilation regiment induces intestinal permeability changes in a rat model. Am J Respir Crit Care Med 2002; 165:A505.
212. Imai Y, Parodo J, kajikawa O,et al. Injurious mechanical ventilation and end-organ epithelial cell apoptosis and organ dysfunction in an experimental model of acute respiratory distress syndrome. JAMA 2003; 289(16):2104–2112.
213. Brower RG, Fessler HE. Mechanical ventilation in acute lung injury and acute respiratory distress syndrome. Clin Chest Med 2000; 21(3):491–510, viii.
214. Slutsky AS, Tremblay LN. Multiple system organ failure. Is mechanical ventilation a contributing factor? Am J Respir Crit Care Med 1998; 157(6, pt 1):1721–1725.

9

Sepsis in the Acute Respiratory Distress Syndrome: Treatment Implications

ARTHUR P. WHEELER and TODD W. RICE

Division of Allergy, Pulmonary and Critical Care Medicine, Department of Medicine, Vanderbilt University School of Medicine, Nashville, Tennessee, U.S.A.

I. Relationship Between Sepsis and Acute Lung Injury

The interrelationship of sepsis (i.e., systemic inflammatory response with presumed infection) and acute lung injury (ALI) is complex. Sepsis, is the most common cause of ALI, accounting for 40–50% of all cases (1,2) and a reciprocal relationship exists in that the lung is the most common site of infection leading to the development of sepsis (3). When an acute organ system dysfunction occurs in patients with sepsis, the syndrome is termed "severe sepsis" (4). ALI is the most common organ dysfunction qualifying patients for the diagnosis of severe sepsis. Consequently, the rapidly increasing incidence of severe sepsis results in evermore cases of lung injury (5). Thus, ALI is often the result of sepsis and by virtue of an acquired vulnerability to infection; ALI victims often develop secondary sepsis (6).

Because pneumonia is the etiology of sepsis in the majority of cases, it is not surprising the lung malfunctions. However, the concurrence of pneumonia and ALI introduces uncertainty as to whether the physiological abnormalities seen represent merely pneumonia or the more diffuse and significant problem of ALI. Patients who develop severe sepsis typically exhibit two or three organ dysfunctions at the time of recognition, but the predominant failing organ is usually the lung (7). Overall, nearly 90% of patients developing severe sepsis have pulmonary dysfunction sufficient to require supplemental oxygen (2) with approximately 40% of patients eventually meeting ARDS criteria (8). Fewer— approximately one third of all patients—will meet ARDS criteria at the time severe sepsis is recognized (9). Not only is the lung the most common organ affected by sepsis, but it is also usually the *first* organ to malfunction (3,7,9). Complaints of dyspnea, tachypnea, and hypoxemia are sentinel findings. The progression from the first signs of lung dysfunction to maximal severity is variable, typically ranging from a few hours to a day (3).

II. Pathophysiological Similarities Between Sepsis and ALI

The pathophysiology of sepsis is substantially more complex than simply excessive inflammation. It also involves an exuberant coagulopathic response and impaired fibrinolysis (10–13). Similar pathophysiology has been described in ALI. Abundant evidence of excessive lung inflammation in ARDS victims exists, including increased numbers of pulmonary leukocytes and inflammatory cytokines (14). Moreover, increased tissue factor expression and fibrin generation lead to capillary thrombosis and alveolar filling (15–18).

In addition to the increased thrombotic tendency, normal fibrinolysis is impaired, as evidenced by elevated plasminogen activator inhibitor-1 levels (15,19,20). Long considered to be a problem predominately of vascular endothelium, it is now clear that ALI results in epithelial dysfunction as well (21) and in this way may predispose to secondary lung infection.

Why the lung is so commonly injured in sepsis remains unclear. In addition to being the most common infection site leading to sepsis, the lung is also the only organ to accept the full cardiac output. The lungs' extensive vascular capillary network presents a huge surface area for endothelial cell exposure to exogenous and endogenous toxins. The lung also has a particularly delicate structure where luxuriantly perfused endothelium and environmentally exposed epithelium are separated by a tiny interstitial space. Furthermore, the lung contains a huge number of macrophages, cells that easily stimulated by both exogenous and endogenous toxins and serve as potent generators of both inflammation and coagulation.

III. Sepsis as a Complication of ALI

Because ALI survivors usually endure a one- to two-week intensive care unit (ICU) stay connected to a mechanical ventilator, they incur significant risk for superimposed infection. Intravenous and urinary catheter–associated infections and ventilator-associated pneumonia (VAP) are the most common infectious problems.

Advanced age, altered mental status, pre-existing lung injury, need for mechanical ventilation, use of a tracheal or gastric tube, and gastric acid suppression have all been reported as risk factors for VAP. Unfortunately, many of these reports fail to account for time on the ventilator (22,23). Animal models suggest excessive lung stretch, especially when coupled with low levels of positive end-expiratory pressure (PEEP), increase susceptibility to infection and bacteremia (24). Mechanical ventilation itself increases the risk of pneumonia among hospitalized patients between 7- and 21-fold (25,26), translating into a 1–3% risk for developing VAP per day of mechanical ventilation (27). In studies using only clinical criteria, the incidence of VAP approaches 70% in ARDS victims (28), 50% higher than in mechanically ventilated patients without ARDS. However, when strict bacteriological criteria are required, the incidence is closer to 20% (29). VAP among patients with ARDS is associated with an increased mortality rate (25,26,30).

As in the lung, distinguishing simple colonization from true infection in the urinary tract can be difficult. Despite the nearly 3% daily incidence of bacteriuria, urinary tract infections rarely cause bacteremia or severe sepsis without obstruction and treatment is usually highly effective (31). Although vascular catheter-related infections may be less common than lung or urinary tact infections, they carry a substantial risk for the development of bacteremia and sepsis. In fact, most episodes of bacteremia in the ICU are now attributed to vascular catheters (32), and up to 70% of colonized central venous catheters result in bacteremia (33). The incidence of severe sepsis when catheter-related bacteremia occurs is significant, and the resulting illness is often costly and lethal (34,35).

IV. Preventing Infection in ALI and ARDS
A. Pneumonia

Due to the relatively high incidence of VAP in patients with ALI and its association with morbidity and mortality, approaches to prevention, early diagnosis, and effective

Table 1 Strategies for Preventing Secondary Infections in Patients with ALI

Ventilator-associated pneumonia
  Hand washing
  Reduce the duration of mechanical ventilation
    Volume and pressure-limited ventilation strategy (1)
    Intermittent bolus dosing of sedation
    Daily spontaneous breathing trials coupled with patient awakening trials (36,37)
  Elevate the head of the bed 30–45° whenever possible (38,39)
  Avoid routine changes of ventilator tubing (40–42)
  Use of closed suctioning systems with ventilator (43,44)
  Subglottic suctioning (45–47)
  Avoid transnasal tubes (i.e., use OG instead of NG, oral ETT instead of nasal ETT)
  Peptic ulcer prophylaxis[a]
  Use of heat–moisture exchange devices (41)[a]
  Use of oral antibiotic paste or nonabsorbable GI antibiotics[a]
  ICU-wide scheduled rotation of antibiotics[a]
  Early enteral feeding[a]
  Immunonutrition[a]

Catheter-related bloodstream infections
  Use peripheral intravenous lines whenever possible (48–50)
  Evaluate continued need for central venous lines daily and remove when not needed
  Central venous catheters placed by experienced operator
  Use cholorhexidine skin decontamination (51)
  Use complete sterile barrier precautions
    Hand washing
    Full body drape
    Long-sleeve gowns
    Sterile gloves
    Nonsterile mask
    Nonsterile cap
  Nurse with checklist to ensure complete sterile barrier precautions used (52)
  Site selection (subclavian preferred over jugular; jugular preferred over femoral) for
    nontunneled catheters (53–56)
  Use tunneled catheters if expected to be needed for prolonged time
  If infected, change catheter via new puncture site; avoid changes of infected catheters over
    guidewires
  Limit frequent entry to catheter or IV tubing system
  Antibiotic/antiseptic-treated catheters (57–62)[a]
  Avoid routine central venous catheter changes (63–65)[a]

Urinary tract infections
  Evaluate the need for the urinary catheter on a daily basis and discontinue as soon as possible
  Keep urinary collection bag well below the level of the bladder
  Antibiotic/antiseptic-coated urinary catheters[a]

[a]Some controversy exists about the effectiveness of these strategies.
Abbreviations: OG, orogastric; NG, nasogastric; ETT, endotracheal tube; GI, gastrointestinal.

treatment, often in the form of "VAP bundles" have become a priority (Table 1) (66,67). Since VAP risk is proportional to time on the ventilator, the simplest method of reducing infection and sepsis risk is to reduce the duration of mechanical ventilation. A safe, economical method to accomplish this goal is to conduct daily spontaneous breathing trials in patients meeting weaning eligibility criteria (36,68). Doing so reduces the average time on the ventilator by several days. Protocols to reduce the use of sedatives facilitate awakening and progression to spontaneous breathing trials are important adjuncts (37,69).

The most common sequence hypothesized for development of pneumonia in ALI is rapid colonization of the upper airway with subsequent aspiration and seeding of the lung days later (70,71). Hence, methods to decrease upper airway colonization and reduce aspiration may be beneficial. Elevating the head of the bed in ventilated patients is a safe and highly effective method of preventing VAP (38,39), but has proven more difficult to implement in practice than one might expect (72). Measures to reduce the oral microbial burden such as regular dental hygiene and disinfectant mouth rinses are simple and beneficial but time consuming (73–76).

Small reports of up to 50% reductions in VAP rates using endotracheal tubes capable of subglottic suctioning are enticing but evidence remains mixed (45,46) and reductions in infection have failed to translate into improved survival or reduced lengths of stay (47). Subglottic suctioning appears most effective in the highest risk patients (e.g., ventilation >5 days), but in practice it is difficult to prospectively identify such patients, requiring use of such tubes in many patients unnecessarily. Another problem is impaction of the secretion clearance channel, rendering the tube ineffective (77). Finally, the higher cost of specialized tubes and failure to demonstrate improvement in survival or lengths of stay have discouraged widespread use (78).

Another source of VAP is contaminated ventilator tubing condensate. The introduction of even a tiny inoculum into the warm moist circuit can result in proliferation of a huge number of organisms. Closed suction systems prevent such seeding (43,44). Paradoxically, frequent replacement of the circuit is associated with higher tubing colonization and subsequent infection rates (40–42). This situation is analogous to intravenous catheters where frequent entry is also associated with increased infection rates. Efforts to prevent "rain out" of water in ventilator tubing have also been tried. Heat–moisture exchange devices (HMEs) have been utilized to maintain the respiratory circuit humidity without using heated humidification. At least one study has shown a reduction in VAP rates using HMEs, but unfortunately these devices have two significant limitations: they introduce dead space into the circuit, and the moisture exchanging properties become less effective as minute ventilation increases (79,80). Heating the ventilator tubing directly is a second approach to prevent condensation. This method has the advantage of not increasing dead space but has yet to gain wide popularity, perhaps because of increased costs in the face of limited data supporting improved outcomes (41,81).

A simple technique to reduce VAP risk is avoidance of transnasal tubes (82). By obstructing ostia, nasal tubes predispose to sinus colonization and inflammation. When VAP develops in nasally intubated patients, the correlation between organisms in the sinuses and the lung is high. Some have even suggested that avoiding tracheal tubes altogether and using noninvasive ventilation could further reduce the VAP risk (83–85). The theoretical appeal of this approach is strong but often negated by the practical problem of being unable to adequately ventilate and oxygenate the ALI victim.

Use of oral antibiotic paste or nonabsorbable gastrointestinal antibiotics (selective digestive tract decontamination) to reduce enteral contamination has been extensively studied but remains controversial. While some studies of surgical patients found benefit, most studies indicate that administration of oral antibiotic paste with or without systemic therapy reduces infection risk temporarily but rapidly increases microbial resistance (86–90). Similarly, neither the administration of aerosolized antibiotics, nor acute vaccination has yet been proven to decrease the incidence of VAP (91,92). Scheduled rotation of antibiotics ICU-wide is another strategy designed to decrease the risk of VAP, particularly that from resistant organisms. The utility of antibiotic class switching remains controversial, and logistical problems in implementing such a strategy are substantial (93–95).

Conflicting data exist regarding the relationship of acid suppression and enteral nutrition practices to VAP risk. Though the evidence is not robust, passage of any device across the lower esophageal sphincter increases the risk of reflux, aspiration, and VAP (96). Drugs used to raise stomach pH to prevent gastrointestinal bleeding have been shown to increase the number of microorganisms in the normally sterile stomach (97). It is argued that if refluxed and aspirated, these organisms can be a source for VAP. Although data suggest that both of these are, and are not, a significant risk for VAP (98,99), on balance, data favor the use of an acid-suppressing drug to decrease the risk of gastrointestinal bleeding coupled with elevation of the head of the bed.

Although several small studies among mostly surgical patients suggest that enteral nutrition reduces the risk of infectious complications among mechanically ventilated patients, the story is complicated and the mechanism of protection speculative. When clinical benefits from enteral nutrition have been demonstrated, they are most commonly limited to reduced VAP or wound infection rates (100,101). In contrast, other studies indicate early enteral feeding may be associated with an increased risk of aspiration and VAP (102–104). Thus, while enteral feeding likely benefits the nutritional status and may reduce infection risks, optimal timing and route for administration are uncertain. Fortunately, a rational if unproven approach is to begin feeding at a relatively low rate as soon as hemodynamic stability is achieved then rapidly increase the rate as tolerated. Unfortunately, there is no standardized definition of "tolerated," and local practice often results in substantial underfeeding compared to projected requirements (105–107). In an attempt to reduce the risks of reflux, aspiration, and pneumonia, some investigators advocate postpyloric feeding. Although this practice may decrease the risk of reflux and aspiration, it has significant technical limitations. On average it takes much longer to achieve tube placement and the tube is often dislodged from its desired position (108–110). It is quite possible that the lower rates of feeding intolerance and aspiration reported with postpyloric feeding are entirely due to delayed initiation or differences in practice. Immunonutrition, or enteral preparations enhanced with glutamine, arginine, omega-3 fatty acids, and/or antioxidants either singly or in combinations, have been associated with reductions in important clinical endpoints, including nosocomial infection (111–115) in small studies of heterogeneous patient populations. Additional information on the utility of specific immunonutritional formulations will come from additional large-scale clinical trials, some of which are currently underway (116,117).

B. Intravenous Catheters

Due to duration of their insertion, location, and frequency of entry, central venous catheters confer a greater risk of bacteremia than short-term peripheral intravenous lines (48–50). Among critically ill patients, up to three quarters of all episodes of bacteremia can be attributed to catheter-related infection (31) and when bloodstream infection occurs, the risk of severe sepsis and death is high and costs significant. (118). Risk factors for catheter-related infections are well accepted (65,119–127) and lead to basic principles for prevention. Central venous catheters have the lowest infection rates if placement is performed by an experienced operator using complete sterile barrier precautions (123). Enhancing adherence to these complete sterile barrier precautions through the use of checklist verification further decreases catheter-site infections and resultant bacteremia (52). Insertion site also influences the risk of infection; femoral insertions are most likely to be infected, with the internal jugular site being next most likely. Because of catheter stability and relative freedom from exposure to bacteria-laden body fluids, the subclavian site has the lowest infection risk (53–56). Body mass index (BMI) may also influence the risk of infection by catheter site. In patients with high BMIs, femoral lines are more likely to become contaminated compared to jugular lines (128). Substantially, less is known about the infection risk of centrally terminating peripherally inserted lines in the critically ill.

During insertion, skin decontamination with chlorhexidine is superior to povidone iodine combinations and is becoming widely accepted (51). Skin should not be shaved. Firmly anchoring the catheter or hub to the patient is important to reduce motion at the skin/catheter interface. Since most line-related infections begin by skin colonization followed by extension along the subcutaneous tract, the "piston-like" movement of an unsecured catheter can act to "inject" organisms along the tract. Nonetheless, it is somewhat surprising that topical antibiotic ointment application at the insertion site has not been shown to be advantageous. However, the use of nonocclusive dressings and minimizing the number of system entries have been shown to reduce the risk of infection (129–133). Although hotly contested, the *routine* use of antiseptic- or antibiotic-impregnated or -coated catheters is not warranted (57–62). Such catheters offer the greatest benefit for those at highest risk of infection (e.g., burn victims or neutropenic patients). Antibiotic/antiseptic-treated catheters have not gained widespread acceptance predominately because of cost–benefit uncertainties. In contrast, permanent or semipermanent tunneled catheters are at a lower risk of infection and should be considered for patients who require long-term central intravenous access (134).

The risk of line colonization and eventual blood stream infection rises exponentially with time after insertion, with a striking inflection point at about seven days (63). Therefore, limiting the duration of catheters to five to seven days is a defensible practice adopted by many. At odds with this practice are clinical trials of catheter-*changing* strategies that have failed to detect benefit from scheduled changes at three or seven days (64,65). Given the many factors influencing catheter-related infection, the decision to replace catheters should balance infection risks, costs, and insertion risks. At the very least, the need for central catheters should be reconsidered on a daily basis and those that are no longer needed should be removed as soon as possible. Overall, a multifaceted approach to catheter insertion combined with care incorporating best care practices can result in dramatic reduction in catheter-associated infections and its resultant morbidity (52,135–138).

C. Urinary Tract Infection

Perhaps the best strategy to prevent development of severe sepsis from urinary infection is to reconsider the need for urinary catheters on a daily basis and promptly removing those that are not essential. When a catheter is needed keeping the urinary collection bag well below the level of the bladder reduces risk by preventing retrograde flow of contaminated urine into the bladder. Studies evaluating the effectiveness of silver- or antibiotic-impregnated urinary catheters are ongoing.

V. Treating Severe Sepsis in ALI and ARDS
A. Antibiotics and Infection Source Control

When sepsis complicates ALI, prompt eradication of source should be undertaken. Areas of localized infection should be drained (e.g., pleural space, abdominal abscess, urinary tract), necrotic tissue excised, and infected foreign bodies (e.g., intravenous catheters, orthopedic hardware) removed. Knowing a specific organism and its sensitivity allows confidence in and simplification of antimicrobial therapy.

Antimicrobial therapy is advocated for the treatment of severe sepsis but it is amazing how little is known about optimal practice. Despite knowledge limitations, widely accepted longstanding recommendations follow. Antibiotic selection should be guided by the presumed site of infection, Gram stain results, suspected or known organisms, resistance patterns in the community, and the presence of individual host factors affecting immune status (139). Relevant cultures should be obtained, preferably before institution of antimicrobials because significantly fewer organisms will be recovered after treatment (140). Obtaining cultures is prudent, even though many patients will remain culture negative from both bloodstream and nonbloodstream sources (9). When the source of infection is known, especially if the etiological organism is definite, narrowly targeted antimicrobial therapy should be used. However, when the offending organism is uncertain, the site of infection is unclear, or perhaps even when the patient is just desperately ill, broader-spectrum antibiotic therapy is prudent. Among patients with bacteremia, appropriate antibiotic therapy may reduce the risk of shock development and the risk of death by as much as 11–50% (141,142). Likewise, failure to provide appropriate antimicrobial therapy within 24–48 hours is associated with a significantly higher mortality (143).

Even after selecting a reasonable empiric antibiotic combination and giving it promptly, antibiotics have significant limitations. Not all microbes will be covered, nor can all possible resistance be anticipated. In large retrospective surveys or prospective clinical trials, the antibiotics prescribed prove inappropriate for the organism(s) eventually isolated in approximately 10% of patients (7,143). For most infections there are a large number of safe, acceptable, and cost-efficient drug combinations, hence dogmatism should be avoided. Clinicians should have a working knowledge of common nosocomial organisms and local resistance patterns and the decision to treat methicillin-resistant staphlycocci or double cover-resistant gram-negative rods should depend on these patterns. By anticipating the likely pathogens infecting the ALI patient, the best initial therapy can be efficiently provided. In most settings this will include coverage for both gram-negative and gram-positive organisms. Although a mainstay in the treatment of severe sepsis, antibiotics are not a panacea and are not sufficient treatment, as evidenced by persistent overall 30–50% mortality despite appropriate antibiotic treatment (9,142).

Except perhaps for brief delays to obtain cultures, it is difficult to think of a reason to deliberately postpone antimicrobial therapy even though there are not and will never be randomized prospective trials proving a temporal effect. In perhaps the most convincing study of antibiotic timing, significant delays in antibiotic administration were evaluated retrospectively in patients with septic shock and each hour of delay was associated with a substantially increased mortality (144). In contrast, despite garnering a great deal of attention from regulatory and quality organizations, accelerated administration of antibiotics for treatment of community-acquired infections appears to have a small effect (145–147). Early broad-spectrum antibiotic therapy is probably good for individual patients with life-threatening infections, but prolonged unnecessary, overly broad coverage is harmful to both the individual patient and the community. Hence, it is very important to narrow or discontinue broad-spectrum antibiotic therapy when cultures identify a single causative organism or when all cultures remain negative after a reasonable period (48–72 hours) of observation. Failure to do so exposes patients to adverse drug reactions, the high cost of antibiotics and breeds resistance. It is probably equally important to question the traditional duration of antimicrobial therapy for many infections. Studies now suggest that arbitrary reductions in duration of therapy (148,149), or perhaps those guided by laboratory tests such as procalcitonin (150) can safely reduce antimicrobial exposure. Unfortunately, in practice, antimicrobial coverage is often not narrowed, tailored, or shortened in duration despite available culture data.

B. Circulatory Support

Expert consensus recommends replacement of intravascular volume in the range of 20 to 30 mL/kg as the initial circulatory support for patients who develop septic shock (151). This recommendation stems from observations that intravascular deficits result from decreased fluid intake, increased venous capacitance, vascular permeability, and fluid losses (i.e., sweating, vomiting, tachypnea). Effective intravascular volume is further reduced by low plasma oncotic pressure from hypoalbuminemia (152,153). Most accept the tenet that volume repletion should provide adequate organ perfusion while avoiding circulatory overload or exacerbating the degree of pulmonary edema. Although clinical indicators of excessive fluid administration including increasing rales, deteriorating oxygenation, and a worsening chest radiograph seem obvious, the optimal metrics for fluid therapy remain uncertain and controversial. Collectively, improved mentation, a rising blood pressure, falling heart rate, increased urine output, reversal of skin mottling, and prolonged capillary refill times are typically used as evidence of improvement. These observations usually correlate with rising central venous pressure and/or pulmonary artery occlusion pressure.

Wide variation exists in vascular pressure monitoring for patients with ALI. Some physicians choose not to routinely monitor intravascular pressures, while others use a central venous catheter (CVC), and historically about half select a pulmonary artery catheter (PAC) (154). Although the PAC may provide additional hemodynamic data (i.e., pulmonary artery occlusion pressure, cardiac output, and mixed venous oxygen), significant concerns exist about the effectiveness of this device. A large case-control study, which found the risk of death among patients receiving a PAC averaged 20–25% higher than for patients without one (155), spurred numerous prospective investigations. In randomized trials of patients with or at risk for ALI, where fluid and vasoactive drug therapy were not rigidly controlled, demonstrated no benefit of a PAC (156–159). Likewise, a large randomized clinical trial conducted by the NIH ARDS Network combining monitoring with a strict fluid management protocol found no benefit of a PAC, but more complications from its insertion (160). Given these data, the routine insertion of a PAC in patients with ALI with or without sepsis cannot be recommended.

Despite the value selected, the fluid volume required to achieve the goal vascular pressure target is surprisingly high. Over the first day, 5 to 10 L of crystalloid or an equivalent amount of colloid is typically required to maintain filling pressure targets (161,162). Initial resuscitation is usually initiated with repeated rapid infusions of 15 mL/kg or more of crystalloid (e.g., isotonic saline or Ringer's solution). Smaller crystalloid boluses are unlikely to alter hemodynamics. Colloids (e.g., albumin) are preferred by some physicians for patients with hypoalbuminemia, severe hypotension with limited vascular access, or renal failure. If albumin is used, sequential doses of 25 to 50 g are usually given. Equivalent vascular volume expansion may be accomplished faster using colloid than crystalloid because of the smaller volume of infusate needed, but the value of this perceived advantage remains unknown. For patients both deficient in soluble clotting proteins and intravascularly volume depleted, fresh frozen plasma provides an alternative resuscitation fluid but incurs the risks of human blood product exposure including infection and transfusion-related acute lung injury (163). A systematic review found a slightly higher mortality associated with colloid resuscitation in critically ill patients (164), and a prospective trial of starch-based colloid therapy was terminated prematurely because of renal toxicity (165). In distinction, toxicity was not seen in a very large randomized clinical trial of albumin versus crystalloid (166) and a posthoc analysis of the subgroup of patients with sepsis suggested a possible mortality benefit of albumin resuscitation. However, in the absence of definitive data showing superiority, the higher cost of colloids dissuade many physicians from routinely using them.

If, after achieving an acceptable filling pressure, hypotension, oliguria, or a low flow state persist, administration of a vasoactive agent is usually undertaken. Although goals for optimal blood pressure and flow are unknown, a mean arterial pressure above 60 to 70 mm Hg and a cardiac index above 2.5 L/min are common targets (167). Obviously these must be individualized: a young, otherwise healthy patient without vascular disease can likely tolerate a significantly lower blood pressure than an elderly chronically hypertensive patient with extensive vascular disease.

The "right" vasoactive agent probably differs for each patient depending on the pathophysiological problem. For example, in patients with low systemic vascular resistance and normal or high cardiac output, agents with predominately vasoconstrictive activity such as norepinephrine or vasopressin are commonly utilized. For patients with mostly impaired cardiac output, a drug possessing β-adrenergic activity, like dobutamine, may be used. Unfortunately, this approach requires a PAC with its attendant risks and costs to measure cardiac output or calculate systemic vascular resistance (SVR). It also presumes that whatever drug strategy is chosen is safe and effective. The major limitation in selecting vasoactive agents is the paucity of head-to-head comparisons in large well-controlled trials. Although personal preference plays a large role, norepinephrine has emerged as the favored vasopressor for many intensivists because it is easily titrated and reliably raises blood pressure even among patients failing substantial doses of dopamine (168–171). Furthermore, observational studies have suggested a survival benefit with its use compared to dopamine (172,173). Dopamine, used for long because of its purported salutary effects on renal function, has now been proven to not have significant renoprotective activity (174) although it does increase blood pressure.

Vasopressin has gained popularity for patients with refractory hypotension due to vasodilatory shock (175). Depletion of pituitary vasopressin and low plasma levels have been reported in hypotensive patients (176). Replacement with low doses of vasopressin has been successful in raising blood pressure and reducing the need for alternative vasopressors. In a large randomized trial of vasopressin versus norepinephrine in volume replete septic shock, no safety concerns were found but no significant differences in important clinical outcomes were observed between groups overall (177). In one subgroup, patients with "less severe septic shock," defined as requiring less than 15 mcg/min of norepinephrine, vasopressin may offer a survival advantage. Although these survival benefits have not been confirmed in a prospective, randomized trial, the demonstrated safety may reasonably prompt some clinicians to use it in this subgroup. Data on vasopressin as a first line vasopressor agent in patients with septic shock are lacking.

Strategies to produce supranormal oxygen delivery in severe sepsis patients are quite controversial. Among high-risk surgical patients, achieving an arbitrary level of oxygen delivery is associated with a reduction in mortality (178–180), but in studies of other patient populations either no benefit has been demonstrated or high oxygen delivery strategies have been harmful (181–183). Interestingly, the studies in which benefit was demonstrated were typically early intervention or "prophylaxis" studies. This observation has resulted in speculation that it may not be sufficient to raise oxygen delivery to a target level but achieving that goal *early* may be critical. Some argue that this principle is responsible for the success of early goal-directed therapy for resuscitation of patients with septic shock (184). In this study of early resuscitation, patients first had central venous pressure restored with fluid. Subsequently, blood pressure was increased above a target using vasoactive agents. Once blood pressure was in the desired range, red blood cells and/or dobutamine were administered if the central venous saturation remained below 70% and the hematocrit was below or above 30%, respectively. This protocol resulted in significant improvements in hospital and 60-day mortality. These findings suggest that early intervention may be essential but have not been widely adopted (185,186).

C. Ventilatory Support

Optimal ventilatory support requires an adequate airway and an Fio_2 and minute ventilation sufficient to maintain a $Pao_2 \geq 60$ mm Hg or hemoglobin saturation $\geq 88\%$. It is now clear that maintaining a near-normal PCO_2 is a much lower priority than once thought provided the pH is not profoundly depressed or specific contraindications to hypercarbia (e.g., increased intracranial pressure) are not present. The traditional approach to ventilation for patients with ALI was to use tidal volumes of 10 to 15 mL/kg of actual body weight. However, excessive alveolar stretch induced by high tidal volumes can produce barotrauma and incite cytokine release contributing to the development of nonpulmonary organ failures. The ARDS Network trial compared a traditional breath size (12 mL/kg) with a lower tidal volume (6 mL/kg of predicted body weight) reduced even further, if necessary, to maintain plateau pressures of <30 cm H_2O (1). Fio_2 and PEEP were adjusted by protocol to maintain hemoglobin saturations between 88% and 95%. This simple inexpensive strategy resulted in a 22% decrease in hospital mortality, an increase in ventilator-free days, and less nonpulmonary organ dysfunction. Large observational studies suggest that use of traditionally higher tidal volumes in patients without ALI is a significant risk factor for developing lung injury (187,188). Therefore, it is rational to use a reduced tidal volume strategy incorporating management of plateau pressures as a starting point for patients with ALI who lack contraindications and it makes sense to use normal tidal volumes in patients without ALI to minimize risk of ALI development.

Although a volume and pressure limited ventilation strategy is slowly being adopted, controversy exists about the use of high levels of PEEP. Animal studies suggested that higher levels of PEEP were protective for ventilator-induced lung injury. However, numerous large, randomized studies in humans have failed to show a mortality benefit from high PEEP applied without customization to the individual patient (189–191). However, these studies also failed to demonstrate harm from the use of high PEEP. Consequently, a recommendation on the appropriate level of PEEP cannot be made until additional studies involving specific patient populations and novel techniques of titrating the PEEP have been completed.

D. Drotrecogin Alfa (Activated)

Severe sepsis is a complex combination of excessive inflammation, coagulation, and impaired fibrinolysis. The interplay of inflammation and abnormal clotting has been recognized for at least 30 years (192,193). Disseminated intravascular coagulation, the most extreme clotting disorder of sepsis, occurs in less than 20% of sepsis victims. However, a more subtle, often subclinical coagulopathy accompanied by impaired fibrinolysis is nearly universal (194). The most common laboratory findings of this process are elevations in d-dimer levels and depletion of circulating protein C.

Along with tissue factor pathway inhibitor and antithrombin III, protein C is one of three native antithrombotic agents. When converted to its active form by a thrombin–thrombomodulin complex, activated protein C has antithrombotic, anti-inflammatory, and profibrinolytic properties. Activated protein C is a key component in controlling septic coagulopathy, as evidenced by the inverse correlation between plasma levels of protein C and morbidity and mortality in septic patients (195–198). Activation of protein C is impaired in severe sepsis 199–201).

Human recombinant activated protein C, available commercially as drotrecogin alfa (activated), produced dose-proportional reductions in d-dimer levels and IL-6, key markers of sepsis-associated coagulopathy and inflammation, in a placebo-controlled Phase II study (202). Based on the Phase II data, a large, randomized, blinded, placebo-controlled, multicenter Phase III study of severe sepsis was conducted (7). Mortality at 28 days was reduced from 31% to 25% by a 96-hour infusion of drotrecogin alfa (activated), representing a 19.4% relative reduction in the risk of death among the 1690 adults enrolled. The salutary effect was remarkably consistent among subgroups, including those stratified by the number of dysfunctional organs, sex, age, site or type of infection, or initial protein C level; a significant departure from other investigational drugs where benefit was confined to small subgroups (203). As expected, the absolute mortality reduction was even larger among the sickest patients, including those with more organ failures, especially shock and respiratory failure, and those with higher modified APACHE II scores at study entry. Similar treatment effects have been observed among similarly ill patients in open label trials (204), but among patients at low risk of death, for whom the drug is not indicated, no benefits were observed (205). In large prospective open label studies and in case series of patients treated in practice, survival benefits appear substantially greater for patients treated in the first 24 hours of illness (204,206). In a subsequent study of the concomitant use of heparin, enoxaparin, or no deep vein thrombosis prophylaxis in severe sepsis patients treated with drotrecogin alfa (activated), heparin or enoxaparin exposure was found to not increase the incidence of bleeding, but was associated with better outcomes suggesting that pharmacological deep venous thrombosis (DVT) prevention should be continued (207) in these patients. Subgroup analysis found that patients receiving DVT chemoprophylaxis at enrollment who were randomized to discontinuing the prophylaxis were especially at risk for death.

Drotrecogin's only recognized toxicity is bleeding. During the 28-day Phase III trial, 30 (3.5%) serious bleeding events occurred among drug-treated patients compared to 17 (2.0%) among placebo recipients. Similar incremental rates of serious bleeding were observed in open label trials of severely ill patients and in blinded trials of patients at low risk of death (204,205). Most serious bleeding occurred during drug infusion. Fortunately, the risk of intracranial hemorrhage was well below 1%. Among treated patients, bleeding episodes were associated with invasive procedures, meningitis, platelet counts <30,000/mL, and significant elevations in prothrombin time. For this reason, drotrecogin should not be given to patients with active hemorrhage or to patients at high risk of serious bleeding, especially into the neuraxis. To minimize bleeding, infusions should be interrupted two hours before invasive procedures and discontinued completely if serious bleeding develops. Infusions may be restarted immediately after minor uncomplicated procedures and 12 hours after surgery provided hemostasis is adequate. There is no antidote for drotrecogin, but the drug is rapidly cleared by plasma enzymes and is completely eliminated within two hours of discontinuing the infusion. Thus, in the event of bleeding, discontinuing the drug rapidly reverses anticoagulation. Drotrecogin very rarely provokes an immunological response, and neutralizing antibody formation, anaphylactoid reactions, or serum sickness have not occurred after infusion.

E. Nutrition and Metabolism

In severe sepsis, nutritional support can be safely deferred for several days. Indeed, feeding the hemodynamically unstable patient can be difficult, and some practitioners have concerns that feeding may precipitate gut ischemia, despite little supporting data. Metabolic changes in the patient with severe sepsis include increases in oxygen consumption, rapid catabolism, lipolysis, hyperglycemia with insulin resistance, and negative nitrogen balance. As a consequence of these alterations, nutritional requirements are high and malnutrition may ensue (208).

Absent contraindications, enteral nutrition is now preferred by most practitioners because it has several potential advantages that include buffering of gastric acid, maintenance of the gut mucosal barrier, avoidance of parenteral nutrition and its complications, and establishment of physiological enteral hormone secretion (209). For patients with severe sepsis, expert consensus groups recommend the following: (1) daily caloric intake of 25 to 30 kcal/kg/usual body weight/day; (2) protein: 1.3 to 2.0 g/kg/day; (3) glucose: 30–70% of total nonprotein calories to maintain serum glucose <225 mg/dL; (4) lipids: 15–30% of total nonprotein calories (210,211). As mentioned previously, increasing the omega-3 to omega-6 fatty acid ratio may have a beneficial immune-enhancing effect (113,114,115). While the proportion can be reduced, omega-6 fatty acids must be provided in amounts sufficient to avoid deficiency of essential fatty acids (generally 1 g/kg/day). A large trial of omega-3 supplemented feeding is currently underway in an attempt to definitively answer this question (117). Since arginine is a precursor to the formation of nitric oxide, it may worsen shock in patients with septic shock. As such, enteral formulas enriched with arginine are not recommended for patients with sepsis (212,213).

The most provocative and interesting nutrition-metabolic development has been the flurry of investigations tightly controlling blood glucose levels. The relationship between high glucose values and poor clinical outcomes among critically ill patients has been recognized for decades but causation is disputed. The sentinel investigation conducted in postoperative patients (214) found that maintaining blood glucose levels below 110 mg/dL reduced blood stream infections by almost half and hospital mortality by approximately 3% absolute. Following this study, there was a rush to institute glucose control protocols in many hospitals, and quality of care was judged against a normoglycemic benchmark. A subsequent study in medical patients suggested benefits might be confined to a subset with longer ICU stays (215). The perceived benefits of tight glucose control have eroded as several subsequent trials either failed to show benefit or found a substantial risk of hypoglycemia (216).

F. Other Supportive Therapies

Gastric stress ulcer prophylaxis to reduce the risk of upper gastrointestinal bleeding is a nearly routine practice in the critically ill (217). Although definitive data are lacking for the severe sepsis population, these patients possess the same risk characteristics as previously studied groups, including prolonged mechanical ventilation, coagulopathy, head injury, burns, and prior ulcer disease. The bleeding risk increases with the number of risk factors present. In perhaps the definitive trial, Cook and coworkers (99) compared sucralfate to an H2-receptor antagonist for the prevention of upper gastrointestinal bleeding in more than 1000 mechanically ventilated patients. Those receiving H2 blockade had a significantly lower rate of gastrointestinal bleeding than those treated with sucralfate. There is little reason to believe that any particular H2 antagonist or proton pump inhibitor is superior to another, hence drug selection can be driven largely by cost considerations. In contrast, traditional antacids represent an expensive, inconvenient, and perhaps more side-effect-prone choice.

Because nearly 30% of critically ill patients will develop a deep venous thrombus or pulmonary embolism during their hospital stay without prophylaxis, essentially all critically ill patients should have some form of prevention administered (218). Both chemical anticoagulants (e.g., heparin or low molecular weight heparin) and mechanical devices such as intermittent pneumatic compression devices are effective if applied early. Overall, the relative reduction in thromboembolism risk exceeds 50% when one of these approaches is chosen. Selection should probably depend on practical issues such as risk of bleeding and presence of lower extremity injuries. Unfortunately, surveys suggest that perhaps as many as two-thirds of critically ill patients do not receive any form of DVT prophylaxis, exposing them to unnecessary thromboembolism risk (219).

Renal failure necessitating dialysis develops in <5% of patients with severe sepsis (2). Even though the need for renal-replacement therapy is uncommon, acute renal failure is a powerful predictor of mortality. Therefore, steps should be taken to maintain renal function during the disease course. These measures include ensuring prompt, adequate hemodynamic resuscitation and avoiding potentially nephrotoxic medications, including contrast media. Renal-replacement therapies for this population include hemodialysis, hemofiltration, isolated ultrafiltration, and peritoneal dialysis (220). Currently the optimal route, timing, and intensity of renal-replacement therapy are unknown, but perhaps daily hemodialysis may be superior to alternate-day therapy, even when controlling for total dialysis dose (221). A recent large, randomized trial done in the Veterans Affairs population demonstrated that intense renal-replacement therapy did not decrease mortality, improve recovery of renal function, or decrease nonrenal organ failures compared to thrice weekly intermittent hemodialysis or standard continuous renal-replacement therapy (222).

Given the average course of illness, anemia is nearly a universal finding in ALI, especially for septic patients. Phlebotomy, bleeding, reduced erythropoietin production, and impaired erythropoiesis all contribute. Transfusions should be judiciously used to restore oxygen-carrying capacity in the nonbleeding patient. A more aggressive transfusion strategy may be more appropriate for the acutely bleeding patient. However, transfusions are not without risk since they can be associated with infection transmission, immunosuppression, transfusion reactions, and volume overload. The most appropriate hemoglobin target for transfusion is unknown but probably lies between the traditional value of 10 g/dL and a bare minimum of 3 to 4 g/dL. With the possible exception of patients with known coronary artery disease or active gastrointestinal bleeding, a restrictive transfusion strategy (i.e., Hgb target of 7 g/dL) is equivalent and may be superior to a liberal strategy (i.e., Hgb target of 10 g/dL) (223). Recombinant human erythropoietin raises hemoglobin values and halves red blood cell transfusion requirements among critically ill patients (224). The optimal dose and schedule are still being determined, but erythropoietin is likely a useful component of an anemia-management program that includes minimizing phlebotomy and lowering traditional hemoglobin values for transfusion. However, recent reports of increased clotting, deep vein thromboses, and myocardial infarctions in cancer patients receiving erythropoietin-stimulating agents have caused some to question its routine use in the ICU (225).

VI. Summary

Severe sepsis is the most common cause of ALI. The onset of lung failure is typically so early in the course of severe sepsis as to preclude any meaningful preventative intervention short of averting infection. Preventing the development of secondary sepsis in patients with established ALI is a more tenable strategy. Measures highly likely to decrease the development of secondary sepsis include closed tracheal suctioning systems, positioning ventilated patients head up, and minimizing the number and duration of central venous and urinary catheters. Avoidance of nasal tubes can also decrease the risk of infection. CVCs should be used only when necessary, and they should be inserted by experienced personnel using full barrier precautions. After insertion, catheters should be entered sparingly, cared for by a trained team, and evaluated daily to see if they are still needed. Reasonable measures to reduce the risk of severe sepsis include minimizing the duration of mechanical ventilation by using a reduced tidal volume strategy, protocolized sedation with daily interruptions, and ventilator weaning protocols.

When sepsis does occur in patients with ALI, source control of the infection, appropriate cultures, and targeted antimicrobial therapy are indicated. Rapid goal-directed fluid and vasopressor therapy probably optimizes survival. Crystalloid infusions followed by norepinephrine now appear to be the most popular therapeutic choices. Routine use of

PACs should be discouraged. Activated human recombinant protein C is a breakthrough life-saving technology for the critically ill patient with severe sepsis at high risk of death and not at significant risk of bleeding. Nutritional support is indicated, probably best delivered enterally, but timing, optimal delivery site, and type of feeding remain uncertain. It is prudent to provide assiduous oral care; DVT and gastrointestinal bleeding prophylaxis; and minimize phlebotomy with a restrictive transfusion strategy, thereby minimizing the number of required blood transfusions.

References

1. The Acute Respiratory Distress Syndrome Network. Ventilation with lower tidal volumes as compared with traditional tidal volumes for acute lung injury and the acute respiratory distress syndrome. N Engl J Med 2000; 342:1301–1308.
2. Wheeler AP. Recent developments in the diagnosis and management of severe sepsis. Chest 2007; 132:1967–1976.
3. Wheeler AP, Bernard GR. Acute lung injury and the acute respiratory distress syndrome: a clinical review. Lancet 2007; 369:1553–1564.
4. Bone RC, Balk RA, Cerra FB, et al. American College of Chest Physicians/Society of Critical Care Medicine Consensus Conference: definitions for sepsis and organ failure and guidelines for the use of innovative therapies in sepsis. Chest 1992; 101:1644–1655.
5. Martin GS, Mannino DM, Eaton S, et al. The epidemiology of sepsis in the United States from 1979 through 2000. N Engl J Med 2003; 348:1546–1554.
6. Stapleton RD, Wang BM, Hudson LD, et al. Causes and timing of death in patients with ARDS. Chest 2005; 128:525–532.
7. Bernard GR, Vincent JL, Laterre PF, et al. Efficacy and safety of recombinant human activated protein C for severe sepsis. N Engl J Med 2001; 344:699–709.
8. Bernard GR, Artigas A, Brigham KL, et al. The American-European Consensus conference on ARDS, definitions, mechanisms, relevant outcomes and clinical trial coordination. Am J Respir Crit Care Med 1994; 149:818–824.
9. Bernard GR, Wheeler AP, Russell JA, et al. The effects of ibuprofen on the physiology and survival of patients with sepsis. N Engl J Med 1997; 336:912–918.
10. Zeerleder S, Hack CE, Wuillemin WA. Disseminated intravascular coagulation in sepsis. Chest 2005; 128:2864–2875.
11. Faust SN, Levin M, Harrison OB, et al. Dysfunction of endothelial protein C activation in severe meningococcal sepsis. N Engl J Med 2001; 345:408–416.
12. Opal SM. Therapeutic rationale for antithrombin III in sepsis. Crit Care Med 2000; 28: S34–S37.
13. Levi M, van der Poll T. Recombinant human activated protein C: current insights into its mechanism of action. Crit Care 2007; 11(Suppl. 5):S3.
14. Ware LB. Pathophysiology of acute lung injury and the acute respiratory distress syndrome. Semin Respir Crit Care Med 2006; 27:337–349.
15. Wygrecka M, Jablonska E, Guenther A, et al. Current view on alveolar coagulation and fibrinolysis in acute inflammatory and chronic interstitial lung diseases. Thromb Haemost 2008; 99:494–501.
16. Idell S. Coagulation, fibrinolysis, and fibrin deposition in acute lung injury. Crit Care Med 2003; 31(Suppl. 4):S213–S220.
17. Levi M, Schultz M. The inflammation-coagulation axis as an important intermediate pathway in acute lung injury. Crit Care 2008; 12:144.
18. Abraham E. Coagulation abnormalities in acute lung injury and sepsis. Am J Respir Mol Cell Biol 2000; 22:401–404.

19. Ware LB, Matthay MA, Parsons PE, et al. Pathogenetic and prognostic significance of altered coagulation and fibrinolysis in acute lung injury/acute respiratory distress syndrome. Crit Care Med 2007; 35:1821–1828.

20. Schultz MJ, Haitsma JJ, Zhang H, et al. Pulmonary coagulopathy as a new target in therapeutic studies of acute lung injury or pneumonia—a review. Crit Care Med 2006; 34:871–877.

21. Bastarache JA, Wang L, Geiser T, et al. The alveolar epithelium can initiate the extrinsic coagulation cascade through expression of tissue factor. Thorax 2007; 62:608–616.

22. Bonten MJ, Kollef MH, Hall JB. Risk factors for ventilator-associated pneumonia: from epidemiology to patient management. Clin Infect Dis 2004; 38:1141–1149.

23. Wolkewitz M, Vonberg RP, Grundmann H, et al. Risk factors for the development of nosocomial pneumonia and mortality on intensive care units: application of competing risks models. Crit Care 2008; 12:R44.

24. Nahum A, Hoyt J, Schmitz L, et al. Effect of mechanical ventilation strategy on dissemination of intratracheally instilled Escherichia coli in dogs. Crit Care Med 1997; 25:1733–1743.

25. Craven DE, Kunches LM, Kilinsky V, et al. Risk factors for pneumonia and fatality in patients receiving continuous mechanical ventilation. Am Rev Respir Dis 1986; 133:792–796.

26. Neiderman MS, Fein AM. The interaction of infection and the adult respiratory distress syndrome. Crit Care Clin 1986; 2:471–495.

27. Cook DJ, Walter SD, Cook RJ, et al. Incidence of and risk factors for ventilator-associated pneumonia in critically ill patients. Ann Intern Med 1998; 129:433–440.

28. Seidenfeld JJ, Pohl DF, Bell RC, et al. Incidence, site, and outcome of infections in patients with adult respiratory distress syndrome. Am Rev Respir Dis 1986; 134:12–16.

29. Sutherland KR, Steinberg KP, Maunder RJ, et al. Pulmonary infection during the acute respiratory distress syndrome. Am J Respir Crit Care Med 1995; 152:550–556.

30. Kollef MH. The prevention of ventilator associated pneumonia. N Engl J Med 1999; 340: 627–634.

31. Saint S. Clinical and economic consequences of nosocomial catheter related bacteruria. Am J Infect Control 2000; 28:68–75.

32. Gosbell IB, Duggan D, Breust M, et al. Infection associated with central venous catheters: a prospective survey. Med J Aust 1995; 162:210–213.

33. Aufwerber E, Ringertz S, Ransjo U. Routine semiquantitative cultures and central venous catheter related bacteremia. APMIS 1991; 99:627–630.

34. Renaud B, Brun-Buisson C. Outcomes of primary and catheter-related bacteremia. A cohort and case-control study in critically ill patients. Am J Respir Crit Care Med 2001; 163: 1584–1590.

35. Rosenthal VD, Guzman S, Migone O, et al. The attributable cost, length of hospital stay, and mortality of central line-associated bloodstream infection in intensive care departments in Argentina: a prospective, matched analysis. Am J Infect Control 2003; 31:475–480.

36. Ely EW, Baker AM, Dunagan DP, et al. Effect of the duration of mechanical ventilation of identifying patients capable of breathing spontaneously. N Engl J Med 1996; 335: 1864–1869.

37. Girard TD, Kress JP, Fuchs BD, et al. Efficacy and safety of a paired sedation and ventilator weaning protocol for mechanically ventilated patients in intensive care (Awakening and Breathing Controlled trial): a randomised controlled trial. Lancet 2008; 371:126–134.

38. Torres A, Anzar R, Fatell JM, et al. Incidence, risk and prognostic factors of nosocomial pneumonia in mechanically ventilated patients. Am Rev Respir Dis 1986; 133:792–796.

39. Drakulovic MB, Torres A, Bauer TT, et al. Supine body position as a risk factor for nosocomial pneumonia in mechanically ventilated patients: a randomized trial. Lancet 1999; 354: 1851–1858.

40. Cook D, Ricard JD, Reeve B, et al. Ventilator circuit and secretion management strategies: a Franco-Canadian survey. Crit Care Med 2000; 28:3547–3554.

41. Kola A, Eckmanns T, Gastmeier P. Efficacy of heat and moisture exchangers in preventing ventilator-associated pneumonia: meta-analysis of randomized controlled trials. Intensive Care Med 2005; 31:5–11.
42. Lacherade JC, Auburitin M, Cerf C, et al. Impact of humidification systems on ventilator-associated pneumonia: a randomized, multicenter trial. Am J Respir Crit Care Med 2005; 172:276–282.
43. Littlewood K, Durbin CG Jr. Evidenced-based airway management. Respir Care 2001; 46:1392–1405.
44. Lorente L, Lecuona M, Martín MM, et al. Ventilator-associated pneumonia using a closed versus an open tracheal suction system. Crit Care Med 2005; 33:115–119.
45. Mahoul PH, Auboyer C, Jospe R, et al. Prevention of nosocomial pneumonia in intubated patients: respective role of mechanical subglottic secretions drainage and stress ulcer prophylaxis. Intensive Care Med 1992; 18:20–25.
46. Valles J, Artigas A, Rello J, et al. Continuous aspiration of subglottic secretions in preventing ventilator associated pneumonia. Ann Intern Med 1995; 122:179–186.
47. Dezfulian C, Shojania K, Collard HR, et al. Subglottic secretion drainage for preventing ventilator-associated pneumonia: a meta-analysis. Am J Med 2005; 118:11–18.
48. National Nosocomial Infections Surveillance (NNIS). System Report, Data Summary from January 1992–June 2001, issued August 2001. Am J Infect Control 2001; 29:404–421.
49. Gil RT, Kruse JA, Thill-Baharozian MC, et al. Triple versus single lumen central venous catheters. A prospective study in a critically ill population. Arch Intern Med 1989; 149: 1139–1143.
50. Raad I, Umphrey J, Kahn A, et al. The duration of placement as a predictor of peripheral and pulmonary arterial catheter infections. J Hosp Infect 1993; 23:17–26.
51. Maki DG, Ringer M, Alvarado CJ. Prospective randomized trial of povidone iodine, alcohol, and chlorhexidine for prevention of infection associated with central venous and arterial catheters. Lancet 1991; 338:339–343.
52. Pronovost P, Needham D, Berenholtz S, et al. An intervention to decrease catheter-related bloodstream infections in the ICU. N Engl J Med 2006; 355:2725–2732.
53. Sitzmann JV, Townsend TR, Siler MC, et al. Septic and technical complications of central venous catheterization. A prospective study of 200 consecutive patients. Ann Surg 1985; 202:766–770.
54. McKinley S, Mackenzie A, Finfer S, et al. Incidence and predictors of central venous catheter related infection in intensive care patients. Anaesth Intensive Care 1999; 27:164–169.
55. Brun-Buisson C, Abrouk F, Legrand P, et al. Diagnosis of central venous catheter-related sepsis. Critical level of quantitative tip cultures. Arch Intern Med 1987; 147:873–877.
56. Merrer J, De Jonghe B, Golliot F, et al. Complications of femoral and subclavian venous catheterization in critically ill patients: a randomized controlled trial. JAMA 2001; 286: 700–707.
57. Darouiche RO, Raad II, Heard SO, et al. A comparison of two anti-microbial impregnated central venous catheters. N Engl J Med 1999; 340:1–8.
58. Maki DG, Stoltz SM, Wheeler S, et al. Prevention of central venous catheter related bloodstream infection by use of an anti-septic impregnated catheter. A randomized controlled trial. Ann Intern Med 1997; 127:257–266.
59. Kamal GD, Pfaller MA, Rempe LE, et al. Reduced intravascular catheter infection by antibiotic bonding. A prospective, randomized, controlled trial. JAMA 1991; 265:2364–2368.
60. Maki DG, Band JD. A comparative study of polyantibiotic and iodophor ointments in prevention of vascular catheter-related infection. Am J Med 1981; 70:739–744.
61. Kalfon P, de Vaumas C, Samba D, et al. Comparison of silver-impregnated with standard multi-lumen central venous catheters in critically ill patients. Crit Care Med 2007; 35: 1032–1039.

62. León C, Ruiz-Santana S, Rello J, et al. Benefits of minocycline and rifampin-impregnated central venous catheters. A prospective, randomized, double-blind, controlled, multicenter trial. Intensive Care Med 2004; 30:1891–1899.

63. Richet H, Hubert B, Nitemberg G, et al. Prospective multicenter study of vascular-catheter-related complications and risk factors for positive central-catheter cultures in intensive care unit patients. J Clin Microbiol 1990; 28:2520–2525.

64. Eyer S, Brummitt C, Crossley K, et al. Catheter related sepsis: prospective randomized study of three methods of long term catheter maintenance. Crit Care Med 1990; 18: 1073–1079.

65. Cobb DK, High KP, Sawyer RG, et al. A controlled trial of scheduled replacement of central venous and pulmonary-artery catheters. N Engl J Med 1992; 327:1062–1068.

66. Resar R, Pronovost P, Haraden C, et al. Using a bundle approach to improve ventilator care processes and reduce ventilator-associated pneumonia. Jt Comm J Qual Patient Saf 2005; 31:243–248.

67. Cocanour CS, Peninger M, Domonoske BD, et al. Decreasing ventilator-associated pneumonia in a trauma ICU. J Trauma 2006; 61:122–130.

68. Girard TD, Ely EW. Protocol-driven ventilator weaning: reviewing the evidence. Clin Chest Med 2008; 29:241–252.

69. Schweickert WD, Gehlbach BK, Pohlman AS, et al. Daily interruption of sedative infusions and complications of critical illness in mechanically ventilated patients. Crit Care Med 2004; 32:1272–1276.

70. Cardenosa-Cendrero JA, Sole-Violan J, Bordes Benitez A, et al. Role of different routes of tracheal colonization in the development of pneumonia in patients receiving mechanical ventilation. Chest 1999; 116:462–470.

71. Safdar, N, Crnich CJ, Maki DG. The pathogenesis of ventilator-associated pneumonia: its relevance to developing effective strategies for prevention. Respir Care 2005;50;725–739.

72. van Nieuwenhoven CA, Vandenbroucke-Grauls C, van Tiel FH, et al. Feasibility and effects of the semirecumbent position to prevent ventilator-associated pneumonia: a randomized study. Crit Care Med 2006; 34:396–402.

73. Koeman M, van der Ven A, Hak E, et al. Oral decontamination with chlorhexidine reduces the incidence of ventilator-associated pneumonia: a randomized, placebo-controlled trial. Am J Respir Crit Care Med 2006; 173:1348–1355.

74. Mori H, Hirasawa H, Oda S, et al. Oral care reduces incidence of ventilator-associated pneumonia in ICU populations. Intensive Care Med 2006; 25:1–7.

75. Baxter AD, Allan J, Bedard J, et al. Adherence to simple and effective measures reduces the incidence of ventilator-associated pneumonia. Can J Anaesth 2005; 52:535–541.

76. Koenig SM, Truwit JD. Ventilator-associated pneumonia: diagnosis, treatment, and prevention. Clin Microbiol Rev 2006; 19:637–657.

77. Diaz E, Rodriguez AH, Rello J. Ventilator-associated pneumonia: issues related to the artificial airway. Respir Care 2005; 50:900–906.

78. Shorr AF, O'Malley PG. Continuous subglottic suctioning for the prevention of ventilator-associated pneumonia: potential economic implications. Chest 2001; 119:228–235.

79. Ricard JD, Le Miere E, Markowicz P, et al. Efficiency and safety of mechanical ventilation with a heat and moisture exchanger changed only once a week. Am J Respir Crit Care Med 2000; 161:104–109.

80. Iotti GA, Olivei MC, Braschi A. Mechanical effects of heat-moisture exchangers in ventilated patients. Crit Care Med 1999; 3:R77–R82.

81. Kirton OC, DeHaven B, Morgan J, et al. A prospective, randomized comparison of an in-line heat moisture exchange filter and heated wire humidifiers: rates of ventilator-associated early-onset (community-acquired) or late-onset (hospital-acquired) pneumonia and incidence of endotracheal tube occlusion. Chest 1997; 112:1055–1059.

82. Rouby JJ, Laurent P, Gosnach M, et al. Risk factors and clinical relevance of nosocomial maxillary sinusitis in the critically ill. Am J Respir Crit Care Med 1994; 150:776–783.

83. Girou E, Schortgen F, Delclaux C, et al. Association of noninvasive ventilation with nosocomial infections and survival in critically ill patients. JAMA 2000; 284:2361–2367.

84. Antonelli M, Conti G, Rocco M, et al. A comparison of noninvasive positive-pressure ventilation and conventional mechanical ventilation in patients with acute respiratory failure. N Engl J Med 1998; 339:429–435.

85. Burns, KEA. Noninvasive positive pressure ventilation as a weaning strategy for intubated adults with respiratory failure. Cochrane Database Syst Rev 2006; 1:1–25.

86. Bergmans DC, Bonten MJ, Gaillard CA, et al. Prevention of ventilator-associated pneumonia by oral decontamination: a prospective, randomized, double-blind, placebo-controlled study. Am J Respir Crit Care Med 2001; 164:382–388.

87. Gastinne H, Wolff M, Delatour F, et al. A controlled trial in intensive care units of selective decontamination of the digestive tract with nonabsorbable antibiotics. N Engl J Med 1992; 326:594–599.

88. Kallet RH, Quinn TE. The gastrointestinal tract and ventilator-associated pneumonia. Respir Care 2005; 50:910–921.

89. Liberati A, D'Amico R, Pifferi S, et al. Antibiotic prophylaxis to reduce respiratory tract infections and mortality in adults receiving intensive care. Cochrane Database Syst Rev 2006; 1:1–54.

90. de Jonge E, Schultz M, Spanjaard L, et al. Selective decontamination of digestive tract in intensive care. Lancet 2003; 362:2119–2120.

91. Claridge JA, Edwards NM, Swanson J, et al. Aerosolized ceftazidime prophylaxis against ventilator-associated pneumonia in high-risk trauma patients: results of a double-blind randomized study. Surg Infect 2007; 8:83–90.

92. MacIntyre NR, Rubin BK. Respiratory therapies in the critical care setting. Should aerosolized antibiotics be administered to prevent or treat ventilator-associated pneumonia in patients who do not have cystic fibrosis? Respir Care 2007; 52:416–421.

93. Kollef MH, Vlasnik J, Sharpless L, et al. Scheduled change of antibiotic classes: a strategy to decrease the influence of ventilator associated pneumonia. Am J Respir Crit Care Med 1997; 156:1040–1048.

94. Gruson D, Hilbert G, Vargas F, et al. Rotation and restricted use of antibiotics in a medical intensive care unit. Impact on the incidence of ventilator-associated pneumonia caused by antibiotic-resistant gram-negative bacteria. Am J Respir Crit Care Med 2000; 162:837–843.

95. Gruson D, Hilbert G, Vargas F, et al. Strategy of antibiotic rotation: long-term effect on incidence and susceptibilities of Gram-negative bacilli responsible for ventilator-associated pneumonia. Crit Care Med 2003; 31:1908–1914.

96. Cook DJ, De Jonghe B, Brochard L, et al. Influence of airway management on ventilator associated pneumonia: evidence from randomized trials. JAMA 1998; 279:781–787.

97. Tryba M. Risk of acute stress bleeding and nosocomial pneumonia in ventilated intensive care unit patients: sucralfate versus antacids. Am J Med 1987; 83:117–124.

98. Cook DJ, Fuller H, Guyatt GH, et al. Risk factors for gastrointestinal bleeding in critically ill patients. N Engl J Med 1994; 330:377–381.

99. Cook DJ, Guyatt GH, Marshall J, et al. A comparison of sucralfate and ranitidine for the prevention of upper gastrointestinal bleeding in patients requiring mechanical ventilation. N Engl J Med 1998; 338:791–797.

100. Heyland DK. Nutritional support in the critically ill patient. A critical review of the evidence. Crit Care Clin 1998; 14:423–440.

101. Heys SD, Walker LG, Smith I, et al. Enteral nutritional supplementation with key nutrients in patients with critical illness and cancer: a meta-analysis of randomized controlled clinical trails. Ann Surg 1999; 229:467–477.

102. Ibrahim EH, Mehringer L, Prentice D, et al. Early versus late enteral feeding of mechanically ventilated patients: results of a clinical trial. JPEN J Parenter Enteral Nutr 2002; 26: 174–181.
103. Kompan L, Vidmar G, Spindler-Vesel A, et al. Is early enteral nutrition a risk factor for gastric intolerance and pneumonia? Clin Nutr 2004; 23:527–532.
104. Reignier J, Thenoz-Jost N, Fiancette M, et al. Early enteral nutrition in mechanically ventilated patients in the prone position. Crit Care Med 2004; 32:94–99.
105. Mentec H, Dupont H, Bocchetti M, et al. Upper digestive intolerance during enteral nutrition in critically ill patients: frequency, risk factors, and complications. Crit Care Med 2001; 29:1955–1961.
106. Krishnan JA, Parce PB, Martinez A, et al. Caloric intake in medical ICU patients: consistency of care with guidelines and relationship to clinical outcomes. Chest 2003; 124: 297–305.
107. Rice TW, Swope T, Bozeman S, et al. Variation in enteral nutrition delivery in mechanically ventilated patients. Nutrition 2005; 21:786–792.
108. Heyland DK, Drover JW, MacDonald S, et al. Effect of post-pyloric feeding on gastroesophageal regurgitation and pulmonary microaspiration: results of a randomized controlled trial. Crit Care Med 2001; 29:1495–1501.
109. Ho KM, Dobb GJ, Webb SA. A comparison of early gastric and post-pyloric feeding in critically ill patients: a meta-analysis. Intensive Care Med 2006; 32:639–649.
110. Marik, PE, Zaloga, GP. Gastric versus post-pyloric feeding: a systematic review. Crit Care 2003; 7:R46–R51.
111. Galban C, Montejo JC, Mesejo A, et al. An immune enhancing enteral diet reduces mortality rate and episodes of bacteremia in septic intensive care unit patients. Crit Care Med 2000; 28:643–648.
112. Gadek J, DeMichele SJ, Karlstad MD, et al. Effect of enteral feeding with eicosapentaenoic acid, gamma linolenic acid, and antioxidants in patients with acute respiratory distress syndrome. Crit Care Med 1999; 27:1409–1420.
113. Beale RJ, Bryg DJ, Bihari DJ. Immunonutrition in the critically ill: a systematic review of clinical outcome. Crit Care Med 1999; 27:2799–2805.
114. Singer P, Theilla M, Fisher H, et al. Benefit of an enteral diet enriched with eicosapentaenoic acid and gamma-linolenic acid in ventilated patients with acute lung injury. Crit Care Med 2006; 34:1033–1038. Erratum in: Crit Care Med 2006; 34:1861.
115. Pontes-Arruda A, Aragão AM, Albuquerque JD. Effects of enteral feeding with eicosapentaenoic acid, gamma-linolenic acid, and antioxidants in mechanically ventilated patients with severe sepsis and septic shock. Crit Care Med 2006; 34:2325–2333.
116. Heyland DK, Novak F, Drover JW, et al. Should immunonutrition become routine in critically ill patients? A systematic review of the evidence. JAMA 2001; 289:944–959.
117. http://clinicaltrials.gov/ct2/show/NCT00609180.
118. Pittet D, Tarara D, Wenzel RP. Nosocomial bloodstream infection in critically ill patients. Excess length of stay, extra costs, and attributable mortality. JAMA 1994; 271:1598–1601.
119. Collignon PJ. Intravascular catheter associated sepsis: a common problem. The Australian Study on Intravascular Catheter Associated Sepsis. Med J Aust 1994; 161:374–378.
120. Coopersmith CM, Rebmann TL, Zack JE, et al. Effect of an education program on decreasing catheter-related bloodstream infections in the surgical intensive care unit. Crit Care Med 2002; 30:59–64.
121. Mermel LA, McCormick RD, Springman SR, et al. The pathogenesis and epidemiology of catheter-related infection with pulmonary artery Swan-Ganz catheters: a prospective study utilizing molecular subtyping. Am J Med 1991; 91:197S–205S.
122. Mermel LA. Prevention of intravascular catheter-related infections. Ann Intern Med 2000; 132:391–402.

123. Raad II, Hohn DC, Gilbreath BJ, et al. Prevention of central venous catheter-related infections by using maximal sterile barrier precautions during insertion. Infect Control Hosp Epidemiol 1994; 15:231–238.

124. Raad I. Intravascular-catheter-related infections. Lancet 1998; 351:893–898.

125. Raad II, Hanna HA. Intravascular catheter-related infections: new horizons and recent advances. Arch Intern Med 2002; 162:871–878.

126. Randolph AG, Cook DJ, Gonzales CA, et al. Tunneling short-term central venous catheters to prevent catheter-related infection: a metaanalysis of randomized, controlled trials. Crit Care Med 1998; 26:1452–1457.

127. Sherertz RJ, Ely EW, Westbrook DM, et al. Education of physicians-in-training can decrease the risk for vascular catheter infection. Ann Intern Med 2000; 132:641–648.

128. Parienti JJ, Thirion M, Megarbane B, et al. Femoral vs. jugular venous catheterization and risk of nosocomial events in adults requiring acute renal replacement therapy. A randomized controlled trial. JAMA 2008; 299:2413–2422.

129. Maki DG, Stolz SS, Wheeler S, et al. A prospective, randomized trial of gauze and two polyurethane dressings for site care of pulmonary artery catheters: implications for catheter management. Crit Care Med 1994; 22:1729–1737.

130. Conly JM, Grieves K, Peters B. A prospective, randomized study comparing transparent and dry gauze dressings for central venous catheters. J Infect Dis 1989; 159:310–319.

131. Maki DG, Botticelli JT, LeRoy ML, et al. Prospective study of replacing administration sets for intravenous therapy at 48- vs 72-hour intervals. 72 hours is safe and cost-effective. JAMA 1987; 258:1777–1781.

132. Eyer S, Brummitt C, Crossley K, et al. Catheter-related sepsis: prospective, randomized study of three methods of long-term catheter maintenance. Crit Care Med 1990; 18: 1073–1079.

133. Snyder RH, Archer FJ, Endy T, et al. Catheter infection. A comparison of two catheter maintenance techniques. Ann Surg 1988; 208:651–653.

134. Timsit JF, Sebille V, Farkas JC, et al. Effect of subcutaneous tunneling on internal jugular catheter-related sepsis in critically ill patients: a prospective randomized multicenter study. JAMA 1996; 276:1416–1420.

135. Eggimann P, Harbarth S, Constantin MN, et al. Impact of a prevention strategy targeted at vascular-access care on incidence of infections acquired in intensive care. Lancet 2000; 355:1864–1868.

136. Bijma R, Girbes AR, Kleijer DJ, et al. Preventing central venous catheter-related infection in a surgical intensive-care unit. Infect Control Hosp Epidemiol 1999; 20:618–620.

137. Berenholtz SM, Pronovost PJ, Lipsett PA, et al. Eliminating catheter-related bloodstream infections in the intensive care unit. Crit Care Med 2004; 32:2014–2020.

138. Snydman DR. Prevention of catheter and intravascular device-related infections: a quality-of-care mandate for institutions and physicians. Mayo Clin Proc 2006; 81:1151–1152.

139. Simon D, Trenholme G. Antibiotic selection for patients with septic shock. Crit Care Clin 2000; 16:215–231.

140. Llewelyn M, Cohen J. Diagnosis of infection in sepsis. Intensive Care Med 2001; 27:510–532.

141. Kreger BE, Craven DH, McCabe WR. Gram-negative bacteremia. Reevaluation of clinical features and treatment of 612 patients. Am J Med 1998; 68:332–343.

142. Pittet D, Thjievent B, Wenzel RP, et al. Bedside prediction of mortality from bacteremic sepsis. A dynamic analysis of ICU patients. Am J Respir Crit Care Med 1996; 153:684–693.

143. Kollef MH, Sherman G, Ward S, et al. Inadequate antimicrobial treatment of infections: a risk factor for hospital mortality among critically ill patients. Chest 1999; 115:462–474.

144. Kumar A, Roberts D, Wood K, et al. Duration of hypotension before initiation of effective antimicrobial therapy is the critical determinant of survival in human septic shock. Crit Care Med 2006; 34:1589–1596.

145. Bartlett JG, Dowell SF, Mandell LA, et al. Practice guidelines for the management of community-acquired pneumonia in adults. Clin Infect Dis 2000; 31:347–382.

146. Houck PM, Bratzler DW, Nsa W, et al. Timing of antibiotic administration and outcomes for Medicare patients hospitalized with community-acquired pneumonia. Arch Intern Med 2004; 164:637–644.

147. Kanwar M, Brar N, Khatib R, et al. Misdiagnosis of community-acquired pneumonia and inappropriate utilization of antibiotics: side effects of the 4-h antibiotic administration rule. Chest 2007; 131:1865–1869.

148. Chastre J, Wolff M, Fagon JY, et al. Comparison of 8 vs. 15 days of antibiotic therapy for ventilator-associated pneumonia in adults: a randomized trial. JAMA 2003; 290:2588–2598.

149. Micek ST, Ward S, Fraser VJ, et al. A randomized controlled trial of an antibiotic discontinuation policy for clinically suspected ventilator-associated pneumonia. Chest 2004; 125:1791–1799.

150. Nobre V, Harbath S, Graf J-D, et al. Use of procalcitonin to shorten antibiotic treatment duration in septic patients. Am J Resp Crit Care Med 2008; 177:498–505.

151. Dellinger RP, Levy MM, Carlet JM, et al. Surviving Sepsis Campaign: International guidelines for management of severe sepsis and septic shock: 2008. Crit Care Med 2008; 36:296–327.

152. Mangialardi RJ, Martin GR, Bernard GR, et al. Hypoproteinemia predicts acute respiratory distress syndrome development, weight gain and death in patients with sepsis. Crit Care Med 2000; 28:3137–3145.

153. Martin GS, Mangialardi RJ, Wheeler AP, et al. Albumin and furosemide therapy in hypoproteinemic patients with acute lung injury. Crit Care Med 2002; 30:2175–2182.

154. Carmichael LC, Dorinsky PM, Higgins S, et al. Diagnosis and therapy of adult respiratory distress syndrome: an international survey. J Crit Care 1996; 11:9–18.

155. Connors AF, Speroff T, Dawson NV, et al. The effectiveness of right heart catheterization in the initial care of critically ill patients. SUPPORT Investigators. JAMA 1996; 276:889–897.

156. Richard C, Warszawski J, Anguel N, et al. Early use of the pulmonary artery catheter and outcomes in patients with shock and acute respiratory distress syndrome: a randomized controlled trial. JAMA 2003; 290:2713–2720.

157. Sandham JD, Hull RD, Brant RF, et al. A randomized, controlled trial of the use of pulmonary-artery catheters in high-risk surgical patients. N Engl J Med 2003; 348:5–14.

158. Rhodes A, Cusack RJ, Newman PJ, et al. A randomized controlled trial of the pulmonary artery catheter in critically ill patients. Intensive Care Med 2002; 28:256–264.

159. Harvey S, Harrison DA, Singer M, et al. Assessment of the clinical effectiveness of pulmonary artery catheters in management of patients in intensive care (PAC-Man): a randomised controlled trial. Lancet 2005; 366:472–477.

160. Wheeler AP, Bernard GR, Thompson BT, et al. Pulmonary-artery versus central venous catheter to guide treatment of acute lung injury. N Engl J Med 2006; 354:2213–2224.

161. Rackow EC, Falk JL, Fein IA, et al. Fluid resuscitation in circulatory shock: a comparison of the cardiorespiratory effects of albumin, hetastarch and saline solutions in patients with hypovolemic and septic shock. Crit Care Med 1983; 11:839–850.

162. Waikar SS, Chertow GM. Crystalloid versus colloids for resuscitation in shock. Curr Opin Nephrol Hypertens 2000; 9:501–504.

163. Cherry T, Steciuk M, Reddy VV, et al. Transfusion-related acute lung injury: past, present, and future. Am J Clin Pathol 2008; 129:287–297.

164. Schierhout G, Roberts I. Fluid resuscitation with colloid or crystalloid solutions in critically ill patients: a systematic review of randomized trials. BMJ 1998; 316:961–964.

165. Brunkhorst FM, Engel C, Bloos F, et al. Intensive insulin therapy and pentastarch resuscitation in severe sepsis. N Engl J Med 2008; 358:125–139.

166. The SAFE Study Investigators. A comparison of albumin and saline for fluid resuscitation in the intensive care unit. N Engl J Med 2004; 350:2247–2256.

167. Vincent JL. Hemodynamic support in septic shock. Intensive Care Med 2001; 27(Suppl. 1): S80–S92.
168. Martin C, Viviand X, Leone M, et al. Effect of norepinephrine on the outcome of septic shock. Crit Care Med 2000; 28:2758–2765.
169. Desjars P, Pinaud M, Bugnon D, et al. Norepinephrine therapy has no deleterious renal effects in human septic shock. Crit Care Med 1989; 17:426–429.
170. Martin C, Papazian L, Perrin G, et al. Norepinephrine or dopamine for the treatment of hyperdynamic septic shock? Chest 1993; 103:1826–1831.
171. Meadows D, Edwards JD, Wilkins RG, et al. Reversal of intractable septic shock with norepinephrine therapy. Crit Care Med 1988; 16:663–666.
172. Levy B, Dusang B, Annane D, et al. Cardiovascular response to dopamine and early prediction of outcome in septic shock: a prospective multiple-center study. Crit Care Med 2005; 33: 2172–2177.
173. Sakr Y, Rheinart K, Vincent JL, et al. Does dopamine administration in shock influence outcome? Results of the sepsis occurrence in acutely ill patients. Crit Care Med 2006; 34:589–597.
174. Bellomo R, Chapman M, Finfer S, et al. Low-dose dopamine in patients with early renal dysfunction: a placebo-controlled randomized trial. Lancet 2000; 356:2139–2143.
175. Landry DW, Oliver JA. The pathogenesis of vasodilatory shock. N Engl J Med 2001; 345: 588–595.
176. Landry DW, Levin HR, Gallant EM, et al. Vasopressin deficiency contributes to the vasodilation of septic shock. Circulation 1997; 95:1122–1125.
177. Russell JA, Walley KR, Singer J, et al. Vasopressin versus norepinephrine infusion in patients with septic shock. N Engl J Med 2008; 358:877–887.
178. Shoemaker WC, Appel PL, Kram HB, et al. Prospective trial of supranormal values of survivors as therapeutic goals in high-risk surgical patients. Chest 1988; 94:1176–1186.
179. Tuchschmidt J, Fried J, Astiz M, et al. Elevation output and oxygen delivery improves outcomes in septic shock. Chest 1992; 102:216–220.
180. Boyd O, Grounds RM, Bennett ED. A randomized clinical trial of the effect of deliberate perioperative increase of oxygen delivery on mortality in high risk surgical patients. JAMA 1993; 270:2699–2707.
181. Yu M, Levy MM, Smith P, et al. Effect of maximizing oxygen delivery on morbidity and mortality rates in critically ill patients: a prospective randomized controlled study. Crit Care Med 1993; 21:830–838.
182. Gattinoni L, Brazzi L, Pelosi P, et al. A trial of goal oriented hemodynamic therapy in critically ill patients. N Engl J Med 1995; 333:1025–1032.
183. Hayes MA, Timmins AC, Yau EHS, et al. Elevation of systemic oxygen delivery in the treatment of critically ill patients. N Engl J Med 1994; 330:1717–1722.
184. Rivers E, Nguyen B, Havstad, et al. Early goal directed therapy in the treatment of severe sepsis and septic shock. N Engl J Med 2001; 345:1368–1377.
185. Huang DT, Clermont G, Dremsizov TT, et al. Implementation of early goal-directed therapy for severe sepsis and septic shock: a decision analysis. Crit Care Med 2007; 35: 2090–2100.
186. Jones AE, Shapiro NI, Roshon M. Implementing early goal-directed therapy in the emergency setting: the challenges and experiences of translating research innovations into clinical reality in academic and community settings. Acad Emerg Med 2007; 14:1072–1078.
187. Gajic O, Dara SI, Mendez JL, et al. Ventilator-associated lung injury in patients without acute lung injury at the onset of mechanical ventilation. Crit Care Med 2004; 32:1817–1824.
188. Gajic O, Frutos-Vivar F, Esteban A, et al. Ventilator settings as a risk factor for acute respiratory distress syndrome in mechanically ventilated patients. Intensive Care Med 2005; 31:922–926.

189. Brower RG, Lankin PN, MacIntyre N, et al. Higher vs. lower positive end-expiratory pressures in patients with the acute respiratory distress syndrome. New Engl J Med 2004; 351:327–336.
190. Meade MO, Cook DJ, Guyatt GH, et al. Ventilation strategy using low tidal volumes, recruitment maneuvers, and high positive end-expiratory pressure for acute lung injury and acute respiratory distress syndrome. JAMA 2008; 299:637–645.
191. Mercat A, Richard JCM, Vielle B, et al. Positive end-expiratory pressure setting in adults with acute lung injury and acute respiratory distress syndrome. A randomized controlled trial. JAMA 2008; 299:646–655.
192. Corrigan JJ Jr, Ray WL, May N. Changes in the blood coagulation system associated with septicemia. N Engl J Med 1968; 279:851–856.
193. Esmon CT. The protein C pathway. Crit Care Med 2000; 28(Suppl. 9):S44–S48.
194. Vervolet MG, Thijs LG, Hack CE. Derangements of coagulation and fibrinolysis in critically ill patients with sepsis and septic shock. Semin Thromb Hemost 1998; 24:33–44.
195. Fourrier F, Chopin C, Goudemand J, et al. Septic shock, multiple organ failure, and disseminated intravascular coagulation: compared patterns of antithrombin III, protein C, and protein S deficiencies. Chest 1992; 101:816–823.
196. Lorente JA, Garcia-Frade LJ, Landin L, et al. Time course of hemostatic abnormalities in sepsis and its relation to outcome. Chest 1993; 103:1536–1542.
197. Powars D, Larsen R, Johnson J, et al. Epidemic meningococcemia and purpura fulminans with induced protein C deficiency. Clin Infect Dis 1993; 17:254–261.
198. Fisher CJ Jr, Yan SB. Protein C levels as a prognostic indicator of outcome in sepsis and related diseases. Crit Care Med 2000; 28(Suppl. 9):S49–S56.
199. Taylor FB Jr, Chang A, Esmon CT, et al. Protein C prevents the coagulopathic and lethal effects of Escherichia coli infusion in the baboon. J Clin Invest 1987; 79:918–925.
200. Taylor FB Jr, Peer GT, Lockhart MS, et al. Endothelial cell protein C receptor plays an important role in protein C activation in vivo. Blood 2001; 97:1685–1688.
201. Taylor FB, Wada H, Kinasewitz G. Description of compensated and uncompensated disseminated intravascular coagulation (DIC) responses (nonovert and overt DIC) in baboon models of intravenous and intraperitoneal Escherichia coli sepsis and in the human model of endotoxemia: toward a better definition of DIC. Crit Care Med 2000; 28(Suppl. 9): S12–S19.
202. Bernard GR, Ely EW, Wright TJ, et al. Safety and dose relationship of recombinant human activated protein C for coagulopathy in severe sepsis. Crit Care Med 2001; 29:2051–2059.
203. Natanson C, Esposito CJ, Banks SM. The sirens' songs of confirmatory sepsis trials: selection bias and sampling error. Crit Care Med 1998; 26:1927–1931.
204. Bernard GR, Margolis BD, Shanies HM, et al. Extended evaluation of recombinant human activated protein C United States trial (ENHANCE US): a single-arm, phase 3B, multicenter study of drotrecogin alfa (activated) in severe sepsis. Chest 2004; 125:2206–2216.
205. Abraham E, Laterre PF, Garg R, et al. Drotrecogin alfa (activated) for adults with severe sepsis and a low risk of death. N Engl J Med 2005; 353:1332–1341.
206. Wheeler A, Steingrub J, Schmidt GA, et al. A retrospective observational study of drotrecogin alfa (activated) in adults with severe sepsis: comparison with a controlled clinical trial. Crit Care Med 2008; 36:14–23.
207. Levi M, Levy M, Williams MD, et al. Xigris and prophylactic heparin evaluation in severe sepsis (XPRESS) Study Group. Prophylactic heparin in patients with severe sepsis treated with drotrecogin alfa (activated). Am J Respir Crit Care Med 2007; 176:483–490.
208. Moriyama S, Okamoto K, Tabria Y, et al. Evaluation of oxygen consumption and resting energy expenditure in critically ill patients with systemic inflammatory response syndrome. Crit Care Med 1999; 27:2133–2136.
209. Kudsk KA, Croce MA, Fabian TC, et al. Enteral vs. parenteral feeding. Effects on septic morbidity after blunt and penetrating abdominal trauma. Ann Surg 1992; 215:503–511.

210. Cerra FB, Benitez MR, Blackburn GL, et al. Applied nutrition in ICU patients. A consensus statement of the American College of Chest Physicians. Chest 1997; 111:769–778.

211. ASPEN Board of Directors. Guidelines for the use of parenteral and enteral nutrition in adult and pediatric patients. J Parenter Enteral Nutr 1993; 17:1SA–26SA.

212. Bertolini G, Iapichino G, Radrizzani D, et al. Early enteral immunonutrition in patients with severe sepsis: results of an interim analysis of a randomized multicentre clinical trial. Intensive Care Med 2003; 29:834–840.

213. Khalil AC, Sevransky JE, Myers DE, et al. Preclinical trial of L-arginine monotherapy alone or with N-acetylcysteine in septic shock. Crit Care Med 2006; 34:2719–2728.

214. Van den Berghe G, Wouters P, Weekersw F, et al. Intensive insulin therapy the surgical intensive care unit. N Engl J Med 2001; 345:1359–1367.

215. Van den Berghe G, Wilmer A, Hermans G, et al. Intensive insulin therapy in the medical ICU. N Engl J Med 2006; 354:449–461.

216. Krinsley J. Glycemic control in critically ill patients: Leuven and beyond. Chest 2007; 132:1–2.

217. Perez J, Dellinger RP. Other supportive therapies in sepsis. Intensive Care Med 2001; 27:S116–S127.

218. Geerts WH, Heit JA, Clagett GP, et al. Prevention of venous thromboembolism. Chest 2001; 119(Suppl. 1):132S–175S.

219. Keane MG, Ingenito EP, Goldhaber SZ. Utilization of venous thromboembolism prophylaxis in the medical intensive care unit. Chest 1994; 106:13–14.

220. Meyer MM. Renal replacement therapies. Crit Care Clin 2000; 16:29–58.

221. Schiffl H, Lang SM, Fischer R. Daily hemodialysis and the outcome of acute renal failure. N Engl J Med 2002; 346:305–310.

222. Palevsky PM, Zhang JH, O'Connor TZ, et al. Intensity of renal support in critically ill patients with acute kidney injury. N Engl J Med 2008; 359(1):7–20.

223. Hebert PC, Wells G, Blajchman MA, et al. A multicenter, randomized, controlled clinical trial of transfusion requirements in critical care. N Engl J Med 1999; 340:409–417.

224. Corwin HL, Gettinger A, Rodriguez RM, et al. Efficacy of recombinant human erythropoietin in the critically ill patient: a randomized, double-blind, placebo controlled trial. Crit Care Med 1999; 27:2346–2350.

225. Bennett CL, Silver SM, Djulbegovic B, et al. Venous thromboembolism and mortality associated with recombinant erythropoietin and darbepoetin administration for the treatment of cancer-associated anemia. JAMA 2008; 299;914–924.

10
Transfusion-Related Acute Lung Injury

MARK R. LOONEY
Department of Medicine, Division of Pulmonary and Critical Care, University of California, San Francisco, California, U.S.A.

OGNJEN GAJIC
Department of Medicine, Division of Pulmonary and Critical Care, Mayo Clinic, Rochester, Minnesota, U.S.A.

I. Introduction and Historical Perspective

Great strides have been made in the safety of allogeneic blood transfusions since their widespread introduction in the early 1900s. Complications such as major blood group incompatibility, bacterial contamination of stored products, and transmission of infectious agents such as the human immunodeficiency virus (HIV) and hepatitis C have plummeted with improved testing and quality assurance in blood banking (1). Accordingly, transfusion-related acute lung injury (TRALI) has emerged as a serious complication of transfusion therapy and the leading cause of transfusion-related fatalities reported to the U.S. Food and Drug Administration (L. Holness, personal communication). Although TRALI was formally described 25 years ago (2), it is very likely that TRALI as a clinical entity has been present since the early days of allogeneic transfusions.

Perhaps the first description of TRALI was by Barnard in 1951 in which a patient who was transfused whole blood developed acute pulmonary edema that was recognized by the authors as being a "hypersensitivity reaction" and not volume overload (3). Various other descriptions in the literature of probable TRALI ensued with terminology such as "pulmonary leukoagglutinin reaction" (4), "noncardiogenic pulmonary edema" (5–7), and "allergic pulmonary edema" (8). In 1983, investigators at the Mayo Clinic published a series of five patients who developed noncardiogenic pulmonary edema after either whole blood or red blood cell (RBC) transfusions and coined the term TRALI (2). Since this publication, there has been an explosion in the literature of suspected TRALI case reports, case series, clinical reviews, and experimental studies.

II. TRALI: Clinical Definition, Presentation, and Incidence

TRALI has been variably defined by investigators and has now benefited from attempts to standardize the clinical definition. There have been two major efforts at a consensus definition: the Canadian Consensus Conference (9) and the National Heart, Lung, and Blood Institute (NHLBI) Working Group definitions (10). Both clinical definitions share a common thread requiring that the standard American-European Consensus Conference (AECC) definition for ALI/ARDS (from all causes) be fulfilled. In brief, the AECC definition requires the acute onset of bilateral pulmonary opacities on chest radiography in conjunction with acute hypoxemia [P:F ratio <300 for ALI; P:F ratio <200 for ARDS (acute respiratory distress syndrome)] and the absence of left heart failure or volume overload (11). In both TRALI definitions, the timing of ALI must be within six hours of blood product transfusion. The selection of the six-hour time point was not completely arbitrary, as the clinical literature supports that the majority of patients develop TRALI within 30 to 60 minutes of blood product challenge and almost always within six hours.

The Canadian Consensus and NHLBI definitions were developed to aid the clinician in making a bedside diagnosis of TRALI. Neither definition considers laboratory testing, such as HLA (human leukocyte antigen) or neutrophil antibody testing. If a patient develops noncardiogenic pulmonary edema temporally related (within six hours) to any blood product transfusion, the diagnosis of TRALI can be assigned. The two definitions diverge when considering other ALI risk factors that may be present, such as sepsis, pneumonia, aspiration, and multiple transfusions. In the presence of these ALI risk factors, the Canadian Consensus definition would assign a diagnosis of "possible" TRALI, while the NHLBI definition requires the clinician to carefully consider the other ALI risk factors and to make a calculated decision as to the risk factor most likely to be related to the development of ALI. Practically speaking, both the exclusion of transfusion-associated circulatory overload (TACO) and the contribution of other credible ALI risk factors can be challenging for the clinician. Diagnostic considerations in TRALI will be discussed in detail later in this chapter.

Inherent in the clinical definition of TRALI is the acute presentation of symptoms. Symptoms such as acute dyspnea, wheezing, coughing, tachycardia, and fever can all accompany the acute pulmonary edema (12). There are no specific signs or symptoms of TRALI that would distinguish it from other causes of ALI. The development of a rash or urticaria would not be typical of TRALI and would point to allergic reactions to the transfused product. Patients may present with either hyper- or hypotension, and it is common for patients, particularly those severely affected, to progress to hypotension soon after presentation. There is a wide spectrum of clinical severity in TRALI ranging from the patient with mild dyspnea and mild oxygen desaturation to the patient who develops fulminant and severe pulmonary edema with pink, frothy pulmonary edema fluid emanating from the lungs. The latter patient often requires high fractions of supplemental oxygen and mechanical ventilation. In fact, in one of the largest series of TRALI patients, 72% of the patients required mechanical ventilation (13).

Of great importance, considering it is an iatrogenic condition, is obtaining an accurate incidence of TRALI. Reports vary in the literature depending on the cohort and cohort size, but the most consistently referenced incidence is 1 in 5000 blood products transfused or 1 in 600 patients transfused (10). It is also estimated that TRALI is fatal in approximately 5% of patients (13), which contrasts strikingly, and favorably, to the roughly 40% mortality in all causes of ALI/ARDS (14). The passive reporting of TRALI fatalities to the U.S. FDA from 2005–2007 has been consistent at approximately 30 cases per year, but in 2008 there was a decrease in TRALI fatalities (L. Holness, personal communication) which could reflect the effects of high-risk donor deferral that will be discussed later in this chapter. Importantly, TRALI is the number one cause of transfusion-associated fatalities and comprises over 50% of all the reported fatalities. Investigators at the Mayo Clinic and the University of California, San Francisco are conducting a prospective, observational trial of TRALI incidence using a comprehensive computerized screening process that should provide a large cohort and an accurate estimation of TRALI incidence.

III.   Blood Transfusions and ALI/ARDS: The Clinical Spectrum

The relationship between transfusion and ALI/ARDS has long been recognized with massive transfusion being one of the strongest underlying risk factors for ALI/ARDS in multiple studies (10). In critically ill patients, however, the development of ALI/ARDS is often attributed to the underlying reason for transfusion ("shock lung due to shock, not to transfusion") and transfusion factors are considered simply a marker of the severity of the underlying illness. While a causal relationship remains elusive to this date, several lines of evidence suggest that transfusion mechanisms play an important role, perhaps as cofactors, in many patients who develop ALI/ARDS temporally related to transfusion (15–17). Because of the complexity of the clinical evaluation of critically-ill patients (18), these potential associations are neither reported nor investigated by transfusion laboratories leading to widespread under-recognition (16).

A.   Observational Studies

Multiple observational studies (19–27) have reported the dose–response relationship with transfusions and both the development and outcome of ALI/ARDS, independent of confounding risk factors. For example, in a recent study from the Mayo Clinic, transfusion, rather than the reason for transfusion was associated with development of ALI/ARDS in the analysis using propensity scores (25). The dose–response association was stronger for plasma-rich blood products, fresh frozen plasma (FFP) and platelets, then for RBCs. It is important to realize that critically ill patients who undergo massive RBC transfusion are universally exposed to non-RBC blood products including FFP and platelet transfusions, potentially further explaining a strong association between massive transfusion and ALI/ARDS (25). Although demonstration of a dose–response relationship is an important feature in establishing causality, the absence of proper accounting for confounding factors, different study populations, and differences in time periods and transfusion exposures preclude meaningful comparisons between these observational studies and limit the ability to determine a causal relationship.

B.   Randomized Clinical Trials

The results of two recent randomized studies also support a possible etiologic role of transfusion factors in the development of ALI/ARDS (22,28). In a multicenter study by the Canadian Critical Care Network, patients randomized to a liberal transfusion strategy had a higher incidence of both ARDS and pulmonary edema, potentially explaining trends toward worse outcome with liberal transfusion (22). In this study, 838 critically ill patients who were admitted to intensive care units for more than 24 hours were randomized to either a liberal strategy (hemoglobin threshold for transfusion 10 g/dL) or restrictive strategy (hemoglobin threshold for transfusion 7 g/dL). On average, the restrictive group received 2.6 units while the liberal group received 5.6 units of red blood cells. ALI/ARDS developed in 11.4% of patients in the liberal group and 7.7% in the restrictive group. The odds ratio for the development of ALI/ARDS was 1.56 (95% CI 0.97–2.49) in patients assigned to the liberal as opposed to the restrictive transfusion group. More recently, patients with blunt trauma randomized to factor VIIa received lower numbers of plasma transfusions and had a significantly lower incidence of ARDS (28). However, these studies were neither designed nor powered to answer the question of causal relationship between transfusion and ALI.

C. The Association Between Specific Donor Characteristics and ALI/ARDS

Look-back studies, case series, and case control studies have reported associations of classic "TRALI" donor and product risk factors and the development of ALI/ARDS in critically ill patients. For example, Kopko and coworkers performed a retrospective review of 36 patient charts in a look-back investigation of transfusion-related fatalities (16). Of the 36 patients who were transfused FFP from one alloimmunized donor (a 54-year-old multiparous female who tested positive with HNA 5b antibody), 13 (36.1%) had transfusion reactions. Of the eight severe reactions involving ALI/ARDS, transfusion was considered in the differential diagnosis of only two. It is reasonable to suspect that transfusion factors played an important role in all eight patients. The adoption of the Canadian Consensus Conference definition (9) facilitated epidemiologic studies of ALI/ARDS temporally related to transfusion. In a recent study of transfused critically ill patients in which the investigators used this definition of TRALI, specific transfusion factors appeared to be independently linked to development of ALI/ARDS (15).

IV. Clinical TRALI Pathogenesis: Donor and Patient Risk Factors

Epidemiologic studies generally support the two principal pathophysiologic mechanisms that were reproduced in preclinical models (transfusion of alloimmunized donor plasma and biologic response modifiers that accumulate during storage) as well as the overall two-hit model of TRALI and ALI/ARDS (29). These two pathogenetic mechanisms may not be mutually exclusive and both seem to require additional predisposing conditions leading to pulmonary endothelial activation (30). In addition to critical illness in general, previous studies identified hematologic malignancies, cardiomyopathy, sepsis, alcohol abuse, and the postoperative state as significant patient-related risk factors for TRALI (13,15,31). These risk factors may serve as the initial priming events ("multiple-hit hypothesis") (29). In a recent review of the pathogenesis of TRALI by Bux and Sachs, the multiple-hit hypothesis has been presented as the "threshold model of TRALI" (29).

With regards to specific products, the risk of TRALI appears to be the highest for platelet transfusions, followed by FFP and packed RBCs (15). This is not surprising, since current platelet preparation and storage is associated with both high plasma volumes as well as with the accumulation of biologic response modifiers that develops during room temperature storage. It is plausible that both mechanisms interact in cases of TRALI after platelet transfusion.

Epidemiologic evidence suggests that high volume plasma transfusion from potentially alloimmunized donors, in particular female donors with multiple pregnancies, plays a role in development of TRALI (13,15–17,32,33). During pregnancy, mothers are typically exposed to alloantigens that can lead to the production of alloantibodies. The rate of alloimmunization correlates directly with parity as described by Insunza and coworkers (34), where the percentage of female donors with antileukocyte antibodies after one, two, or three prior pregnancies was approximately 9%, 18%, and 23%, respectively. In the original case series of TRALI, Popovsky and Moore (2) found antileukocyte antibodies in 85% of the donors whose blood was implicated in the development of TRALI.

The strongest evidence yet for the role of multiparous donors in the pathogenesis of TRALI comes from a recent clinical trial (32). In a randomized cross-over design, 100 patients requiring at least two units of FFP were infused FFP from both nulliparous and multiparous donors. After receiving the unit of multiparous FFP, patients were found to have a greater decrease in their Pao_{22}/Fio_2 ratio and increased levels of circulating TNF-α. Further evidence regarding the role of specific donor factors in development of ALI/ARDS after transfusion comes from a recent U.K. study, in which the investigators observed a significant decrease in development of ALI/ARDS in patients undergoing repair of ruptured abdominal aneurysms after the introduction of predominantly male-donor FFP in this country (17).

However, some investigators have reported contradictory findings (31,35) and it has become increasingly clear that plasma transfusion from potentially alloimmunized donors may not be the only important epidemiologic risk factor. Biological response modifiers such as proinflammatory cytokines (interleukin [IL]-6, IL-8, and tumor necrosis factor [TNF]-α) and lysophosphatidylcholines (lyso-PCs) are known to accumulate during storage of cellular blood products and the effect of "storage lesion" has been put forward as an alternative mechanism for TRALI development (36,37). In the study by Silliman and coworkers no association was observed between donor antibodies and development of TRALI (31). Instead, the levels of neutrophil priming activity increased with the duration of storage time of the transfused units in the patients who ultimately developed TRALI (31). It is believed that the primary culprits in the development of these circulating inflammatory mediators present in stored blood are residual leukocytes. However, in a recent clinical trial the development of ALI/ARDS after trauma was unaffected by the transfusion of leukoreduced as opposed to nonleukoreduced RBCs (38).

In a recent prospective study, Mayo Clinic researchers used the Canadian Consensus Conference definition to investigate the incidence, risk factors, and outcome of ALI/ARDS that develops within six hours after the transfusion of blood products in patients admitted to the medical ICU (15). Seventy-four of 901 patients (8%) developed ALI/ARDS within six hours of transfusion. Patients with sepsis, liver disease, and a history of chronic alcohol abuse were more likely than other patients to develop ALI/ARDS, as were patients who received plasma-rich blood products, blood products from female donors, and larger volumes of plasma from female donors. Donors to patients who subsequently developed ALI/ARDS had a higher number of pregnancies and tested positive for antileukocyte antibodies more often than donors to patients who did not develop ALI/ARDS (Table 1). IL-8 concentrations and storage age of RBC products did not differ between patients who developed ALI/ARDS and matched controls, but the concentration of lyso-PC was significantly higher in blood products given to ALI/ARDS case subjects than to control subjects (Table 1).

In summary, epidemiologic data support a TRALI mechanism that requires specific antigen–antibody pairing between the donor and recipient as well as achieving a certain concentration threshold of antileukocyte antibodies to initiate neutrophil priming and activation leading to an overwhelming inflammatory response resulting in alveolar-capillary membrane damage in a predisposed patient. The amount or concentration of passively transferred antibodies is likely an important determinant of the severity of the reaction (39). The exact concentration or threshold amount of these antibodies remains to be elucidated. It is doubtful, however, that a single mechanism explains the entire process and it is likely that in many instances there is interplay amongst several mechanisms. Pre-existing endothelial activation likely serves to potentiate the antigen–antibody reaction. The genetic and environmental patient predispositions, etiologic versus biomarker role of HLA and HNA antibodies, and the exact role of "storage lesion" and biologic response

Table 1 Specific Donor and Product-Related Risk Factors Associated with the Development of TRALI in Medical Critically Ill Patients

Variable	Adjusted odds ratio (95% CI)	*P*-value
Any high plasma volume components (FFP or platelets)	2.78 (1.21, 6.38)	0.016
Number of units	1.11 (0.99, 1.25)	0.086
Number of units from female donors	1.51 (1.08, 2.12)	0.016
Amount of male plasma (L)	1.60 (0.76, 3.37)	0.215
Amount of female plasma (L)	5.09 (1.37, 18.85)	0.015
Amount of plasma from female donors with at least one pregnancy (L)	9.48 (1.38, 65.35)	0.022
Number of pregnancies among donors	1.19 (1.05, 1.34)	0.007
Number of HLA class I + units	1.70 (0.94, 3.09)	0.098
Number of HLA class II + units	3.08 (1.15, 8.25)	0.025
Number of GIF + units	4.85 (1.32, 17.86)	0.018
Mean LysoPC 16 (per 10 umol/L)	1.16 (1.02, 1.32)	0.022

Source: From Ref. 15.
Abbreviation: GIF, granulocyte immunofluorescence.

modifiers have yet to be determined. While the evidence of a causal relationship between transfusion and ALI/ARDS remains limited, the burden of the problem forces an early implementation of potential preventive strategies including a restrictive transfusion policy and the avoidance of plasma from donors with a high likelihood of alloimmunization.

V. Experimental TRALI

Experimental studies on ALI/ARDS have significantly advanced our understanding of the mechanisms of injury development and have identified critical pathways that might be amenable to pharmacologic intervention. Although no pharmacotherapy exists for ALI/ARDS, successful intervention in the future will undoubtedly be linked to advances in clinical and laboratory-based research. For example, the clinical trials investigating the life-saving low tidal volume ventilation protocols in ALI/ARDS were rooted solidly in relevant animal models (40).

TRALI has been modeled in vitro (41), in isolated, perfused animal lung preparations (37,39,42,43), and in vivo in mice (44). These model systems have made significant contributions to the current understanding of TRALI pathogenesis. Seeger and coworkers described an isolated, perfused rabbit lung model in which a human antineutrophil antibody (HNA-3a), human neutrophils (HNA-3a$^+$), and rabbit plasma with complement were added to the perfusate resulting in an increase in lung weight and vascular permeability (43). This model has been updated by Sachs and coworkers in which a mouse, monoclonal antihuman neutrophil antibody (HNA-2a) produces lung edema and vascular permeability in the absence of complement and through direct activation of neutrophils (39). Silliman has made critical contributions to the biologically active lipid hypothesis of TRALI through both isolated, perfused lung studies in rats (37,42) and in vitro modeling (41). When plasma from RBCs or platelets on the day of outdate is added to the perfusate of rat lungs that have been primed with systemic lipopolysaccharide, an increase in lung

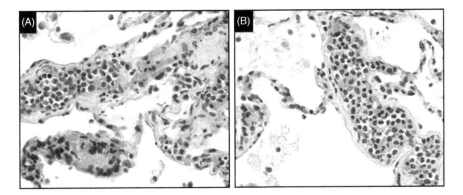

Figure 1 Lung histological sections from a patient who died from TRALI. (**A**) and (**B**) reveal interstitial and alveolar pulmonary edema and neutrophil aggregates in the microvasculature. H&E × 180. *Source*: From Ref. 45.

edema and pulmonary artery pressures is observed. Importantly, lyso-PCs can be isolated from these stored, cellular products and the perfusion of these lipids also produces lung injury. Lyso-PCs can prime and activate the neutrophil, which appears to be an essential cellular mediator of injury in experimental TRALI.

Other investigators have established an in vivo model of antibody-mediated TRALI in mice (44). The challenge of mice with MHC I monoclonal antibody produces an increase in pulmonary edema and lung vascular permeability at two hours and is associated with peripheral blood neutropenia. Neutrophils are sequestered in the lung microcirculation and neutrophil depletion protects mice from this model of TRALI. Neutrophil engagement of bound MHC I antibody is essential as mice lacking Fc gamma receptors are protected from injury. A recent report of a patient, who died of TRALI after an FFP transfusion, reinforces the central role of lung neutrophil sequestration in the pathogenesis of TRALI (Fig. 1) (45).

These experimental models have importantly implicated neutrophils, HLA and neutrophil antibodies, and lyso-PCs in TRALI pathogenesis. These studies have also complemented clinical series implicating HLA and neutrophil antibodies in the pathogenesis of TRALI and helped to strengthen blood-banking initiatives protecting transfused recipients from exposure to these agents.

VI. Diagnosis of TRALI

The diagnosis of TRALI in the ICU is difficult. In addition to acute bleeding, critically ill patients are often transfused with blood products to correct coagulopathies, to decrease the risk of bleeding during interventional procedures, or are transfused with RBCs to improve the oxygen delivery during the early resuscitation of septic shock (46). Diagnosing TRALI in these situations is problematic because ALI/ARDS is often attributed to the underlying condition that precipitated the transfusion of the blood product. Clinically, TRALI is indistinguishable from other causes of ALI/ARDS presenting as an acute permeability pulmonary edema. Physiologic abnormalities include the acute onset of hypoxemia, with

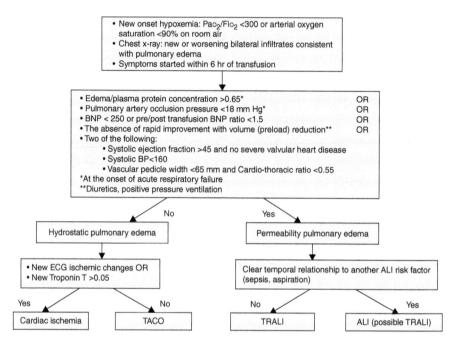

Figure 2   Differential diagnosis of post-transfusion acute pulmonary edema. *Source*: From Ref. 18.

a Pao_2/Fio_2 ratio less than 300 mm Hg and decreased pulmonary compliance (9,10). Laboratory findings for TRALI are nonspecific and may include acute transient neutropenia (9,10).

While the application of a standardized definition can help to differentiate acute lung injury (ALI) from hydrostatic pulmonary edema (TACO), distinguishing TRALI from other causes of ALI/ARDS such as sepsis, trauma, aspiration, pneumonia or ventilator-associated lung injury, is all but impossible solely on clinical grounds when one or more of these conditions is present. The differential diagnosis of ALI/ARDS other than TRALI is beyond the scope of this chapter, and, most importantly, these conditions do not necessarily exclude transfusions as an etiologic factor in cases where multiple factors may interact.

Bedside clinical information is of paramount importance in order to develop an adequate differential diagnosis of pulmonary transfusion reactions. Figure 2 outlines a clinical approach to acute pulmonary edema after transfusion (18). It is important to consider in the differential diagnosis other clinical entities associated with transfusion that can manifest respiratory symptoms similar to TRALI, most importantly TACO. While signs of fluid overload are usually present prior to transfusion, transfusion may precipitate acute hydrostatic pulmonary edema (18). Septic transfusion reactions can be associated with hypotension and ALI/ARDS, and bronchospasm and laryngeal edema can accompany allergic transfusion reactions. In addition, dyspnea may be a prominent feature of acute febrile and hemolytic reactions.

The differentiation between post-transfusion ALI and hydrostatic pulmonary edema (TRALI vs. TACO) is challenging since the clinical and radiological manifestations are often similar (47). The cause of edema may only be determined posthoc based on the clinical course and response to therapy (18). In addition, the two conditions may coexist with about 25% of patients with ALI/ARDS having a component of hydrostatic pulmonary edema (18). Noninvasive echocardiography and B-type natriuretic peptide measurements may aid in the differential diagnosis and invasive techniques such as right heart catheterization are sometimes helpful. In patients with an endotracheal tube in place, high protein concentration in the edema fluid, if sampled within the first hour of intubation, may help in differentiating ALI from hydrostatic pulmonary edema (18).

Given the complexity of the differential diagnosis of pulmonary transfusion reactions, it is important that bedside clinicians and transfusion medicine specialists work together in the assessment of patients suspected of having a pulmonary transfusion reaction. In the instances where, after thorough review, it appears that the patient has clinical evidence of both ALI and circulatory overload, the case should be classified as ALI with appropriate implications for prognosis and donor/product management. A systematic standardized approach to the assessment of pulmonary transfusion reactions will not only enhance the proper diagnosis and treatment of individual patients but will also allow blood centers to take appropriate actions regarding product safety and donor management.

VII. Treatment and Prevention of TRALI

The treatment of the TRALI patient implicitly requires ruling out the contribution of other ALI risk factors and also volume overload. TRALI can range widely in severity with some patients requiring only low-flow oxygen to others requiring mechanical ventilation (13) with high fractions of oxygen and high levels of positive end-expiratory pressure. Case reports even describe the use of extracorporeal membrane oxygenation in the most severe TRALI cases with refractory hypoxemia (48). If mechanical ventilation is required, we would recommend a low tidal volume (6 mL/kg, predicted body weight) and plateau pressure-limiting (<30 cm H_2O) approach that has been shown to lower mortality in all causes of ALI/ARDS (40).

It is also essential to determine as best as possible the volume status of the patient. TRALI can be associated with significant hypotension, especially after the indiscriminant use of diuretics (49). Diuretic therapy should be administered cautiously in the acute setting of TRALI, since the severely affected patient is often volume depleted from the increased lung vascular permeability. Diuretic therapy in ALI/ARDS has been shown to decrease time on mechanical ventilation, but the diuretic therapy was administered with the guidance of central venous pressure monitoring and at least 12 hours after the resolution of shock state (50).

Available evidence does not justify routine administration of corticosteroid therapy in the acute phase of ALI/ARDS (51), although the duration of ventilation may be favorably affected in cases that persist beyond the first week (52). It should be considered that the mortality of TRALI patients is low and that with supportive care most patients will be liberated from mechanical ventilation within 96 hours (13). Since the presentation of TRALI can be fulminant and severe, caring for the suspected TRALI patient much like the trauma patient with the "golden hour" approach is advisable. This involves careful attention to supporting hemodynamics, oxygenation, and using lung protective mechanical ventilation.

The prevention of TRALI has garnered much attention recently as there has been greater clarity on the pathogenesis of this condition. If investigation of a TRALI case reveals a donor with a HLA or neutrophil antibody that matches the recipient's antigen, this individual donor is generally removed from the donor pool. Given the association of female donors with TRALI cases, the U.K. National Blood Service initiated in 2003 the diversion of female blood donations away from FFP and platelet concentrates. The American Association of Blood Banks has also recommended the diversion of FFP and platelets from donors likely to be alloimmunized (53). Practically, blood banks are either diverting all females from FFP donation or using screening questions addressing pregnancy history and previous transfusions. Time will tell if these policy changes in the United Kingdom and the United States will lead to a decreased incidence of TRALI, although the Serious Hazards of Transfusion service in the United Kingdom has published a decrease in passively reported cases without a negative impact on the transfusion availability (54). The prudent use and avoidance of unnecessary transfusions remain the cornerstones for both TRALI prevention and availability of this precious resource.

VIII. Future Directions

We await the outcome of the donor management prevention strategies initiated in the United Kingdom and the United States. It may take some time to ascertain clear trends in the incidence of TRALI given the passive reporting systems in place. An active screening system, such as that being used at the Mayo Clinic and the University of California, San Francisco may eventually be most informative in determining the impact of the donor procurement strategies affecting FFP and platelet products. Other considerations include the screening of potentially alloimmunized donors for HLA or neutrophil antibodies using rapid, bead-based assays. The role of solvent-detergent–treated FFP, washed RBC and platelet products, and specific platelet additive solutions remains to be investigated.

IX. Summary

TRALI is an important cause of iatrogenic injury in hospitalized patients and it contributes to the majority of transfusion-associated deaths. Clinical and experimental evidence implicate donor HLA and neutrophil antibodies and biologically active lipids that accumulate in stored, cellular blood products. The host response to the passive transfusion of these mediators seems to prominently involve neutrophilic inflammation in the lung microcirculation. Treatment is supportive and similar to other forms of ALI/ARDS. Deferral of donors at high risk for alloimmunization may decrease the incidence of this serious complication of transfusion therapy.

References

1. Dodd RY. Current risk for transfusion transmitted infections. Curr Opin Hematol 2007; 14(6):671–676.
2. Popovsky MA, Abel MD, Moore SB. Transfusion-related acute lung injury associated with passive transfer of antileukocyte antibodies. Am Rev Respir Dis 1983; 128(1):185–189.
3. Barnard RD. Indiscriminate transfusion: a critique of case reports illustrating hypersensitivity reactions. N Y State J Med 1951; 51(20):2399–2402.

4. Ward HN. Pulmonary infiltrates associated with leukoagglutinin transfusion reactions. Ann Intern Med 1970; 73(5):689–694.

5. Carilli AD, Ramanamurty MV, Chang YS, et al. Noncardiogenic pulmonary edema following blood transfusion. Chest 1978; 74(3):310–312.

6. Culliford AT, Thomas S, Spencer FC. Fulminating noncardiogenic pulmonary edema. A newly recognized hazard during cardiac operations. J Thorac Cardiovasc Surg 1980; 80(6): 868–875.

7. Hashim SW, Kay HR, Hammond GL, et al. Noncardiogenic pulmonary edema after cardiopulmonary bypass. An anaphylactic reaction to fresh frozen plasma. Am J Surg 1984; 147(4):560–564.

8. Kernoff PB, Durrant IJ, Rizza CR, et al. Severe allergic pulmonary oedema after plasma transfusion. Br J Haematol 1972; 23(6):777–781.

9. Kleinman S, Caulfield T, Chan P, et al. Toward an understanding of transfusion-related acute lung injury: statement of a consensus panel. Transfusion 2004; 44(12):1774–1789.

10. Toy P, Popovsky MA, Abraham E, et al. Transfusion-related acute lung injury: definition and review. Crit Care Med 2005; 33(4):721–726.

11. Bernard GR, Artigas A, Brigham KL, et al. The American-European Consensus Conference on ARDS. Definitions, mechanisms, relevant outcomes, and clinical trial coordination. Am J Respir Crit Care Med 1994; 149(3, pt 1):818–824.

12. Looney MR, Gropper MA, Matthay MA. Transfusion-related acute lung injury: a review. Chest 2004; 126(1):249–258.

13. Popovsky MA, Moore SB. Diagnostic and pathogenetic considerations in transfusion-related acute lung injury. Transfusion 1985; 25(6):573–577.

14. Rubenfeld GD, Caldwell E, Peabody E, et al. Incidence and outcomes of acute lung injury. N Engl J Med 2005; 353(16):1685–1693.

15. Gajic O, Rana R, Winters JL, et al. Transfusion-related acute lung injury in the critically ill: prospective nested case-control study. Am J Respir Crit Care Med 2007; 176(9): 886–891.

16. Kopko PM, Marshall CS, MacKenzie MR, et al. Transfusion-related acute lung injury: report of a clinical look-back investigation. JAMA 2002; 287(15):1968–1971.

17. Wright SE, Snowden CP, Athey SC, et al. Acute lung injury after ruptured abdominal aortic aneurysm repair: the effect of excluding donations from females from the production of fresh frozen plasma. Crit Care Med 2008; 36(6):1796–1802.

18. Gajic O, Gropper MA, Hubmayr RD. Pulmonary edema after transfusion: how to differentiate transfusion-associated circulatory overload from transfusion-related acute lung injury. Crit Care Med 2006; 34(Suppl. 5):S109–S113.

19. Pepe PE, Potkin RT, Reus DH, et al. Clinical predictors of the adult respiratory distress syndrome. Am J Surg 1982; 144(1):124–130.

20. Hudson LD, Milberg JA, Anardi D, et al. Clinical risks for development of the acute respiratory distress syndrome. Am J Respir Crit Care Med 1995; 151(2, pt 1):293–301.

21. Silverboard H, Aisiku I, Martin GS, et al. The role of acute blood transfusion in the development of acute respiratory distress syndrome in patients with severe trauma. J Trauma 2005; 59(3):717–723.

22. Hebert PC, Wells G, Blajchman MA, et al. A multicenter, randomized, controlled clinical trial of transfusion requirements in critical care. Transfusion Requirements in Critical Care Investigators, Canadian Critical Care Trials Group. N Engl J Med 1999; 340(6):409–417.

23. Gajic O, Dara SI, Mendez JL, et al. Ventilator-associated lung injury in patients without acute lung injury at the onset of mechanical ventilation. Crit Care Med 2004; 32(9):1817–1824.

24. Gong MN, Thompson BT, Williams P, et al. Clinical predictors of and mortality in acute respiratory distress syndrome: potential role of red cell transfusion. Crit Care Med 2005; 33(6):1191–1198.

25. Khan H, Belsher J, Yilmaz M, et al. Fresh-frozen plasma and platelet transfusions are associated with development of acute lung injury in critically ill medical patients. Chest 2007; 131(5):1308–1314.
26. Croce MA, Tolley EA, Claridge JA, et al. Transfusions result in pulmonary morbidity and death after a moderate degree of injury. J Trauma 2005; 59(1):19–23.
27. Zilberberg MD, Carter C, Lefebvre P, et al. Red blood cell transfusions and the risk of acute respiratory distress syndrome among the critically ill: A cohort study. Crit Care 2007; 11(3):R63.
28. Boffard KD, Riou B, Warren B, et al. Recombinant factor VIIa as adjunctive therapy for bleeding control in severely injured trauma patients: two parallel randomized, placebo-controlled, double-blind clinical trials. J Trauma 2005; 59(1):8–15; discussion 15–18.
29. Bux J, Sachs UJ. The pathogenesis of transfusion-related acute lung injury (TRALI). Br J Haematol 2007; 136(6):788–799.
30. Silliman CC, Kelher M. The role of endothelial activation in the pathogenesis of transfusion-related acute lung injury. Transfusion 2005; 45(Suppl. 2):109S–116S.
31. Silliman CC, Boshkov LK, Mehdizadehkashi Z, et al. Transfusion-related acute lung injury: epidemiology and a prospective analysis of etiologic factors. Blood 2003; 101(2):454–462.
32. Palfi M, Berg S, Ernerudh J, et al. A randomized controlled trial of transfusion-related acute lung injury: is plasma from multiparous blood donors dangerous? Transfusion 2001; 41(3):317–322.
33. Rana R, Fernandez-Perez ER, Khan SA, et al. Transfusion-related acute lung injury and pulmonary edema in critically ill patients: a retrospective study. Transfusion 2006; 46(9):1478–1483.
34. Insunza A, Romon I, Gonzalez-Ponte ML, et al. Implementation of a strategy to prevent TRALI in a regional blood centre. Transfus Med 2004; 14(2):157–164.
35. Toy P, Hollis-Perry KM, Jun J, et al. Recipients of blood from a donor with multiple HLA antibodies: a lookback study of transfusion-related acute lung injury. Transfusion 2004; 44(12):1683–1688.
36. Silliman CC, Paterson AJ, Dickey WO, et al. The association of biologically active lipids with the development of transfusion-related acute lung injury: a retrospective study. Transfusion 1997; 37(7):719–726.
37. Silliman CC, Voelkel NF, Allard JD, et al. Plasma and lipids from stored packed red blood cells cause acute lung injury in an animal model. J Clin Invest 1998; 101(7):1458–1467.
38. Watkins TR, Rubenfeld GD, Martin TR, et al. Effects of leukoreduced blood on acute lung injury after trauma: a randomized controlled trial. Crit Care Med 2008; 36(5):1493–1499.
39. Sachs UJ, Hattar K, Weissmann N, et al. Antibody-induced neutrophil activation as a trigger for transfusion-related acute lung injury in an ex vivo rat lung model. Blood 2006; 107(3):1217–1219.
40. ARDS Network. Ventilation with lower tidal volumes as compared with traditional tidal volumes for acute lung injury and the acute respiratory distress syndrome. The Acute Respiratory Distress Syndrome Network. N Engl J Med 2000; 342(18):1301–1308.
41. Wyman TH, Bjornsen AJ, Elzi DJ, et al. A two-insult in vitro model of PMN-mediated pulmonary endothelial damage: requirements for adherence and chemokine release. Am J Physiol Cell Physiol 2002; 283(6):C1592–C1603.
42. Silliman CC, Bjornsen AJ, Wyman TH, et al. Plasma and lipids from stored platelets cause acute lung injury in an animal model. Transfusion 2003; 43(5):633–640.
43. Seeger W, Schneider U, Kreusler B, et al. Reproduction of transfusion-related acute lung injury in an ex vivo lung model. Blood 1990; 76(7):1438–1444.
44. Looney MR, Su X, Van Ziffle JA, et al. Neutrophils and their Fcγ receptors are essential in a mouse model of transfusion-related acute lung injury. J Clin Invest 2006; 116(6):1615–1623.
45. Cherry T, Steciuk M, Reddy VV, et al. Transfusion-related acute lung injury: past, present, and future. Am J Clin Pathol 2008; 129(2):287–297.

46. Rivers E, Nguyen B, Havstad S, et al. Early goal-directed therapy in the treatment of severe sepsis and septic shock. N Engl J Med 2001; 345(19):1368–1377.
47. Skeate RC, Eastlund T. Distinguishing between transfusion related acute lung injury and transfusion associated circulatory overload. Curr Opin Hematol 2007; 14(6):682–687.
48. Nouraei SM, Wallis JP, Bolton D, et al. Management of transfusion-related acute lung injury with extracorporeal cardiopulmonary support in a four-year-old child. Br J Anaesth 2003; 91(2):292–294.
49. Levy GJ, Shabot MM, Hart ME, et al. Transfusion-associated noncardiogenic pulmonary edema. Report of a case and a warning regarding treatment. Transfusion 1986; 26(3):278–281.
50. Wiedemann HP, Wheeler AP, Bernard GR, et al. Comparison of two fluid-management strategies in acute lung injury. N Engl J Med 2006; 354(24):2564–2575.
51. Bernard GR, Luce JM, Sprung CL, et al. High-dose corticosteroids in patients with the adult respiratory distress syndrome. N Engl J Med 1987; 317(25):1565–1570.
52. Steinberg KP, Hudson LD, Goodman RB, et al. Efficacy and safety of corticosteroids for persistent acute respiratory distress syndrome. N Engl J Med 2006; 354(16):1671–1684.
53. Strong DM, Lipton KS. American Association of Blood Banks Association Bulletin #06–07. Available online at: http://www.bpro.or.jp/publication/pdf_jptrans/us/us200611en.pdf. Accessed February 25, 2008.
54. Serious Hazards of Transfusion Annual Report 2006. Available online at: http://www.shotuk.org/SHOT_report_2006.pdf. Accessed March 25, 2008.

11
Mechanisms of Fibroproliferation in Acute Lung Injury

DANIELLE MORSE
Division of Pulmonary and Critical Care Medicine, Brigham and Women's Hospital, Harvard Medical School, Boston, Massachusetts, U.S.A.

CAROL FEGHALI-BOSTWICK
Division of Pulmonary, Allergy and Critical Care Medicine, University of Pittsburgh School of Medicine, Pittsburgh, Pennsylvania, U.S.A.

I. Introduction

In a landmark 1967 article published in Lancet, Ashbaugh and coworkers formally introduced the medical community to the syndrome of "acute respiratory distress in adults," or ARDS (1). This article described a pattern of clinical findings common to patients with respiratory failure due to a wide range of inciting injuries. ARDS was characterized histologically as protein-rich pulmonary edema with neutrophilic infiltration and hemorrhage (2,3). Over the ensuing two decades, distinct pathological phases in the development of ARDS were described, including an initial exudative phase characterized by cell injury and vascular leak (4), and a later "fibroproliferative" phase. The fibroproliferative phase was defined by chronic inflammation, fibrosis, and neovascularization (2,5). The dividing line between the acute exudative phase and the late fibroproliferative phase is not easily demarcated, and in the absence of lung biopsy tissue, this division must largely be inferred from chronicity. For the purposes of clinical trials, the term "persistent ARDS" has been used to describe patients meeting the criteria for ARDS and requiring mechanical ventilation seven or more days (6). It is presumed that persistent impairment of gas exchange and poor lung compliance more than one week after onset of ARDS correlates with progressive fibrosis (4). Variability among individuals exists, however, with some patients demonstrating relatively little fibrosis and others evincing ongoing neutrophilic inflammation well beyond the first week after symptom onset (7,8). It is therefore perhaps more accurate to consider exudation, inflammation, cell necrosis, and fibroproliferation as overlapping facets of the response to acute lung injury rather than as temporally distinct phases.

Although fibrosis dominates during the later phase of ARDS, there are indications that the initiation of fibrosis occurs early in the course of disease. Active transforming growth factor-β_1 (TGF-β_1), a master regulator of fibrosis, can be detected in bronchoalveolar lavage (BAL) fluid from patients with ARDS within 24 hours of diagnosis (9). A marker of collagen turnover, type III procollagen peptide, is also elevated in BAL fluid of patients with ARDS within the first day of recognized disease. An argument may therefore be made that treatment strategies for ARDS should target fibroproliferation from the outset. Fibrosing alveolitis is present in most patients dying with ARDS (3,10), and although there is no proven correlation between the extent of fibrosis and mortality, there is some suggestion that the presence of fibrosis portends a poorer outcome. In lung biopsy specimens obtained from 25 consecutive patients with ARDS, those with evidence of fibrosis (64%) had a significantly higher mortality rate than those without fibrosis (7). Given the association between prolonged dependence on mechanical ventilation and the predominance of fibroproliferative changes on lung biopsy, it is not unreasonable to suppose that prevention of fibrosis could lead to improved survival. A second rationale for targeting fibrosis in ARDS would be to improve recovery of lung function in the longer term. Survivors of ARDS continue to have exercise limitation and abnormal lung function, indicating a degree of irreversible lung impairment (11,12). Poor recovery of pulmonary function correlates with a prolonged course of mechanical ventilation and more severe cumulative lung injury scores, suggesting that patients with worse fibrosis have the poorest outcomes (11).

Understanding of the pathobiology of fibrosis in ARDS could have benefits beyond targeted therapies for this specific patient population. A remarkable feature of fibroproliferation in ARDS is the trend toward long-term physiologic stability or improvement. This contrasts with most chronic fibrotic lung diseases, where declining lung function is the rule. Studies of survivors of ARDS report mild abnormalities in spirometry that tend to improve or remain stable over time (12–14). Of 109 survivors of ARDS evaluated 3, 6, and 12 months after discharge from the intensive care unit, lung volume and spirometric measurements had normalized by six months, although carbon monoxide diffusion capacity remained low throughout the 12-month follow-up. None of the patients required supplemental oxygen at the 12-month time point (12). In contrast, individuals with idiopathic pulmonary fibrosis or history of occupational lung fibrosis generally experience progressive declines in lung function (15,16). Elucidation of the mechanisms by which lung fibrosis regresses or resolves in survivors of ARDS could shed light on the reasons for progression of fibrosis in other disease settings.

II. Pathological Features of the Fibroproliferative Phase of Lung Injury

The exudative phase of ARDS is characterized histologically by diffuse alveolar damage, and these changes typically persist through the first week of disease (17). Dominant features of this phase include proteinaceous edema, hyaline membranes, neutrophilic infiltration, and focal areas of epithelial necrosis (3,18). The endothelium may also be denuded in places with associated fibrin clot. The pathology of the exudative phase is described in detail in chapter 10. By the second week after symptom onset, the exudates take on a more organized appearance, and fibrosis can be appreciated microscopically. Alveolar type II epithelial cells, which occupy only 5% of the normal alveolar surface area, replicate in order to repopulate a basement membrane that has been denuded of type I cells (10,17). During this phase, alveolar exudate and apoptotic cells may be cleared, but frequently there is persistence of an alveolar provisional matrix consisting of fibrin, fibronectin, and hyaluronan fragments. Fibroblasts migrate into this fibrinous exudate and begin to convert the exudate into granulation tissue; this in turn is progressively replaced by collagen fibrils, beginning with type III collagen and followed by type I collagen (19). In addition, fibroblasts within the alveolar wall deposit matrix locally, resulting in thickened, fibrotic alveolar septa (17). Beyond three or four weeks from the onset of ARDS, the lungs may take on a cobblestoned gross appearance due to progressive scarring. The lung architecture becomes distorted, with alveolar walls composed primarily of collagenous connective tissue and irregular enlargement of the air spaces (10). A typical example of this histology is shown in Figure 1.

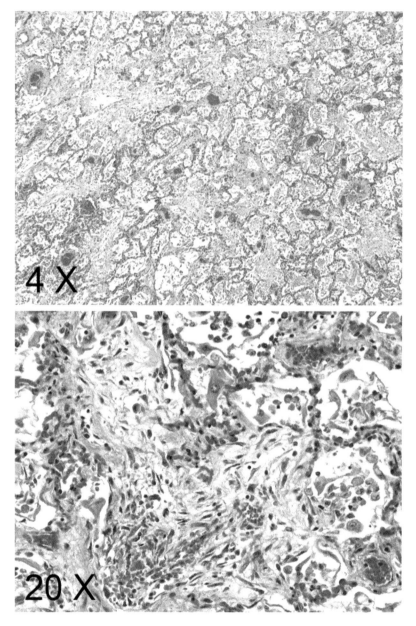

Figure 1   Histological features of the fibroproliferative phase.

The interstitial edema characteristic of early ARDS results from endothelial cell injury and vascular leak. Although microscopic evidence of endothelial injury may be subtle early in the course of ARDS (20), vascular abnormalities are prominent during the fibroproliferative phase (21). Thromboemboli are frequently present, as is fibrocellular intimal proliferation (21). Dilation of the capillary bed or a decline in capillary number may occur during the fibrotic phase of ARDS. Larger arteries demonstrate intimal proliferation and fibrosis resulting in reduced luminal areas, a contributing factor to the development of pulmonary hypertension in late stage ARDS.

A. Epithelial Injury and Repair

Diffuse alveolar damage is the hallmark of ARDS, and extensive epithelial necrosis is a prominent feature. Although type I and type II epithelial cells are present in similar numbers in the lung, the type I epithelial cells populate approximately 95% of the alveolar surface due to their extremely attenuated cytoplasmic extensions (22). It has been suggested that type II pneumocytes are more resistant to cell death than are type I pneumocytes (17), and certainly type I cells bear the brunt of losses due to necrosis in the setting of acute lung injury. Death of type I cells may be associated with loss of the alveolar basement membrane, which is thought to negatively impact the lung's ability to recapitulate normal architecture (23). The alveolar epithelial type II cell normally proliferates slowly, but following epithelial injury, the rate of proliferation increases to cover areas of denuded alveolar basement membrane. During successful lung repair, type II cells then differentiate into type I cells, restoring normal function. Epithelial cell proliferation is controlled by epithelial growth factors, including keratinocyte and hepatocyte growth factors (KGF and HGF) (22). The regulation of type II cell differentiation toward a type I phenotype in vivo is yet poorly understood, but the nature of the extracellular matrix and the presence or absence of epithelial growth factors have been implicated (23).

Clues to the relationship between epithelial repair and fibrosis have been sought in chronic fibrotic disorders such as idiopathic pulmonary fibrosis. Lungs from patients with idiopathic pulmonary fibrosis exhibit evidence of loss of type I epithelial cells and proliferation of type II pneumocytes (24). It is not clear whether the increased number of cuboidal epithelial cells seen in idiopathic pulmonary fibrosis results from a failure of differentiation toward a type I phenotype or ongoing epithelial turnover. Evidence exists to support both continual epithelial proliferation in response to injury (24) and abnormal epithelial cell differentiation, possibly in response to transforming growth factor (TGF-β) (25). Failure of type II cell repair and re-epithelialization has been correlated with the development of pulmonary fibrosis in a number of disease models (26), and the presence of an intact epithelium has been shown to inhibit fibroblast proliferation and matrix production (27). It is therefore reasonable to postulate that by encouraging successful epithelial repair, the progression of lung fibrosis in chronic and acute disease settings might be averted. Supplementation of epithelial-specific growth factors has been tested in animal models of lung injury and fibrosis on the theory that enhanced pneumocyte proliferation could lead to more rapid and effective lung repair (28). One of the most extensively tested growth factors is keratinocyte growth factor (KGF), which is known to induce type II cell hyperplasia. Pretreatment with KGF has been shown to protect the lung in a variety of animal lung injury models (29–31), although interestingly, the protection afforded by KGF in the setting of acute lung injury appears to be due to activation of epithelial cell survival pathways as opposed to increased cell proliferation (29–31). Further work remains to be done in unraveling the precise mechanisms by which the balance of growth factors in the fibroproliferative phase of ARDS affects lung re-epithelialization, but it is becoming increasingly apparent that failure of epithelial repair and dysregulation of alveolar type II cell differentiation influence the ultimate development of pulmonary fibrosis (32). The behavior of type II epithelial cells is therefore an important but relatively understudied determinant of the progression of lung fibrosis.

B.   The Fibroblast: Central Player in the Fibroproliferative Phase

Fibrosis associated with ARDS is characterized by accumulation of extracellular matrix molecules, particularly fibrillar collagens, and the fibroblast is the main cell responsible for the production of extracellular matrix components. Fibroblasts are not a homogeneous population, and in the last decade the concept of phenotypic diversity has emerged (33). Rates of proliferation, actin filament expression, and matrix production differ among fibroblasts isolated from different individuals and from subpopulations of fibroblasts isolated from the same individual (33). There is some controversy as to whether phenotypic alterations of fibroblasts in certain individuals predispose them to progressive fibrosis independent of persistent external signals. One study showed that in a small number of individuals with acute lung injury and fibrosis ($n = 3$), the rate of ex vivo mesenchymal cell proliferation was higher than that of individuals with normal lungs. This difference persisted through multiple passages, suggesting a stable, intrinsic difference in cellular behavior as opposed to a reversible response to extracellular signals (34). The investigators reported that the immediate early cell division cycle genes c-fos and c-jun were constitutively expressed in cells derived from injured lungs but not from control lungs (34). It is likely that fibroblast behavior is altered in response to early environmental signals in ARDS even if these behaviors are not reversed by removal of the cells from their extracellular milieu. Fibroblast mitogenic activity has been shown to be increased in BAL fluid from patients with ARDS relative to control patients (35,36). A significant proportion of the bioactivity was ascribed to platelet-derived growth factor (PDGF) and related peptides (36).

Additional controversy exists regarding the source of mesenchymal matrix-producing cells in fibrotic lung disease. Most studies have addressed this issue in the context of chronic fibrosis, and therefore the relevance to fibroproliferation in ARDS is unclear. Epithelial cells have been shown to have the capacity to transdifferentiate into mesenchymal cells in a process called epithelial-mesenchymal transition (EMT) (37,38). EMT has been observed in response to epithelial cell injury in a number of tissues, and type II pneumocytes have the capacity to develop a mesenchymal phenotype in vitro (38). The extent to which this process contributes to lung fibrosis is unknown. Recent studies have further suggested that repair of injured lung epithelium may be driven by cells derived from outside the lung. Fibrocytes, which are bone marrow-derived blood cells expressing type I collagen, are recruited to the lung in animal models of lung fibrosis (39) and in human disease (40). Whether such cells contribute to fibrosis in the setting of acute lung injury is unknown.

Although fibroblasts may be derived from other cell types or sources outside of the lung (such as the bone marrow), there is no question that activation of local lung fibroblasts by specific factors contributes significantly to fibrogenesis. Interstitial fibroblasts are activated to migrate, proliferate, and secrete extracellular matrix proteins in response to myriad

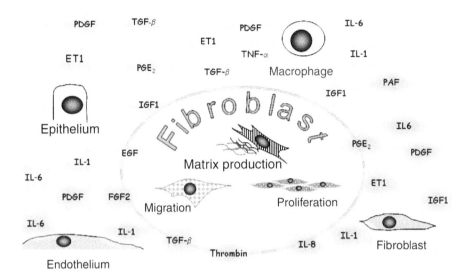

Figure 2 Schematic of representative growth factors affecting fibroblast behaviors in the setting of fibroproliferative ARDS. Growth factors are derived from various cellular components of the lung, not all of which are represented in the schematic. *Abbreviations*: PDGF, platelet-derived growth factor; IL-6, interleukin-6; IL-1, interleukin-1; TGF-β, transforming growth factor-β; ET1, endothelin-1; FGF2, fibroblast growth factor-2; PGE$_2$, prostaglandin E$_2$; IGF1, insulin-like growth factor-1; PAF, platelet activating factor; EGF, epidermal growth factor.

external stimuli (Fig. 2). Reduced apoptosis of fibroblasts and decreased degradation of extracellular matrix components may also contribute to the progression of fibrosis. Stimuli that activate fibroblasts include factors such as TGF-β, TGF-α, tumor necrosis factor (TNF)-α, PDGF, insulin-like growth factor (IGF), and proinflammatory cytokines among others. Several of these factors have been measured in BAL fluid of ARDS patients and found to be elevated (reviewed in Bellingan 2002) (41). One of the markers of fibroblast activation is the expression of α-smooth muscle actin, a component of the actin–myosin complex. Such fibroblasts are often referred to as myofibroblasts, cells capable of speeding wound repair by contracting the edges of the wound. Myofibroblasts are important contributors to the progression of lung fibrosis, and they are present in the early phase of ARDS (42). BAL fluid from ARDS patients has been shown to induce myofibroblast differentiation; this effect was partially reversible by treatment with a TGF-β$_1$ receptor inhibitor (42). Myofibroblasts have been shown to express high level of collagen and other matrix molecules as well as cytokines and chemokines capable of modulating the inflammatory and fibrotic response (43,44). This cell type is therefore capable of promoting repair or fibrosis by a number of mechanisms beyond its ability to contract a wound.

While contractile cells such as myofibroblasts have the capacity to exert mechanical tension on the repairing lung parenchyma, it is also true that external mechanical forces are capable of influencing cell behavior. The lung is subjected to tensile stress throughout the respiratory cycle, and the influence of stretch, pressure, and shear force on clinical outcomes in mechanically ventilated patients has been an area of considerable research interest (45). Although the effect of mechanical forces on fibroblast behavior has long been recognized in other organs such as skin (46), relatively little is known about the relationship between mechanical forces and lung fibrosis. Changes in cell surface stresses can lead to remodeling of focal adhesions, and cell stretch along with signaling via integrins has been shown to alter matrix and protease production by fibroblasts (47,48). Mechanical forces can also induce direct secretion of various growth factors that accelerate the remodeling of the matrix, such as TGF-β (49). It is likely that lung stretch and local mechanical forces modulate extracellular matrix production and remodeling in the fibroproliferative phase of ARDS, although the nature and magnitude of this effect remain to be elucidated.

III. Mediators of Tissue Remodeling in Lung Injury

The role of growth factors and cytokines in orchestrating tissue remodeling has been explored mainly through the use of BAL fluid from patients with ARDS. Several of these factors are not unique to ARDS and likely contribute to the pathogenesis of other fibrotic lung disorders such as idiopathic pulmonary fibrosis. Secreted proteins may induce disparate effects in different cell types, and also represent a mechanism by which various cell types can "cross-talk." The best-studied mediator of fibrosis is TGF-β, the archetypical profibrotic growth factor. It is produced by many cell types and is remarkably pleiotropic in its actions (50). TGF-β is produced in latent form, noncovalently associated with latency-associated peptide (LAP). This complex is in turn associated with latent transforming growth factor β-binding protein, a family of fibrillin-like extracellular matrix proteins thought to modulate TGF-β bioavailability and targeting to the extracellular matrix (50). Activation of TGF-β in vivo is accomplished primarily via the epithelial cell integrin αvβ6 (51). This integrin releases TGF-β from LAP, allowing active TGF-β to bind to cell surface receptors. Mice lacking the β6 integrin do not develop lung fibrosis in response to bleomycin (51), and blocking antibodies to integrin αvβ6 also reduce fibrosis in the bleomycin model, confirming the importance of this integrin in the regulation of TGF-β (52).

Active TGF-β exerts myriad biological actions varying by cell type and disease setting, making its precise functions challenging to define. For example, TGF-β causes or growth arrest or apoptosis in epithelial cells (53), whereas fibroblasts are stimulated by TGF-β to express matrix proteins and α-smooth muscle actin and may have increased proliferation (42,54). TGF-β plays a central role in immunity, generally (although not uniformly) dampening the inflammatory response by leukocytes (55). Although precise mechanisms remain to be clarified, there is no doubt regarding the importance of TGF-β in promoting fibrosis. TGF-β is highly expressed in virtually all fibrotic conditions, including fibroproliferative ARDS. Overexpression of constitutively active TGF-β in the lung is sufficient to cause fibrosis (56), and neutralization of TGF-β abrogates progression of fibrosis in models of lung, liver, kidney, and pancreatic fibrosis, among others (57).

The identification of additional mediators of lung injury and tissue remodeling in BAL fluid has taken advantage of more recently developed proteomic approaches. One such approach identified an increase in the levels of a novel factor, insulin-like growth factor binding protein (IGFBP-3), that can modulate epithelial cell survival and production of extracellular matrix by fibroblasts (58,59). In patients with early ARDS or at risk for the development of ARDS, IGF-I and IGFBP-3 levels are elevated in BAL fluid. IGF-I and its receptor, IGF-IR, have also been shown to be elevated in lung tissues from patients with fibroproliferative ARDS (60). The cellular sources of IGF-I and IGF-IR were identified as alveolar and interstitial macrophages and mesenchymal cells. Levels of IGF-I correlate with increases in collagens I and III in the lung tissues (60); IGF-I also contributes to fibroblast survival, potentially enabling the progression of fibrosis (58)

Endothelin-1 (ET-1) is a factor that is increased in the plasma of patients with ARDS; it may contribute to the pulmonary hypertension seen in some patients with ARDS (61). The increased ET-1 levels were due to increased production of endothelin as well as decreased degradation of this vasoconstricting peptide in the pulmonary vasculature (62). Cellular sources of ET-1 in ARDS lung tissues included vascular endothelial cells and smooth muscle cells, epithelial cells, and alveolar macrophages (63). Since ET-1 acts as a mitogen for smooth muscle cells and an inducer of matrix production, increased levels can contribute to the proliferative and fibrotic phase of ARDS.

Mediators such as HGF and KGF are found in BAL fluid of patients with ARDS; these are secreted by fibroblasts but predominantly affect epithelial cell responses (64), promoting proliferation of alveolar type II epithelial cells.

The balance of matrix metalloproteases (MMPs) and tissue inhibitors of metallo-proteases (TIMP) may also be important in the fibrotic and repair phase of ARDS. MMPs are a large class of proteinases with the ability to cleave fibrillar collagens as well as other matrix components. MMPs may also degrade nonmatrix proteins and thus have been implicated in the activation and shedding of a wide array of biologically active molecules (65). Individual MMP family members have varying substrate specificity and variable susceptibility to inhibition by TIMPs. Many different MMPs and inhibitors (TIMPs) exist, and the range of synergistic or antagonistic mechanisms of action of the MMP family make it difficult to reach broad conclusions regarding their role in fibroproliferative ARDS. Levels of gelatinases and TIMP are increased in ARDS BAL fluid (Ricou 1996) (66), suggesting that collagen-degrading enzymes are active in ARDS but increased TIMP levels may alter the balance in patients with sustained fibrosis. Mechanistic studies will be required to better define the role of each family member in the pathogenesis of acute lung injury and fibrosis.

IV. Fibroproliferative Markers as Predictors of Outcome/Mortality

Although mediators of fibroproliferation have been studied primarily in order to gain insight into mechanisms of disease and as targets of potential therapy, there is also interest in developing markers for diagnosis and prognosis. Attempts have been made to correlate the levels of several of the factors discussed above with patient outcomes. TGF-β, the master regulator of fibrosis, is elevated in BAL fluid of ARDS patients and levels have been associated with ventilator-free and ICU-free day (54). Detection of KGF in BAL fluid of ARDS patients has been associated with the detection of type III procollagen peptide and correlated with poor prognosis (67). Persistently increased plasma levels of TNF-α, IL-1β, IL-6, and IL-8 predicted low likelihood of survival in patients with ARDS (68). Yet another factor associated with poor outcome in ARDS is circulating angiopoietin-2, which is believed to contribute to pulmonary permeability edema and severity of ARDS (69). Increased levels of vascular endothelial growth factor in lung epithelial lining fluid predict a better outcome and are inversely correlated with lung injury score (70,71). Despite such observations, a single marker that accurately predicts outcome in ARDS in a specific and sensitive manner is still not available; it is likely to be some time before a clinically useful marker becomes available.

V. Conclusions

Despite recent improvements in treatment for ARDS, the human cost in terms of morbidity and mortality remains high. Further research is needed to identify predictors of outcome and effective therapeutic interventions. Since ARDS is a complication of disparate disease processes, it is unsurprising that numerous mediators of injury and remodeling have been implicated in the pathogenesis of fibroproliferative ARDS. No single treatment is likely to be efficacious, and tailored treatment approaches may be required to halt ongoing injury and to prevent aberrant tissue remodeling. Furthermore, although many of the mediators discussed above have been implicated in progression of fibrosis, most are also natural components of our body's defense against infection and response to injury. Inhibiting the action of these mediators may result in unforeseen complications and this should be undertaken with caution and with an awareness of the complex interplay of the signaling molecules and cell types involved in lung repair.

References

1. Ashbaugh DG, Bigelow DB, Petty TL, et al. Acute respiratory distress in adults. Lancet 1967; 2:319–323.
2. Bernard GR. Acute respiratory distress syndrome: a historical perspective. Am J Respir Crit Care Med 2005; 172:798–806.
3. Lamy M, Fallat RJ, Koeniger E, et al. Pathologic features and mechanisms of hypoxemia in adult respiratory distress syndrome. Am Rev Respir Dis 1976; 114:267–284.
4. Hudson LD, Hough CL. Therapy for late-phase acute respiratory distress syndrome. Clin Chest Med 2006; 27:671–677; abstract ix–x.
5. Gattinoni L, Bombino M, Pelosi P, et al. Lung structure and function in different stages of severe adult respiratory distress syndrome. JAMA 1994; 271:1772–1779.
6. Steinberg KP, Hudson LD, Goodman RB, et al. Efficacy and safety of corticosteroids for persistent acute respiratory distress syndrome. N Engl J Med 2006; 354:1671–1684.
7. Martin C, Papazian L, Payan MJ, et al. Pulmonary fibrosis correlates with outcome in adult respiratory distress syndrome. A study in mechanically ventilated patients. Chest 1995; 107: 196–200.
8. Goodman RB, Strieter RM, Martin DP, et al. Inflammatory cytokines in patients with persistence of the acute respiratory distress syndrome. Am J Respir Crit Care Med 1996; 154: 602–611.
9. Fahy RJ, Lichtenberger F, McKeegan CB, et al. The acute respiratory distress syndrome: a role for transforming growth factor-beta 1. Am J Respir Cell Mol Biol 2003; 28:499–503.
10. Fukuda Y, Ishizaki M, Masuda Y, et al. The role of intraalveolar fibrosis in the process of pulmonary structural remodeling in patients with diffuse alveolar damage. Am J Pathol 1987; 126:171–182.
11. McHugh LG, Milberg JA, Whitcomb ME, et al. Recovery of function in survivors of the acute respiratory distress syndrome. Am J Respir Crit Care Med 1994; 150:90–94.
12. Herridge MS, Cheung AM, Tansey CM, et al. One-year outcomes in survivors of the acute respiratory distress syndrome. N Engl J Med 2003; 348:683–693.

13. Heyland DK, Groll D, Caeser M. Survivors of acute respiratory distress syndrome: relationship between pulmonary dysfunction and long-term health-related quality of life. Crit Care Med 2005; 33:1549–1556.
14. Orme J Jr, Romney JS, Hopkins RO, et al. Pulmonary function and health-related quality of life in survivors of acute respiratory distress syndrome. Am J Respir Crit Care Med 2003; 167:690–694.
15. Ohlson CG, Bodin L, Rydman T, et al. Ventilatory decrements in former asbestos cement workers: a four year follow up. Br J Ind Med 1985; 42:612–616.
16. Gross TJ, Hunninghake GW. Idiopathic pulmonary fibrosis. N Engl J Med 2001; 345:517–525.
17. Tomashefski JF Jr. Pulmonary pathology of acute respiratory distress syndrome. Clin Chest Med 2000; 21:435–466.
18. Katzenstein AL, Bloor CM, Leibow AA. Diffuse alveolar damage—the role of oxygen, shock, and related factors. A review. Am J Pathol 1976; 85:209–228.
19. Raghu G, Striker LJ, Hudson LD, et al. Extracellular matrix in normal and fibrotic human lungs. Am Rev Respir Dis 1985; 131:281–289.
20. Albertine KH. Ultrastructural abnormalities in increased-permeability pulmonary edema. Clin Chest Med 1985; 6:345–369.
21. Tomashefski JF Jr, Davies P, Boggis C, et al. The pulmonary vascular lesions of the adult respiratory distress syndrome. Am J Pathol 1983; 112:112–126.
22. Uhal BD. Cell cycle kinetics in the alveolar epithelium. Am J Physiol 1997; 272:L1031–L1045.
23. Ingbar DH. Mechanisms of repair and remodeling following acute lung injury. Clin Chest Med 2000; 21:589–616.
24. Selman M, Pardo A. Role of epithelial cells in idiopathic pulmonary fibrosis: from innocent targets to serial killers. Proc Am Thorac Soc 2006; 3:364–372.
25. Zhang F, Nielsen LD, Lucas JJ, et al. Transforming growth factor-beta antagonizes alveolar type II cell proliferation induced by keratinocyte growth factor. Am J Respir Cell Mol Biol 2004; 31:679–686.
26. Kuwano K. Involvement of epithelial cell apoptosis in interstitial lung diseases. Intern Med 2008; 47:345–353.
27. Adamson IY, Young L, Bowden DH. Relationship of alveolar epithelial injury and repair to the induction of pulmonary fibrosis. Am J Pathol 1988; 130:377–383.
28. Ware LB, Matthay MA. Keratinocyte and hepatocyte growth factors in the lung: roles in lung development, inflammation, and repair. Am J Physiol Lung Cell Mol Physiol 2002; 282:L924–L940.
29. Yi ES, Williams ST, Lee H, et al. Keratinocyte growth factor ameliorates radiation- and bleomycin-induced lung injury and mortality. Am J Pathol 1996; 149:1963–1970.
30. Plantier L, Marchand-Adam S, Antico VG, et al. Keratinocyte growth factor protects against elastase-induced pulmonary emphysema in mice. Am J Physiol Lung Cell Mol Physiol 2007; 293:L1230–L1239.
31. Gomperts BN, Belperio JA, Fishbein MC, et al. Keratinocyte growth factor improves repair in the injured tracheal epithelium. Am J Respir Cell Mol Biol 2007; 37:48–56.
32. Selman M, King TE, Pardo A. Idiopathic pulmonary fibrosis: prevailing and evolving hypotheses about its pathogenesis and implications for therapy. Ann Intern Med 2001; 134:136–151.
33. Ramos C, Montano M, Garcia-Alvarez J, et al. Fibroblasts from idiopathic pulmonary fibrosis and normal lungs differ in growth rate, apoptosis, and tissue inhibitor of metalloproteinases expression. Am J Respir Cell Mol Biol 2001; 24:591–598.
34. Chen B, Polunovsky V, White J, et al. Mesenchymal cells isolated after acute lung injury manifest an enhanced proliferative phenotype. J Clin Invest 1992; 90:1778–1785.
35. Marshall RP, Bellingan G, Webb S, et al. Fibroproliferation occurs early in the acute respiratory distress syndrome and impacts on outcome. Am J Respir Crit Care Med 2000; 162: 1783–1788.

36. Snyder LS, Hertz MI, Peterson MS, et al. Acute lung injury. Pathogenesis of intraalveolar fibrosis. J Clin Invest 1991; 88:663–673.
37. Kim KK, Kugler MC, Wolters PJ, et al. Alveolar epithelial cell mesenchymal transition develops in vivo during pulmonary fibrosis and is regulated by the extracellular matrix. Proc Natl Acad Sci U S A 2006; 103:13180–13185.
38. Willis BC, Borok Z. TGF-beta-induced EMT: Mechanisms and implications for fibrotic lung disease. Am J Physiol Lung Cell Mol Physiol 2007; 293:L525–L534.
39. Hashimoto N, Jin H, Liu T, et al. Bone marrow-derived progenitor cells in pulmonary fibrosis. J Clin Invest 2004; 113:243–252.
40. Mehrad B, Burdick MD, Zisman DA, et al. Circulating peripheral blood fibrocytes in human fibrotic interstitial lung disease. Biochem Biophys Res Commun 2007; 353:104–108.
41. Bellingan GJ. The pulmonary physician in critical care * 6: the pathogenesis of ALI/ARDS. Thorax 2002; 57:540–546.
42. Synenki L, Chandel NS, Budinger GR, et al. Bronchoalveolar lavage fluid from patients with acute lung injury/acute respiratory distress syndrome induces myofibroblast differentiation. Crit Care Med 2007; 35:842–848.
43. Phan SH, Zhang K, Zhang HY, et al. The myofibroblast as an inflammatory cell in pulmonary fibrosis. Curr Top Pathol 1999; 93:173–182.
44. Zhang K, Rekhter MD, Gordon D, et al. Myofibroblasts and their role in lung collagen gene expression during pulmonary fibrosis. A combined immunohistochemical and in situ hybridization study. Am J Pathol 1994; 145:114–125.
45. The Acute Respiratory Distress Syndrome Network. Ventilation with lower tidal volumes as compared with traditional tidal volumes for acute lung injury and the acute respiratory distress syndrome. N Engl J Med 2000; 342:1301–1308.
46. Eckes B, Krieg T. Regulation of connective tissue homeostasis in the skin by mechanical forces. Clin Exp Rheumatol 2004; 22:S73–S76.
47. Lambert CA, Soudant EP, Nusgens BV, et al. Pretranslational regulation of extracellular matrix macromolecules and collagenase expression in fibroblasts by mechanical forces. Lab Invest 1992; 66:444–451.
48. Torday JS, Rehan VK. Mechanotransduction determines the structure and function of lung and bone: a theoretical model for the pathophysiology of chronic disease. Cell Biochem Biophys 2003; 37:235–246.
49. Suki B, Ito S, Stamenovic D, et al. Biomechanics of the lung parenchyma: critical roles of collagen and mechanical forces. J Appl Physiol 2005; 98:1892–1899.
50. Border WA, Noble NA. Transforming growth factor beta in tissue fibrosis. N Engl J Med 1994; 331:1286–1292.
51. Munger JS, Huang X, Kawakatsu H, et al. The integrin alpha v beta 6 binds and activates latent TGF beta 1: a mechanism for regulating pulmonary inflammation and fibrosis. Cell 1999; 96:319–328.
52. Horan GS, Wood S, Ona V, et al. Partial inhibition of integrin alpha(v)beta6 prevents pulmonary fibrosis without exacerbating inflammation. Am J Respir Crit Care Med 2008; 177:56–65.
53. Lee CG, Kang HR, Homer RJ, et al. Transgenic modeling of transforming growth factor-beta(1): role of apoptosis in fibrosis and alveolar remodeling. Proc Am Thorac Soc 2006; 3:418–423.
54. Budinger GR, Chandel NS, Donnelly HK, et al. Active transforming growth factor-beta1 activates the procollagen I promoter in patients with acute lung injury. Intensive Care Med 2005; 31:121–128.
55. Letterio JJ, Roberts AB. Regulation of immune responses by TGF-beta. Annu Rev Immunol 1998; 16:137–161.
56. Sime PJ, Xing Z, Graham FL, et al. Adenovector-mediated gene transfer of active transforming growth factor-beta1 induces prolonged severe fibrosis in rat lung. J Clin Invest 1997; 100: 768–776.

57. Prud'homme GJ. Pathobiology of transforming growth factor beta in cancer, fibrosis and immunologic disease, and therapeutic considerations. Lab Invest 2007; 87:1077–1091.
58. Schnapp LM, Donohoe S, Chen J, et al. Mining the acute respiratory distress syndrome proteome: identification of the insulin-like growth factor (IGF)/IGF-binding protein-3 pathway in acute lung injury. Am J Pathol 2006; 169:86–95.
59. Pilewski JM, Liu L, Henry AC, et al. Insulin-like growth factor binding proteins 3 and 5 are overexpressed in idiopathic pulmonary fibrosis and contribute to extracellular matrix deposition. Am J Pathol 2005; 166:399–407.
60. Krein PM, Sabatini PJ, Tinmouth W, et al. Localization of insulin-like growth factor-I in lung tissues of patients with fibroproliferative acute respiratory distress syndrome. Am J Respir Crit Care Med 2003; 167:83–90.
61. Langleben D, DeMarchie M, Laporta D, et al. Endothelin-1 in acute lung injury and the adult respiratory distress syndrome. Am Rev Respir Dis 1993; 148:1646–1650.
62. Druml W, Steltzer H, Waldhausl W, et al. Endothelin-1 in adult respiratory distress syndrome. Am Rev Respir Dis 1993; 148:1169–1173.
63. Albertine KH, Wang ZM, Michael JR. Expression of endothelial nitric oxide synthase, inducible nitric oxide synthase, and endothelin-1 in lungs of subjects who died with ARDS. Chest 1999; 116:101S–102S.
64. Quesnel C, Marchand-Adam S, Fabre A, et al. Regulation of hepatocyte growth factor secretion by fibroblasts in patients with acute lung injury. Am J Physiol Lung Cell Mol Physiol 2008; 294:L334–L343.
65. Parks WC, Shapiro SD. Matrix metalloproteinases in lung biology. Respir Res 2001; 2:10–19.
66. Ricou B, Nicod L, Lacraz S, et al. Am Matrix metalloproteinases and TIMP in acute respiratory distress syndrome. J Respir Crit Care Med. 1996; 154:346–352.
67. Stern JB, Fierobe L, Paugam C, et al. Keratinocyte growth factor and hepatocyte growth factor in bronchoalveolar lavage fluid in acute respiratory distress syndrome patients. Crit Care Med 2000; 28:2326–2333.
68. Meduri GU, Headley S, Kohler G, et al. Persistent elevation of inflammatory cytokines predicts a poor outcome in ARDS. Plasma IL-1 beta and IL-6 levels are consistent and efficient predictors of outcome over time. Chest 1995; 107:1062–1073.
69. Van der Heijden M, van Nieuw Amerongen GP, Koolwijk P, et al. Angiopoietin-2, permeability oedema, occurrence and severity of ALI/ARDS in septic and non-septic critically ill patients. Thorax 2008; 63:903–909.
70. Thickett DR, Armstrong L, Millar AB. A role for vascular endothelial growth factor in acute and resolving lung injury. Am J Respir Crit Care Med 2002; 166:1332–1337.
71. Koh H, Tasaka S, Hasegawa N, et al. Vascular endothelial growth factor in epithelial lining fluid of patients with acute respiratory distress syndrome. Respirology 2008; 13:281–284.

12

Current Approaches and Recent Advances in the Genetic Epidemiology of Acute Lung Injury/Acute Respiratory Distress Syndrome

MICHELLE NG GONG

Department of Medicine, Critical Care Medicine, Montefiore Medical Center, and Department of Epidemiology and Population Health, Albert Einstein College of Medicine, Bronx, New York, U.S.A.

DAVID C. CHRISTIANI

Department of Medicine, Pulmonary and Critical Care Unit, Massachusetts General Hospital, Harvard Medical School, and Department of Environmental Health, Harvard School of Public Health, Boston, Massachusetts, U.S.A.

I. Introduction

Acute* lung injury and acute respiratory distress syndrome (ALI/ARDS) is a devastating form of respiratory failure characterized by intense inflammation and increased permeability in the lungs that usually develops in response to a major insult such as sepsis, trauma, pneumonia, burns, and multiple transfusions (1). In the United States, ALI/ARDS is now recognized to be more prevalent than initially thought with an age-adjusted incidence of 86.2/100,000 person-years with a mortality of 38.5% and significant morbidity among the survivors (2).

Despite the common occurrence of sepsis and trauma, only a minority of patients with these precipitants develop ALI (3,4). Our current understanding of why some patients develop and die from ALI while others do not is incomplete. Recently, discoveries about genetic regulation of innate immunity and the inflammatory response have raised the question of whether the multiple polymorphic alleles of genes that encode for cytokines and other mediators of inflammation may result in phenotypic differences in host inflammatory response. These differences may account for some of the observed heterogeneity in individual susceptibility to, and survival in, ARDS.

Genetic epidemiology, as applied to common, complex diseases, is a relatively new discipline that seeks to determine the role of genetic factors and their interactions with the environment in the occurrence of the disease or its outcome within a population. (5) Although genetic determinants to the development of and outcome in ALI/ARDS have only been considered recently, there has been an explosion of studies in this field in the last few years. As potential targets, genes hold several advantages over protein markers of lung injury especially with regard to possible prevention. Because of the invariant nature of the genome, there is inherently less variability to the determination of genotypes than

*This work has been supported by RO1 HL60710, RO1 HL086667, and RO1 HL084060.

for protein markers. The time variation of many of the protein markers before and during critical illness means that the window of opportunity for assessment must be consistent and is likely to be narrow. In addition, regional differences in cytokine expression and concentrations in some biomarkers in ALI like TNF-α mean that biomarkers may be best measured from alveolar fluid (6). But measurements from the lungs are invasive, prone to technical variation, and not always appropriate for severely hypoxemic ARDS patients or for the nonintubated at-risk patients. However, DNA for genotype assessment can be obtained easily from peripheral blood samples and thus can be performed safely for any patient. Another advantage of genetic assessment is that any true genetic association with the disease is unlikely to be epiphenomena to lung injury. Any variation in a protein marker may be a product of developing lung injury rather than the cause of it. The genotype of an individual precedes the lung injury and the precipitant to lung injury. Thus, any true genetic association gives more support to the biological causality of the gene or its product in the development of ALI/ARDS and therefore, may be more appropriate to target in future prevention and treatment.

In the following sections, we will review the recently published studies in the genetic epidemiology of ALI/ARDS and discuss the relative strengths and limitations of the current approach with a focus toward the implications for future prevention and treatment.

II. Candidate Gene Studies in the Genetic Epidemiology of ALI/ARDS

A.   Selection of Candidate Gene

Thus far, all studies on the genetic epidemiology of ALI, thus far, have used the candidate gene approach that focuses on specific genes whose products have been well characterized as biologically important in the pathogenesis, manifestation, or progression of ALI/ARDS. The candidate gene approach is hypothesis driven and founded upon current knowledge of the disease process. The validity of the candidate genes rests upon the evidence supporting its selection as a candidate in ALI/ARDS (Fig. 1). The strongest candidates for investigation are those genes that have been linked to ALI or related conditions in prior association studies or in animal models of the disease, especially if the association was with a polymorphism with known functional consequences. If such studies are not yet available, then the biologic plausibility of the candidate gene in the pathogenesis of lung injury as evidenced by functional studies in animal models and in in vivo samples from ALI patients becomes central. This requirement is also important if the study supporting the first criteria was based upon association studies. More recently, functional genomics have contributed to the confirmation of previously suspected genes and the discovery of novel genes in the genetic susceptibility to ALI. This approach has proven to be effective and successful in the investigation of the genetic susceptibility to ALI/ARDS. Ultimately even with appropriately chosen candidate genes, the success of genetic association studies in ALI will still rely upon sound study design, inclusion of appropriate study population, accurate phenotyping of patients, and assessment of important clinical factors that affect the development of ALI (see sec. "Study Design"). Therefore, sound clinical studies of ALI populations are needed to inform the design of genetic association studies in ALI.

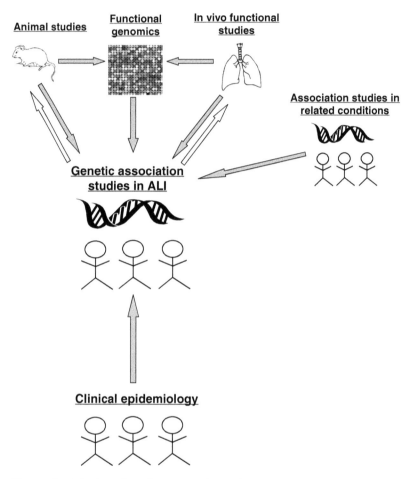

Figure 1 Selection of candidate genes in studies in acute lung injury. Candidate genes in many studies were selected on the basis of prior genetic association with related conditions such as sepsis, pneumonia, or neonatal distress syndrome. Others were selected on the basis of animal and in vivo studies involving plasma or bronchoalveolar fluid of small number of patients that indicate the importance of their gene product or function in ALI. More recently, functional genomics have revealed previously suspected and unsuspected novel genes that are differentially expressed in ALI. Coupled with supportive functional studies in animal models and in vivo studies of samples from ALI patients, these findings have led to their examination in genetic association studies in ALI. These genetic association studies are informed by clinical epidemiology studies in ALI in terms of possible gene–environment interactions and potential confounders. In return, there is bidirectional translational where findings from genetic association studies have lead back to animal models and in vivo studies to better define the role of the genes in ALI and the pathophysiologic mechanisms behind certain gene–environment interactions.

A.1. Candidates from Prior Association Studies of Related Syndromes

The selection of many of the candidate genes in recently published studies was supported by previously published reports in other similar conditions such as neonatal respiratory distress syndrome in *surfactant protein-B* (*SFTPB*) and sepsis for the *tumor necrosis factor-α* (*TNF-α*), *interleukin-10* (*IL-10*), *mannose binding lectin-2* (*MBL-2*), and *interleukin-6* (*IL-6*) genes. Genetic contribution to susceptibility to severe infection has important implications for ALI. Sepsis is the leading cause of ALI/ARDS and is associated with worse mortality than ALI secondary to other etiologies (3,7). Bacterial infection is frequently found in ARDS patients with one autopsy study indicating a prevalence of 98% (8). Most fatal cases of ARDS die from refractory infection and sepsis, not from respiratory failure (9). Conversely, several candidate genes found to be associated with ARDS (the *+1580CT* polymorphisms in the *SFTP-B* gene, the *T-1001G* and *C-1543T* polymorphisms in the *pre-B cell colony-enhancing factor* (*PBEF*) gene, and the *codon 54* polymorphism in the *MBL-2* gene) were also found to be associated with increased risk for sepsis or septic shock in the same population (10–12). Overall these results suggest that genes and polymorphisms that have been implicated in sepsis are strong candidate genes in ALI/ARDS.

Recent studies also suggest that genes found to be important in multiple noncritical illnesses may also be valid candidates to investigate in ALI/ARDS. The implication of a particular gene in multiple diseases is an indication of the functional importance of that gene and its associated pathway. Since that the pathophysiologic pathways found to be important in ALI such as inflammation, coagulation, and oxidative stress have also been implicated in chronic pulmonary and other diseases, it is not surprising that the same genes may be important in many different conditions. This phenomenon has been described as the "common variant/multiple disease" hypothesis and is an extension of the common variant/common disease hypothesis (13). Indeed, many of the genes found to be important in ARDS such as *angiotensin converting enzyme* (*ACE*), *TNF-α, myosin light chain kinase* (*MYLK*), and *PBEF* have been implicated in cardiovascular disease, rheumatoid arthritis, asthma, and type 2 diabetes (14–17).

A.2. Functional Studies for Discovery of Novel Candidate Genes

More recently, novel candidate genes in ALI have been identified from functional genomic studies in animals and humans that established their biological plausibility in lung injury. Using gene expression microarray profiling and sophisticated bioinformatics on samples from different animal models of stretch and lipopolysaccharide-induced lung injury, Garcia and his coworkers have identified a number of previously suspected and novel genes that were differentially expressed in ALI (18,19). *PBEF* was one of the previously unsuspected genes found to be upregulated in these studies. Further in vivo functional studies indicated that PBEF protein expression was also increased in the lungs, bronchoalveolar lavage fluid, and serum of patients with ALI. After identifying two common promoter SNPs in the *PBEF* gene, Ye and coworkers found that the variant of the *T-1001G* polymorphism was associated with increased risk of sepsis-induced ALI compared to healthy controls while the variant *C-1543T* polymorphism was associated with a protective effect in sepsis-induced ALI compared to healthy adults (11). Using similar techniques, pre-elafin was recently identified as a novel candidate in the development of ALI/ARDS (20,21).

Others have identified potential candidate genes by examining animals with variable susceptibility to ALI. Either by using quantitative trait locus analysis of traits such as median survival time after cross breeding strains of mice found to be resistant to lung injury with mice that are very susceptible (22,23) or by comparing the differentially upregulated genes in rats that are resistant to rats that are susceptible to lung injury (24), previously studied candidate genes such as *SFTPB* and *ACE* and previously unsuspected novel genes have been identified as potential candidate genes in ALI.

B.   Genotyping and Analyses of Candidate Genes

After the selection of the candidate genes, there are two approaches to genotyping and investigation. The direct approach focuses on genotyping specific polymorphisms, often single nucleotide polymorphisms (SNPs), in the candidate gene that are thought to be functional either because of linkage with other disease processes or because of its known effect on altering the levels, function, or effectiveness of the gene. This approach was used most frequently initially in the investigation of genetic susceptibility to ALI. Such an approach is very effective for hypothesis testing but is limited to only previously studied polymorphisms on a gene.

More recently, studies in ALI have used the indirect approach for genotyping the candidate genes. In the indirect approach, all common SNPs in the gene (>1% in a sample population) are examined regardless of whether the SNPs have any functional significance. Often these SNPs are examined individually and in combinations with other SNPs on the same gene as a haplotype. A haplotype refers to two or more SNPs that are linked and tend to be inherited together in block. Multilocus haplotypes can be viewed as a signature pattern of allelic variation on a gene that capture and characterize all polymorphisms within the haplotype block. A functional or disease polymorphism may be one of the loci genotyped or it may reside within the haplotype block and it will be captured by the haplotype. Thus, the haplotype would serve as a surrogate marker for the functional polymorphism that is truly linked to the disease state. As such, some argue that haplotype analyses could identify a functional or disease loci better than a single polymorphism especially if the penetrance is low as would be expected in complex diseases and syndromes like ARDS (25,26). Haplotype analyses can also be more efficient in large epidemiology studies since genotyping can be confined to the minimum number of SNPs that define that haplotype block (haplotype-tagging SNPs) (27). Haplotype analyses can also capture *cis*-interaction between SNPs. If one polymorphism increases the risk of disease only in the presence of another polymorphism in the same gene, haplotype analysis will be able to discern this while analysis of the polymorphisms separately will not. Lastly, haplotype analysis can help localize the disease locus to within the haplotype block in the gene that may help focus the search for functional variants in subsequent studies. Such an approach was used in the investigation of *inhibitor kappa B-alpha* (*NFKBIA*), *vascular endothelial growth factor* (*VEGF*), *PBEF*, and *MYLK* (11,28–30).

Together, these studies have justified the candidate gene approach in the search for genetic determinants of ALI/ARDS. The candidate gene approach in the investigation of the genetic epidemiology of ALI is an excellent application of bidirectional translational (31). The "benchside" work may occur before the association study to lend support to its selection as a candidate gene as was the case with the *PBEF* and *MLCK* genes (11,30). Alternatively, the finding of an association between a gene and ALI can often lead to additional functional studies to better define the role of the gene in the disease (Fig. 1). For example, after an association between the *D* allele in the *ACE* gene and ARDS was reported, greater support for the role of ACE in lung injury was established when the loss of ACE activity in ACE knockout mice was found to protect against lung injury (32). In contrast, mice deficient in ACE 2, a homolog of ACE, were more susceptible to sepsis and endotoxin-induced lung injury. But inactivation of the ACE gene reduced the injury seen in these ACE 2 knockout mice. These results lend greater strength to the biological plausibility of ACE in the development of ARDS.

C. Study Design

Given the high mortality rate of ARDS and the generally late age of onset, traditional family-based approaches in genetic epidemiology are either not feasible or impractical. Rather studies in ALI/ARDS have established the unrelated cohort or case-control study as an effective design in the investigation of the genetic determinants of ALI/ARDS. These studies require the delineation of a non-ARDS control group and focus on whether the gene variant of interest is associated with the ARDS cases at a significantly higher frequency than among the non-ARDS controls. These association studies are the most sensitive and powerful of all of the study designs described thus far in detecting common, low penetrant (i.e., low relative risk), susceptibility genes in complex disease (5). However, association studies have been criticized, as well. The most common and troubling criticisms are inconsistency and lack of replication. This heterogeneity is due to a number of factors. First, the epidemiologic quality of genetic studies that are published is quite variable (33). Other factors include the lack of power in some studies (type II errors) and the lack of control for confounders such as population differences or gene–environment interaction. However, as is true in any case-control design in epidemiology, the strength of the study depends entirely on the proper selection of cases and controls and on the appropriate accounting of potential confounders, power and type I error (34). The following section will focus on the features of genetic case-control design as illustrated by studies in ALI. Table details some of these features and the results of recent genetic epidemiology studies in ALI/ARDS.

C.1. Phenotyping of Cases and Controls

As with any case-control study, the choice and phenotype of cases and controls are central to the design, strength, validity, and generalizability of the study. Depending on whether the focus is on susceptibility or outcome, the case definition will differ. Genetic epidemiology studies examining outcomes in ALI/ARDS usually use mortality or ventilator-free days. However, the outcome of ALI/ARDS in genetic susceptibility studies is more heterogeneous and prone to misclassification, since there is no definitive diagnostic test. The American-European Consensus Conference (AECC) criteria serve as an uniformly accepted guideline for defining lung injury but is not very specific (35). Because of variability in the interpretation of the radiologic criteria (36), difficulty excluding heart failure, and use of a cutoff in the Pao_2/Fio_2 ratio of 300 mm Hg in a continuum of hypoxemic respiratory failure, some inevitable random misclassification of cases and controls will occur which tend to bias results toward the null hypothesis. Care must be taken to assess carefully the rigors by which the cases adhere to the ALI/ARDS criteria. Even still, misclassification will occur and large, well phenotyped sample sizes will be needed to detect an association.

Table 1 Summary of Published Genetic Epidemiology Studies in ALI/ARDS

Potential pathway	Gene	References	Patient population		Major findings	
			Case	Controls	Susceptibility to ALI/ARDS	Outcomes in ALI/ARDS
Endothelial function and permeability	Vascular endothelial growth factor (VEGF)	(43)	117 Caucasians with AECC defined ARDS	137 healthy Caucasians 103 EA with respiratory failure	+936CT and +936TT genotype associated with ↑ susceptibility to ARDS compared to both control groups	+936CT and +936TT genotypes associated with greater severity of illness in ARDS but no association with ARDS mortality was found
		(28)	394 Caucasians with AECC defined ARDS from a cohort of ICU patients with sepsis, trauma, aspiration, and massive transfusion	859 Caucasians from same cohort of ICU patients admitted with sepsis, trauma, aspiration, and massive transfusions who did not develop ARDS	No statistically significant association with development of ARDS found	T allele of +936CT SNP and haplotype were associated with lower plasma VEGF levels and increased mortality in ARDS
	Myosin light chain kinase (MLCK)	(30)	92 Caucasians with sepsis-related AECC defined ALI; 46 African-Americans sepsis-related AECC defined ALI	114 Caucasians with sepsis; 85 healthy Caucasians; 51 AA with sepsis; 61 healthy African-Americans	One SNP and one haplotype associated with ALI in Caucasians compared to septic controls; 2 haplotypes associated with ALI in African-Americans compared to septic controls	Not examined

Inflammatory and anti-inflammatory cytokine	Clara cell protein-16 (CC16)	(40)	117 Germans with AECC defined ARDS	373 healthy German newborns	No association found	Not examined
	Interleukin-6 (IL-6)	(71)	96 Caucasians with AECC defined ARDS	88 Caucasians with non-ARDS respiratory failure 174 Caucasians after heart surgery 1906 healthy Caucasian males	No association found	Variant C allele of −174 GC promoter SNP and −174CC genotype correlated with serum IL-6 levels and was associated with survival in ARDS and in non-ARDS with respiratory failure
		(72)	67 Spaniards with severe sepsis and ALI	96 healthy population-based Spanish controls	Haplotype was associated with increased susceptibility to sepsis-related ALI	Not examined
	Interleukin-10 (IL-10)	(52)	211 Caucasians with AECC defined ARDS from a cohort of ICU patients with sepsis, trauma, aspiration, and massive transfusion	429 Caucasians from same cohort of ICU patients admitted with sepsis, trauma, aspiration, and massive transfusions who did not develop ARDS	−1082GG genotype was associated with ARDS but only in the presence of significant interaction between genotype and age	−1082GG genotype associated with less organ failure and lower mortality in ARDS

(Continued)

Table 1 Summary of Published Genetic Epidemiology Studies in ALI/ARDS (Continued)

Potential pathway	Gene	References	Patient population		Major findings	
			Case	Controls	Susceptibility to ALI/ARDS	Outcomes in ALI/ARDS
		(73)	49 Caucasians with severe trauma and acute respiratory failure defined as need for mechanical ventilation and Pao$_2$/Fio$_2$ < 200	51 Caucasians with severe trauma without acute respiratory failure	−1082GG genotype was associated with less acute respiratory failure	Not examined
	Macrophage inhibitory factor (MIF)	(74)	90 Caucasians with sepsis 61 AA with sepsis	113 Caucasians with sepsis 69 AA with sepsis	Haplotypes in 3′ region associated with sepsis and sepsis-induced ALI	Not examined
	Pre-B cell colony-enhancing factor (PBEF)	(11)	87 Caucasians with sepsis-related AECC defined ALI	100 Caucasians with sepsis 84 healthy Caucasians	Compared to healthy controls, variant G1001 allele and 1001G:1543C haplotype were associated with ↑ susceptibility to ALI while the variant T1543 allele was associated with ↓ susceptibility to ALI No association seen in comparison to septic controls	No association between variant G1001 allele and ARDS mortality

		Cases	Controls		
	(44)	375 Caucasians with AECC defined ARDS from a cohort of ICU patients with sepsis, trauma, aspiration, and massive transfusion	787 Caucasians from same cohort of ICU patients admitted with sepsis, trauma, aspiration, and massive transfusions who did not develop ARDS	Variant *G1001* allele and *1001G:1543C* haplotype were associated with ↑ susceptibility to ALI in septic and noninfectious risks for ARDS. Variant *T1543* allele was not associated with ARDS	*T1543* variant and associated *1001T:1543T* haplotype were associated with decreased ARDS mortality
Tumor necrosis factor-α (TNFA) Tumor necrosis factor-β (TNFB)	(51)	237 Caucasians with AECC defined ARDS from a cohort of ICU patients with sepsis, trauma, aspiration, and massive transfusion	476 Caucasians from same cohort of ICU patients admitted with sepsis, trauma, aspiration, and massive transfusions who did not develop ARDS	*−308A TNFA* allele and *−308A:TNFB1* haplotype were associated with ↑ susceptibility to ARDS in direct pulmonary injury. No association with ARDS found for *TNFB1/2*	Increasing ARDS mortality with increasing number of *−308A* alleles with greatest mortality found in younger patients carrying the *−308A* allele
Transcription factors for inflammation	(29)	382 Caucasians with AECC defined ARDS from a cohort of ICU patients with sepsis, trauma, aspiration, and massive transfusion	828 Caucasians from same cohort of ICU patients admitted with sepsis, trauma, aspiration, and massive transfusions who did not develop ARDS	Haplotype of promoter SNPs, *−881A/G*, *−826C/T*, *−297C/T*, was associated with increased ARDS	Not examined
Inhibitor kappa B-alpha (NFKBIA)					

(Continued)

Table 1 Summary of Published Genetic Epidemiology Studies in ALI/ARDS (Continued)

Potential pathway	Gene	References	Patient population		Major findings	
			Case	Controls	Susceptibility to ALI/ARDS	Outcomes in ALI/ARDS
	Nuclear factor E2-related factor 2 (Nrf2)		15 Caucasians and 15 AA with trauma associated AECC defined ALI	30 Caucasians and 30 AA with trauma matched with on ancestry and injury severity score	A allele of −617CA SNP was associated with decreased expression and binding affinity and increased risk of ARDS after trauma	Not examined
Innate immunity	*Mannose binding lectin-2 (MBL-2)*	(12)	212 Caucasians with AECC defined ARDS from a cohort of ICU patients with sepsis, trauma, aspiration, and massive transfusion	442 Caucasians from same cohort of ICU patients admitted with sepsis, trauma, aspiration, and massive transfusions who did not develop ARDS	Homozygotes for variant *codon 54B* allele was associated with greater severity of illness and ↑ susceptibility to ARDS	Homozygotes for variant *codon 54B* allele was associated with greater daily organ failures and ↑ ARDS mortality
Pulmonary function and gas exchange	*Surfactant protein-B (SFTPB)*	(42)	15 Germans with AECC defined ARDS	21 healthy Americans	Variant insertion/deletion allele in intron 4 associated with ↑ susceptibility to ARDS	Not examined
		(75)	72 Caucasians with AECC defined ARDS from a cohort of ICU patients with sepsis, trauma, aspiration, and massive transfusion	117 Caucasians from same cohort of ICU patients admitted with sepsis, trauma, aspiration, and massive transfusions who did not develop ARDS	Variant insertion/deletion allele in intron 4 associated with ↑ susceptibility to ARDS and ↑ susceptibility to severe direct pulmonary injury like pneumonia in women	Not examined

Gene/function	Ref.	Subjects	Findings	Variant
		242 Caucasians with AECC defined ARDS from a cohort of ICU patients with sepsis, trauma, aspiration, and massive transfusion	—	insertion/deletion allele in intron 4 associated with ↑ ARDS mortality. No association with +1580CT SNP and ARDS mortality
	(41)	52 German patients with AECC defined ARDS 46 healthy German adults 25 Caucasians with trauma, pneumonia, and heart failure	C allele in the +1580CT SNP in codon 131 and the +1580CC genotype were associated with ↑ susceptibility to ARDS compared to both control groups	Not examined
	(10)	12 Caucasians and AA with ARDS from pneumonia 390 Caucasians and AA with pneumonia	+1580CC genotype was associated with ↑ susceptibility to respiratory failure, septic shock, and ARDS	No association with mortality in pneumonia. ARDS mortality not specifically examined
Vasomotor tone and function *Angiotensin converting enzyme (ACE)*	(76)	96 Caucasians with AECC defined ARDS 88 Caucasians with non-ARDS respiratory failure 174 Caucasians after heart surgery 1906 healthy Caucasians males	Deletion (D)allele and DD genotype with I/D polymorphism in intron 16 associated with ↑ susceptibility to ARDS	Increasing mortality in ARDS associated with increasing number of D alleles carried

(Continued)

Table 1 Summary of Published Genetic Epidemiology Studies in ALI/ARDS (Continued)

Potential pathway	Gene	References	Patient population		Major findings	
			Case	Controls	Susceptibility to ALI/ARDS	Outcomes in ALI/ARDS
		(77)	17 Chinese patients with AECC defined ARDS from SARS	123 Chinese patients with SARS 326 healthy Chinese individuals	No association found	Not examined
		(78)	101 Chinese patients in MICU with AECC defined ARDS from mostly sepsis or pneumonia	138 Chinese patients in MICU with respiratory failure 210 healthy Chinese controls	No association found	Increased mortality in ARDS associated with *D* allele in intron 16
		(79)	84 Caucasians with AECC defined ARDS	200 healthy Caucasian blood donors	No association with I/D and *AGT(-6)A/G* polymorphisms	*DD* genotype was associated with increased mortality in ARDS. No association with *AGT(-6)A/G* polymorphism
		(80)	120 Spanish patients with AECC defined ARDS from sepsis	92 Spanish patients with sepsis 92 Spanish nonseptic ICU patients 364 healthy subjects from Canarian population	No associations found	No associations found

| Iron ion homeostasis | Ferritin light chain (FTL) Hemeoxygenase 2 (HMOX2) | (81) | 104 Caucasian patients with AECC defined ARDS | 193 healthy Caucasian blood donors | GG genotype of −3381 FTL SNP associated with ARDS from extrapulmonary injury. A allele of +4775A/G SNP and associated haplotypes of HMOX2 were associated with decreased ARDS from direct pulmonary injury | Not examined |
| Coagulation and fibrinolysis | Factor V Leiden | (82) | 106 Caucasian Germans with AECC defined ARDS | None | Not examined | Carriers of the Factor V Leiden mutation had decreased mortality in ARDS |

Abbreviations: SNP, single nucleotide polymorphism; SARS, severe acute respiratory syndrome; EA, European-Americans; MICU, Medical Intensive Care Unit.

It is important to note that in molecular epidemiology studies, factors important in susceptibility studies may not be important in prognostication of outcomes and vice versa. For example, mutations in the *BRCA1* gene, now known to be important in DNA repair, are associated with increased susceptibility to developing early onset breast or ovarian cancer. But the *BRCA1* gene is not associated with differences in breast cancer recurrence or disease-free survival after therapy, even though *BRCA1*-associated breast cancer tends to present at a more advanced stage (37).

The choice of controls in case-control studies is equally important although often neglected. In case-controls studies, controls are intended to represent the population that is at risk for the disease. In other words, they should not have the disease at the time of selection but, under the study design, they would have been included as a case if they did develop the disease (38). Since ALI/ARDS has been found to be commonly under diagnosed (39), the same screening procedures to determine ALI/ARDS should be applied to the controls to ensure that they do not also have the condition. However, the most common problem is the selection of controls that are not at risk for the disease, making comparisons with the cases difficult. The controls in many of the earlier studies in ALI/ARDS were healthy individuals or hospitalized patients without a clear prior injury placing them at risk for ALI (40–43). As discussed before, genes associated with sepsis make strong candidate genes for ALI, but because sepsis is also the leading precipitant for ALI, one must be careful to avoid confounding from genetic association with the predisposing injury. When the controls are healthy or have conditions that are different from the precipitating injuries in the ARDS cases, any association found between a candidate gene and ALI/ARDS may actually be due to an association between the polymorphism and the risk condition for ALI/ARDS such as sepsis. It is important to use at-risk individuals with similar conditions as the cases to avoid this confounding bias. In the initial investigation of the *PBEF* gene, the variants *T-1001G* and *C-1543T* alleles were associated with ALI only after comparing ALI patients to healthy individuals. Thus, it was not clear whether the variant *T-1001G* and *C-1543T* alleles were associated with ALI or to the severe sepsis that placed the patients at risk for ALI (11). In a subsequent study in a different cohort of patients with sepsis, trauma, aspiration, and multiple transfusions, the variant *T-1001G* but not the *C-1543T* allele was confirmed to be associated with ARDS compared to at-risk individuals (44). This association was present even among patients with noninfectious etiologies of ARDS, extending the generalizability of the genetic association.

However, one potential issue with using at-risk controls is that the patients are not drawn randomly from the general population. Rather they are selected to be controls on the basis of their critical illness (i.e., at-risk) status. If the genotype of interest is associated with critical illness, then the genotype frequency may deviate from that predicted by random mating (Hardy Weinberg Equilibrium) (45). Indeed, such was the case with the −1082GA *IL-10* and *MBL-2* polymorphisms. In such cases, extra efforts are needed to exclude deviation from Hardy Weinberg Equilibrium from genotype or recording error. Such efforts include repeat genotyping, blinding of personnel or validation of genotyping in a different population.

C.2. Race and Genetic Epidemiology of ALI/ARDS

Recently, the role of race in critical illnesses has been explored. African-Americans have been demonstrated to have a higher incidence of ARDS mortality than Caucasians and Hispanics (46). Some have raised questions about whether genetic variability may explain such racial differences in ALI/ARDS. A gene that truly influences disease susceptibility should be associated with the disease in all racial groups. But the frequency of the disease genotype and the size of the effect may vary with different racial groups. For example, the *MLCK* gene was found to be associated with variable susceptibility to developing sepsis-induced ALI in both European American Caucasians and in African-Americans (30). But Caucasians and African-American differed in the linkage disequilibrium between SNPs, in the haplotype block definition, in the haplotypes found to be associated with ALI and in the size of the odds ratio found. However, the similar location of the race-specific at-risk haplotypes in Caucasians and African-Americans suggests that the true disease associated variant may be located within the 5' region of the gene. There may be several reasons for such differences in the prevalence of the at-risk genotype and effect size in different ethnic groups. The examined SNP may be in linkage disequilibrium with the disease locus and the extent of linkage disequilibrium and hence, the haplotype blocks and frequencies may differ between racial groups (47). Additionally, there may be modifying genes that interact with *MYLK* or there may be multiple susceptibility loci within or near the gene that may have different frequencies in different populations. Lastly, clinical factors (such as the presence of comorbid disease like diabetes, susceptibility to different risks for ALI like sepsis or trauma, and alcohol abuse) that may modify any effect of the at-risk genotype may be different in different population. Thus, any genotype analysis should be restricted to one racial group or account for race by stratification or adjustment for ancestry informative markers to avoid confounding from differences in ethnic groups (population stratification).

After stratifying by major racial groups, additional methods to adjust for population stratification may not be necessary, especially for studies conducted in the United States. Wacholder and coworkers demonstrated that, among Caucasians, bias from population stratification is small and decreases as the number of ethnic subgroups within the Caucasian population increases (48). This may be especially pertinent for U.S. Caucasians, the group that tends to be composed of many different ethnic subgroups. Similar results were found with African-Americans when there are large numbers of ethnic subgroups (49). Consistent with these stimulation studies, Gao and coworkers found evidence for ethnic differences within their African-Americans subjects, but adjusting for these differences did not significantly change the associations between haplotypes and SNPs in the *MLCK* gene and ALI except for one SNP, in which the association was actually strengthened (30).

C.3. Gene–Environment Interaction

The role of the environment is particularly critical in determining the genetic determinants in a complex disorder. Common gene variants may have no influence on the risk of disease unless there is concomitant exposure to a particular environmental insult. Such interaction is important in understanding and interpreting the genetic contribution to complex diseases like ALI. Recently, there is growing evidence to suggest potential gene–environment interaction by age and the initial precipitant for ARDS.

Age is an important factor in genetic epidemiology studies. Age-varying genetic associations have been found and validated recently in multiple populations and are now thought to contribute to inconsistent genetic association studies for complex disease (50). Potential age-varying genetic associations have been found in genetic epidemiology studies of ALI/ARDS. Among the 212 patients with ARDS, the *−308A* allele in the *TNF-α* gene was associated with more daily organ dysfunction and increased 60-day mortality in ARDS (OR_{adj} 3.5, 95% CI 1.4–8.6), but the effect was strongest among those 117 ARDS patients younger than median age of 67 (OR_{adj} 14.9, 95% CI 3.0–74; $p < 0.001$) (51). In the same cohort of critically ill at-risk patients, the *IL-10* −*1082GG* genotype was associated with increased susceptibility to ARDS in critically ill patients ($p < 0.001$) but only in the presence of a statistically significant interaction between age and the −*1082GG* genotype ($p < 0.001$) (52). The −*1082GG* genotype was protective against ARDS among the elderly (OR_{adj} 0.63, 95% CI 0.34–1.2) but not among the younger patients (OR 1.7, 95% CI 0.89–3.2). Overall, these results suggest a possible age-dependent genetic susceptibility to developing and dying from ARDS.

One of the most important gene–environment interactions in ALI/ARDS is from the initial injury that predisposed to the development of lung injury. SFTPB is essential for the surface tension lowering properties of pulmonary surfactant, which is known to be dysfunctional in ALI/ARDS. The *C* allele of +*1580CT SNP* was found to be associated with ARDS, but this association was confined to those patients with "idiopathic" insults which consisted of mostly direct pulmonary injuries like pneumonia (41). No associations were found with the group of patients with exogenic ARDS that consisted of mostly patients with extrapulmonary causes of ARDS (10). Although healthy controls were used, a subsequent study using ARDS cases and controls with community acquired pneumonia confirmed this association between the *C* allele and ARDS, suggesting that the +*1580C* allele is associated with ALI/ARDS and not with severe pneumonia. Together, these studies suggest that the *SFTPB* gene may be important in ARDS susceptibility in direct pulmonary injuries like pneumonia. There may also be a role for this gene in susceptibility to direct pulmonary injury such as severe pneumonia that places them at risk for ALI/ARDS. The role of the *SFTPB* gene with other etiologies of lung injury is not yet clear.

A similar gene–environment interaction was found with the −*308GA* polymorphisms in the *TNF-α* gene (51). No association was found between the variant −*308A* allele and ARDS compared to other critically ill non-ARDS controls with sepsis, aspiration, massive transfusion, or trauma. However, after stratifying by the site of injury, the −*308A* allele was associated with decreased odds of developing ARDS among those with direct pulmonary injury (OR_{adj} 0.52, 95% CI 0.30–0.91) but a nonsignificant increased odds of ARDS in indirect pulmonary injury (OR_{adj} 1.7, 95% CI 0.93–3.2) with evidence for significant effect modification ($p = 0.01$).

The reasons for these interactions remain unclear. The risk of ARDS is very different in direct pulmonary injuries compared to indirect pulmonary injuries (53). Certainly, the inflammatory response and the radiologic, histologic, and mechanical properties of the lung differ depending on whether the site of infection or the etiology of ARDS is pulmonary or extrapulmonary (54,55). It is also possible that the difference between direct and indirect pulmonary injury is due to the differences in the underlying risk factor such as sepsis, aspiration, or massive transfusion. The cytokine profile and inflammatory markers between ARDS patients and at-risk non-ARDS patients differ depending on whether their predisposing injury was sepsis, trauma, acute pancreatitis, or massive transfusion (56). More recently, different patterns of gene expression was found in rats models of ALI depending on whether lung injury was induced by high tidal volume ventilation or intravenous lipopolysaccharide (57). Alternatively, the interaction may reflect different heterogeneity in the diagnosis of ALI. The AECC criterion for diagnosis of ALI was found to be more sensitive in patients with indirect pulmonary injury compared to direct pulmonary injury (35). While these interactions need to be confirmed in larger studies, the above findings indicate important gene–environment interactions in the genetic susceptibility to developing ALI/ARDS that depends on the risk factor that predisposes the individual to lung injury.

Defining these gene–environment interactions is important. Many of the polymorphisms identified in ARDS are commonly found in the population. With their persistence in the genome throughout human evolution and the lethality of ARDS, it is unlikely that these polymorphisms are universally detrimental. It is likely that these variants may be detrimental in some situations and benign or even beneficial in others. Failure to examine the role of environmental exposure can lead to decreased sensitivity in detecting an association between the gene of interest and the disease and to inconsistent findings from different studies (58,59).

D. Power, Type I Error, and Replication

Statistical power is extremely important in genetic association studies of complex disease. Power to detect an association depends upon the size of the effect, the population frequency of the genotype, and the sensitivity of the analysis deployed. Some of the negative studies in genetic epidemiology in ALI are likely due to the lack of adequate power (40). This is especially important when there may be phenotype misclassification and gene–gene or gene–environment interaction. Currently, most ALI/ARDS studies are relatively small for genetic epidemiology studies that make it difficult to examine for interactions.

Type I error is the likelihood of a false positive finding. Although a *p*-value or a type I error rate of 5% is generally accepted, one may be more likely to find an association by chance alone if multiple comparisons of different genetic loci to the development of disease are performed. While adjustment for multiple comparisons is ideal, it is not entirely clear what the best strategy is. While many studies report *p*-values adjusting for false discovery rate as suggested by Benjamin and Hochberg (60), this and other similar methods may not be appropriate for candidate gene approach as it does not account for the fact that the candidate gene was selected for investigation because of high prior suspicion for its role in ALI. Others have started using a Bayesian or semi-Bayesian approach to incorporate the prior probability of finding an association to calculate the probability of a false positive finding for any associations detected (61,62). Such as technique can be used to select for the candidate genes that have a low likelihood of being false positive and that should be pursued with confirmatory studies or functional studies. Alternatively, such techniques have been used to better interpret genome-wide association studies or pathway-based studies that involve large number of genes, some that may be suspected to be important in the disease of interest and many without any prior suspicion (63).

Ultimately, the likelihood of a cause and effect relationship underlying any genetic association will depend on the reproducibility of well-designed studies in different populations and in the strength of the biological rationale behind the selection of that gene for analysis. While troublesome to classical geneticist, the need to confirm studies is common in epidemiology. Any population study needs to be replicated for different populations in adequately powered studies. But how should one define replication for a gene association study? Some have argued that the replication of genetic association studies should be viewed at the level of the gene in different populations rather than a specific variant, haplotype, or effect (64). Indeed, many of the most well-replicated asthma susceptibility genes are based upon an association with different functional variants within the same gene or opposing alleles at the same SNP in different populations or subpopulations (65). It is likely that the same kind of replication results will be seen in ALI.

III. Future Directions

While the candidate gene approach has been successful, it is limited to previously examined genes and it is dependent upon the strength of the evidence supporting the role of the gene in ALI/ARDS. However, it is likely that other undiscovered genes may be involved and that multiple genes may interact in an additive or multiplicative fashion (epistaxis). Consequently, there has been much interest in genome-wide association studies (GWASs) in ALI. The technical aspect of this approach is becoming more realistic as the cost of high-throughput genotyping is decreasing. GWAS has the ability to examine large number of SNPs distributed throughout the genome. Hence, the major advantage of GWAS is the ability to detect disease association with known and previously unsuspected genes.

Potential limitations with genome-wide testing in ALI/ARDS include power and multiple testing. With increasing number of SNPs examined in genome-wide testing, many SNPs will have low pretest probability and the risk of false positives from multiple testing is quite substantial. Although ARDS is now recognized as more common than initially thought, the high mortality associated with ALI means that there are fewer prevalent cases than other complex genetic disorders like breast cancer or diabetes. In addition, it is likely that an estimated relative risk in ALI will be modest (except maybe in subgroups of patients). It is estimated that under current methods for multiple testing adjustments, as many as 1000 cases and 1000 controls will be needed to detect modest estimates in a case-control GWAS (66,67). If we consider that in ALI/ARDS gene–environment interactions are likely, the sample size requirements will increase further. Thus, it will be very important that any GWAS in ALI as well as any confirmatory study be sufficiently powered.

Besides the approaches described above, other approaches that may be useful for ALI/ARDS are a candidate pathway-based association study where particular focus is placed on SNPs that blanket only those genes in a particular pathway (inflammation or coagulation, for example) that are highly likely to be important in ALI/ARDS. Utilizing this approach, the number of SNPs examined is limited, resulting in a lower cost and a reduction in the number of multiple comparisons made. Because a large number of genes in the same or related pathways are examined concurrently, gene–gene interactions can be examined. Such an approach have already been done in other diseases such as age-related macular degeneration (68) and lung cancer (69). A number of genetic databases and analytical software designed to characterize genes according to specific biological pathways are now available. Using one such system, Ingenuity Pathway Analysis, Loza and coworkers constructed 17 interrelated functional pathways important in the various aspects of inflammation including the development of immune cells, signaling of immune cells to sites of injury, activation and modulation of inflammatory response, and resolution of immune response (70). From these pathways, 1027 inflammation-associated candidate genes were identified for pathway analysis.

With improving technology, GWAS and pathway-based association studies will become more common but the candidate gene approach will still be instrumental in the genetic epidemiology of ALI. Any genes found to be important in ALI in GWAS will need to be further investigated using the candidate gene approach with finer mapping of the gene to better characterize the variation in the gene, to confirm the gene's association with ALI in a different population, and to examine for potential gene–environment interactions. In addition, additional functional studies of the high-risks genotypes will be necessary to better understand the role of the top candidate genes in the development and outcome of ALI.

IV. Conclusions

The application of genetic epidemiology and genomics to the study of ALI/ARDS is still in its infancy. Optimal study designs and approaches are still being debated and the large prospective cohorts that will be necessary to examine gene–environment interaction and to confirm prior findings are being developed. In the near future, we can look forward to more comprehensive gene association studies either with GWAS or with pathway-based genetic association studies. There will be technological and analytic challenges to the proper study of genetic determinants of ALI/ARDS that will benefit from a multifaceted approach. However, the ultimate goal in epidemiology is in the intervention and prevention of disease on the population level. Unlike other risk factors for ARDS, genotype allows for the prospective determination of individuals at high risk for the development of or mortality from ALI. This knowledge will be important in the design of future preventive and therapeutic trials. In addition, knowledge of genetic risk factors with high population attributable risk can help focus preventive and therapeutic trials in ways that will have the greatest population impact. Lastly, knowledge of gene–environmental interaction allows for the targeting of high-risk individuals and, more importantly, offers them an opportunity to reduce their overall risk by the modulation of their environment. Despite these possibilities, there will be significant barriers to the translation of genetic epidemiology studies and genomics to preventive and therapeutic interventions. In oncology where there is a longer history of genetic and molecular epidemiology studies, genetic tests are now available commercially to conduct individualized risk assessment and tailored therapy. While significant challenges lay ahead, there is a similar potential for such individualized risk assessment and therapy in critical care medicine and a multifaceted approach involving animal models and large, well phenotyped studies will be crucial to this goal.

References

1. Ware LB, Matthay MA. The acute respiratory distress syndrome. N Engl J Med 2000; 342:1334–1349.
2. Rubenfeld GD, Caldwell E, Peabody E, et al. Incidence and outcomes of acute lung injury. N Engl J Med 2005; 353:1685–1693.
3. Hudson LD, Milberg JA, Anardi D, et al. Clinical risks for development of the acute respiratory distress syndrome. Am J Respir Crit Care Med 1995; 151:293–301.
4. Fowler AA, Hamman RF, Good JT, et al. Adult respiratory distress syndrome: risk with common predispositions. Ann Intern Med 1983; 98:593–597.
5. Khoury MJ, Yang Q. The future of genetic studies of complex human diseases: an epidemiologic perspective. Epidemiology 1998; 9:350–354.
6. Suter PM, Suter S, Girardin E, et al. High bronchoalveolar levels of tumor necrosis factor and its inhibitors, interleukin-1, interferon, and elastase, in patients with adult respiratory distress syndrome after trauma, shock, or sepsis. Am Rev Respir Dis 1992; 145:1016–1022.
7. Zilberberg MD, Epstein SK. Acute lung injury in the medical icu: comorbid conditions, age, etiology, and hospital outcome. Am J Respir Crit Care Med 1998; 157:1159–1164.

8. Bell RC, Coalson JJ, Smith JD, et al. Multiple organ system failure and infection in adult respiratory distress syndrome. Ann Intern Med 1983; 99:293–298.

9. Ferring M, Vincent JL. Is outcome from ARDS related to the severity of respiratory failure? Eur Respir J 1997; 10:1297–1300.

10. Quasney MW, Waterer GW, Dahmer MK, et al. Association between surfactant protein b +1580 polymorphism and the risk of respiratory failure in adults with community-acquired pneumonia. Crit Care Med 2004; 32:1115–1119.

11. Ye SQ, Simon BA, Maloney JP, et al. Pre-b-cell colony-enhancing factor as a potential novel biomarker in acute lung injury. Am J Respir Crit Care Med 2005; 171:361–370.

12. Gong MN, Zhou W, Thompson, BT, et al. Mannose binding lectin-2 gene and acute respiratory distress syndrome. Crit Care Med 2007; 35(1):48–56.

13. Gao L, Tsai YJ, Grigoryev DN, et al. Host defense genes in asthma and sepsis and the role of the environment. Curr Opin Allergy Clin Immunol 2007; 7:459–467.

14. Gao L, Grant AV, Rafaels N, et al. Polymorphisms in the myosin light chain kinase gene that confer risk of severe sepsis are associated with a lower risk of asthma. J Allergy Clin Immunol 2007; 119:1111–1118.

15. Zhang YY, Gottardo L, Thompson R, et al. A visfatin promoter polymorphism is associated with low-grade inflammation and type 2 diabetes. Obesity (Silver Spring) 2006; 14:2119–2126.

16. Niu T, Chen X, Xu X. Angiotensin converting enzyme gene insertion/deletion polymorphism and cardiovascular disease: therapeutic implications. Drugs 2002; 62:977–993.

17. Lee YH, Ji JD, Song GG. Tumor necrosis factor-alpha promoter -308 a/g polymorphism and rheumatoid arthritis susceptibility: a metaanalysis. J Rheumatol 2007; 34:43–49.

18. Nonas SA, Finigan JH, Gao L, et al. Functional genomic insights into acute lung injury: role of ventilators and mechanical stress. Proc Am Thorac Soc 2005; 2:188–194.

19. Meyer NJ, Garcia JG. Wading into the genomic pool to unravel acute lung injury genetics. Proc Am Thorac Soc 2007; 4:69–76.

20. Tejera P, Wang Z, Zhai R, et al. Genetic Polymorphisms of Peptidase Inhibitor 3 (Elafin) are Associated with ARDS. Am J Respir Cell Mol Biol. 2009 Feb 27. [Epub ahead ofprint] PubMed PMID: 19251943.

21. Wang Z, Beach D, Su L, et al. A genome-wide expression analysis in blood identifies pre-elafin as a biomarker in ARDS. Am J Respir Cell Moi Bio. 2008 June;38;(6):724–732. Epub 2008 Jan 18. PubMed PMID: 18203972; PubMed Central PMCID: PMC2396250.

22. Prows DR, McDowell SA, Aronow BJ, et al. Genetic susceptibility to nickel-induced acute lung injury. Chemosphere 2003; 51:1139–1148.

23. Prows DR, Hafertepen AP, Winterberg AV, et al. Reciprocal congenic lines of mice capture the aliq1 effect on acute lung injury survival time. Am J Respir Cell Mol Biol 2008; 38:68–77.

24. Nonas SA, Moreno-Vinasco L, Ma SF, et al. Use of consomic rats for genomic insights into ventilator-associated lung injury. Am J Physiol Lung Cell Mol Physiol 2007; 293:L292–L302.

25. Pritchard JK, Cox NJ. The allelic architecture of human disease genes: common disease-common variant . . . Or not? Hum Mol Genet 2002; 11:2417–2423.

26. Schork N. The future of genetic case-control studies. In: Rao DC, Province MA, eds. Genetic Dissection of Complex Traits. San Diego, CA: Academic Press, 2001:191–212.

27. Cardon LR, Abecasis GR. Using haplotype blocks to map human complex trait loci. Trends Genet 2003; 19:135–140.

28. Zhai R, Gong MN, Zhou W, et al. Genotypes and haplotypes of the VEGF gene are associated with higher mortality and lower VEGF plasma levels in patients with ARDS. Thorax 2007; 62:718–722.

29. Zhai R, Zhou W, Gong MN, et al. Inhibitor kappaB-alpha haplotype GTC is associated with susceptibility to acute respiratory distress syndrome in Caucasians. Crit Care Med 2007; 35:893–898.

30. Gao L, Grant A, Halder I, et al. Novel polymorphisms in the myosin light chain kinase gene confer risk for acute lung injury. Am J Respir Cell Mol Biol 2006; 34:487–495.

31. Burnham EL. Translational Research: Basic Concepts and the Importance of Heterogeneity. 2006 [cited 2009 8/29/2009]. Available online at: http://www.thoracic.org/sections/clinical-information/critical-care/critical-care-research/translational-research.html.

32. Imai Y, Kuba K, Rao S, et al. Angiotensin-converting enzyme 2 protects from severe acute lung failure. Nature 2005; 436:112–116.

33. Bogardus ST Jr, Concato J, Feinstein AR. Clinical epidemiological quality in molecular genetic research: the need for methodological standards. JAMA 1999; 281:1919–1926.

34. Boffetta P. Molecular epidemiology. J Intern Med 2000; 248:447–454.

35. Esteban A, Fernandez-Segoviano P, Frutos-Vivar F, et al. Comparison of clinical criteria for the acute respiratory distress syndrome with autopsy findings. Ann Intern Med 2004; 141: 440–445.

36. Rubenfeld GD, Caldwell E, Granton J, et al. Interobserver variability in applying a radiographic definition for ARDS. Chest 1999; 116:1347–1353.

37. Brekelmans CT, Seynaeve C, Menke-Pluymers M, et al. Survival and prognostic factors in brca1-associated breast cancer. Ann Oncol 2006; 17:391–400.

38. Hennekens CH, Buring JE. Case-control studies. In: Hennekens CH, Buring JE, eds. Epidemiology in medicine. Boston, MA: Little, Brown and Company, 1987:132–152.

39. Ferguson ND, Frutos-Vivar F, Esteban A, et al. Acute respiratory distress syndrome: under-recognition by clinicians and diagnostic accuracy of three clinical definitions. Crit Care Med 2005; 33:2228–2234.

40. Frerking I, Sengler C, Gunther A, et al. Evaluation of the -26 g>a cc16 polymorphism in acute respiratory distress syndrome. Crit Care Med 2005; 33:2404–2406.

41. Lin Z, Pearson C, Chinchilli V, et al. Polymorphisms of human SP-A, SP-B, and SP-D genes: association of sp-b thr131ile with ards. Clin Genet 2000; 58:181–191.

42. Max M, Pison U, Floros J. Frequency of SP-B and SP-A1 gene polymorphisms in acute respiratory distress syndrome (ARDS). Appl Cardiopulm Pathophysiol 1996; 6:111–118.

43. Medford AR, Keen LJ, Bidwell JL, et al. Vascular endothelial growth factor gene polymorphism and acute respiratory distress syndrome. Thorax 2005; 60:244–248.

44. Bajwa EK, Yu C, Gong MN, et al. PBEF gene polymorphisms and risk of developing ARDS. Crit Care Med 2007; 35(5):1290–1305.

45. Li C. Large Random Mating Population. First Course in Population Genetics. Pacific Grove, CA: Boxwood Press, 1976:1–15.

46. Moss M, Mannino DM. Race and gender differences in acute respiratory distress syndrome deaths in the united states: an analysis of multiple-cause mortality data (1979–1996). Crit Care Med 2002; 30:1679–1685.

47. Gabriel SB, Schaffner SF, Nguyen H, et al. The structure of haplotype blocks in the human genome. Science 2002; 296:2225–2229.

48. Wacholder S, Rothman N, Caporaso N. Population stratification in epidemiologic studies of common genetic variants and cancer: quantification of bias. J Natl Cancer Inst 2000; 92: 1151–1158.

49. Wang Y, Localio R, Rebbeck TR. Evaluating bias due to population stratification in case-control association studies of admixed populations. Genet Epidemiol 2004; 27:14–20.

50. Lasky-Su J, Lyon HN, Emilsson V, et al. On the replication of genetic associations: timing can be everything! Am J Hum Genet 2008; 82:849–858.

51. Gong MN, Zhou W, Williams PL, et al. –308 GA and TNFB polymorphisms in acute respiratory distress syndrome. Eur Respir J 2006; 26:382–389.

52. Gong MN, Zhou W, Williams PL, et al. Interleukin-10 polymorphism in position –1082 and acute respiratory distress syndrome. Eur Respir J 2006; 27(4):674–681.

53. Gong MN, Thompson BT, Williams P, et al. Clinical predictors of and mortality in acute respiratory distress syndrome: potential role of red cell transfusion. Crit Care Med 2005; 33:1191–1198.

54. Pelosi P, D'Onofrio D, Chiumello D, et al. Pulmonary and extrapulmonary acute respiratory distress syndrome are different. Eur Respir J Suppl 2003; 42:48 s–56 s.

55. Negri EM, Hoelz C, Barbas CS, et al. Acute remodeling of parenchyma in pulmonary and extrapulmonary ARDS. An autopsy study of collagen-elastic system fibers. Pathol Res Pract 2002; 198:355–361.

56. Parsons PE, Eisner MD, Thompson BT, et al. Lower tidal volume ventilation and plasma cytokine markers of inflammation in patients with acute lung injury. Crit Care Med 2005; 33:1–6; discussion 230–232.

57. dos Santos CC, Okutani D, Hu P, et al. Differential gene profiling in acute lung injury identifies injury-specific gene expression. Crit Care Med 2008; 36:855–865.

58. Khoury MJ, Beaty TH. Applications of the case-control method in genetic epidemiology. Epidemiol Rev 1994; 16:134–150.

59. Andrieu N, Goldstein AM. Epidemiologic and genetic approaches in the study of gene-environment interaction: an overview of available methods. Epidemiol Rev 1998; 20:137–147.

60. Benjamini Y, Hochberg Y. Controlling the false discovery rate: a practical and powerful approach to multiple testing. J R Stat Soc Series B Stat Methodol 1995; 57:289–300.

61. Wacholder S, Chanock S, Garcia-Closas M, et al. Assessing the probability that a positive report is false: an approach for molecular epidemiology studies. J Natl Cancer Inst 2004; 96:434–442.

62. Wakefield J. A Bayesian measure of the probability of false discovery in genetic epidemiology studies. Am J Hum Genet 2007; 81:208–227.

63. Samani NJ, Erdmann J, Hall AS, et al. Genomewide association analysis of coronary artery disease. N Engl J Med 2007; 357:443–453.

64. Neale BM, Sham PC. The future of association studies: gene-based analysis and replication. Am J Hum Genet 2004; 75:353–362.

65. Ober C, Hoffjan S. Asthma genetics 2006: the long and winding road to gene discovery. Genes Immun 2006; 7:95–100.

66. Gail MH, Pfeiffer RM, Wheeler W, et al. Probability of detecting disease-associated single nucleotide polymorphisms in case-control genome-wide association studies. Biostatistics 2008; 9:201–215.

67. Nannya Y, Taura K, Kurokawa M, et al. Evaluation of genome-wide power of genetic association studies based on empirical data from the HapMap project. Hum Mol Genet 2007; 16:2494–2505.

68. Dinu V, Miller PL, Zhao H. Evidence for association between multiple complement pathway genes and AMD. Genet Epidemiol 2007; 31:224–237.

69. Engels EA, Wu X, Gu J, et al. Systematic evaluation of genetic variants in the inflammation pathway and risk of lung cancer. Cancer Res 2007; 67:6520–6527.

70. Loza MJ, McCall CE, Li L, et al. Assembly of inflammation-related genes for pathway-focused genetic analysis. PLoS ONE 2007; 2:e1035.

71. Marshall RP, Webb S, Hill MR, et al. Genetic polymorphisms associated with susceptibility and outcome in ARDS. Chest 2002; 121:68 S–69 S.

72. Flores C, Ma SF, Maresso K, et al. Il6 gene-wide haplotype is associated with susceptibility to acute lung injury. Transl Res 2008; 152:11–17.

73. Schroeder O, Schulte KM, Schroeder J, et al. The -1082 interleukin-10 polymorphism is associated with acute respiratory failure after major trauma: a prospective cohort study. Surgery 2008; 143:233–242.

74. Gao L, Flores C, Fan-Ma S, et al. Macrophage migration inhibitory factor in acute lung injury: expression, biomarker, and associations. Transl Res 2007; 150:18–29.

75. Gong MN, Wei Z, Xu LL, et al. Polymorphism in the surfactant protein-B gene, gender, and the risk of direct pulmonary injury and ARDS. Chest 2004; 125:203–211.

76. Marshall RP, Webb S, Bellingan GJ, et al. Angiotensin converting enzyme insertion/deletion polymorphism is associated with susceptibility and outcome in acute respiratory distress syndrome. Am J Respir Crit Care Med 2002; 166:646–650.

77. Chan KC, Tang NL, Hui DS, et al. Absence of association between angiotensin converting enzyme polymorphism and development of adult respiratory distress syndrome in patients with severe acute respiratory syndrome: a case control study. BMC Infect Dis 2005; 5:26.

78. Jerng JS, Yu CJ, Wang HC, et al. Polymorphism of the angiotensin-converting enzyme gene affects the outcome of acute respiratory distress syndrome. Crit Care Med 2006; 34:1001–1006.

79. Adamzik M, Frey U, Sixt S, et al. ACE I/D but not AGT (-6)A/G polymorphism is a risk factor for mortality in ARDS. Eur Respir J 2007; 29:482–488.

80. Villar J, Flores C, Perez-Mendez L, et al. Angiotensin-converting enzyme insertion/deletion polymorphism is not associated with susceptibility and outcome in sepsis and acute respiratory distress syndrome. Intensive Care Med 2008; 34:488–495.

81. Lagan AL, Quinlan GJ, Mumby S, et al. Variation in iron homeostasis genes between patients with acute respiratory distress syndrome and healthy controls. Chest 2008; 133(6):1302–1311.

82. Adamzik M, Frey UH, Riemann K, et al. Factor v Leiden mutation is associated with improved 30-day survival in patients with acute respiratory distress syndrome. Crit Care Med 2008; 36:1776–1779.

13
Gene Expression Profiling and Biomarkers in ARDS

JUDIE HOWRYLAK
Division of Pulmonary and Critical Care Medicine, Brigham and Women's Hospital,
Harvard Medical School, Boston, Massachusetts, U.S.A.

AUGUSTINE M. K. CHOI
Division of Pulmonary and Critical Care Medicine, Brigham and Women's Hospital,
Harvard Medical School, Boston, Massachusetts, U.S.A.

I. Genomic and Proteomic Approaches to the Study of ARDS

Although the cute respiratory distress syndrome (ARDS) was described 40 years ago, the advances in diagnostic and treatment options have been progressing slowly. Part of the reason for this slow pace is due to the difficulty in establishing a method for the unbiased diagnosis of this syndrome. Currently, the diagnosis of ARDS/acute lung injury (ALI) is clinical, and is described according to the American-European Consensus Conference (AECC) definition by a series of clinical findings including acute onset, severe hypoxemia, the presence of bilateral pulmonary infiltrates, and no evidence of heart failure (1). However, there are several problems with the current clinical criteria for diagnosis. One problem is that there has been found to be a large degree of interobserver variability in applying the radiographic criteria to the diagnosis of ARDS (2). This large degree of variability makes it difficult to identify subsets of patients with the potential to benefit from more targeted therapy, and also makes it difficult to select patients for ongoing clinical trials. Furthermore, the difficulty in identifying patients with the disease makes it difficult to further the understanding of the pathogenesis of this disease in certain groups of patients, such as those with sepsis, trauma, pancreatitis, and certain types of surgery. Another problem with the AECC clinical diagnosis of ARDS is that attempts to validate the clinical criteria by comparison with pathologic findings have revealed that the accuracy of the clinical diagnosis is only moderate when compared to the pathologic diagnosis of diffuse alveolar damage (3).

Due to the difficulty in establishing a definitive diagnosis for ARDS/ALI, and improving the understanding of the clinical pathogenesis of the disease, interest has recently developed in using approaches from bioinformatics and computational biology to improve diagnosis and further the understanding of the pathogenesis of the disease.

Bioinformatics is defined by the NIH working definitions of bioinformatics and computational biology as research, development, or application of computational tools and approaches for expanding the use of biological, medical, behavioral, or health data, including those to acquire, store, organize, archive, analyze, or visualize such data. Conversely, computational biology involves the use of mathematical and computational approaches to address theoretical and experimental questions in biology. In short, bioinformatics involves developing tools for the analysis of biomedical data whereas computational biology involves the development of hypotheses to be answered using the tools of bioinformatics.

One of the ways in which computational biology may be used to study ARDS/ALI is through the analysis of high-throughput data, such as that obtained from gene expression microarrays, proteomic studies, and ChIP-on-chip data. Such high-throughput data provide an additional source of information that may be used to augment earlier studies where only clinical data such as physical exams and radiographic studies were available. One of the advantages of high-throughput data over more traditional low-throughput methods of obtaining gene expression and protein levels, such as northern blots, and ELISA assays is that high-throughput methods provide a more comprehensive source of information that allows for the collection of thousands of gene expression and protein levels from a single collection of tissue from a patient. Such information may then be used for biomarker detection to improve disease diagnosis, and also for more hypothesis-generating attempts to uncover additional pathogenetic information. Several high throughput approaches will be described in the following Sections.

II.   The Detection of Biomarkers in Patients with ARDS/ALI

A biomarker is a genetic, protein, or other chemical indicator of a disease process that has been used to improve disease diagnosis and/or assess the severity and outcome of a disease. One of the goals of biomarker detection in ARDS patients is to improve disease diagnosis. In other fields, the use of biomarker has helped to improve the diagnosis of diseases with the potential for high morbidity and mortality when untreated. For example, in the field of cardiology, the discovery of troponin as a biomarker for acute myocardial infarction has helped to standardize its diagnosis (4).

Because the AECC criteria for the diagnosis of ARDS leave room for error, one of the difficulties with biomarker studies has been the determination of an appropriate gold standard against which to compare the chosen biomarker. One way to avoid dealing with a gold standard is to correlate the chosen biomarker with a particular clinical outcome. There have been numerous studies to identify biomarkers for ARDS (5–26). A variety of single-center studies have found correlated levels of factors such as von Willebrand factor (19), interleukin-8 (27), transforming growth factor-α (28), and type III procollagen (29) with adverse clinical outcomes such as disease severity or mortality.

III.   The Use of Microarrays and the Study of ARDS/ALI

Recently, the development of microarray technology has provided a means for the identification of not just one biomarker for a particular disease process, but rather a number of biomarkers sometimes referred to as a profile. Gene expression profiling studies have been used to better understand the pathogenesis of lung injury in numerous animal studies. For example, several recent studies of ventilator-induced lung injury have identified differentially expressed genes among animals with and without lung injury (30–36). There have also been several studies performed in animal models attempting to elucidate specific gene expression patterns present in different subtypes of ARDS/ALI (34,37–40). For example, in one recent study completed in a rat model, three different forms of ALI were created, including lipopolysaccharide, hemorrhagic shock/resuscitation, and high-volume ventilation (38). It was found that unique gene expression patterns characterized ALI caused by different insults. Although this study was performed in an animal model, it demonstrates the heterogeneity of ALI. In this respect, the search for biomarkers in ARDS/ALI may in fact allow us not only to diagnose the disorder, but also to distinguish different subtypes of it by way of the presence of different chemical properties.

All of the studies mentioned in the previous paragraph were performed in animal models, such as mice and rats (37,38,41–43). The problem with performing biomarker studies for ARDS/ALI in mice is that it is now well known that ARDS/ALI in humans is characterized by regional variation in the cellular and mechanical behavior of the lungs (44,45), a phenomenon that is not observed in mouse models of lung injury. Thus, we may conclude that the search for biomarkers of clinical utility for ARDS/ALI may best be obtained through translational research in humans.

There have been a small number of microarray studies of human subjects with ARDS/ALI, attempting to identify biomarkers. One such study (46) involved the recruitment of study subjects admitted to the intensive care unit (ICU) with at least one risk factor for ARDS, including (1) sepsis, (2) septic shock, (3) trauma, (4) pneumonia, (5) aspiration, (6) massive transfusion of packed red blood cells (PRBCs: defined as >8 units of PRBC during the 24 hours before admission). During their time in the ICU, subjects were followed for the development of ARDS. Subjects who developed symptoms of ARDS consistent with the American-European Consensus Conference (AECC) criteria (1) were identified as ARDS cases, while subjects who did not meet the AECC criteria were identified as control cases. Blood samples were obtained from each study subject in the acute stage of disease (within three days of ARDS diagnosis) and the recovery stage (collected within the six-day period between three days before and three days after ICU discharge) and microarrays were performed on collected samples. Subsequent microarray analysis involved comparing samples from each patient during the acute and recovery stages of disease in order to identify potential biomarkers for ARDS. This study was able to identify several novel genes that appeared to be associated with ARDS, most notably, pre-elafin.

The above study highlights many of the difficulties associated with using gene expression including the variable course of disease progression among study subjects, which makes standardization of blood collection times difficult, and the difficulty in obtaining large numbers of critically ill study subjects for microarray analysis. When the number of genes being assayed by microarray analysis far exceeds the number of study subjects, there is an increased risk that the differential gene expression observed within the population studies may not be generalized to a larger population. However, there are many obstacles to the search for biomarkers in ARDS/ALI. For instance, as stated above, obtaining an adequate number of samples from a critically ill population can be challenging. In addition, one of the most significant obstacles stems from the fact that ARDS/ALI defines a clinical syndrome, and thus is often caused by different insults. Thus, different insults may lead to different forms of ARDS/ALI that may be defined by different gene expression profiles and hence different biomarkers.

IV. Using Classification to Identify Genomic and Proteomic Markers for ARDS

As noted in the preceding sections of this chapter, there have been many previous studies utilizing both high- and low-throughput techniques attempting to identify biomarkers for

ARDS. One limitation of low-throughput approaches is that a particular marker must be chosen in advance to be assayed as a potential biomarker. An advantage of high-throughput approaches is that a particular marker does not need to be chosen in advance of the biomarker assay. Indeed, the high-throughput assay may be performed on two groups of subjects, that is, those with and without ARDS and may lead to the identification of numerous differentially expressed genomic and proteomic disease markers.

Along with the identification of numerous differentially expressed genomic and proteomic markers comes the need to elucidate and clarify the often massive amounts of information obtained. Such efforts are carried out using a variety of newly developed data mining techniques. Data mining involves the use of techniques that attempt to extract the underlying patterns from large sets of data in an unbiased fashion. Some of the more common techniques will be described along with their potential application to the analysis of ARDS.

One such data mining method is known as classification. Classification methods for disease diagnosis have been gaining increased popularity in medical literature, particularly in studies of cancer diagnosis. The term classification derives from the fact that this approach attempts to partition patients into two or more disease groups. Traditionally, this approach used clinical criteria as a means of classification, but increasingly, high-throughput data from genomic and proteomic experiments are being used in an attempt to achieve a more systematic and unbiased method of disease diagnosis.

There are two main functions for classification analysis in medicine. Those functions are class prediction and class discovery (47). In class prediction, mathematical methods are used to predict the disease state of each patient in a set of patients. Class prediction may be used to distinguish between multiple disease states, but is most commonly used to distinguish between two disease states. Another name for class prediction is supervised learning. In the class discovery, accumulated data are analyzed in order to find patterns that distinguish one particular disease state from another. Class discovery is often used to uncover heterogeneity in a patient population. For example, in a population of patients, class discovery may be used to determine underlying patterns of gene expression that distinguish between multiple disease states. Such clusters may then be correlated with clinical findings to uncover novel disease states. Another name for class discovery is clustering, or unsupervised learning.

V. Class Prediction

Class prediction takes places in two stages. In order to complete both stages of class prediction, it is often necessary to first partition the set of available patients into two groups, a training group and a test group. The first stage of such an analysis is the training phase. The training group of patients is used for this initial analysis. In this phase, after gene expression levels are obtained, a mathematical formula is determined from the different gene expression levels obtained from each group of patients that allows for the best possible separation between each disease group. This is accomplished through the use of a specific classification algorithm, or set of instructions for completing a specific task. Multiple different classification algorithms exist, including such well-known algorithms as logistic regression, Naïve Bayes, k-nearest neighbor, support vector machine, neural networks, and decision trees. All of the aforementioned algorithms are similar with respect to their ability to classify different diseases, yet differ in terms of their mathematical foundations.

The second stage of class prediction is the test phase. The test group of patients is used for this analysis. In this stage the classification algorithm, along with the formula that was learned in the training step is used to partition the test group of patients into specific disease classes. The specific disease classifications determined by the classification algorithm are then compared to true disease classifications in order to determine the error rate of the particular classification algorithm.

Typically several different classification algorithms are used when attempting to perform class prediction for a particular set of patients. The reason for this has to do with the difference in the mathematical basis of each algorithm. For example, some algorithms, such as logistic regression and support vector machine, develop formulas that will create a linear separation between groups of patients. Conversely, algorithms such as Naïve Bayes, *k*-nearest neighbor, neural networks, and decision trees will create a nonlinear separation between groups of patients. If the gene expression data for different patient groups are linearly separable, algorithms that create a linear separation between different classes of patients will lead to a lower prediction error rate than algorithms that create nonlinear separations between different patient classes. If the gene expression data for different patient groups are not linearly separable, the nonlinear algorithms will lead to a lower prediction error rate. Unfortunately, it is impossible to predict in advance whether the gene expression data will be linearly or nonlinearly separable, and thus it is impossible to predict which classification algorithm will work best for a particular set of patients. Therefore, it is often necessary to train a mixture of linear and nonlinear classification algorithms in order to find the one that will lead to the lowest prediction error rate during the test phase of classification.

In a classification analysis, after the training and test phases are performed for a group of patients, it is necessary to perform an internal validation step. This step is necessary because when training and testing of a classification algorithm takes place, what develops is a classifier that works well in classifying the particular set of patients used to train and test the algorithm. However, in such a case, the classifier will often not work as well in classifying other groups of patients not included in the initial training and testing of the classifier. When a classifier is able to classify one set of patients well, but not other sets, the classifier is biased, and considered to be "overfitted" to a particular set of patients. Internal validation can help to offset this type of overfitting.

Internal validation can take many different forms, but commonly involves cross validation. Cross validation is performed by taking the initial group of patients and removing a subset of those patients. For example, in the case of leave-one-out cross validation, one patient is removed from the initial group of patients. After this removal, the remainder of the patients are used to train the classifier. Then the classifier is tested on the patient that was removed from the initial group. This process is repeated, each time removing a different patient from the set of patients used to train the classifier until all of the patients have been left out of the training set at least once (Fig. 1). This type of cross validation can help to reduce bias and overfitting in classification analysis. In cases where too many patients are present to perform leave-one-out cross validation, other forms of cross validation may be used, such as leave-two-out or leave-ten-out cross validation, where two or ten patients are left out of each train/test cycle respectively.

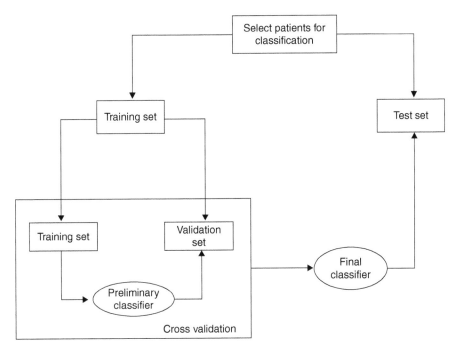

Figure 1 Flowchart representing the step in the process of developing a method of patient classification from high-throughput data. After initially selecting the group of patients to be used for a classification analysis, the group is split into a training set and a test set. The training itself is then split into a smaller training and validation set, and multiple iterations of cross validation are performed to develop a final classifier that is used to classify the test set of patients.

Methods of internal validation, such as leave-one-out cross validation, may help to reduce bias and overfitting in a classification analysis; however, external validation is also needed to ensure that such an analysis is unbiased. External validation using the mathematical formula obtained from training and cross validation of the initial set of patients is used to classify an independently obtained set of patients. Ideally, the independently obtained set of patients would be recruited from a different institution than the initial set of patients. However, obtaining sets of patients from different institutions is often not possible, and in such cases it is necessary to split the initial set of patients into two groups: a training group of patients on which the classifier will be trained and cross validated, and a test group of patients on which the classifier will be used to predict the class of each patient. Splitting the initial set of patients will only work if the total number of patients is high. The actual number of patients required for such an analysis is not exactly known. However, including more patients in the training set will help to reduce bias in development of the classifier. Reducing bias will, in turn, help to decrease the error rate in classification of the test set of patients (Fig. 2).

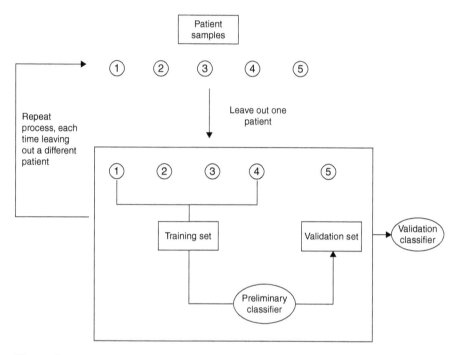

Figure 2 The process of leave-one-out cross validation (LOOCV). Each gray circle represents gene expression information from a particular patient. Depicted is a single iteration of LOOCV where gene expression information for patient 6 is left out of the initial training set, and used as part of the validation set. Subsequent iterations would leave out genes 1, 2, 3, 4, and 5 respectively. The combined results of each iteration of LOOCV lead to development of the validated classifier that can then be used to classify a test set of patients.

VI. Using Class Prediction to Uncover Biomarkers for ARDS/ALI

A class prediction analysis might also be extended to the case of patients with ARDS/ALI. Since ARDS/ALI is a particularly heterogeneous population, it will be necessary for a large number of patients to be collected for training. Ideally, a test set of patients would be obtained from a separate institution. After the patients are recruited, biologic material must be taken from each patient. Such material might be peripheral blood, and/or bronchoalveolar lavage fluid, and/or lung edema fluid. In selecting biologic material, it is important to consider the primary reason for undertaking most class prediction studies. That is, since the goal of most class prediction studies is to improve upon diagnostic criteria, and to develop new forms of screening for disease, it is important to select biologic material that is easy to obtain from patients, and may be obtained in a relative noninvasive way.

After the set of patients and biologic material is obtained, patients must be labeled as having either ARDS/ALI or not having ARDS/ALI. As was discussed in the introduction, in order to label patients as having ARDS/ALI or not having ARDS/ALI, it is necessary to rely on the clinical definitions, which are not completely reliable as there is a wide range of intraobserver variability in diagnosis. In a study seeking to improve upon the current clinical criteria, it is best to avoid the clinical criteria themselves as a gold standard when labeling the patients as ARDS/ALI or not ARDS/ALI.

Thus, it is necessary to determine an alternative gold standard for labeling the patients for classification analysis. One possible alternative is to label the patients based upon clinical outcome as opposed to ARDS/ALI versus not ARDS/ALI. The selection of outcome to correlate with patient labels is likely to be the most challenging aspect of class prediction in the ARDS/ALI population. One possible outcome is among ventilated patients in the ICU, patients may be labeled according to those who are successfully extubated, and those who are not successfully extubated. Undoubtedly, such labels will not necessarily correspond to the current ARDS/ALI versus not ARDS/ALI clinical criteria, but rather might correspond to new, more clinically useful criteria.

Selection based upon outcomes is challenging for several reasons. One reason is that ARDS/ALI is the end result of a wide variety of insults ultimately leading to lung injury, such as sepsis, pancreatitis, trauma, surgery, and transfusion. If the variety of causes leading to ARDS/ALI is not controlled for in a classification analysis, the results of such an analysis are likely to lead to patients being classified on the basis of the particular insult leading to ARDS/ALI as opposed to ARDS/ALI itself.

For example, suppose there is a group of ICU patients some of whom have sepsis, and some of whom have pancreatitis. Suppose that peripheral blood is obtained from all patients in the study, and microarray analysis is performed. The first step in a class prediction analysis is to split this group of patients into a training set and a test set. After the set of patients is split, the next step in class prediction is to label each patient based on outcome. Suppose the patients are to be labeled based upon whether or not they are successfully extubated within a certain time frame.

After this, the training step is performed to determine a mathematical formula for patient classification. Ideally, during this step, the classification algorithm develops such that genes that are differentially expressed between different clinical outcomes are weighted as more important in classification than those genes which are not differentially expressed between the different clinical outcomes, in this case the success of extubation. However, if the patient groups differ in other respects, such as in terms of different predisposing factors for ARDS/ALI, such differences might lead to differences in levels of gene expression. Differences in the levels of gene expression could then lead to ambiguity in development of the classification algorithm, and thus lead to increased errors in classification of the test set of patients.

A. Class Discovery

The second function of classification analysis is class discovery, or clustering. Clustering is also known as unsupervised learning. This type of analysis is useful when the goal is to identify subgroups of patients within a large heterogeneous group. For example, ARDS/ALI often represents a heterogeneous group of patients, and the syndrome is often the end result of a varied group of potential insults, including sepsis, trauma, pancreatitis, and surgery. Suppose one wished to examine whether the gene expression patterns of a group of patients with ARDS/ALI could be grouped into different clusters based on different clinical factors.

In order to carry out such an analysis, one would first need to identify a large group of patients with ARDS/ALI. As with class prediction, it is unclear what the minimum number of patients should be for such an analysis. However, with increasing heterogeneity, it is often necessary to increase the number of patients to decrease the risk of random fluctuation in gene expression levels that might interfere with the identification of valid differential gene expression changes that correspond to different clinical groups. Furthermore, as with class prediction, because there is intraobserver variability in the diagnosis of ARDS/ALI, the actual selection of patients with the diagnosis of ARDS/ALI for inclusion into the group of patients to be clustered may be subject to errors that could obscure the end results of cluster analysis. The problem of intraobserver variability could be minimized by increasing the number of patients selected for cluster analysis.

After the patients are selected, a clustering algorithm is run. There are different clustering algorithms available, all of which differ in terms of their mathematical foundations. However, all clustering algorithms are similar in their attempts to group patients with the most similar gene expression patterns into similar clusters (Fig. 3). For most clustering algorithms, it is necessary to select the number of clusters in advance.

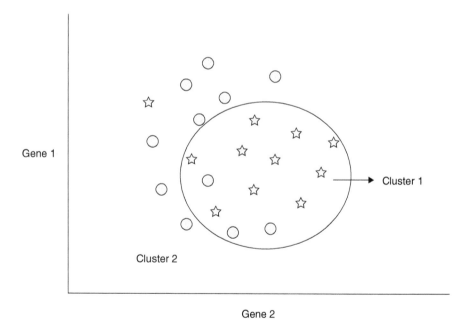

Figure 3 Example of clustering. The two different shapes in the figure represent two different classes of patients to be clustered. Vertical and horizontal dimensions correspond to different levels of gene expression for two genes. In the case where patients are clustered based on the expression levels of hundreds of genes, one may envision this process taking place in hundreds of dimensions.

Often this is done by clustering the group of patients several different times with different numbers of clusters, and then checking whether the clusters correspond to specific clinical criteria.

VII. The Use of Additional High-Throughput Methods for the Identification of Biomarkers for ARDS/ALI

Currently, microarray analysis provides one of the most commonly use high-throughput methods for identifying biomarkers of disease. However, additional high-throughput methods for identifying biomarkers exist beyond gene expression profiling. For example, high-throughput assays exist to identify levels of proteins like cytokines present in human samples, such as blood, urine, or pulmonary edema fluid from patients with ARDS/ALI (48). Other methods that may help to identify potential biomarkers for disease include mass-spectrometry techniques such as surface-enhanced laser desorption/ionization (SELDI) and matrix-assisted laser desorption/ionization (MALDI). SELDI may be used to detect proteins in tissue samples, such as blood, urine, or pulmonary edema fluid. One advantage to mass-spectrometry techniques like MALDI is that they allow for the identification of peptides and sugars in addition to proteins as potential biomarkers. Furthermore, because there are many more proteins in existence than genes in the human genome, mass-spectrometry techniques provide the opportunity to identify many more potential disease biomarkers.

The same methods of class prediction and class discovery that were used to explore gene expression profiles as potential biomarkers may be used with proteins, and other metabolites. In fact, multiple biologic assays may be run on the same samples of blood, urine, or fluid to detect levels of gene expression, protein, and other metabolites and then subsequently combined for class prediction or class discovery analyses. One problem that arises with such a combined approach is that such a large number of high-throughput assays require an increasingly complex computational analysis, requiring more computer memory and CPU time for completion.

In addition, in the field of biomarker discovery, more information is not always better. That is, when combining levels of gene expression, proteins, and other metabolites, the potential for differential levels of expression between different classes being due to random chance increases, and thus the potential for type-1 error increases. Furthermore, the increased number of potential biomarkers to be analyzed may obscure the presence of any true biomarkers that may exist. For example, suppose that there is one particular gene that allows one to best distinguish between two particular classes of patients. The patients will best be classified when the expression level of that gene is examined. However, if the expression level of another, irrelevant gene is present, the irrelevant gene may diminish the ability to distinguish between the two classes (Fig. 4). This phenomenon is often referred to as the curse of dimensionality, with each gene contributing one dimension to the analysis.

One way to lessen the curse of dimensionality is to perform a series of filtering steps prior to classification in order to reduce the number of genes (dimensions). One way in which this may be done is on the basis of fold-change between genes. That is, gene expression levels from each class of patients are compared, and those genes with

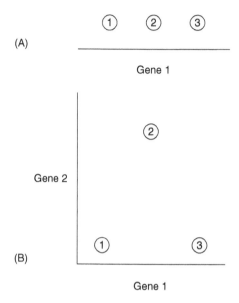

(A)

Gene 1

Gene 2

(B)

Gene 1

Figure 4   The curse of dimensionality. In both figures, the gray circles represent three different patients. Suppose that gene 1 represents a clinically relevant gene, and gene 2 represents a
clinically irrelevant gene. (**A**) Expression levels of gene 1 are represented along the horizontal
axis. In this case, when observing levels of gene 1 alone, patient 1 is physically closer to
patient 2 than patient 3. (**B**) Expression levels of gene 1 are represented along the horizontal
axis and expression levels of gene 2 are represented along the vertical axis. In this case, it
may be seen that when observing the combination of expression levels of gene 1 and gene 2,
patient 1 is physically closer to patient 3 than patient 2. Thus, the presence of gene 2, which is
clinically irrelevant, may obscure the distance between patient 1 and patient 2 in terms of the
more clinically relevant gene 1.

less than a specified fold-change between them are filtered out and not used for further
analysis. Often, after removing some genes on the basis of fold-change, it is necessary
to perform additional filtering. This is because most of the classification algorithms work
best if the number of genes (dimensions) is less than the number of samples. However, in
clinical studies with a limited number of patients, this is often not possible, and the best
that can be done is to decrease the number of genes in the analysis to a certain "optimum"
number.

   Another straightforward method for performing further gene selection is to use a
"greedy" algorithm. A greedy algorithm is one in which the best solution is chosen at each
intermediate stage of the process with the goal result being the best overall solution. For
example, in the case of gene selection, a greedy algorithm might proceed according to the
following steps. First, genes with less than a prespecified fold-change would be filtered out
and not used for further analysis. Then, with the remaining genes for each patient class,
a hypothesis test, such as a *t*-test or Mann–Whitney Wilcoxon test may be performed
to determine a test statistic for each gene. These test statistics should then be ranked

in descending order. After the list of ranked test statistics for each gene is determined, starting with the most highly ranked gene, the classification analysis is performed on the training and validation sets, and an error rate of classification is computed. Then multiple classification analyses are performed, each time adding the next highest ranked gene by test statistic. When this type of analysis has been performed for each gene, the genes used to determine the classifier with the lowest error rate are selected as the optimal "gene signature." This signature is then used to classify the test set and determine the overall classification accuracy.

VIII. Using Gene Expression Profiles to Understand the Pathogenesis of ARDS/ALI

Another application of gene expression data from patients with ARDS/ALI is to improve the understanding of the pathogenesis of the disease. As described above, class prediction and class discovery allow us to determine markers that would provide the potential to improve diagnosis and to uncover disease subgroups for ARDS/ALI patients respectively. However, the biomarkers uncovered by classification analysis do not provide information about disease pathogenesis. Genes from gene expression profiling experiments identified by classification analysis serve as markers for particular disease phenotypes used for either class prediction or class discovery. Such genes may be involved in disease pathogenesis, but the classification analysis itself does not provide information regarding the relationship between such genes and disease pathogenesis. To determine such a relationship, it is necessary to perform a different type of analysis. The type of analysis necessarily falls under the rubric of systems biology, which refers to an integrative approach to networks of complex interactions in biological systems.

One systems biology approach that may be particularly effective in uncovering relationships between differentially expressed genes in disease pathogens is the development of gene correlation networks. Gene correlation networks may be constructed by determining the pairwise correlations between genes. Typically, if the pairwise correlation between two genes is above a certain threshold, then the genes are considered to be linked in a functionally significant way (49).

For example, suppose we have a population of patients with ARDS/ALI that we wish to analyze by using a correlation network. The way this would be done is by first obtaining gene expression profiles from each patient through the use of microarrays. After microarrays are obtained, the patients are divided into two groups, such as patients with ARDS/ALI and patients without ARDS/ALI, or patients meeting other similarly dichotomous clinical criteria. After this, the pairwise correlation coefficients of genes within each group are calculated. Genes with correlation coefficients above some predetermined threshold are considered to be functionally related. Also, genes with correlation coefficients below some predetermined threshold are inversely functionally related. The ideal size of the threshold is not known, and the size may be modified to create networks of correlated genes that are large enough to be potentially biologically meaningful, yet small enough to exclude genes that may be related purely by random chance.

After functionally related sets of genes are determined by developing correlation networks, it remains to discover the nature of the functional relationships between genes within networks. It is possible that many of the genes included in a network have similar transcriptional regulation, and thus may operate together as part of a signaling pathway. This would represent a direct link between genes. However, this is not always the case with genes linked within a network because it is also possible that genes may be indirectly linked to each other. That is, the genes may have expression levels that move in similar directions, such as increased/decreased expression, but are involved in different pathways. For the case of ARDS/ALI patients, the different pathways might both be involved in inflammation, and thus have genes that become upregulated in the case of ARDS/ALI.

One step in determining the functional relationships between genes in a network is by learning the functional annotations of each gene in the network. Often from a microarray analysis, there will be multiple networks available for further study. The functional annotations may be obtained by using a database such as Gene Ontology (http://www.geneontology.org/index.shtml), or DAVID (http://david.abcc.ncifcrf.gov/home.jsp). Once the functional annotations for the genes within a particular network have been obtained, they can be examined to see whether genes from a similar pathway are included in the network. This finding would suggest that genes within a network might be regulated by a similar transcription factor.

Other observations that may be made from the descriptive information provided by gene correlation networks are in terms of the connectivity of the network. That is, how correlated each of the genes in the network are to each other. For example, suppose that one or two of the genes in the network are highly correlated with each of the other genes in the network (Fig. 5). Such genes would be considered to be highly connected, implying the possibility that the highly connected genes may act as transcription factor that regulates the transcription of the other genes in the network. Such a hypothesis could then be validated with pre-existing data from the literature regarding particular signaling pathways, or by performing experiments to uncover new signaling relationships. Conversely, genes in a correlation network might not have a high connectivity (Fig. 6). This type of connectivity implies a "series-type" relationship between the genes in the network. That is, the genes in the network appear to act sequentially on one another, implying that the correlation network may function as a signal transduction cascade (Fig. 6).

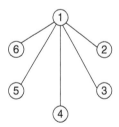

Figure 5 Gene correlation network with one gene of high connectivity. Each of the circles represents a gene in a network of six genes. The lines represent correlations or relationships between genes. In this case, expression levels of gene 1 correlate with expression levels of each of the other genes in the network, suggesting that gene 1 may act as a transcription factor to regulate the expression levels of the other genes in the network.

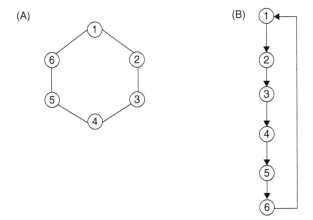

Figure 6 Gene correlation network with minimal connectivity. (**A**) Each of the circles represents a gene in a network of six genes. The lines represent correlations or relationships between genes. In this case, the expression level of each gene in the network is correlated with the expression level of two other genes. Such a network might correspond to the signal transduction cascade represented in (**B**). It should be noted that the network in part (**A**) does not provide any information about which gene is at the beginning of the signal transduction cascade, and the order could be different from that represented above. Information regarding the specific ordering must be obtained experimentally.

The development of gene correlation networks is somewhat similar to the class discovery clustering methods discussed in the preceding section. Both methods involve identifying groups of genes with similar gene expression profiles. However, one important difference between the two is that the class discovery methods only provide information regarding which genes may be grouped together. This information is absolute. That is, either the genes are clustered together, or they are not. Thus, it is often difficult to derive functional relationships from this type of data, and the most useful application of class discovery clustering has been in the identification of biomarkers for disease subgroups. Conversely, the information from gene correlation networks can vary in terms of magnitude. Genes may be more or less highly correlated with each other. Furthermore, genes may also be negatively correlated, which suggests potential negative regulatory relationships between them.

References

1. Bernard GR, Artigas A, Brigham KL, et al. The American-European Consensus Conference on ARDS. Definitions, mechanisms, relevant outcomes, and clinical trial coordination. Am J Respir Crit Care Med 1994; 149:818–824.
2. Rubenfeld GD, Caldwell E, Granton J, et al. Interobserver variability in applying a radiographic definition for ARDS. Chest 1999; 116:1347–1353.
3. Esteban A, Fernandez-Segoviano P, Frutos-Vivar F, et al. Comparison of clinical criteria for the acute respiratory distress syndrome with autopsy findings. Ann Intern Med 2004; 141:440–445.

4. Katus HA, Remppis A, Neumann FJ, et al. Diagnostic efficiency of troponin T measurements in acute myocardial infarction. Circulation 1991; 83:902–912.
5. Ware LB. Prognostic determinants of acute respiratory distress syndrome in adults: impact on clinical trial design. Crit Care Med 2005; 33:S217–S222.
6. Flori HR, Ware LB, Glidden D, et al. Early elevation of plasma soluble intercellular adhesion molecule-1 in pediatric acute lung injury identifies patients at increased risk of death and prolonged mechanical ventilation. Pediatr Crit Care Med 2003; 4:315–321.
7. Greene KE, Ye S, Mason RJ, et al. Serum surfactant protein-A levels predict development of ARDS in at-risk patients. Chest 1999; 116:90S–91S.
8. Rubin DB, Wiener-Kronish JP, Murray JF, et al. Elevated von Willebrand factor antigen is an early plasma predictor of acute lung injury in nonpulmonary sepsis syndrome. J Clin Invest 1990; 86:474–480.
9. Goodman RB, Pugin J, Lee JS, et al. Cytokine-mediated inflammation in acute lung injury. Cytokine Growth Factor Rev 2003; 14:523–535.
10. Parsons PE, Moss M. Early detection and markers of sepsis. Clin Chest Med 1996; 17:199–212.
11. Pittet JF, Mackersie RC, Martin TR, et al. Biological markers of acute lung injury: prognostic and pathogenetic significance. Am J Respir Crit Care Med 1997; 155:1187–1205.
12. McClintock D, Zhuo H, Wickersham N, et al. Biomarkers of inflammation, coagulation and fibrinolysis predict mortality in acute lung injury. Crit Care 2008; 12:R41.
13. Ware LB, Matthay MA, Parsons PE, et al. Pathogenetic and prognostic significance of altered coagulation and fibrinolysis in acute lung injury/acute respiratory distress syndrome. Crit Care Med 2007; 35:1821–1828.
14. McClintock DE, Ware LB, Eisner MD, et al. Higher urine nitric oxide is associated with improved outcomes in patients with acute lung injury. Am J Respir Crit Care Med 2007; 175:256–262.
15. Parsons PE, Matthay MA, Ware LB, et al. Elevated plasma levels of soluble TNF receptors are associated with morbidity and mortality in patients with acute lung injury. Am J Physiol Lung Cell Mol Physiol 2005; 288:L426–L431.
16. Ware LB, Eisner MD, Thompson BT, et al. Significance of von Willebrand factor in septic and nonseptic patients with acute lung injury. Am J Respir Crit Care Med 2004; 170: 766–772.
17. Prabhakaran P, Ware LB, White KE, et al. Elevated levels of plasminogen activator inhibitor-1 in pulmonary edema fluid are associated with mortality in acute lung injury. Am J Physiol Lung Cell Mol Physiol 2003; 285:L20–L28.
18. Ware LB, Fang X, Matthay MA. Protein C and thrombomodulin in human acute lung injury. Am J Physiol Lung Cell Mol Physiol 2003; 285:L514–L521.
19. Ware LB, Conner ER, Matthay MA. von Willebrand factor antigen is an independent marker of poor outcome in patients with early acute lung injury. Crit Care Med 2001; 29: 2325–2331.
20. Verghese GM, McCormick-Shannon K, Mason RJ, et al. Hepatocyte growth factor and keratinocyte growth factor in the pulmonary edema fluid of patients with acute lung injury. Biologic and clinical significance. Am J Respir Crit Care Med 1998; 158:386–394.
21. Madtes DK, Rubenfeld G, Klima LD, et al. Elevated transforming growth factor-alpha levels in bronchoalveolar lavage fluid of patients with acute respiratory distress syndrome. Am J Respir Crit Care Med 1998; 158:424–430.
22. Clark JG, Milberg JA, Steinberg KP, et al. Type III procollagen peptide in the adult respiratory distress syndrome. Association of increased peptide levels in bronchoalveolar lavage fluid with increased risk for death. Ann Intern Med 1995; 122:17–23.
23. Pugin J, Verghese G, Widmer MC, et al. The alveolar space is the site of intense inflammatory and profibrotic reactions in the early phase of acute respiratory distress syndrome. Crit Care Med 1999; 27:304–312.

24. Greene KE, Wright JR, Steinberg KP, et al. Serial changes in surfactant-associated proteins in lung and serum before and after onset of ARDS. Am J Respir Crit Care Med 1999; 160:1843–1850.

25. Moss M, Gillespie MK, Ackerson L, et al. Endothelial cell activity varies in patients at risk for the adult respiratory distress syndrome. Crit Care Med 1996; 24:1782–1786.

26. Meduri GU, Kohler G, Headley S, et al. Inflammatory cytokines in the BAL of patients with ARDS. Persistent elevation over time predicts poor outcome. Chest 1995; 108: 1303–1314.

27. Miller EJ, Cohen AB, Nagao S, et al. Elevated levels of NAP-1/interleukin-8 are present in the airspaces of patients with the adult respiratory distress syndrome and are associated with increased mortality. Am Rev Respir Dis 1992; 146:427–432.

28. Chesnutt AN, Kheradmand F, Folkesson HG, et al. Soluble transforming growth factor-alpha is present in the pulmonary edema fluid of patients with acute lung injury. Chest 1997; 111:652–656.

29. Chesnutt AN, Matthay MA, Tibayan FA, et al. Early detection of type III procollagen peptide in acute lung injury. Pathogenetic and prognostic significance. Am J Respir Crit Care Med 1997; 156:840–845.

30. Altemeier WA, Matute-Bello G, Frevert CW, et al. Mechanical ventilation with moderate tidal volumes synergistically increases lung cytokine response to systemic endotoxin. Am J Physiol Lung Cell Mol Physiol 2004; 287;L533–L542; erratum appears in Am J Physiol Lung Cell Mol Physiol. 2005; 288(4):L771.

31. Simon BA, Easley RB, Grigoryev DN, et al. Microarray analysis of regional cellular responses to local mechanical stress in acute lung injury. Am J Physiol Lung Cell Mol Physiol 2006; 291:L851–L861.

32. Hong S-B, Huang Y, Moreno-Vinasco L, et al. Essential role of pre-B-cell colony enhancing factor in ventilator-induced lung injury. Am J Respir Crit Care Med 2008; 178:605–617.

33. Dolinay T, Wu W, Kaminski N, et al. Mitogen-activated protein kinases regulate susceptibility to ventilator-induced lung injury. PLoS One 2008; 3:e1601.

34. Nonas SA, Vinasco LM, Ma SF, et al. Use of consomic rats for genomic insights into ventilator-associated lung injury. Am J Physiol Lung Cell Mol Physiol 2007; 293:L292–L302.

35. Copland IB, Kavanagh BP, Engelberts D, et al. Early changes in lung gene expression due to high tidal volume. Am J Respir Crit Care Med 2003; 168:1051–1059.

36. Grigoryev DN, Ma S-F, Irizarry RA, et al. Orthologous gene-expression profiling in multi-species models: search for candidate genes. Genome Biol 2004; 5:R34.

37. Feinman R, Deitch EA, Aris V, et al. Molecular signatures of trauma-hemorrhagic shock-induced lung injury: hemorrhage- and injury-associated genes. Shock 2007; 28:360–368.

38. dos Santos CC, Okutani D, Hu P, et al. Differential gene profiling in acute lung injury identifies injury-specific gene expression. Crit Care Med 2008; 36:855–865.

39. Kim DJ, Park SH, Sheen MR, et al. Comparison of experimental lung injury from acute renal failure with injury due to sepsis. Respiration 2006; 73:815–824.

40. Mallakin A, Kutcher LW, McDowell SA, et al. Gene expression profiles of Mst1r-deficient mice during nickel-induced acute lung injury. Am J Respir Cell Mol Biol 2006; 34:15–27.

41. Gharib SA, Liles WC, Matute-Bello G, et al. Computational identification of key biological modules and transcription factors in acute lung injury. Am J Respir Crit Care Med 2006; 173:653–658.

42. Jeyaseelan S, Chu HW, Young SK, et al. Transcriptional profiling of lipopolysaccharide-induced acute lung injury. Infect Immun 2004; 72:7247–7256.

43. Sun H-C, Qian X-M, Nie S-N, et al. Serial analysis of gene expression in mice with lipopolysaccharide-induced acute lung injury. Chin J Traumatol 2005; 8:67–73.

44. Gattinoni L, Caironi P, Pelosi P, et al. What has computed tomography taught us about the acute respiratory distress syndrome? Am J Respir Crit Care Med 2001; 164:1701–1711.

45. Puybasset L, Cluzel P, Chao N, et al. A computed tomography scan assessment of regional lung volume in acute lung injury. The CT Scan ARDS Study Group. Am J Respir Crit Care Med 1998; 158;1644–1655.
46. Wang Z, Beach D, Su L, et al. A genome-wide expression analysis in blood identifies pre-elafin as a biomarker in ARDS. Am J Respir Cell Mol Biol 2008; 38:724–732.
47. Golub TR, Slonim DK, Tamayo P, et al. Molecular classification of cancer: class discovery and class prediction by gene expression monitoring. Science 1999; 286:531–537.
48. Rouquette A-M, Desgruelles C, Laroche P. Evaluation of the new multiplexed immunoassay, FIDIS, for simultaneous quantitative determination of antinuclear antibodies and comparison with conventional methods. Am J Clin Pathol 2003; 120:676–681.
49. Butte AJ, Tamayo P, Slonim D, et al. Discovering functional relationships between RNA expression and chemotherapeutic susceptibility using relevance networks. Proc Natl Acad Sci U S A 2000; 97:12182–12186.

14

Resolution of Alveolar Edema: Mechanisms and Relationship to Clinical Acute Lung Injury

LORRAINE B. WARE
Division of Allergy, Pulmonary and Critical Care Medicine, Department of Medicine, Vanderbilt University, Nashville, Tennessee, U.S.A.

MICHAEL A. MATTHAY
Pulmonary and Critical Care Medicine and Cardiovascular Research Institute, University of California, San Francisco, California, U.S.A.

I. Introduction

Studies of epithelial fluid transport by the distal pulmonary epithelium have provided important new insights into the resolution of acute pulmonary edema, a common clinical problem. For many years, it was believed that differences in hydrostatic and protein osmotic pressures (Starling forces) accounted for the removal of excess fluid from the airspaces of the adult lung. Until the early 1980s, there were no satisfactory adult animal models to study the resolution of alveolar edema, and the isolation and culture of alveolar epithelial type II cells was just becoming a useful experimental method. In the early 1980s, new work provided evidence that fluid balance in the lung was regulated by active ion transport mechanisms (1–3), setting the stage for a rapid advance in our understanding of lung epithelial ion and fluid transport. This chapter discusses the regulation of lung fluid balance by active transport mechanisms across both the alveolar and distal airway epithelium of the mature lung, in both animals with conditions resembling acute lung injury or respiratory distress syndrome and in patients with acute lung injury (ALI), acute respiratory distress syndrome (ARDS), and cardiogenic pulmonary edema. Some of the information and perspectives in this chapter has been included in a recent review (4) and in a prior version of this chapter (5). Another recent review by Davis and Matalon (6) focuses on recent advances in the function of sodium and fluid transport under pathological conditions. A review of fetal and newborn lung fluid balance is beyond the scope of this chapter, although several excellent articles by Strang, Olver, Walters, Bland, and other investigators are available (7–9).

II. Mechanisms of Alveolar Epithelial Fluid Absorption

The general model for transepithelial fluid movement is that active salt transport generates a minisomotic pressure gradient that draws water across a tight epithelial barrier. This paradigm is probably correct for fluid clearance from the distal airspaces of the lung (10,11). The results of several in vivo studies have demonstrated that changes in hydrostatic or protein osmotic pressures cannot account for the removal of excess fluid from the distal airspaces (12–15). Furthermore, pharmacological inhibitors of sodium transport reduce the rate of fluid clearance in the lungs of several different species, including humans (14,16–21). In addition, there is good evidence that epithelial cells isolated from the distal airspaces actively transport sodium and other ions (10). More recent evidence indicates that under some conditions alveolar epithelial cells also secrete chloride both in vivo and in vitro and that movement of chloride significantly impacts net sodium and chloride transport and alveolar fluid clearance (22). In addition, several functional water channels, aquaporins, have been identified in alveolar epithelial cells; however, in contrast to the kidney, aquaporins do not seem to play a significant role in fluid movement across the normal or injured alveolar epithelium.

A. Structure of the Distal Pulmonary Epithelia

Although the large surface area of the alveoli favors the hypothesis that most fluid reabsorption occurs at the alveolar level, active fluid reabsorption may occur across all of the different segments of the pulmonary epithelium of the distal airspaces of the lung. The exact contribution of each of the anatomical segments of the distal airspaces to fluid reabsorption is not firmly established. The human lung consists of a series of highly branched hollow tubes that end blindly in the alveoli, with the conducting airways (the cartilaginous trachea, bronchi, and the membranous bronchioles) occupying the first 16 airway generations. The airways and alveoli, approximately 1.4 and 143 m^2 in the adult human lung (23), respectively, constitute the interface between lung parenchyma and the external environment and are lined by a continuous epithelium. The distal airway epithelium is composed of terminal respiratory and bronchiolar units with polarized epithelial cells that have the capacity to transport sodium and chloride, including ciliated Clara cells and nonciliated cuboidal cells. The alveoli are composed of a thin alveolar epithelium (0.1–0.2 μm) that covers 99% of the airspace surface area in the lung and contains thin, squamous type I cells and cuboidal type II cells (23,24). The alveolar type I cell covers 95% of the alveolar surface (23). The close apposition between the alveolar epithelium and the vascular endothelium facilitates efficient exchange of gases, but also forms a tight barrier to movement of liquid and proteins from the interstitial and vascular spaces, thus assisting in maintaining relatively dry alveoli (25).

The tight junctions are critical structures for the barrier function of the alveolar epithelium. Ion transporters and other membrane proteins are asymmetrically distributed on opposing cell surfaces, conferring vectorial transport properties to the epithelium. Physiological studies of the barrier properties of tight junctions in the alveolar epithelium indicate that diffusion of water-soluble solutes between alveolar epithelial cells is much slower than through the intercellular junctions of the adjacent lung capillaries (26). Based on tracer fluxes of small water-soluble solutes across the air/blood barrier of the distal airspaces, the effective pore radii were 0.5 to 0.9 nm in the distal respiratory epithelium and 6.5 to 7.5 nm in the capillary endothelium. Removal of large quantities of soluble protein from the airspaces appears to occur primarily by restricted diffusion (27,28), although there is evidence for some endocytosis and transcytosis of albumin across alveolar epithelium (29). Overall, the movement of protein across the normally tight alveolar epithelial barrier is very slow (30).

The alveolar epithelial type II cell is responsible for the secretion of surfactant as well as vectorial transport of sodium and chloride from the apical to the basolateral surface. Sodium uptake occurs on the apical surface, partly through amiloride-sensitive and amiloride-insensitive channels. Subsequently, sodium is pumped actively from the basolateral surface into the lung interstitium by Na,K-ATPase. An epithelial sodium channel (ENaC) that participates in sodium movement across the cell apical membrane was cloned from the colon of salt-deprived rats and characterized in 1994 (31), and work by other investigators has provided new insight into the molecular and biochemical basis for both sodium and chloride uptake in alveolar epithelial cells (32–34) (see details below).

Although the difficulty of studying alveolar type I cells in culture has hindered progress in assessing their capacity for ion transport and the role they may play in vectorial fluid transport across the alveolar epithelium, there is now evidence that alveolar type I cells participate in vectorial salt transport in the lung. On the basis of studies in freshly isolated type I cells, it is known that these cells have a high osmotic permeability to water with expression of aquaporin 5 on the apical surface (35). Although immunocytochemical studies in the intact lung by some investigators failed to demonstrate the presence of Na,K-ATPase in type I cells (36), more recent studies have reported the presence of the α_1 and α_2 subunits of Na,K-ATPase in type-1 like cells in vitro (37). The presence of the Na,K-ATPase could be consistent with a role for this cell in vectorial fluid transport, although Na,K-ATPase may also be needed to maintain cell volume. Recent studies of freshly isolated alveolar type I cells from rats demonstrated that these cells express the Na,K-ATPase α_1 and β_1 subunit isoforms, but not the α_2 subunit (38). In addition, there is evidence for expression of all the subunits of ENaC in freshly isolated alveolar type I cells from two laboratories (38,39) as well as in situ in the rat lung (38). Sodium uptake can be partially inhibited by amiloride in freshly isolated rat alveolar type I cells and patch clamp studies of isolated rat type I alveolar cells suggest that type I cells contain functional ENaC, pimozide-sensitive cation channels, K(+) channels, and the cystic fibrosis transmembrane regulator (CFTR) (40).

The alveolar epithelium comprises 99% of the surface area of the lung, a finding that suggests that removal of edema fluid from the lung might primarily occur across the alveolar epithelium. However, it has been demonstrated that the distal airway epithelium actively transports sodium, a process that depends on amiloride inhibitable uptake of sodium on the apical surface and extrusion of sodium through a basolateral Na,K-ATPase (41). In support of the potential role of distal airway cells is evidence that Clara cells actively absorb sodium and transport from an apical to basal direction (42). Also, there are new data on the role of CFTR in upregulating cAMP fluid clearance (43–45). This information provides support for a possible role of distal airway epithelia in fluid clearance since CFTR is expressed abundantly in distal airway epithelial cells of both adult and fetal cells (46). Thus, even though their surface area is limited, a contribution from distal airway epithelia to the overall fluid transport is probable, especially since cells from the distal airway epithelium primarily transport salt from the apical to the basolateral surface. The contribution of distal airway epithelia needs to be better defined.

B. Fluid Transport in the Lung

Several innovative experimental methods have been used to study fluid and protein transport from the distal airspaces of the intact lung, including isolated perfused lung preparations, in situ lung preparations, surface fluorescence methods, and intact lung preparations in living animals for short time periods (30–240 minutes) or for extended time periods

(24–144 hours). The advantages and disadvantages of these preparations have been reviewed in some detail (11,47).

In vivo evidence that active ion transport could account for the removal of alveolar edema fluid across the distal pulmonary epithelium of the mature lung was first obtained in studies of anesthetized, ventilated sheep (3). In those studies, the critical discovery was that isosmolar fluid clearance of salt and water occurred in the face of a rising concentration of protein in the airspaces of the lung, whether the instilled solution was autologous serum or an isosmolar protein solution. The initial protein concentration of the instilled protein solution was the same as the circulating plasma. After four hours, the concentration of the protein had risen from approximately 6.5 to 8.4 g/100 mL, while the plasma protein concentration was unchanged. In longer term studies in unanesthetized, spontaneously breathing sheep, alveolar protein concentrations increased to very high levels. After 12 and 24 hours, the alveolar protein concentration increased to 10.2 and 12.9 g/100 mL, respectively (48). The overall rise in protein concentration was equivalent to an increase in distal airspace protein osmotic pressure from 25 to 65 cm H_2O.

Other studies in the intact lung have supported the hypothesis that removal of alveolar fluid requires active transport processes. For example, elimination of ventilation to one lung did not change the rate of fluid clearance in sheep, thus ruling out changes in transpulmonary airway pressure as a major determinant of fluid clearance, at least in the uninjured lung (49). Furthermore, if active ion transport were responsible for fluid clearance, then fluid clearance should be temperature dependent. In an in situ perfused goat lung preparation, the rate of fluid clearance progressively declined as temperature was lowered from 37 to 18°C (50). Similar results were obtained in perfused rat lungs (51) and ex vivo human lung studies (19) in which hypothermia inhibited sodium and fluid transport.

Additional evidence for active ion transport was obtained in intact animals with the use of amiloride, an inhibitor of sodium uptake by the apical membrane of alveolar epithelium and distal airway epithelium. Amiloride inhibited 40–70% of basal fluid clearance in sheep, rabbits, rats, guinea pigs, mice, and in the human lung (4). Amiloride also inhibited sodium uptake in distal airway epithelium from sheep and pigs (52). To further explore the role of active sodium transport, experiments were designed to inhibit Na,K-ATPase. It has been difficult to study the effect of ouabain in intact animals because of cardiac toxicity. However, in the isolated rat lung, ouabain inhibited >90% of fluid clearance (53,54). Subsequently, following the development of an in situ sheep preparation for measuring fluid clearance in the absence of blood flow, it was reported that ouabain inhibited 90% of fluid clearance over a four-hour period (49).

C.   Sodium Transport in Cultured Alveolar Epithelial Cells

The success in obtaining high-purity cultures of alveolar epithelial type II cells from rats made it possible to study the transport properties of these cells and relate the results to the findings in the intact lung studies. The initial studies showed that when type II cells were cultured on a nonporous surface such as plastic, they would form a continuous confluent layer of polarized cells after two to three days (1,2). Interestingly, after three to five days, small domes of fluid could be appreciated from where the substratum was detached. The domes were thought to result from active ion transport from the apical to the basal surface with water following passively since they were inhibited by the replacement of sodium by another cation or by pharmacological inhibitors of sodium transport, such as amiloride and ouabain (55). More detailed information on the nature of ion transport across alveolar type II cells was obtained by culturing these cells on porous supports and mounting them in Ussing chambers and measuring short circuit current and ion flux under voltage clamp conditions. Further details are available in a recent review (4).

III. Regulation of Epithelial Fluid Transport

Until recently, most studies focused primarily on the active transport of sodium as the primary determinant for regulating catecholamine-dependent transport across distal pulmonary epithelium. New evidence indicates that cAMP-stimulated uptake of either chloride or bicarbonate may be an important mechanism for regulating fluid clearance across distal lung epithelium (43–46,56–59). Therefore, this section is divided into the effects of catecholamines on fluid transport based primarily on studies that examined the effects of sodium transport inhibitors and the more recent work on the role of chloride.

A. Upregulation of Fluid Transport by Catecholamine-Dependent Mechanisms

Studies in newborn animals indicate that endogenous release of catecholamines, particularly epinephrine, may stimulate reabsorption of fetal lung fluid from the airspaces of the lung (9,16,60). In most adult mammal species, stimulation of β_2-adrenergic receptors by either salmeterol, terbutaline, or epinephrine increases fluid clearance (4). This stimulatory effect occurs rapidly after intravenous administration of epinephrine or instillation of terbutaline into the alveolar space and is completely prevented by either a nonspecific β_2-receptor antagonist, propranolol, or in rats by a specific β_2-antagonist.

The increased fluid clearance by β_2-agonists can be prevented by amiloride, indicating that the stimulation was related to an increased transepithelial sodium transport. In anesthetized ventilated sheep, terbutaline-induced stimulation of fluid clearance was associated with an increase in lung lymph flow, a finding that reflected removal of some of the alveolar fluid volume to the interstitium of the lung (14). Although terbutaline also increased pulmonary blood flow, this effect was not important since control studies with nitroprusside, an agent that increased pulmonary blood flow, did not increase fluid clearance. Other studies have demonstrated that β-adrenergic agonists increased fluid clearance in several animal species, as well as in human lung (9,19,61).

Based on studies of the resolution of alveolar edema in humans, it has been difficult to quantify the effect of catecholamines on the rate of fluid clearance (62). However, studies of fluid clearance in the isolated human lung have demonstrated that β-adrenergic agonist therapy increases fluid clearance, and the increased fluid clearance can be inhibited with propranolol or amiloride (19,61,63). Subsequent studies showed that long-acting lipid-soluble β-agonists are more potent than hydrophilic β-agonists in the ex vivo human lung (61). The magnitude of the effect is similar to that observed in other species, with a β-agonist-dependent doubling of fluid clearance over baseline levels. These data are particularly important because aerosolized β-agonist treatment in some patients with pulmonary edema might accelerate the resolution of alveolar edema (64,65).

What has been learned about the basic mechanisms that mediate the catecholamine-dependent upregulation of sodium transport in the lung? Based on in vitro studies, it was proposed that an increase in intracellular cAMP resulted in increased sodium transport across alveolar type II cells by an independent upregulation of the apical sodium-conductive pathways and the basolateral Na,K-ATPase. Proposed mechanisms for upregulation of sodium transport proteins by cAMP include augmented sodium channel open probability, increases in Na,K-ATPase α subunit phosphorylation, delivery of more ENaC channels to the apical membrane, and more Na,K-ATPases to the basolateral cell membrane (4).

B. CFTR in cAMP-Mediated Upregulated Fluid Transport

While most experimental studies have attributed a primary role for active sodium transport in the vectorial transport of salt and water from the apical to the basal surface of the alveolar epithelium of the lung, a definitive role for chloride transport, especially in mediating the cAMP-mediated upregulation of fluid clearance across distal lung epithelium, has only recently been confirmed. One older study of cultured alveolar epithelial cells concluded that vectorial transport of chloride across alveolar epithelium occurs by a paracellular route under basal conditions and perhaps by a transcellular route in the presence of cAMP stimulation (66). Another study of cultured alveolar epithelial type II cells suggested that cAMP-mediated apical uptake of sodium might depend on an initial uptake of chloride (56). A more recent study of cultured alveolar type II cells under apical air interface conditions reported that β-adrenergic agonists produced acute activation of apical chloride channels with enhanced sodium absorption (57). However, the results of these studies were considered to be inconclusive by some investigators (67–69), partly because the data depend on cultured cells of an uncertain phenotype. Furthermore, studies of isolated alveolar epithelial type II cells do not address the possibility that vectorial fluid transport may be mediated by several different epithelial cells including alveolar epithelial type I cells as well as distal airway epithelial cells.

In order to define the role of chloride transport in the active transport of salt and water across the distal pulmonary epithelium of the lung, two groups have used in vivo lung studies to define the mechanisms and pathways that regulate chloride transport during the absorption of fluid from the distal airspaces of the lung. This approach may be important because studies in several species, as already discussed, have indicated that distal airway epithelia are capable of ion transport (52,70,71) and both ENaC and CFTR are expressed in alveolar and distal airway epithelia (72–76).

Both inhibition and ion substitution studies demonstrated that chloride transport was necessary for basal fluid clearance. In the first group of studies (59), rabbits administered Na^+ methane sulfonate were observed to have a significantly ($p < 0.05$) decreased AFC compared to the control group (i.e., rabbits that were instilled with NaCl) at 60 and 120 minutes postinstillation. Rabbits instilled with Na^+ methane sulfonate and forskolin demonstrated a negative alveolar fluid clearance (AFC) (i.e., fluid secretion into the alveolar space) at 60 minutes postinstillation. These studies provided evidence for the coupled transcellular movement of Na and Cl both under basal and cAMP-activated conditions and indicate that under some conditions (absence of chloride in the alveolar space) chloride secretion may occur. In a later study (46), this group provided evidence that agents that increase cAMP stimulate either chloride or bicarbonate secretion across confluent monolayers of distal airway cells isolated from the lungs of matured fetal rats.

In more definitive studies, the potential role of CFTR under basal and cAMP-stimulated conditions was tested using intact lung studies in which CFTR was not functional because of failure in trafficking of CFTR to the cell membrane, the most common human mutation in cystic fibrosis (ΔF508 mice). The results supported the hypothesis that CFTR was essential for cAMP-mediated upregulation of isosmolar fluid clearance from the distal airspaces of the lung because fluid clearance could not be increased in the ΔF508 mice with either β-agonists or forskolin, unlike the wild-type control mice (43). Additional studies using pharmacological inhibition of CFTR in both the mouse and human lung with glibenclamide or with a novel CFTR inhibitor, CFTR$_{inh}$-172, supported the same conclusion, namely that chloride uptake and CFTR-like transport are required for cAMP-stimulated fluid clearance from the distal airspaces of the lung (43,44,77). Overexpression of CFTR via an adenoviral vector also led to increased alveolar epithelial fluid transport that was dependent on intact expression of β-adrenergic receptors (45). The data in these studies provide additional evidence that the absence of CFTR prevents cAMP-upregulated fluid clearance from the distal airspaces of the lung, a finding that is similar to work on the importance of CFTR in mediating cAMP-stimulated sodium absorption in human sweat ducts (78). Because CFTR is distributed throughout the distal pulmonary epithelium in distal airway epithelium as well at the alveolar level (40,79,80), the data also suggest that the cAMP-mediated upregulated reabsorption of pulmonary edema fluid may occur across distal airway epithelium as well as at the level of the alveolar epithelium. Additional studies indicated that the lack of CFTR results in a greater accumulation of pulmonary edema in the presence of a hydrostatic stress, thus demonstrating the potential physiological importance of CFTR in upregulating fluid transport from the distal airspaces of the lung (43). Finally, one other group has provided some evidence that alveolar liquid secretion under basal conditions might depend on CFTR (81).

C. Catecholamine-Independent Regulation

In the last few years, several interesting catecholamine-independent mechanisms have been identified that can upregulate fluid transport across the distal airspaces of the lung as well as in cultured alveolar type II cells. These mechanisms are explored in a review in some detail (4). Hormonal factors, such as glucocorticoids, can upregulate transport by transcriptional mechanisms (76,82–85), while thyroid hormone increases alveolar epithelial fluid transport through upregulation of Na,K-ATPase activity (86–89). Some growth factors can work by either a transcriptional or direct membrane effect or by enhancing the number of alveolar type II cells (90). The vasoactive agent, dopamine, upregulates alveolar fluid clearance (91–93) by increasing recruitment of the Na,K-ATPase from intracellular endosomal compartments to the plasma membrane of alveolar epithelial cells (94,95). Dopamine also activates amiloride-sensitive Na channels in type I alveolar epithelial cells (96). In addition, proteolytic activity can regulate the activity of ENaC and potentially increase fluid clearance across the distal airway epithelium (97). New work has also established that adenosine may regulate alveolar fluid clearance through G-protein coupled receptors that activate or inhibit adenyl cyclase (98).

There is growing evidence that inflammatory mediators can modulate alveolar epithelial fluid transport (99). The proinflammatory cytokine, tumor necrosis factor (TNF)-α, can rapidly upregulate lung epithelial sodium uptake and fluid transport through the activity of its lectin-like domain, although interaction of TNF-α with its receptor TNFR1 inhibits alveolar fluid clearance (100). The proinflammatory cysteinyl leukotriene, leukotriene D4, has also been shown to increase alveolar epithelial fluid transport both in vitro and in the isolated perfused rat lung through increased activity and membrane localization of the Na,K-ATPase (101). Finally, transforming growth factor-beta (TGF-β), a critical mediator of ALI in several animal models (102), decreased sodium uptake by primary rat and human alveolar epithelial cells in vitro through decreases in ENaC expression (103). Intratracheal administration of TGF-β in rats inhibited the amiloride-sensitive fraction of distal lung epithelial fluid transport at a dose that was not associated with any increase in epithelial protein permeability. Taken together, these findings indicate that proinflammatory pathways may have significant impact on mechanisms of alveolar fluid clearance and the resolution of alveolar edema.

IV. Mechanisms That Impair Vectorial Fluid Transport

Several mechanisms have been identified that can impair fluid transport from the distal airspaces of the lung. This section will discuss how hypoxia, anesthetics, and reactive oxygen and nitrogen species may affect the resolution of pulmonary edema under clinically relevant conditions. The next section will review mechanisms that impair fluid transport under specific pathological conditions.

A. Hypoxia

Hypoxia may occur during residence or recreation at high altitudes and under a variety of pathological conditions associated with acute and chronic respiratory disease. Therefore, it is important to understand the effect of hypoxia on the ion and fluid transport capacity of the lung epithelium. In anesthetized rats, as well as in isolated perfused rat lungs, hypoxia decreases alveolar fluid clearance by inhibition of both ENaC and Na,K-ATPase activity (104–108). Hypoxia increased α-ENaC and β$_1$-Na,K-ATPase mRNA transcripts with little increase or no change in protein amounts, suggesting a post-translational mechanism such as a direct change of sodium transporter protein activity or protein internalization (108). This latter hypothesis was supported by the normalization of fluid clearance by a cAMP agonist (terbutaline), which is known to increase the trafficking of sodium transporter proteins from the cytoplasm to the membrane (109,110). A recently published article demonstrated that terbutaline increases the activity of ENaC in alveolar epithelial type II cells by increasing the traffic of ENaC subunits to the apical cell membrane under hypoxic conditions (111). In addition, multiple studies have now shown that acute hypoxia promotes endocytosis of the Na,K-ATPase from the alveolar epithelial cell plasma membrane to intracellular compartments, inhibiting Na,K-ATPase activity (112,113).

B. Anesthetics

In alveolar epithelial cells, the halogenated anesthetics affect sodium and fluid transport at the physiological level as well as on a cellular level. In the rat, halothane and isoflurane decrease fluid clearance by inhibition of the amiloride-sensitive component. This effect was rapidly reversible after cessation of halothane exposure (114). Unlike the rat, the ability of the rabbit to clear fluid from the alveolar space through an amiloride-sensitive pathway is not decreased by halothane (115). In vitro, exposure to a low concentration of halothane (1%) for a short time (30 minutes) induced a reversible decrease in Na,K-ATPase activity and amiloride-sensitive ^{22}Na influx in rat alveolar type II cells (116). However, a recent patch clamping study in two human alveolar epithelial cell lines found that short term (<30 minutes) direct exposure to halothane and other halogenated anesthetics *increased* the amiloride-sensitive inward current suggesting that the effects of halothane are not uniform across species (117). Further studies are needed to better understand the effects of halogenated anesthetics on alveolar fluid clearance in the human lung.

Lidocaine is widely used in patients with acute cardiac disorders and has also been recently implicated as a possible cause of pulmonary edema following liposuction. In experimental studies in rats, either intravenous or intra-alveolar lidocaine reduced fluid clearance in rats by 50% (118). Since lidocaine did not inhibit ENaC when expressed in oocytes, it seems that the inhibitory effect on vectorial fluid transport was primarily on the basal surface of alveolar epithelial cells, either through an effect on the activity of Na,K-ATPase or through an indirect effect through blockade of potassium channels, a well-known property of lidocaine (119). The effect of lidocaine was completely reversible with β_2-agonist therapy (118).

C. Reactive Oxygen and Nitrogen Species

Under several pathological conditions, in response to proinflammatory cytokines, activated neutrophils and macrophages can localize in the lung and migrate into the airspaces of the lung and release reactive oxygen species by the membrane-bound enzyme complex NADPH oxidase and nitric oxide (NO) via the calcium-insensitive iNOS form of NO synthase. Reactive oxygen–nitrogen intermediates can modulate alveolar fluid clearance (120). NO decreased Isc across cultured rat type II cells without affecting transepithelial resistance. NO also inhibited 60% of amiloride-sensitive Isc across type II cell monolayers following permeabilization of the basolateral membrane with amphotericin B (121). NO reacted with superoxide (O_2) to form peroxynitrite ($ONOO^-$), a potent oxidant and nitrating species that directly oxidizes a wide spectrum of biological molecules, such as DNA constituents, lipids, and proteins (10). Boluses of peroxynitrite (0.5–1 mM) into suspensions of freshly isolated type II cells from rabbits decreased amiloride-inhibitable sodium uptake to 68% and 56% of control values without affecting cell viability (122). Some investigators reported that products of macrophages, including NO, can downregulate sodium transport in fetal distal lung epithelium stimulated with endotoxin (123,124). Also, another study indicated that a generator of peroxynitrite (3-morpholinosydnonime) inhibited the amiloride-sensitive whole cell conductance in *Xenopus* oocytes expressing the three cloned subunits of ENaC (125). The data indicate that oxidation of critical amino acids residues in ENaC protein is probably responsible for this effect. This evidence matches well with other studies that have shown that protein nitration and oxidation by reactive oxygen and nitrogen species have been associated with diminished function of a variety of important proteins present in the alveolar space, including α_1-proteinase inhibitor (126) and surfactant protein A (127–129). Indeed intratracheal instillation of DETANONOate, a substance that decomposed to release NO, in the alveolar spaces of rabbits resulted in significant downregulation of amiloride-sensitive transport (130) and aminoguanidine, an inhibitor of iNOS, which restored alveolar fluid resorption that was inhibited by hemorrhagic shock (131). On the other hand, endogenously produced NO may play an important role in the regulation of sodium transporters in vivo as shown by the fact that iNOS(−/−) mice (132) and alveolar epithelial cells treated with iNOS inhibitors (133) lack amiloride-sensitive AFC transport.

V.   Alveolar Fluid Transport Under Pathological Conditions

Fluid clearance from the distal airspaces of the lung has been measured in mechanically ventilated patients with acute respiratory failure from pulmonary edema as well as in several animal models designed to simulate clinically relevant pathological conditions.

A.   Clinical Studies

Studies of fluid clearance have been done in intubated, ventilated patients by measuring the concentration of total protein in sequential samples of undiluted pulmonary edema fluid aspirated from the distal airspaces of the lung with a standard suction catheter passed through the endotracheal tube into a wedged position in the distal airways of the lung (28,62,128,134–136). This method for measuring fluid clearance in patients was adapted from the method for aspirating fluid from the distal airspaces of the lung in experimental studies in small and large animals (11,14). The clinical procedure has been validated in patients by demonstrating that there is a relationship between fluid clearance and the improvement in oxygenation and the chest radiograph (62,134).

In patients with severe hydrostatic pulmonary edema, there was net fluid clearance in the majority of the patients during the first four hours following endotracheal intubation and the onset of positive pressure ventilation (134). The rate of fluid clearance in these patients varied between maximal (>14% per hour) in 38% and submaximal (3–14% per hour) in 37%. Overall, 75% of the patients had intact fluid clearance. There was no significant correlation between the levels of fluid clearance and endogenous plasma levels of epinephrine, although twice as many of the patients with intact fluid clearance received aerosolized β-adrenergic therapy as those with impaired fluid clearance, but this difference did not reach statistical significance, perhaps because the total number of studied patients was modest. The inability to transport edema fluid from the distal airspaces of the lung in 25% of the patients was not simply related to elevated pulmonary vascular pressures. Several mechanisms could downregulate fluid transport in these patients including elevated levels of atrial natriuretic factor (137,138) or the presence of ouabain-like substances in the circulation (139–141) or damage to Na transporters by reactive oxygen–nitrogen intermediates (see above).

Experimental studies have provided some insight into the mechanisms that may downregulate fluid transport from the distal airspaces of the lung in the presence of elevated pulmonary vascular hydrostatic pressures (see below). Because hydrostatic pulmonary edema is associated with an uninjured epithelial barrier, the studies of hydrostatic pulmonary edema provide an important comparison group to the patients with pulmonary edema from ALI because some degree of morphological or functional injury to the epithelial barriers probably occurs in most lung injuries (see below).

The majority of patients with increased permeability edema and ALI have impaired alveolar epithelial fluid transport, a finding associated with more prolonged respiratory failure and a higher mortality (Fig. 1). In contrast, a minority of patients can remove alveolar edema fluid rapidly, and these patients have a higher survival rate (62,135,136). These results indicate that a functional, intact distal lung epithelium is associated with a better prognosis in patients with ALI, thus supporting the hypothesis that the degree of injury to the distal lung epithelium is an important determinant of the outcome in patients with increased permeability pulmonary edema from ALI.

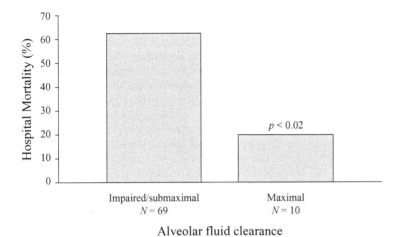

Alveolar fluid clearance

Figure 1 Hospital mortality (y-axis) plotted against two groups of patients with acute lung injury or the acute respiratory distress syndrome: those with maximal fluid clearance (>14% per hour) and those with impaired or submaximal fluid clearance (<14% per hour). The columns represent percent hospital mortality in each group. Hospital mortality of patients with maximal fluid clearance was significantly less ($p < 0.02$). *Abbreviations*: N, number of patients. *Source*: From Ref. 136.

What are the mechanisms that may impair fluid clearance from the airspaces of the lung? Some patients have pathological (142) and biochemical (143,144) evidence of injury to the alveolar epithelium. There are also some clinical data that a decrease in fluid clearance may be associated with higher levels of nitrate and nitrite in pulmonary edema fluid, a finding that supports the hypothesis that nitration and oxidation of proteins essential to the epithelial fluid transport may occur in some patients with lung injury, depressing their ability to remove alveolar edema fluid (128) (see next section).

B. Experimental Studies of Hypovolemic Shock

Hypovolemic shock from blood loss is an important clinical problem following major trauma. Short-term studies in rats that simulated acute hemorrhagic shock with a 30% loss of blood volume resulted in a sharp rise in endogenous levels of plasma epinephrine, a finding associated with a doubling of fluid clearance from the distal airspaces of the lung (145,146). The effect was inhibited by propranolol and partially inhibited by amiloride.

When hypovolemic shock, however, was prolonged for four to five hours in rats, the results were markedly different. Under these conditions, there was no increase in fluid transport from the airspaces of the lung, even when β_2-adrenergic agonists were instilled into the distal airspaces. This result prompted a series of experiments to discover the mechanisms that downregulate fluid clearance after prolonged hemorrhagic shock in rats. The initial studies established that the mechanism was neutrophil dependent (147). Further studies established that the process involves α-adrenergic activity and release of oxidant radicals with interleukin-1β in the airspaces (148,149), probably from neutrophils that accumulate in the lung after the onset of hemorrhagic shock. Finally, recent work has indicated that an increase in the expression of iNOS in the lung and release of NO, probably in part from alveolar macrophages, diminishes the capacity of the alveolar epithelium to actively transport fluid from the airspaces after severe hemorrhage. Second, NO inhibits the upregulation of alveolar epithelial fluid transport by cAMP-dependent mechanisms by directly affecting the function of the β_2-adrenergic receptor and adenylcyclase. Third, shock-mediated release of NO in the airspaces of the lung depends in part on the activation and nuclear translocation of NFκB (131). However, another study found no difference in AFC between iNOS(+/+) and iNOS(−/−) mice exposed to hyperoxia for 55 hours (132). A potential explanation for this discrepancy is the existence of significant levels of oxidizing and nitrating species in the lungs of iNOS(−/−) mice exposed to oxidant stress (150) generated by the interaction of neutrophil myeloperoxidase with nitrite and hydrogen peroxide.

The results of these experimental studies may have important clinical implications for explaining the susceptibility to pulmonary edema in some patients following major trauma. Since, as already discussed, in vitro studies demonstrated that peroxynitrate can directly impair the function of sodium channels (121,122,125,151–153), these in vivo studies fit well with one clinical study that reported an inverse relationship between elevated levels of nitrate and nitrite and the rate of fluid clearance in patients with pulmonary edema (128). Also, one prior study identified nitrotyrosine (the stable byproduct of peroxynitrite reactions with tyrosine residues) in the lungs of patients with the ARDS (154) as well as in alveolar macrophages isolated from patients with ARDS-induced acute respiratory failure (155,156).

C. Experimental Studies of Infection

The effects of endotoxemia and bacteremia on lung vascular permeability were well described in studies in sheep several years ago (157,158). However, the impact on the function of the alveolar epithelial barrier was not addressed in those studies. Subsequent work has indicated that the acute shock produced by severe bacteremia in rats markedly increases plasma epinephrine levels, as in hemorrhagic shock, and the elevated epinephrine levels markedly upregulate the fluid transport capacity of the distal lung epithelium (159). Thus, it is possible that in the short-term, upregulation of fluid clearance may protect the airspaces against alveolar flooding when there is an increase in lung vascular permeability and accumulation of interstitial edema. In fact, one study in sheep demonstrated that lung vascular permeability can be augmented markedly with intravenous endotoxin with a rise in protein-rich lung lymph flow, but this effect was not associated with a change in lung epithelial permeability to protein and no change in the capacity of the alveolar epithelium to remove alveolar fluid (160). These studies were done over 4 and 24 hours in sheep, and in some of the studies both intra-alveolar and intravenous endotoxin was administered, but in all cases the epithelial barrier remained intact and capable of transporting alveolar fluid normally.

However, when large doses of live bacteria (*Pseudomonas aeruginosa*) were given to sheep, there was an increase in both lung endothelial and epithelial permeability to protein in the sheep that had developed the most severe shock (161). These sheep had alveolar flooding and their capacity to remove alveolar fluid was impaired, similar to the findings in humans who develop severe permeability pulmonary edema with septic shock (162). The mechanisms for injury to the epithelial barrier probably depend on both neutrophil-dependent release of injurious proteases and reactive oxygen species as well as the bacterial exoproducts (see below). In one study, gram-negative bacteria that produced proteases increased alveolar epithelial barrier permeability to protein by altering epithelial basolateral surface permeability while the non–protease-producing strains only increased lung vascular permeability (163). It should be noted that the contribution of neutrophils to alveolar epithelial and endothelial injury depends on the originating insult: for example, neutopenic rabbits exposed to hyperoxia have similar levels of AFC as neutrophil-replete ones (164).

In sharp contrast to intra-alveolar endotoxin, live bacteria increased alveolar epithelial barrier permeability and decreased fluid transport in sheep (160). Further studies indicated that the products of *P. aeruginosa* were important in determining the extent of injury. For example, exoenzyme S and phospholipase *C* mediated injury to the epithelial barrier in rabbits with a decrease in vectorial fluid transport. Subsequent studies indicated that bacterial pneumonia may progress to septic shock when the infecting gram-negative organism generates proinflammatory cytokines in the airspaces of the lung that are released into the circulation when bacterial-mediated injury results in sufficient injury to the distal lung epithelial barrier (165). Several experimental studies have indicated that active and passive immunization against *P. aeruginosa* antigens can prevent epithelial injury in sheep (166) and in mice (167).

Recent data also indicate that influenza virus infection (A/PR/8/34) can specifically alter epithelial ion transport by inhibiting amiloride-sensitive sodium current across mouse tracheal epithelium (168) and rat alveolar epithelial type II cells (169). In the mouse tracheal epithelium, the inhibitory effect of the influenza virus was caused by binding the viral hemagglutinin to a cell-surface receptor, which then activated phospholipase C and protein kinase C. Influenza-mediated reduction of the open probability of ENaC channels in rat alveolar type II cells was also blocked by a phospholipase C inhibitor as well as by PP2, a Src inhibitor and GF-109203X, a protein kinase C inhibitor (169). It is well known that protein kinase C can reduce ENaC activity (170). As further evidence that influenza virus infection can reduce lung fluid clearance, Chen and coworkers showed that intratracheal administration of influenza virus produced a rapid inhibition of amiloride-sensitive lung fluid transport (169). Finally, there is new data that respiratory syncytial virus can induce insensitivity to β-adrenergic agonists based on in vivo studies in mice (171). Given the importance of sodium channels in vectorial transport of fluid in distal airway epithelia and in the alveoli, these results provide a new mechanism that may explain the accumulation of alveolar edema fluid in patients with viral pneumonia and ALI.

D. Experimental Studies of Hyperoxia

Several investigators have used hyperoxia as a model to study the effect of ALI on epithelial ion and fluid transport in the lung, in part because the injury develops over two to five days in rats and mice, and pathologically resembles clinical ALI with both endothelial and epithelial injury in association with an influx of neutrophils and protein-rich pulmonary edema.

However, the results of these studies have not been uniform, in part because of variations in the duration of O_2 exposure, the exact level of hyperoxia, and the use of rats or mice. For example, exposure of rats or rabbits to 100% O_2 at one atmosphere for two to four days results in extensive injury to both the endothelial and alveolar epithelial barriers (172–174). On the other hand, exposure of these animals to <85% O_2 results in sublethal injury and development of resistance to a subsequent exposure to hyperoxia or any oxidant stress (175,176). Administration of 85% O_2 for seven days increased the level of αENaC protein, and both inward and outward sodium currents were stimulated in patch clamps of isolated alveolar type II cells (177). Subsequently, another study from the same group showed increased expression and activity of amiloride-inhibitable sodium channels in alveolar type II cells of rats exposed to 85% O_2 for seven days followed by 100% O_2 for four days. Both the number and the open probability of the L-type sodium channels (25 pS) were increased (25). Another group also studied the effect of 85% O_2 for seven days in rats and found that amiloride-inhibitable sodium uptake was greater in hyperoxic rats than in control rats and that ouabain decreased active sodium transport to a greater percentage in the hyperoxic rats, suggesting an upregulation of Na,K-ATPase activity after subacute hyperoxia (54,178–180). In other studies, exposure to 100% O_2 for 48 hours produced moderate interstitial lung edema but no impairment of basal or cAMP-stimulated fluid transport (181–183). However, when exposure was prolonged to 64 hours, one group of investigators reported decreased transport in rats, an effect that seemed to be related to decreased gene expression of α_1 Na,K-ATPase subunits (184). Other studies found that there was rapid upregulation of mRNA for α_1 and β_1 subunits of Na,K-ATPase as well as antigenic protein shortly after prolonged exposure to >97% O_2 in rats for 60 hours (185), suggesting the induction of the Na,K-ATPase could occur as a protective mechanism. In the same vein, intratracheal administration of phenamil, an irreversible blocker of sodium channels, in rats exposed to hyperoxia worsened pulmonary edema as compared to sham-instilled animals, indicating that sodium reabsorption plays an important role in limiting edema in oxidant injury (186). Similar findings were reported by Stern and coworkers (187) in a thiourea model of lung injury in which upregulation of Na,K-ATPase gene expression and protein occurred after initial injury and was associated with recovery from the pulmonary edema. Other studies have reported that hyperoxia does not seem to produce a clear change in sodium and fluid transport during the period of hyperoxia (188–190). However, one recent study in mice showed that basal and cAMP-stimulated alveolar fluid clearance declines as lung water rises after 48 to 72 hours of hyperoxia (191).

Interestingly, one group of investigators reported that pretreatment of rats with aerosolized adenoviral β_1 Na,K-ATPase upregulated fluid transport and also made the rats resistant to the lethal effects of hyperoxia (180). This represented the first evidence that gene therapy could potentially be used to produce a sustained upregulation of fluid transport in the lung in the presence of a pathological condition. Furthermore, gene transfer of both α_1 and β_1 Na,K-ATPase decreases edema formation induced by thiourea in rats (187). An earlier study had shown that administration of the adenoviral β_1 Na,K-ATPase gene, but not the α_1 Na,K-ATPase, would increase fluid transport in normal rats (192).

VI. Conclusions

Several major advances have been made in the basic understanding of the mechanisms that regulate the reabsorption of edema fluid in the alveoli and the distal lung epithelia with characterization of sodium, chloride, and water transport pathways under both physiological and pathological conditions. However, as discussed in a recent review (4), several fundamental issues require additional study.

Alveolar type I and type II cells and distal airway epithelial cells, such as Clara cells, are implicated in sodium and fluid transport but their contribution in both physiological and pathological conditions are not well defined. Innovative approaches are needed to determine the contribution of these cells. Alveolar type I cells cover 95% of the alveolar surface area and the recent demonstration of the presence of water channels and ENaC expression in those cells suggests a role for these cells in net fluid clearance. More studies are needed to assess the differential contribution of alveolar type I and II cells to net fluid transport.

Another important area of research is the characterization of the sodium transporters involved in sodium and fluid reabsorption and their regulation. Amiloride-sensitive sodium transport is one of the major pathways for sodium entry across distal epithelial cells but several questions remain unsolved. For example, are the molecular and biophysical characteristics of these channels in vitro representative of their in vivo characteristics, and how are these channels regulated during physiological and pathological conditions? The mechanisms that regulate the trafficking of ENaC and Na,K-ATPases between the cytoplasm and the membrane need to be better evaluated also in distal lung epithelia. Increased insertion of transport proteins seems to be an important mechanism for increasing sodium and fluid transport under pathological conditions and may potentially contribute to regulating the clearance of edema fluid from distal airspaces of the lung. In addition to amiloride-sensitive sodium transport, a characterization of ion transporters involved in amiloride-insensitive sodium transport needs to be better defined. Also, the contribution of pathways for chloride reabsorption under basal and stimulated conditions needs to be determined with particular attention to the role of CFTR under cAMP-stimulated conditions.

As discussed in a recent review (4), recent advances have been made with transgenic mice models to define the role of sodium and water channels in the lung fluid balance. Knockout of the three subunits of ENaC clearly established the preponderant role of α compared to β and γENaC in alveolar transepithelial sodium absorption. Similarly, the knockout mice for several aquaporin-type water channels have revealed that in the lung these channels are not essential for water transport. However, a genomic disruption of genes that are expressed during development or in multiple tissue types complicates the phenotypic analysis. A solution to this problem may be provided by conditional knockouts. This system permits control of the timing for cell-specific expression of specific proteins, thereby circumventing both embryonic lethality and confounding effects of complex adaptive responses that can occur when the physiological observations follow the gene knockout events by days or weeks. In this system, gene expression is regulated temporally and spatially using cell-specific promoters, such as SP-C for alveolar type II cells, in combination with a regulatory on–off system. This approach may provide an opportunity to advance the understanding of the role of sodium and fluid transport during pathological conditions during the reabsorption of edema from the distal airspaces of the lung.

The rate of edema reabsorption from the distal airspaces of the lung can be estimated in ventilated, critically ill patients with acute pulmonary edema. In conjunction with progress in experimental studies of lung fluid balance under clinically relevant pathological conditions, further studies should be done to test the potential role of catecholamine-dependent and independent therapies that might enhance the resolution of clinical pulmonary edema, both hydrostatic pulmonary edema and ALI edema. Some of the therapies that might be tested for treatment of clinical lung injury, such as β_2-agonist treatment, might directly improve lung epithelial vectorial ion transport and therefore net fluid clearance, thus hastening the resolution of pulmonary edema. Therapies that may enhance the recovery of the injured alveolar epithelium may also result in more rapid restoration of alveolar fluid clearance (193).

References

1. Goodman BE, Crandall ED. Dome formation in primary cultured monolayers of alveolar epithelial cells. Am J Physiol 1982; 243(1):C96–C100.
2. Mason RJ, William MC, Widdicombe JH, et al. Transepithelial transport by pulmonary alveolar type II cells in primary culture. Proc Natl Acad Sci U S A 1982; 79:6033–6077.
3. Matthay MA, Landolt CC, Staub NC. Differential liquid and protein clearance from the alveoli of anesthetized sheep. J Appl Physiol 1982; 53:96–104.
4. Matthay MA, Folkesson HG, Clerici C. Lung epithelial fluid transport and the resolution of pulmonary edema. Physiol Rev 2002; 82:569–600.
5. Matthay MA, Fang X, Clerici C, et al. Resolution of alveolar edema: mechanisms and relationship to clinical acute lung injury. In: Matthay MA, ed. Acute Respiratory Distress Syndrome. New York: Marcel Dekker, 2003:409–438.
6. Davis IC, Matalon S. Epithelial sodium channels in the adult lung–important modulators of pulmonary health and disease. Adv Exp Med Biol 2007; 618:127–140.
7. Barker PM, Markiewicz M, Parker KA, et al. Synergistic action of triiodothyronine and hydrocortisone on epinephrine-induced reabsorption of fetal lung liquid. Pediatr Res 1990; 27(6):588–591.
8. Bland RD. Loss of liquid from the lung lumen in labor: more than a simple "squeeze". Am J Physiol Lung Cell Mol Physiol 2001; 280(4):L602–L605.
9. Walters DV, Olver RE. The role of catecholamines in lung liquid absorption at birth. Pediatr Res 1978; 12(3):239–242.
10. Matalon S, O'Brodovich H. Sodium channels in alveolar epithelial cells: molecular characterization, biophysical properties, and physiological significance. Annu Rev Physiol 1999; 61:627–661.
11. Matthay MA, Folkesson HG, Verkman AS. Salt and water transport across alveolar and distal airway epithelia in the adult lung. Am J Physiol 1996; 270:L487–L503.
12. Basset G, Crone C, Saumon G. Fluid absorption by rat lung in situ: pathways for sodium entry in the luminal membrane of alveolar epithelium. J Physiol 1987; 384:325–345.
13. Berthiaume Y, Broaddus VC, Gropper MA, et al. Alveolar liquid and protein clearance from normal dog lungs. J Appl Physiol 1988; 65:585–593.
14. Berthiaume Y, Staub NC, Matthay MA. Beta-adrenergic agonists increase lung liquid clearance in anesthetized sheep. J Clin Invest 1987; 79:335–343.
15. Effros RM, Mason GR, Hukkanen J, et al. New evidence for active sodium transport from fluid-filled rat lungs. J Appl Physiol 1989; 66(2):906–919.
16. Finley N, Norlin A, Baines D, et al. Alveolar epithelial fluid clearance is mediated by endogenous catecholamines at birth in Guinea pigs. J Clin Invest 1998; 101:972–981.
17. Norlin A, Finley N, Abedinpour P, et al. Alveolar liquid clearance in the anesthetized ventilated guinea pig. Am J Physiol 1998; 274:L235–L243.
18. O'Brodovich H, Hannam V, Seear M, et al. Amiloride impairs lung water clearance in newborn guinea pigs. J Appl Physiol 1990; 68(4):1758–1762.
19. Sakuma T, Okinawa G, Nakada T, et al. Alveolar fluid clearance in the resected human lung. Am J Respir Crit Care Med 1994; 150:305–310.

20. Smedira N, Gates L, Hastings R, et al. Alveolar and lung liquid clearance in anesthetized rabbits. J Appl Physiol 1991; 70:1827–1835.

21. Fukuda N, Folkesson HG, Matthay MA. Relationship of interstitial fluid volume to alveolar fluid clearance in mice: ventilated versus in situ studies. J Appl Physiol 2000; 89:672–679.

22. Folkesson HG, Matthay MA. Alveolar epithelial ion and fluid transport: recent progress. Am J Respir Cell Mol Biol 2006; 35(1):10–19.

23. Weibel ER. Lung morphometry and models in respiratory physiology. In: Chang HK, Paiva M, eds. Respiratory Physiology: An Analytical Approach. New York: Dekker, 1989:xv, 869 p.

24. Staub NC, Albertine KH. The structure of thelungs relative to their principal function. In: Murray JF, Nadel JA, eds. Textbook of Respiratory Medicine. Philadelphia, PA: W. B. Saunders, 1988:12–36.

25. West JB, Mathieu-Costello O. Strength of the pulmonary blood-gas barrier. Respir Physiol 1992; 88(1–2):141–148.

26. Schneeberger EE, Karnovsky MJ. The influence of intravascular fluid volume on the permeability of newborn and adult mouse lungs to ultrastructural protein tracers. J Cell Biol 1971; 49:319–334.

27. Hastings RH, Grady M, Sakuma T, et al. Clearance of different-sized proteins from the alveolar space in humans and rabbits. J Appl Physiol 1992; 73:1310–1316.

28. Hastings RH, Wright JR, Albertine KH, et al. Effect of endocytosis inhibitors on alveolar clearance of albumin, immunoglobulin G, and SP-A in rabbits. Am J Physiol 1994; 266(5, pt 1):L544–L552.

29. Berthiaume Y, Albertine KH, Grady M, et al. Protein clearance from the air spaces and lungs of unanesthetized sheep over 144h. J Appl Physiol 1989; 67:1887–1897.

30. Hastings RH, Folkesson HG, Matthay MA. Mechanisms of alveolar protein clearance in the intact lung. Am J Physiol Lung Cell Mol Physiol 2004; 286(4):L679–L689.

31. Canessa CM, Schild L, Buell G, et al. Amiloride-sensitive epithelial Na^+ channel is made of three homologous subunits. Nature 1994; 367(6462):463–467.

32. O'Brodovich H, Canessa C, Ueda J, et al. Expression of the epithelial Na^+ channel in the developing rat lung. Am J Physiol 1993; 265(2, pt 1):C491–C496.

33. Yue G, Russell WJ, Benos DJ, et al. Increased expression and activity of sodium channels in alveolar type II cells of hyperoxic rats. Proc Natl Acad Sci U S A 1995; 92:8418–8422.

34. Berthiaume Y, Matthay MA. Alveolar edema fluid clearance and acute lung injury. Respir Physiol Neurobiol 2007; 159(3):350–359.

35. Dobbs LG, Gonzalez R, Matthay MA, et al. Highly water-permeable type I alveolar epithelial cells confer high water permeability between the airspace and vasculature in rat lung. Proc Natl Acad Sci U S A 1998; 95:2991–2996.

36. Schneeberger EE, McCarthy KM. Cytochemical localization of Na^+-K^+-ATPase in rat type II pneumocytes. J Appl Physiol 1986; 60(5):1584–1589.

37. Ridge KM, Rutschman DH, Factor P, et al. Differential expression of Na-K-ATPase isoforms in rat alveolar epithelial cells. Am J Physiol 1997; 273(1, pt 1):L246–L255.

38. Borok Z, Liebler JM, Lubman RL, et al. Na transport proteins are expressed by rat alveolar epithelial type I cells. Am J Physiol Lung Cell Mol Physiol 2002; 282(4):L599–L608.

39. Johnson MD, Widdicombe JH, Allen L, et al. Alveolar epithelial type I cells contain transport proteins and transport sodium, supporting an active role for type I cells in regulation of lung liquid homeostasis. Proc Natl Acad Sci U S A 2002; 99(4):1966–1971.

40. Johnson MD, Bao HF, Helms MN, et al. Functional ion channels in pulmonary alveolar type I cells support a role for type I cells in lung ion transport. Proc Natl Acad Sci U S A 2006; 103(13):4964–4969.

41. Inglis SK, Corboz MR, Taylor AE, et al. Regulation of ion transport across porcine distal bronchi. Am J Physiol 1996; 270(2, pt 1):L289–L297.

42. Van Scott MR, Chinet TC, Burnette AD, et al. Purinergic regulation of ion transport across nonciliated bronchiolar epithelial (Clara) cells. Am J Physiol 1995; 269(1, pt 1):L30–L37.
43. Fang X, Fukuda N, Barbry P, et al. Novel role for CFTR in fluid absorption from the distal airspaces of the lung. J Gen Physiol 2002; 119(2):199–207.
44. Fang X, Song Y, Hirsch J, et al. Contribution of CFTR to apical-basolateral fluid transport in cultured human alveolar epithelial type II cells. Am J Physiol Lung Cell Mol Physiol 2006; 290(2):L242–L249.
45. Mutlu GM, Adir Y, Jameel M, et al. Interdependency of beta-adrenergic receptors and CFTR in regulation of alveolar active Na^+ transport. Circ Res 2005; 96(9):999–1005.
46. Lazrak A, Thome U, Myles C, et al. cAMP regulation of $Cl(-)$ and $HCO(-)(3)$ secretion across rat fetal distal lung epithelial cells. Am J Physiol Lung Cell Mol Physiol 2002; 282(4):L650–L658.
47. Saumon G, Basset G. Electrolyte and fluid transport across the mature alveolar epithelium. J Appl Physiol 1993; 74:1–15.
48. Matthay MA, Berthiaume Y, Staub NC. Long-term clearance of liquid and protein from the lungs of unanesthetized sheep. J Appl Physiol 1985; 59:928–934.
49. Sakuma T, Pittet JF, Jayr C, et al. Alveolar liquid and protein clearance in the absence of blood flow or ventilation in sheep. J Appl Physiol 1993; 74(1):176–185.
50. Serikov VB, Grady M, Matthay MA. Effect of temperature on alveolar liquid and protein clearance in an in situ perfused goat lung. J Appl Physiol 1993; 75(2):940–947.
51. Rutschman DH, Olivera W, Sznajder JI. Active transport and passive liquid movement in isolated perfused rat lungs. J Appl Physiol 1993; 75(4):1574–1580.
52. Ballard ST, Taylor AE. Bioelectric properties of proximal bronchiolar epithelium. Am J Physiol 1994; 267(1, pt 1):L79–L84.
53. Basset G, Crone C, Saumon G. Significance of active ion transport in transalveolar water absorption: a study on isolated rat lung. J Physiol 1987; 384:311–324.
54. Olivera W, Ridge K, Wood LD, et al. Active sodium transport and alveolar epithelial Na-K-ATPase increase during subacute hyperoxia in rats. Am J Physiol 1994; 266(5, pt 1):L577–L584.
55. Goodman BE, Fleisher RS, Crandall ED. Evidence for active sodium transport by cultured monolayers of pulmonary alveolar epithelial cells. Am J Physiol 1982; 245:C78–C83.
56. Jiang X, Ingbar DH, O'Grady SM. Adrenergic stimulation of Na^+ transport across alveolar epithelial cells involves activation of apical Cl- channels. Am J Physiol 1998; 275:C1610–C1620.
57. Jiang X, Ingbar DH, O'Grady SM. Adrenergic regulation of ion transport across adult alveolar epithelial cells: effects on Cl- channel activation and transport function in cultures with an apical air interface. J Membr Biol 2001; 181(3):195–204.
58. O'Grady SM, Jiang X, Ingbar DH. Cl- channel activation is necessary for stimulation of Na transport in adult alveolar epithelial cells. Am J Physiol Lung Cell Mol Physiol 2000; 278(2):L239–L244.
59. Nielsen VG, Duvall MD, Baird MS, et al. cAMP activation of chloride and fluid secretion across the rabbit alveolar epithelium. Am J Physiol 1998; 275:L1127–L1133.
60. Brown MJ, Olver RE, Ramsden CA, et al. Effects of adrenaline and of spontaneous labour on the secretion and absorption of lung liquid in the fetal lamb. J Physiol 1983; 344:137–152.
61. Sakuma T, Folkesson HG, Suzuki S, et al. Beta-adrenergic agonist stimulated alveolar fluid clearance in ex vivo human and rat lungs. Am J Respir Crit Care Med 1997; 155:506–512.
62. Matthay MA, Wiener-Kronish JP. Intact epithelial barrier function is critical for the resolution of alveolar edema in humans. Am Rev Respir Dis 1990; 142:1250–1257.
63. Ware LB, Fang X, Wang Y, et al. Selected contribution: mechanisms that may stimulate the resolution of alveolar edema in the transplanted human lung. J Appl Physiol 2002; 93:1869–1874.

64. Sartori C, Allemann Y, Duplain H, et al. Salmeterol for the prevention of high-altitude pulmonary edema. New Engl J Med 2002; 346:1631–1636.
65. Perkins GD, McAuley DF, Thickett DR, et al. The beta-agonist lung injury trial (BALTI): a randomized placebo-controlled clinical trial. Am J Respir Crit Care Med 2006; 173(3): 281–287.
66. Kim KJ, Cheek JM, Crandall ED. Contribution of active Na^+ and Cl- fluxes to net ion transport by alveolar epithelium. Respir Physiol 1991; 85(2):245–256.
67. Lazrak A, Nielsen VG, Matalon S. Mechanisms of increased $Na(^+)$ transport in ATII cells by cAMP: we agree to disagree and do more experiments. Am J Physiol Lung Cell Mol Physiol 2000; 278(2):L233–L238.
68. Widdicombe JH. How does cAMP increase active Na absorption across alveolar epithelium? Am J Physiol Lung Cell Mol Physiol 2000; 278(2):L231–L232.
69. Widdicombe JH. Yet another role for the cystic fibrosis transmembrane conductance regulator. Am J Respir Cell Mol Biol 2000; 22(1):11–14.
70. Al-Bazzaz FJ. Regulation of Na and Cl transport in sheep distal airways. Am J Physiol 1994; 267(2, pt 1):L193–L198.
71. Ballard ST, Schepens SM, Falcone JC, et al. Regional bioelectric properties of porcine airway epithelium. J Appl Physiol 1992; 73(5):2021–2027.
72. Farman N, Talbot CR, Boucher R, et al. Noncoordinated expression of alpha-, beta-, and gamma-subunit mRNAs of epithelial Na^+ channel along rat respiratory tract. Am J Physiol 1997; 272(1, pt 1):C131–C141.
73. Gaillard D, Hinnrasky J, Coscoy S, et al. Early expression of beta- and gamma-subunits of epithelial sodium channel during human airway development. Am J Physiol Lung Cell Mol Physiol 2000; 278:L177–L184.
74. Kreda SM, Gynn MC, Fenstermacher DA, et al. Expression and localization of epithelial aquaporins in the adult human lung. Am J Respir Cell Mol Biol 2001; 24(3): 224–234.
75. Pitkanen OM, Smith D, O'Brodovich H, et al. Expression of alpha-, beta-, and gamma-hENaC mRNA in the human nasal, bronchial, and distal lung epithelium. Am J Respir Crit Care Med 2001; 163(1):273–276.
76. Renard S, Voilley N, Bassilana F, et al. Localization and regulation by steroids of the alpha, beta and gamma subunits of the amiloride-sensitive Na^+ channel in colon, lung and kidney. Pflugers Arch 1995; 430(3):299–307.
77. Sakuma T, Gu X, Wang Z, et al. Stimulation of alveolar epithelial fluid clearance in human lungs by exogenous epinephrine. Crit Care Med 2006; 34(3):676–681.
78. Reddy MM, Light MJ, Quinton PM. Activation of the epithelial Na^+ channel (ENaC) requires CFTR Cl- channel function. Nature 1999; 402(6759):301–304.
79. Engelhardt JF, Zepeda M, Cohn JA, et al. Expression of the cystic fibrosis gene in adult human lung. J Clin Invest 1994; 93(2):737–749.
80. Brochiero E, Dagenais A, Prive A, et al. Evidence of a functional CFTR $Cl(-)$ channel in adult alveolar epithelial cells. Am J Physiol Lung Cell Mol Physiol 2004; 287(2): L382–L392.
81. Lindert J, Perlman CE, Parthasarathi K, et al. Chloride-dependent secretion of alveolar wall liquid determined by optical-sectioning microscopy. Am J Respir Cell Mol Biol 2007; 36(6):688–696.
82. Norlin A, Baines DL, Folkesson HG. Role of endogenous cortisol in basal liquid clearance from distal air spaces in adult guinea-pigs. J Physiol 1999; 519(pt 1):261–272.
83. Folkesson H, Matthay M. Dexamethasone upregulates epithelial liquid clearance in anesthetized ventilated rats (Abstract). FASEB J 1997; 11:A561.
84. Noda M, Suzuki S, Tsubochi H, et al. Single dexamethasone injection increases alveolar fluid clearance in adult rats. Crit Care Med 2003; 31(4):1183–1189.

85. Dagenais A, Denis C, Vives MF, et al. Modulation of alpha-ENaC and alpha1-Na$^+$-K$^+$-ATPase by cAMP and dexamethasone in alveolar epithelial cells. Am J Physiol Lung Cell Mol Physiol 2001; 281(1):L217–L230.

86. Bhargava M, Runyon MR, Smirnov D, et al. Triiodo-l-thyronine rapidly stimulates alveolar fluid clearance in normal & hyperoxia injured lungs. Am J Respir Crit Care Med 2008; 178(5):506–512.

87. Lei J, Mariash CN, Ingbar DH. 3,3′,5-Triiodo-L-thyronine up-regulation of Na,K-ATPase activity and cell surface expression in alveolar epithelial cells is Src kinase- and phospho-inositide 3-kinase-dependent. J Biol Chem 2004; 279(46):47589–47600.

88. Lei J, Nowbar S, Mariash CN, et al. Thyroid hormone stimulates Na-K-ATPase activity and its plasma membrane insertion in rat alveolar epithelial cells. Am J Physiol Lung Cell Mol Physiol 2003; 285(3):L762–L772.

89. Bhargava M, Lei J, Mariash CN, et al. Thyroid hormone rapidly stimulates alveolar Na,K-ATPase by activation of phosphatidylinositol 3-kinase. Curr Opin Endocrinol Diabetes Obes 2007; 14(5):416–420.

90. Wang Y, Folkesson HG, Jayr C, et al. Alveolar epithelial fluid transport can be simultaneously upregulated by both KGF and beta-agonist therapy. J Appl Physiol 1999; 87: 1852–1860.

91. Barnard M, Olivera W, Rutschman D, et al. Dopamine stimulates sodium transport and liquid clearance in rat lung epithelium. Am J Respir Crit Care Med 1997; 156:709–714.

92. Barnard ML, Ridge KM, Saldias F, et al. Stimulation of the dopamine 1 receptor increases lung edema clearance. Am J Respir Crit Care Med 1999; 160:982–986.

93. Chamorro-Marin V, Garcia-Delgado M, Touma-Fernandez A, et al. Intratracheal dopamine attenuates pulmonary edema and improves survival after ventilator-induced lung injury in rats. Crit Care 2008; 12(2):R39.

94. Ridge KM, Dada L, Lecuona E, et al. Dopamine-induced exocytosis of Na,K-ATPase is dependent on activation of protein kinase C-epsilon and -delta. Mol Biol Cell 2002; 13(4):1381–1389.

95. Bertorello AM, Komarova Y, Smith K, et al. Analysis of Na$^+$,K$^+$-ATPase motion and incorporation into the plasma membrane in response to G protein-coupled receptor signals in living cells. Mol Biol Cell 2003; 14(3):1149–1157.

96. Helms MN, Self J, Bao HF, et al. Dopamine activates amiloride-sensitive sodium channels in alveolar type I cells in lung slice preparations. Am J Physiol Lung Cell Mol Physiol 2006; 291(4):L610–L618.

97. Hughey RP, Carattino MD, Kleyman TR. Role of proteolysis in the activation of epithelial sodium channels. Curr Opin Nephrol Hypertens 2007; 16(5):444–450.

98. Factor P, Mutlu GM, Chen L, et al. Adenosine regulation of alveolar fluid clearance. Proc Natl Acad Sci U S A 2007; 104(10):4083–4088.

99. Ware LB. Modulation of alveolar fluid clearance by acute inflammation. The plot thickens. Am J Respir Crit Care Med 2004; 169:332–333.

100. Braun C, Hamacher J, Morel DR, et al. Dichotomal role of TNF in experimental pulmonary edema reabsorption. J Immunol 2005; 175(5):3402–3408.

101. Sloniewsky DE, Ridge KM, Adir Y, et al. Leukotriene D4 activates alveolar epithelial Na, K-ATPase and increases alveolar fluid clearance. Am J Respir Crit Care Med 2003; 169(3): 407–412.

102. Pittet J-F, Griffiths MJD, Geiser T, et al. TGF-b is a critical mediator of acute lung injury. J Clin Invest 2001; 107:1537–1544.

103. Frank J, Roux J, Kawakatsu H, et al. Transforming growth factor-beta1 decreases expression of the epithelial sodium channel alphaENaC and alveolar epithelial vectorial sodium and fluid transport via an ERK1/2-dependent mechanism. J Biol Chem 2003; 278:43939–43950.

104. Litvan J, Briva A, Wilson MS, et al. Beta-adrenergic receptor stimulation and adenoviral overexpression of superoxide dismutase prevent the hypoxia-mediated decrease in Na,K-ATPase and alveolar fluid reabsorption. J Biol Chem 2006; 281(29):19892–19898.

105. Tomlinson LA, Carpenter TC, Baker EH, et al. Hypoxia reduces airway epithelial sodium transport in rats. Am J Physiol 1999; 277(5, pt 1):L881–L886.

106. Carpenter TC, Schomberg S, Nichols C, et al. Hypoxia reversibly inhibits epithelial sodium transport but does not inhibit lung ENaC or Na-K-ATPase expression. Am J Physiol Lung Cell Mol Physiol 2003; 284(1):L77–L83.

107. Suzuki S, Noda M, Sugita M, et al. Impairment of transalveolar fluid transport and lung $Na^{(+)}$-$K^{(+)}$-ATPase function by hypoxia in rats. J Appl Physiol 1999; 87(3): 962–968.

108. Vivona ML, Matthay M, Chabaud MB, et al. Hypoxia reduces alveolar epithelial sodium and fluid transport in rats: reversal by beta-adrenergic agonist treatment. Am J Respir Cell Mol Biol 2001; 25(5):554–561.

109. Butterworth MB, Helman SI, Els WJ. cAMP-sensitive endocytic trafficking in A6 epithelia. Am J Physiol Cell Physiol 2001; 280(4):C752–C762.

110. Snyder PM. Liddle's syndrome mutations disrupt cAMP-mediated translocation of the epithelial $Na^{(+)}$ channel to the cell surface. J Clin Invest 2000; 105(1):45–53.

111. Planes C, Blot-Chabaud M, Matthay MA, et al. Hypoxia and beta 2-agonists regulate cell surface expression of the epithelial sodium channel in native alveolar epithelial cells. J Biol Chem 2002; 277(49):47318–47324.

112. Dada LA, Chandel NS, Ridge KM, et al. Hypoxia-induced endocytosis of Na,K-ATPase in alveolar epithelial cells is mediated by mitochondrial reactive oxygen species and PKC-zeta. J Clin Invest 2003; 111(7):1057–1064.

113. Zhou G, Dada LA, Sznajder JI. Regulation of alveolar epithelial function by hypoxia. Eur Respir J 2008; 31(5):1107–1113.

114. Rezaiguia-Delclaux S, Jayr C, Luo DF, et al. Halothane and isoflurane decrease alveolar epithelial fluid clearance in rats. Anesthesiology 1998; 88(3):751–760.

115. Nielsen VG, Baird MS, Geary BT, et al. Halothane does not decrease amiloride-sensitive alveolar fluid clearance in rabbits. Anesth Analg 2000; 90(6):1445–1449.

116. Molliex S, Crestani B, Dureuil B, et al. Effects of halothane on surfactant biosynthesis by rat alveolar type II cells in primary culture. Anesthesiology 1994; 81(3):668–676.

117. Roch A, Shlyonsky V, Goolaerts A, et al. Halothane directly modifies Na^+ and K^+ channel activities in cultured human alveolar epithelial cells. Mol Pharmacol 2006; 69(5): 1755–1762.

118. Laffon M, Jayr C, Barbry P, et al. Lidocaine induces a reversible decrease in alveolar epithelial fluid clearance in rats. Anesthesiology 2002; 96(2):392–399.

119. Butterworth JFT, Strichartz GR. Molecular mechanisms of local anesthesia: a review. Anesthesiology 1990; 72(4):711–734.

120. Song W, Matalon S. Modulation of alveolar fluid clearance by reactive oxygen-nitrogen intermediates. Am J Physiol Lung Cell Mol Physiol 2007; 293(4):L855–L858.

121. Guo Y, Duvall D, Crow JP, et al. Nitric oxide inhibits Na absorption across cultures of alveolar type II monolayers. Am J Physiol 1998; 274:L369–L377.

122. Hu P, Ischiropoulos H, Beckman JS, et al. Peroxynitrite inhibition of oxygen consumption and sodium transport in alveolar type II cells. Am J Physiol 1994; 266:L628–L634.

123. Compeau CG, Rotstein OD, Tohda H, et al. Endotoxin-stimulated alveolar macrophages impair lung epithelial Na^+ transport by an L-Arg-dependent mechanism. Am J Physiol 1994; 266(5, pt 1):C1330–C1341.

124. Ding JW, Dickie J, O'Brodovich H, et al. Inhibition of amiloride-sensitive sodium-channel activity in distal lung epithelial cells by nitric oxide. Am J Physiol 1998; 274(3, pt 1):L378–L387.

125. DuVall MD, Zhu S, Fuller CM, et al. Peroxynitrite inhibits amiloride-sensitive Na^+ currents in Xenopus oocytes expressing alpha beta gamma-rENaC. Am J Physiol 1998; 274(5, pt 1):C1417–C1423.
126. Moreno JJ, Pryor WA. Inactivation of alpha I-proteinase inhibitor by peroxynitrite. Chem Res Toxicol 1992; 5:425–431.
127. Zhu S, Basiouny KF, Crow JP, et al. Carbon dioxide enhances nitration of surfactant protein A by activated alveolar macrophages. Am J Physiol Lung Cell Mol Physiol 2000; 278:L1025–L1031.
128. Zhu S, Ware LB, Geiser T, et al. Increased levels of nitrate and surfactant protein A nitration in the pulmonary edema fluid of patients with acute lung injury. Am J Respir Crit Care Med 2001; 163:166–172.
129. Zhu S, Kachel DL, Martin WJN, et al. Nitrated SP-A does not enhance adherence of *Pneumocystis carinii* to alveolar macrophages. Am J Physiol 1998; 275:L1031–L1039.
130. Nielsen VG, Baird MS, Chen L, et al. DETANONOate, a nitric oxide donor, decreases amiloride-sensitive alveolar fluid clearance in rabbits. Am J Respir Crit Care Med 2000; 161(4, pt 1):1154–1160.
131. Pittet JF, Lu LN, Morris DG, et al. Reactive nitrogen species inhibit alveolar epithelial fluid transport after hemorrhagic shock in rats. J Immunol 2001; 166:6301–6310.
132. Hardiman K, Lindsey JR, Matalon S. Lack of amiloride-sensitive transport across alveolar and respiratory epithelium of iNOS (−/−) mice in vivo. Am J Physiol Lung Cell Mol Physiol 2001; 281:L722–L731.
133. Hardiman KM, McNicholas-Bevensee CM, Fortenberry J, et al. Regulation of amiloride-sensitive $Na(^+)$ transport by basal nitric oxide. Am J Respir Cell Mol Biol 2004; 30(5):720–728.
134. Verghese GM, Ware LB, Matthay BA, et al. Alveolar epithelial fluid transport and the resolution of clinically severe hydrostatic pulmonary edema. J Appl Physiol 1999; 87:1301–1312.
135. Ware LB, Golden JA, Finkbeiner WE, et al. Alveolar epithelial fluid transport capacity in reperfusion lung injury after lung transplantation. Am J Respir Crit Care Med 1999; 159:980–988.
136. Ware LB, Matthay MA. Alveolar fluid clearance is impaired in the majority of patients with acute lung injury and the acute respiratory distress syndrome. Am J Respir Crit Care Med 2001; 163:1376–1383.
137. Campbell AR, Folkesson HG, Berthiaume Y, et al. Alveolar epithelial fluid clearance persists in the presence of moderate left atrial hypertension in sheep. J Appl Physiol 1999; 86(1):139–151.
138. Olivera W, Ridge K, Wood LDH, et al. ANF decreases active sodium transport and increases alveolar epithelial permeability in rats. J Appl Physiol 1993; 75:1581–1586.
139. De Angelis C, Riscazzi M, Salvini R, et al. Isolation and characterization of a digoxin-like immunoreactive substance from human urine by affinity chromatography. Clin Chem 1997; 43:1416–1420.
140. Ferrandi M, Manunta P, Balzan S, et al. Ouabain-like factor quantification in mammalian tissues and plasma: comparison of two independent assays. Hypertension 1997; 30:886–896.
141. Ferri C, Bellini C, Coassin S, et al. Plasma endogenous digoxin-like substance levels are dependent on blood O2 in man. Clin Sci 1994; 87:447–451.
142. Bachofen M, Weibel ER. Alterations of the gas exchange apparatus in adult respiratory insufficiency associated with septicemia. Am Rev Respir Dis 1977; 116:589–615.
143. Newman V, Gonzalez RF, Matthay MA, et al. A novel alveolar type I cell-specific biochemical marker of human acute lung injury. Am J Respir Crit Care Med 2000; 161:990–995.
144. Calfee CS, Ware LB, Eisner MD, et al. Plasma receptor for advanced glycation end-products and clinical outcomes in acute lung injury. Thorax 2008; 63:1083–1089.

145. Modelska K, Matthay MA, McElroy MC, et al. Upregulation of alveolar liquid clearance after fluid resuscitation for hemorrhagic shock in rats. Am J Physiol 1997; 276: L844–L857.

146. Pittet JF, Brenner TJ, Modelska K, et al. Alveolar liquid clearance is increased by endogenous catecholamines in hemorrhagic shock in rats. J Appl Physiol 1996; 81(2):830–837.

147. Modelska K, Matthay MA, Brown LAS, et al. Inhibition of beta-adrenergic dependent alveolar epithelial clearance by oxidant mechanisms after hemorrhagic shock in rats. Am J Physiol 1999; 276:L844–L857.

148. Laffon M, Lu LN, Modelska K, et al. Alpha-adrenergic blockade restores normal fluid transport capacity of alveolar epithelium after hemorrhagic shock. Am J Physiol 1999; 277(4, pt 1):L760–L768.

149. Le Tulzo Y, Shenkar R, Kaneko D, et al. Hemorrhage increases cytokine expression in lung mononuclear cells in mice: involvement of catecholamines in nuclear factor-kappaB regulation and cytokine expression. J Clin Invest 1997; 99(7):1516–1524.

150. Hickman-Davis JM, Lindsey JR, Matalon S. Cyclophosphamide decreases nitrotyrosine formation and inhibits nitric oxide production by alveolar macrophages in mycoplasmosis. Infect Immun 2001; 69(10):6401–6410.

151. Bauer ML, Beckman JS, Bridges RJ, et al. Peroxynitrite inhibits sodium uptake in rat colonic membrane vesicles. Biochim Biophys Acta 1992; 1104(1):87–94.

152. Haddad IY, Ischiropoulos H, Holm BA, et al. Mechanisms of peroxynitrite-induced injury to pulmonary surfactants. Am J Physiol 1993; 265(6, pt 1):L555–L564.

153. Matalon S, Hu P, Ischiropoulos H, et al. Peroxynitrite inhibition of oxygen consumption and ion transport in alveolar type II pneumocytes. Chest 1994; 105(Suppl. 3):74S.

154. Haddad IY, Pataki G, Hu P, et al. Quantitation of nitrotyrosine levels in lung sections of patients and animals with acute lung injury. J Clin Invest 1994; 94:2407–2413.

155. Baldus S, Castro L, Eiserich JP, et al. Is * NO news bad news in acute respiratory distress syndrome? Am J Respir Crit Care Med 2001; 163(2):308–310.

156. Sittipoint C, Steinberg KP, Ruzinski JT, et al. Nitric oxide and nitrotyrosine in the lungs of patients with acute respiratory distress syndrome. Am J Respir Crit Care Med 2001; 163:503–510.

157. Brigham KL, Meyrick B. Endotoxin and lung injury. Am Rev Respir Dis 1986; 133:913–927.

158. Brigham KL, Woolverton WC, Blake LH, et al. Increased sheep lung vascular permeability caused by Pseudomonas bacteremia. J Clin Invest 1974; 54:792–804.

159. Pittet JF, Wiener-Kronish JP, McElroy MC, et al. Stimulation of lung epithelial liquid clearance by endogenous release of catecholamines in septic shock in anesthetized rats. J Clin Invest 1994; 94:663–671.

160. Wiener-Kronish JP, Albertine KH, Matthay MA. Differential responses of the endothelial and epithelial barriers of the lung in sheep to Escherichia coli endotoxin. J Clin Invest 1991; 88:864–875.

161. Pittet JF, Wiener-Kronish JP, Serikov V, et al. Resistance of the alveolar epithelium to injury from septic shock in sheep. Am J Respir Crit Care Med 1995; 151:1093–1100.

162. Rubin DB, Wiener-Kronish JP, Murray JF, et al. Elevated von Willebrand factor antigen is an early plasma predictor of acute lung injury in nonpulmonary sepsis. J Clin Invest 1990; 86:474–480.

163. Pittet JF, Kudoh I, Wiener-Kronish JP. Endothelial exposure to Pseudomonas aeruginosa proteases increases the vulnerability of the alveolar epithelium to a second injury. Am J Respir Cell Mol Biol 1998; 18(1):129–135.

164. Laughlin MJ, Wild L, Nickerson PA, et al. Effects of hyperoxia on alveolar permeability of neutropenic rabbits. J Appl Physiol 1986; 61(3):1126–1131.

165. Kurahashi K, Kajikawa O, Sawa T, et al. Pathogenesis of septic shock in Pseudomonas aeruginosa pneumonia. J Clin Invest 1999; 104:743–750.

166. Pittet JF, Matthay MA, Pier G, et al. Pseudomonas aeruginosa-induced lung and pleural injury in sheep. Differential protective effect of circulating versus alveolar immunoglobulin G antibody. J Clin Invest 1993; 92(3):1221–1228.

167. Sawa T, Yahr TL, Ohara M, et al. Active and passive immunization with the Pseudomonas V antigen protects against type III intoxication and lung injury. Nat Med 1999; 5(4): 392–398.

168. Kunzelmann K, Beesley AH, King NJ, et al. Influenza virus inhibits amiloride-sensitive Na$^+$ channels in respiratory epithelia. Proc Natl Acad Sci U S A 2000; 97(18):10282–10287.

169. Chen XJ, Seth S, Yue G, et al. Influenza virus inhibits ENaC and lung fluid clearance. Am J Physiol Lung Cell Mol Physiol 2004; 287(2):L366–L373.

170. Guggino WB, Guggino SE. Amiloride-sensitive sodium channels contribute to the woes of the flu. Proc Natl Acad Sci U S A 2000; 97(18):9827–9829.

171. Davis IC, Xu A, Gao Z, et al. Respiratory syncytial virus induces insensitivity to beta-adrenergic agonists in mouse lung epithelium in vivo. Am J Physiol Lung Cell Mol Physiol 2007; 293(2):L281–L289.

172. Matalon S, Egan EA. Effects of 100% O$_2$ breathing on permeability of alveolar epithelium to solute. J Appl Physiol 1981; 50(4):859–863.

173. Matalon S, Cesar MA. Effects of 100% oxygen breathing on the capillary filtration coefficient in rabbit lungs. Microvasc Res 1985; 29(1):70–80.

174. Freeman BA, Young SL, Crapo JD. Liposome-mediated augmentation of superoxide dismutase in endothelial cells prevents oxygen injury. J Biol Chem 1983; 258(20):12534–12542.

175. Hayatdavoudi G, O'Neil JJ, Barry BE, et al. Pulmonary injury in rats following continuous exposure to 60% O$_2$ for 7 days. J Appl Physiol 1981; 51(5):1220–1231.

176. Baker RR, Holm BA, Panus PC, et al. Development of O$_2$ tolerance in rabbits with no increase in antioxidant enzymes. J Appl Physiol 1989; 66(4):1679–1684.

177. Haskell J, Yue G, Benos D, et al. Upregulation of sodium conductive pathways in alveolar type II cells in sublethal hyperoxia. Am J Physiol 1994; 266:L30–L37.

178. Sznajder J, Olivera W, Ridge K, et al. Mechanisms of lung liquid clearance during hyperoxia in isolated rat lungs. Am J Resp Crit Care Med 1995; 151:1519–1525.

179. Gonzalez-Flecha B, Evelson P, Ridge K, et al. Hydrogen peroxide increases Na$^+$/K($^+$)-ATPase function in alveolar type II cells. Biochim Biophys Acta 1996; 1290(1):46–52.

180. Factor P, Dumasius V, Saldias F, et al. Adenovirus-mediated transfer of an Na$^+$/K$^+$-ATPase beta1 subunit gene improves alveolar fluid clearance and survival in hyperoxic rats. Hum Gene Ther 2000; 11(16):2231–2242.

181. Garat C, Meignan M, Matthay MA, et al. Alveolar epithelial fluid clearance mechanisms are intact after moderate hyperoxic lung injury in rats. Chest 1997; 111:1381–1388.

182. Lasnier JM, Wangensteen OD, Schmitz LS, et al. Terbutaline stimulates alveolar fluid resorption in hyperoxic lung injury. J Appl Physiol 1996; 81:1783–1789.

183. Saldias F, Comellas A, Ridge KM, et al. Isoproterenol increases edema clearance in rat lungs exposed to hyperoxia. J Appl Physiol 1999; 87:30–36.

184. Olivera WG, Ridge KM, Sznajder JI. Lung liquid clearance and Na,K-ATPase during acute hyperoxia and recovery in rats. Am J Respir Crit Care Med 1995; 152(4, pt 1):1229–1234.

185. Nici L, Dowin R, Gilmore-Hebert M, et al. Response of rat type II pneumocyte Na,K-ATPase to hyperoxic injury. Chest 1991; 99(Suppl. 3):31S–33S.

186. Yue G, Matalon S. Mechanisms and sequelae of increased alveolar fluid clearance in hyperoxic rats. Am J Physiol 1997; 272:L407–L412.

187. Stern M, Ulrich K, Robinson C, et al. Pretreatment with cationic lipid-mediated transfer of the Na$^+$K$^+$-ATPase pump in a mouse model in vivo augments resolution of high permeability pulmonary oedema. Gene Ther 2000; 7(11):960–966.

188. Borok Z, Mihyu S, Fernandes VF, et al. KGF prevents hyperoxia-induced reduction of active ion transport in alveolar epithelial cells. Am J Physiol 1999; 276(6, pt 1):C1352–C1360.

189. Carter EP, Wangensteen OD, Dunitz J, et al. Hyperoxic effects on alveolar sodium resorption and lung Na-K-ATPase. Am J Physiol 1997; 273(6, pt 1):L1191–L1202.

190. Carter EP, Wangensteen OD, O'Grady SM, et al. Effects of hyperoxia on type II cell Na-K-ATPase function and expression. Am J Physiol 1997; 272(3, pt 1):L542–L551.

191. Looney MR, Esmon CT, Matthay MA. The role of coagulation pathways and treatment with activated protein C in hyperoxic lung injury in mice. Thorax 2008; 64(2):114–20. .

192. Factor P, Saldias F, Ridge K, et al. Augmentation of lung liquid clearance via adenovirus-mediated transfer of a Na,K-ATPase beta1 subunit gene. J Clin Invest 1998; 102(7):1421–1430.

193. Ware LB, Matthay MA. Keratinocyte and hepatocyte growth factors in the lung: roles in lung development, inflammation and repair. Am J Physiol Lung Cell Mol Physiol 2002; 282:L924–L940.

15

Lung Vascular Dysfunction and Repair in Acute Lung Injury: Role of the Endothelial Cytoskeleton

GABRIEL D. LANG, EDDIE T. CHIANG, and JOE G. N. GARCIA

Department of Medicine, Section of Pulmonary and Critical Care Medicine, Pritzker School of Medicine, University of Chicago, Chicago, Illinois, U.S.A.

I. Introduction and Overview of Lung Endothelial Cell Barrier Regulation

A single layer of mesenchymal-derived, nonfenestrated lung microvascular endothelial cells (ECs) serves as a semipermeable cellular barrier between the lung interstitium and the pulmonary circulation. The large surface area of the lung microvasculature is well suited for regulating multiple key biologic processes (including lung fluid balance and solute transport between vascular compartments). Since the pulmonary circulation receives the entire cardiac output, it is also well positioned to sense mechanical, chemical, and cellular injury by inhaled or circulating substances. During conditions of intense lung inflammation such as observed in acute lung injury (ALI) or acute respiratory distress syndrome (ARDS), the large surface area becomes a liability and provides the opportunity for profound vascular permeability and alveolar flooding, critical and defining features of common and devastating inflammatory lung disorders primarily caused by sepsis, pneumonia, and trauma (1,2).

A key concept of the dynamically regulated lung EC barrier is the notion that two general pathways, transcellular and paracellular, describe the movement and flow of fluid, macromolecules, and leukocytes into the interstitium (and subsequently the alveolar air spaces) to produce clinically significant pulmonary edema during inflammatory lung processes (Fig. 1). The transcellular pathway utilizes a tyrosine kinase–dependent, gp60-mediated transcytotic albumin route, an active process of albumin transport in which endocytic vessels fuse with the endothelium in response to surface glycoprotein (gp60) receptor ligation (3). However, there is general consensus that the primary mode of fluid and transendothelial leukocyte trafficking occurs by the paracellular pathway as shown by the elegant electron microscopy studies of Majno and Palade (4,5) who demonstrated lung EC rounding and paracellular gap formation at sites of active inflammation within the lung vasculature. Disruption in the integrity of the EC monolayer is now recognized as a cardinal feature of inflammation, ischemia reperfusion injury, and angiogenesis and occurs in response to a variety of mechanical stress factors, inflammatory mediators, and activated neutrophil products (reactive oxygen species, proteases, cationic peptides). The dramatic cell shape change, which results in paracellular gap formation, implicates the direct involvement of endothelial structural components comprised of cytoskeletal proteins (microfilaments and microtubules).

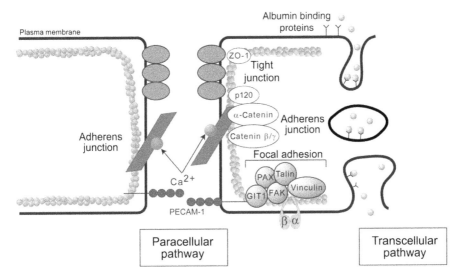

Figure 1 Schematic representation of molecular pathways of endothelial permeability and transendothelial transport. Shown is the *transcellular pathway* of vesicular (nondiffusive) transport with endothelial cell surface expression of albumin-binding proteins that bind albumin. ECs form vesicles containing albumin bound to albumin-binding proteins. The vesicle membrane fuses with the abluminal cell membrane, and albumin bound to binding protein and free albumin are extruded to the abluminal side. Also shown is the *paracellular pathway* of diffuse transport at intercellular junctions where edemagenic agents induce cytoskeletal contraction and cell retraction producing paracellular gaps and increased vascular permeability. Also illustrated are tight and adherens junctions of EC and interactions of linking proteins that form junctions. Cell–cell connections include tight junctions composed of transmembrane occluding proteins linked to the actin cytoskeleton by the zona occludens family (ZO-1); adherens junctions mediated by Ca^{2+}-dependent association of cadherin proteins in turn linked to the α-, β-, and γ-catenin complex; and platelet-endothelial cell adhesion molecule-1 (PECAM-1)–associated junctions. Cell-matrix tethering is maintained by focal adhesion plaques composed of α- and β-integrin transmembrane proteins linked to the actin cytoskeleton by a complex of proteins, including talin, paxillin, vinculin, talin, and focal adhesion kinase (FAK).

A useful paradigm to understand cytoskeletal influences on vascular barrier regulation is the tensegrity model that addresses the balance of competing contractile forces (which generate centripetal tension) and adhesive cell–cell and cell–matrix tethering forces (which promote monolayer integrity) (Fig. 2). This equilibrium is intimately influenced by the dynamic microfilamentous actin-based endothelial cytoskeleton via a variety of actin-binding proteins (capping, nucleating, and severing proteins) that are critical participants in cytoskeletal rearrangement and tensile force generation as well as in the regulation of endothelial junctional stability (6). During states of increased vascular permeability, spatially driven alterations in the cytoskeleton result in cell rounding, disruption of junctional integrity and focal adhesion complexes, paracellular gap formation, and increased vascular permeability (7,8). Barrier restorative processes likewise utilize

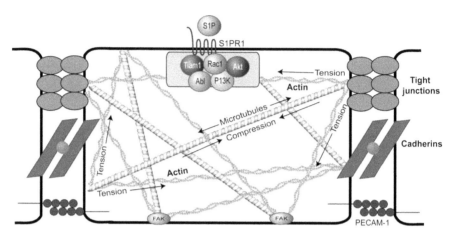

Figure 2 Tensegrity model addresses the balance of competing contractile forces (which generate centripetal tension) and adhesive cell–cell and cell–matrix tethering forces (which promote monolayer integrity) involving both microtubule and microfilament components. Endothelial cells maintain tight connections with each other and the underlying matrix to tilt the balance toward increased barrier integrity.

a carefully choreographed dynamic rearrangement of the cytoskeleton that restores the integrity of the endothelial monolayer (9).

Thus, although once perceived as a passive cellular barrier, ECs are now recognized as a highly dynamic tissue contributing to the multiple dimensions of EC function including interactions with a number of barrier-regulatory effectors via the endothelial cytoskeleton. The duration and outcome of inflammatory disease processes depends upon the balance between the severity of endothelial injury caused by adhesive biophysical forces, mechanical shear stress (10), or receptor ligation by specific inflammatory mediators and the efficiency of endogenous repair mechanisms to restore vascular integrity (1,2). In this chapter, we will address the role of cytoskeletal rearrangements in key regulatory mechanisms that contribute to increased pulmonary vascular permeability and define novel strategies designed to enhance the integrity of the lung vascular endothelium (11).

II. EC Cytoskeleton Components—Overview

It is now well accepted that dynamic cytoskeletal elements—actin, microtubules, and intermediate filaments—are key elements of vascular barrier regulation. The vast majority of the studies contributing to this recognition have focused on agonist-mediated signaling to the actomyosin cytoskeleton with subsequent effects on lung vascular barrier-regulatory properties. Historically viewed as separate and distinct cytoskeletal systems, microtubules and actin filaments are now known to interact functionally during dynamic cellular processes. The microtubule scaffolding complex (12,13), with a central role of tubulin dynamics, actively contributes to cytoskeletal rearrangement and in transducing competing barrier-regulatory forces, often in close collaboration with microfilament elements. Much less is known about intermediate filaments, an enigmatic component of the EC cytoskeleton consisting of dimer-structured alpha helical proteins that combine to form fibrils. Intermediate filament proteins are expressed in a specific manner with vimentin the primary intermediate filament protein found in EC. The role of intermediate filaments in regulating EC barriers represents a fertile area for future investigations as only limited information is available (14,15). Nevertheless, cytoskeletal constituents together provide the capacity for dynamic regulation of cell shape and as a consequence of moment-to-moment adaptation to an ever changing vascular environment.

III. EC Cytoskeleton Components—Actin and Myosin Microfilaments

Actin, a globular protein with a centrally located ATP-binding site, is critical to many cellular processes including cell motility, cell division, cell signaling, and as we and others have shown, EC permeability (16–18). G-actin reversibly assembles to form polymerized actin fibers called filamentous-actin (F-actin), conferring strength to structural elements regulating cell shape, particularly when accompanied by phosphorylated myosin. Dynamic remodeling of actin filaments within peripherally distributed cortical bands is essential for maintenance of endothelial integrity and basal barrier function with inhibition of actin polymerization (cytochalasin D) directly increasing EC permeability (17). Edemagenic agents initiate dramatic cytoskeletal rearrangement characterized by the loss of peripheral actin filaments with a concomitant increase in organized actin cables that span the cell, known as "stress fibers." Critically involved in regulating the spatial locale and level of actin cycling (polymerization–depolymerization) are numerous actin-binding proteins that serve as cross-linking/bundling proteins, polymerization/depolymerization proteins, and capping/severing proteins (Table 1) (16).

One key actin-binding protein and central regulator of the EC contractile apparatus is the Ca^{2+}/calmodulin-dependent nonmuscle isoform of myosin light chain kinase (nmMLCK). Phosphorylation of the substrate myosin light chain (MLC) by nmMLCK is central to paracellular gap formation and increased permeability by many edemagenic agents including thrombin (6) and vascular endothelial growth factor (VEGF) (54), both in vitro and in preclinical models of inflammatory lung injury. Studies with nmMLCK knockout mice reveal protection from sepsis-induced ALI and the Garcia lab has shown that nmMLCK knockout mice, as well as mice treated with an inhibitory peptide that reduces MLCK activity, are protected against ventilator-induced lung injury (55). In addition, we have shown that genetic variants (single nucleotide polymorphisms) in *MYLK*, the gene on chromosome 3q21 encoding MLCK, confer significant susceptibility to sepsis and ALI (56), as well as contribute to risk of severe asthma in African-Americans, another inflammatory lung disorder (57). Numerous studies have shown that increased levels of nmMLCK tyrosine phosphorylation, by either p60src kinase, c-abl kinase, or vanadate, an inhibitor of tyrosine phosphatases, increase kinase activity and modulate causes of EC barrier responses (16,24,58,59). Diperoxovanadate, a potent tyrosine phosphatase inhibitor, also increased nmMLCK activity, stress fibers, and EC contraction via activation of p60src tyrosine kinase. The nmMLCK isoform binds cortactin, another actin-binding protein and EC barrier regulator that localizes to numerous cortical structures within cells (24). The SH3 domain in cortactin binds the proline-rich areas in nmMLCK (6,9,25) with this interaction enhancing cortical actin formation and tensile strength. The central region of cortactin binds and cross-links actin filaments, with its C-terminus site for p60src

Table 1 Actin-Binding Proteins Involved in Endothelial Cell Barrier Regulation

Cross-linking/bundling protein family	Function	Molecular mass kDa
Spectrin	Cross-links F-actin in cell periphery. Stimulates myosin II ATPase activity. Links surface receptors to cortical actin filaments. Maintains plasma membrane integrity (19,20)	260/240
α-Actinin	Reorganizes actin cytoskeleton in cell movement. Links actin to plasma membrane and integrins. Part of focal adhesion plaque. Attaches actin to a variety of intracellular structures. Binds vinculin, nebulin, clathrin, and B1 integrins (7,8,21)	100
Fimbrin	Links actin cytoskeleton to vimentin network at sites of cell adhesion. Present in F-actin-rich adhesion structures as well as microvilli. Calcium regulated (22,23)	68
Cortactin	Cross-links actin in cell periphery. Involved in actin rearrangement. Substrate for Abl and Src modulated tyrosine phosphorylation-associated cytoskeletal rearrangement. Tyrosine phosphorylation of cortactin is critical to EC barrier enhancement (9,24,25,26)	80
Filamin	Participates in vascular permeability. Reorganizes peripheral actin. Anchors various transmembrane proteins to actin cytoskeleton. Regulated by cAMP-dependent PKA-mediated phosphorylation and Ca^{2+} CaM kinase (27,28–30)	280
Polymerization/depolymerization proteins		
Cofilin	Depolymerizing activity increased by Rho inactivation. Involved in actin disruption. Regulates actin reorganization in response to extracellular stimuli (31–33)	20
HSP-27	Target of p38 MAP kinase to produce cell contraction. Phosphorylation attenuates its inhibitory effect on actin polymerization (34,35)	27
VASP	Key actin regulator at cell–cell and cell–matrix sites. Involved in cell junctional activity. Required for normal actomyosin contractility and the response to shear stress. Involved in barrier-strengthening effects of cAMP and Rac (36,37)	45
Profilin	Induces actin bundling and tethering in focal adhesions. Participates in EC migration and angiogenesis. Link between the plasma membrane and extracellular signaling (22,38)	14
Arp 2/3	Critical effector in actin polymerization. Binds directly to cortactin to promote actin polymerization and stabilization (39,40)	215
Capping/severing proteins		
Gelsolin	Activation produces F-actin filament disintegration. Gelsolin helps restructure the actin cytoskeleton for motility. It severs, caps, and nucleates actin filaments (41,42)	83

Table 1 Actin-Binding Proteins Involved in Endothelial Cell Barrier Regulation (*Continued*)

Cross-linking/ bundling protein family	Function	Molecular mass kDa
Miscellaneous ABPs		
MLCK (nonmuscle isoform)	Ca^{2+} -calmodulin-dependent kinase. Regulated by Ser/Thr/Tyr phosphorylation. Key EC and epithelial regulatory protein. Involved in both stress fiber and cortical actin formation (16,43,44)	210
Caldesmon	Binds both actin and myosin. Serves as a nuclear switch for regulation of actomyosin contraction. Phosphorylation by ERK p38 MAPK and PKC facilitates actomyosin contraction. Involved in MLCK independent mechanisms of stress fiber formation (45,46)	77
Vinculin	Binds actin at adherens junction sites and stabilizes cellular adhesions. Involved in thrombin-induced barrier regulation. Substrate for PKC (47–49)	130
Catenins	Peripheral cytoplasmic proteins that interact with E-cadherin. Mediate binding of E-cadherin to microfilaments. Also connect cadherin to actin (50,51)	80, 88, 102
Coronin	Found in crown shaped, actin dense area on the cell's dorsal surface. May be a G-protein messenger that is directly coupled to the cytoskeleton. Cells lacking coronin are defective in cytokinesis and cell motility (52)	55
Paxillin	A focal adhesion protein that interacts with vinculin. Links actin to plasma membrane. It is tyrosine phosphorylated (53)	68

kinase-mediated phosphorylation that reduces cross-linking activity. Tyrosine phosphorylation of cortactin by p60src potentiates and stabilizes actin polymerization, as well as strengthens cortactin–nmMLCK interactions (60) and is a key step in a sequence of events that produce cytoskeletal changes, reassembly of adherens junctions, and barrier restoration during lung inflammation.

The activity of other actin-binding proteins is also tightly regulated by serine/threonine or tyrosine phosphorylation. For example, cofilin, an actin depolymerizer, is inhibited by Rho-GTPase pathway activation and ROCK-mediated phosphorylation (61) whereas the actin-binding protein, HSP27, is altered by phosphorylation by p38 mitogen-activated protein kinase (MAPK) that reverses HSP27-induced inhibition of actin polymerization, and produces stress fibers (62,63). Caldesmon, an actin-binding protein that functions to facilitate actomyosin interaction, also serves as a substrate for p38 MAPK and protein kinase C (PKC), a family of 12 serine/threonine kinases (64–66). Both kinases phosphorylate caldesmon thereby interfering with actomyosin interaction, EC contraction, stress fiber formation, and EC permeability (45,46,66,67). Furthermore, caldesmon regulation of actomyosin occurs through the actin-binding proteins filamin and gelsolin, which are cross-linking proteins that exert their effects through the small GTPase Rho, a signaling cascade critical to EC stress fiber formation and cellular contraction. These proteins provide further evidence of the importance of actin in regulating EC permeability.

The formation of cytoplasmic stress fibers, critical to cellular contraction and increased intracellular tension, occurs via the coordinate activation of nmMLCK and Rho that together increase the level of phosphorylated MLC in a spatially distinct manner. The resultant increases in actin stress fiber formation and actomyosin cellular contraction disrupt the barrier-regulatory balance with tethering forces and destabilize cytoskeletal-junctional linkages, culminating in increased vascular permeability. Direct inhibition of either nmMLCK (6,68) or Rho kinase, as well as Ca^{2+}/calmodulin antagonism, attenuates agonist-induced MLC phosphorylation, gap formation, and barrier dysfunction as well as the increased vascular permeability observed in many models of lung edema. Rho kinase inhibits the myosin-associated phosphatase that dephosphorylates MLC and leads to cell relaxation (24). This sequence of events is best seen in the cellular responses to thrombin, a protease activated on the surface of injured endothelium and found prominently in the microthrombi of the pulmonary vasculature in ALI patients. Thrombin-induced EC activation, via cleavage of its proteinase-activated receptor (PAR-1), elicits a transient increase in intracellular Ca^{2+} that leads to nmMLCK activation and MLC phosphorylation as well as involvement of Rho that phosphorylates the myosin-binding subunit of MLC phosphatase via Rho kinase thereby inhibiting phosphatase activity and allowing levels of MLC phosphorylation to accumulate. The integrated response increases contractility, formation of intercellular gaps, associated with disruption in the integrity of paracellular adherens junctions and reorganization of focal adhesion plaques and dysregulation of endothelial permeability (69,70).

IV.   EC Cytoskeleton Components—Microtubules

Microtubules are 25-nm polymers of α- and β-tubulin that form a lattice network of rigid hollow rods spanning the cell in a polarized fashion from the nucleus to the periphery while undergoing frequent assembly and disassembly (71,72). Important functions of microtubules include intracellular transport of vesicles and organelles, as well as signal transduction and cytoskeletal structure. In addition, microtubules act in concert with the actin cytoskeleton to promote EC barrier integrity. Microtubules and actin filaments exhibit complex, but intimate functional interactions during dynamic cellular processes (71–74). Microtubule disruption with agents such as nocodazole or vinblastine induces rapid assembly of actin filaments and focal adhesions, isometric cellular contraction that correlates with the level of MLC phosphorylation, increased permeability across EC monolayers, and increased transendothelial leukocyte migration, events that can be reversed or attenuated by microtubule stabilization with paclitaxel (73,74). The mechanisms involved in these effects are poorly understood but are likely to be mediated through interaction with actin filaments, suggesting significant microfilament–microtubule crosstalk.

Disruption of microtubules causes actin cytoskeletal remodeling, cell contraction, and decreased transendothelial resistance through a Rho-kinase-induced phosphorylation of MLC phosphatase (11,73). Nocadozole causes formation of stress fibers and myofilament assembly accompanied by increases in MLC phosphorylation, remodeling of adherens junctions (75,76), and barrier disruption (73). Microtubules play a significant role in TNF-α-induced EC permeability further highlighting the interaction between microtubules and actin filaments in regulating EC barrier function. TNF-α decreases stable tubulin content and dissolves the peripheral microtubule network, causing the formation of actin stress fibers and paracellular gaps through the p38 MAPK pathway (77), an MLCK-independent mechanism of EC permeability (74). Microtubule stabilization with paclitaxel inhibits the formation of stress fibers and preserves cellular shape and intercellular contacts (74). Although these effects are poorly understood, microfilament–microtubule crosstalk represents an intriguing area of EC barrier regulation (74,78).

V.   EC Cytoskeleton Components—Intermediate Filaments

Intermediate filaments (IFs) represent the third major element involved in EC cytoskeletal structure. Despite greater diversity than the highly conserved components of either actin microfilaments or microtubules, IF proteins share a common dimer structure containing two parallel alpha helices that combine to form polar fibrils that associate with an array of IF-binding proteins while connecting to the nuclear envelope, peripheral cell junctions, and other cytoskeletal components. IF proteins are expressed in a highly cell-specific manner with vimentin serving as the primary IF protein found in EC and other cells of mesenchymal origin. Although these data suggest potential roles for IF in EC cytoskeletal structure and barrier function, these effects are likely to be subtle and subject to compensation by biologic redundancy and the function of IFs in EC barrier regulation are much less understood (16). IFs were defined on the basis of their 10- to 12-nm filament structure, which distinguished them from 7-nm microfilament and 25-nm microtubules. Assembly of IFs is a complex process likely highly regulated by signaling cascades associated with cell motility. Vimentin is a dynamic structure undergoing constant assembly/disassembly, as well as anterograde and retrograde movements. Microtubule-based movement of IF are likely critical for assembly and maintenance of the vimentin IF network (79,80). The physical and dynamic properties of vimentin network in the vascular EC are likely important in regulation of cell shape and resistance to hemodynamic stress that accompanies blood flow and resistance to shear strain, physiological changes regulated by the IF cytoskeleton and IF-associated proteins that serve as internal scaffolding for EC, linked to the plasma membrane, and to junctional contacts. Vimentin protein expression is higher in macrovascular EC lining vessels subjected to the highest hemodynamic strain, such as the aorta, compared to microvascular EC lining vessels under less shear stress. Vimentin knockout mice develop normally without gross blood vessel abnormalities, but reduced mesenteric artery vessel dilation in response to flow (79,80). Downstream responses to flow may be the result of intracellular mechano-signaling events triggered by deformation of the IF cytoskeleton. Changes in unidirectional laminar flow results in rapid adaptation of the EC vimentin network with directional displacement within minutes of initial exposure. As noted with microfilaments and microtubules, over a period of hours, cytoskeletal filaments align themselves in the direction of flow with significantly larger change in the vimentin distribution around the nucleus compared with displacement occurring in the cytosol closer to the substrate. These observed spatial changes may be a means of distribution of local shear force transmission throughout the cell and therefore convey cell-signaling messages via a mechano-signaling pathway.

Finally, we have previously demonstrated that barrier-regulatory agonists induce vimentin phosphorylation occurs rapidly in EC (81), and vimentin disassembly results in dramatic alteration of actin and microtubule filaments in cultured cells. The role of vimentin in EC structure and resultant barrier function, however, remains unclear but again is likely related to responses to mechanical stress. Along with microfilaments, vimentin IF likely have a structural/functional role in EC focal contact organization inserting into focal contacts composed of $\alpha v\beta 3$ and $\alpha 6\beta 4$ laminin-binding integrins in microvascular ECs. Vimentin IFs in EC both stabilize and regulate the size of focal contacts allowing regulation of cell–matrix adhesion and resistance to flow (82). Thus, vimentin IFs are likely critical for maintaining the structural integrity of EC under shear stress, and may also be a conduit for signaling cascades triggered by mechanical force, again an exciting area for future examination.

VI. Mechanical Stress and EC Barrier Regulation
Vascular ECs withstand constant mechanical shear force of blood flow and can adapt in response to acute and chronic changes in hemodynamic forces. In addition, lung vascular EC are exposed to widely varying levels of cyclic stretch, a mechanical stress particularly relevant to critically ill patients receiving mechanical ventilation. Importantly, in addition to activation of the EC contractile apparatus by receptor-mediated pathways, mechanical signals are also transduced to the EC cytoskeleton (10,83). Nuclear magnetic resonance techniques have demonstrated that cell surface proteoglycans behave as viscoelastic anionic polymers, undergoing shear-dependent conformational changes that may function as blood flow sensors to transduce signals into EC (84). Components of the glycocalyx, such as heparan sulfate proteoglycans and sialoproteins, modulate cell–cell and cell–matrix adhesions via effects on the cytoskeleton and alter EC barrier properties (85–87). Syndecan is a heparan sulfate proteoglycan known to influence cytoskeletal organization, cell–cell adhesion, and motility (86) and mediates cationic peptide–induced signaling that leads to EC cytoskeletal rearrangement and barrier dysfunction (85). Cationic peptide–mediated EC barrier dysfunction was associated with syndecan-1 and syndecan-4 clustering and actin stress fiber formation; whereas removal of cell surface heparan sulfated proteoglycans attenuated these responses (85). Thus, the glycocalyx may represent not only sensors for mechanical stress and cytoskeletal rearrangement, but also endothelial surface-binding domains for inflammatory cationic peptides as well. This provides potential mechanistic insight for the recent observations that neutrophil-derived cationic peptides are responsible for the increase in vascular permeability produced during EC interaction with activated neutrophils (88,89).

Mechanical ventilation with excessive tidal volumes is known to cause ventilator-induced lung injury (VILI), a clinically important entity (90) which like ALI, is characterized by vascular leakiness and inflammation. We mimicked EC biophysical alterations during mechanical ventilation and exposed EC grown on a flexible substrate to a vacuum applied to generate mechanical stress elicited by in vitro cyclic stretch (91). The cyclic stretch is proportional to the degree of vacuum pressure, either to a physiologic (5% cyclic stretch) or pathologic (18% cyclic stretch). Interestingly, EC exposure to 5% cyclic stretch, a physiologically relevant value, revealed a barrier-protective effect and nearly complete restoration of monolayer integrity and peripheral redistribution of focal adhesions and cortactin within minutes after thrombin challenge (91). These data are consistent with clinical observations in VILI, a condition characterized by increased vascular permeability (92). EC exposed to 18% radial stretch for 48 hours did not demonstrate any breach in monolayer integrity evaluated histologically or by measurements of transmonolayer electrical resistance (TER) under basal conditions. However, cyclic stretch-preconditioned EC demonstrated greater paracellular gap formation with increase gap surface area in response to thrombin that correlated with increased levels of MLC phosphorylation (83). Additionally, our findings were associated with significant changes in the expression of genes related to regulation of the cytoskeleton (including MLCK) and proinflammatory genes as determined by expression profiling (93). High tidal volume mechanical ventilation increases mortality in patients with ARDS compared to low tidal volume strategies (94,95), likely related to the increased cytokine release, increased permeability and the development of a proinflammatory state, findings directly related to the degree of mechanical stress exposure (96).

VII. Structural and Junctional Elements of the Endothelial Barrier

The EC barrier is maintained by multiple components including the negatively charged glycocalyx comprised of membrane-bound proteoglycans and glycoproteins that coat the luminal surface. Specific members of the glycocalyx include a number of bioactive elements such as various cell adhesion molecules and mediators of coagulation and fibrinolysis (tissue factor and plasminogen) (60). A second major contributor to the intact cellular barrier is the tight apposition of individual ECs with neighboring cells via intercellular junctions (tight junctions and adherens junctions) that collectively contribute to basal endothelial barrier function (Fig. 1). As noted above, dynamic equilibrium exists between EC contractile forces and the adhesive protein-cytoskeletal linkages with cell–cell and cell–matrix interactions necessary for proper barrier function. Intercellular contacts between ECs are predominantly adherens junctions or tight junctions, both of which link ECs to the actin cytoskeleton to provide mechanical stability and mediate signal transduction (16). Specific components of the focal adhesion complex, that is, the integrin-based linkage between the extracellular matrix and the endothelial cytoskeleton provides strong tethering of the endothelium to the vessel wall and thus enhanced barrier integrity.

Adherens junctions (AJs) are composed of cadherins that bind catenin family intracellular proteins (primarily β-catenin) via the cadherin's cytoplasmic tail, which bind to the actin cytoskeleton of ECs. Between the cell–cell junction, the extracellular portion of the cadherin binds to a cadherin from adjacent EC in a calcium-dependent manner. The primary adhesive protein in human AJs is vascular endothelial cadherin (VE-cadherin), which is a critical regulator of permeability, neutrophil transmigration, interstitial edema, and actin remodeling. The MAPK pathway plays a role in regulating the EC AJ as MAPK inhibitors abolish VEGF-mediated VE-cadherin rearrangement and EC monolayer permeability (66). VE-cadherin-mediated permeability is catenin dependent and the resultant cytoskeletal connection is extremely important in the maintenance of junctional strength and paracellular permeability (97). The phosphorylation status of β-catenin is the primary determinant of the adhesive strength of AJs with tyrosine phosphorylation producing junctional protein dissociation from the cytoskeleton (97). ECs are treated with pervanadate and results in hyper-phosphorylation of catenins and partial dissociation of the catenin–cadherin complex and decreased cell–cell adhesion (98,99). Furthermore, thrombin causes dissociation of the tyrosine phosphatase SHP2 from VE–cadherin complexes resulting in increased tyrosine phosphorylation of catenins and destabilization of AJs (100).

Tight junctions, or zona occludens, are areas that surround the entire apical perimeter of adjacent cells and are formed by the fusion of the outer layers of the plasma membranes. These associations are sufficiently tight as to form a virtually impermeable barrier to fluid (101,102) and are comprised of occludins, claudins, and junctional adhesion molecules coupled to cytoplasmic proteins (Fig. 1) (103). The transmembrane occluding proteins are linked to the EC actin cytoskeleton by the zona occludens family (ZO-1). Alterations in tight junctions appear to be signaled through the MAPK pathway since both VEGF- and H_2O_2-mediated occluden dissociation is attenuated by MAPK inhibitors (103,104). Lung EC barrier regulation involves signaling between the cytoskeleton and adhesion complexes as well as signaling to the extracellular matrix (ECM). Focal adhesions are attachments of ECs to the underlying ECM and are mediated by ECM proteins (i.e., collagen, fibronectin, laminin, etc.), integrins, and cytoplasmic adhesion plaques (containing vinculin, talin, paxillin) (105,106). Integrins couple the ECM to the cytoskeleton and transmit signals from the surrounding environment and play a key role in the formation of cell adhesion complexes that attach to the actin cytoskeleton via the cytoskeletal proteins actin, vinculin, talin, and α-actinin. Focal adhesions, primarily through integrins, form a bridge for bidirectional signal transduction between the actin cytoskeleton and the cell–matrix interface. Disruptions of the integrin-ECM connection can increase EC permeability (107,108) and integrins modulate EC permeability to shear stress and inflammatory mediators (97). Integrin-ECM binding stimulates tyrosine phosphorylation of proteins such as paxillin, cortactin, and focal adhesion kinase (FAK), as well as calcium influx (109,110). FAK is the principal kinase that catalyzes the downstream reactions of integrin engagement and focal adhesion assembly (97) with FAK activity regulated by tyrosine phosphorylation mediated by the Src family. Activation of FAK through tyrosine phosphorylation produces cell contraction and increased EC barrier permeability.

VIII. Bioactive Agonists That Increase Lung Vascular Permeability

A. Thrombin and TNF-α

A variety of agonists, cytokines, growth factors, and mechanical forces alter pulmonary vascular barrier properties and serve to increase vascular permeability (12,16,18,54,59,83,88,111). As noted above, the serine protease, thrombin, represents an ideal model for the examination of agonist-mediated lung endothelial activation and barrier dysfunction as thrombin evokes numerous EC responses that regulate hemostasis, thrombosis, and is recognized as an important mediator in the pathogenesis of ALI (16). Thrombin increases EC leakiness to macromolecules by ligating and proteolytically cleaving the extracellular NH2-terminal domain of the thrombin receptor, a member of the family of proteinase-activated receptors (PARs) (27,112,113). The cleaved NH2-terminus, acting as a tethered ligand, activates the receptor and initiates a number of downstream effects, including cytoskeletal rearrangement (Fig. 3). In vivo studies detailed events that followed thrombin infusion into the pulmonary artery of the chronically instrumented lung lymph sheep model initiating a cascade of events that culminate in intravascular coagulation, inflammation, and vascular leak (114–116). Naturally occurring agonists, such as the cytokines TNF-α and IL-1β, have a prominent effect early in ALI, causing microthrombosis, and eliciting a cascade of inflammatory signals that result in capillary endothelial production of P-selectin, an adhesion molecule that enhances leukocyte-EC migration

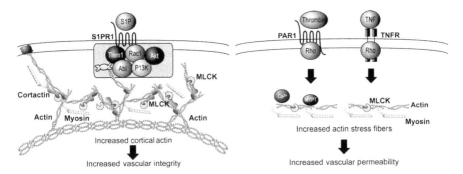

Figure 3 Thrombin and S1P signaling pathways leading to cytoskeletal rearrangement and barrier regulation. The left panel depicts S1PR1 ligation that induces Rac-dependent recruitment of key targets to lipid rafts that signal to Rac-dependent cortical actin formation and enhanced barrier integrity. The right panel shows thrombin or TNF-α receptor ligation elicits a signaling sequence that involves: Ca^{2+} increases, Rho/ROCK inhibition of the myosin phosphatase known as MYPT1, MLC phosphorylation, stress fiber formation, cellular contraction, paracellular gaps, and increased EC permeability.

(64,117,118) and actin reorganization, and paracellular gap formation (119). TNF-α also increases tyrosine phosphorylation of VE-cadherin leading to increased paracellular gaps in human lung endothelium (118).

B. PBEF

In contrast to the vast information available addressing TNF-α and lung vascular permeability, much less is known about pre-B-cell colony enhancing factor (PBEF), a relatively unknown cytokine discovered via high-throughput functional genomic approaches to identify novel ALI candidate genes (120,121). We previously demonstrated PBEF as a novel biomarker in sepsis and sepsis-induced ALI with genetic variants conferring ALI susceptibility (120,121). Furthermore, PBEF is highly expressed in polymorphonuclear leukocytes (PMNs) of sepsis subjects with expression upregulated by mechanical force and inflammatory cytokines and is involved in EC barrier regulation (120–122). We explored the mechanistic participation of PBEF in ALI and VILI and demonstrated that recombinant human PBEF (rhPBEF) is a direct neutrophil chemotactic factor and elicits marked increases in BAL PMNs and PMN chemoattractants (KC and MIP-2) after intratracheal injection in mice (123), changes accompanied by modest increases in lung vascular and alveolar permeability. We also observed dramatic increases in BAL PMNs, BAL protein, and cytokine levels (IL-6, TNF-α, KC) in rhPBEF- and VILI-challenged mice (123). Gene expression profiling identified induction of ALI- and VILI-associated gene modules, and heterozygous PBEF(±) mice were significantly protected (reduced BAL protein, BAL IL-6 levels, peak inspiratory pressures) when exposed to a model of severe VILI and exhibited significantly reduced expression of VILI-associated gene expression modules. Finally, strategies to reduce PBEF availability (neutralizing antibody) resulted in significant protection from VILI. These studies implicate PBEF as a key inflammatory mediator intimately involved in both the development and severity of ventilator-induced ALI.

C. Angiotensin II

The role of the renin-angiotensin system in pulmonary vascular regulation is now well recognized with angiotensin II, a key component of the renin-angiotensin system, generated primarily by angiotensin converting enzyme (ACE) from angiotensin I and its effects are mediated through angiotensin type I (AT-1) and type II (AT-2) receptors that are expressed in the normal lung. The pulmonary endothelium represents a major site of ACE expression and angiotensin II production with ACE2, a homolog of ACE, expressed in the lung that inactivates angiotensin II leading to the downstream generation of angiotensin 1 to 7 that acts through AT-2 receptors to induce vasodilatation. Although components of the renin-angiotensin system have been implicated in a variety of lung diseases including pulmonary hypertension and fibrotic lung diseases, the system has been strongly linked to the pathophysiology of pulmonary vascular leak syndromes. For example, ACE2 serves as the receptor for the coronavirus, first identified in 2003, responsible for severe acute respiratory syndrome (124,125) with a mortality rate >50% in the elderly. ACE and AT-2 serve a protective role in ARDS while ACE2, angiotensin II, and AT-1 mediate lung edema and injury associated with ARDS. A role for ACE via angiotensin II (Ang II) and/or bradykinin in ALI was proposed (126). We assessed whether ACE and therefore, Ang II and/or bradykinin, are implicated in inflammation and apoptosis by mechanical ventilation as been suggested. Reductions in ACE activity by captopril attenuated the inflammatory response and apoptosis whereas blocking bradykinin receptors did not attenuated the anti-inflammatory and antiapoptotic effects of captopril (127). Captopril did not attenuate ACE activity or necrosis indicating that inflammation and apoptosis in VILI is due to ACE-mediated Ang II production (128).

D. VEGF

New blood vessel formation, or angiogenesis, is a complex process involving EC activation, migration, maturation, and remodeling and is defined by the generation of new capillaries by EC either by sprouting or by splitting from pre-existing vessels. Sprouting angiogenesis involves EC detachment from the basement membrane, migration, and subsequent proliferation, tube formation, and, finally, functional maturation of the new vessel (129). While the mode of angiogenesis may vary according to the organ involved or the initiating angiogenic signals, nonsprouting is the primary process in lung vascular development (130). A number of angiogenic factors are now recognized as capable of activating EC including ECM proteins and their integrin receptors (131). VEGF is key in vasculogenesis as mice lacking the VEGF receptor, Flt-1, fail to develop fully functional blood vessels (132). Inhibition of VEGF is a promising therapeutic strategy in the management of patients with advanced malignancies (133). Pulmonary hypertension is a devastating disease with many similarities to neoplastic processes and is characterized by aberrant angiogenesis with VEGF serving as a target in pulmonary hypertension (134,135). VEGF increases EC permeability and is associated with pathological angiogenesis and embryonic vasculogenesis. Pulmonary EC may be especially sensitive to the effects of VEGF as VEGF levels are highest in the lungs and plasma VEGF was increased in patients with ARDS compared to the other groups (136). VEGF increases cytosolic calcium and levels of MLC phosphorylation at high doses and VEGF inhibition decreases EC permeability (136,137).

E. Angiopoietin

Additional angiogenic factor with barrier-regulatory properties includes angiopoietin 1 (ANG-1) and 2 (ANG-2) that are critical for normal vascular development. The ANG family is comprised of vascular growth factors that are ligands to the family of tyrosine kinases that are selectively expressed in the vascular endothelium. VEGF induces EC differentiation and migration, while ANG-1 stabilizes vascular networks (96,138,139). ANG-1 and ANG-4 modulate EC permeability by altering the state of AJs and specifically inhibit vascular leakage in response to VEGF or other barrier-disruptive agents, as well as promoting vessel maturation. ANG-2 antagonizes ANG-1 and promotes barrier dysregulation by blocking the ability of ANG-1 to activate its receptor (96).

IX. Strategies to Restore Vascular Barrier Integrity

A. MLCK Inhibitors

Historically, cyclic nucleotides have represented the sole strategy for retarding the edema phase observed in inflammatory lung syndromes possibly via cAMP-dependent protein kinases that phosphorylate proteins such as MLCK and inhibit F-actin reorganization (43,140–142). Increases in cellular cAMP also prevent the increase in Ca^{2+} and isotype-specific PKC activation, downstream signals regulating permeability (142). Prior studies highlighted the role of nmMLCK as an essential element of inflammatory response with polymorphisms that alters ALI susceptibility. We examined nmMLCK as a molecular target involved in increase of lung epithelial and EC barrier permeability utilizing genetically engineered mice and complementary strategies to reduce nmMLCK activity or expression. Both MLC kinase inhibition (membrane-permeant oligopeptide, PIK) and silencing of nmMLCK expression in the lung significantly attenuate endotoxin-induced lung permeability and inflammation. We also targeted pulmonary vessels and used ACE antibody-conjugated liposomes with nmMLCK siRNA as cargo in murine VILI model, again with significant attenuation of VILI lung injury. Furthermore, nmMLCK$^{-/-}$ knock-out mice were significantly protected when exposed to a model of severe VILI. Thus, the multidimensional cytoskeletal protein, nmMLCK, represents an attractive target for reducing lung vascular permeability and lung inflammation in the critically ill.

B. Sphingosine 1-Phosphate

The interface between EC barrier regulation and angiogenesis is an exciting area of vascular biology. Our initial studies determined that sphingosine 1-phosphate (S1P), a sphingolipid generated by sphingosine kinase action on sphingosine, directly activates EC and is the most potent EC chemotactic agent present in serum and is ultimately involved in angiogenesis and vascular hemostasis through its ability to evoke various cell-specific responses (143,144–149). In the setting of coagulation, S1P is abundantly released from platelets and, via its pleiotropic effects, potentially contributes to new blood vessel formation. This is evidenced by in vivo studies that establish S1P as remarkably effective in avian chorioallantoic membranes (150), in Matrigel-implanted plugs in mice (147,151), and in the avascular mouse cornea (145).

In contrast to VEGF-induced increases in EC permeability, we were the first to report that another angiogenic factor (S1P) can also produce EC barrier restoration and enhancement (152). S1P strongly enhances TER across human EC monolayers and signif-icantly attenuates thrombin-induced barrier disruption (149,152) while rapidly restoring barrier integrity in the isolated perfused murine lung (153). A single intravenous dose of S1P, given one hour after intratracheal endotoxin administration, produced highly signif-icant reductions in multiple indices of inflammatory lung injury, including vascular leak, as demonstrated in both murine (153,154) and canine (154) models of ALI. Furthermore, S1P is a major serum component released by platelets and represents a key mechanism by which platelets nurture the microcirculation and preserve vascular integrity (155).

S1P elicit numerous cellular responses via ligation of cell surface G protein-coupled receptors (Gi and G12/13) of the endothelial differentiation gene (Edg) family of receptors (147,151,156). The primary S1P receptors expressed in EC are Edg1 (S1PR1) and Edg3 (S1PR3) (148,152,157). We demonstrated that S1PR1 is the critical S1P receptor for bar-rier enhancement (149,158) mediated by small GTPase Rac1-mediated signaling pathway leading to cytoskeletal rearrangement with increased cortical peripheral actin resulting in increased endothelial junctional integrity and focal adhesion strength (53,143,149,159) (Fig. 3). Rac inactivates cofilin, an actin-binding protein with actin severing capabili-ties and leads to the translocation of cortactin, which as noted above is an actin-binding protein that stimulates actin polymerization and stabilizes actin filaments (152,160) and via binding to MLCK localizes to the site of cortical actin polymerization (9,161). The p21-associated Ser/Thr kinase 1 (PAK1) is an important downstream Rac target (152) as its binding to Rac results in the phosphorylation and activation of LIM kinase and the sub-sequent inactivation of the LIM kinase target, cofilin (162), events that are consistent with EC barrier enhancement. Interestingly, S1P at elevated concentrations (>5 uM) results in Edg3 or S1PR3-dependent RhoA-mediated signaling and increased barrier permeability (161,163). As a result, we are excited about the potential utility of FTY720, an unphos-phorylated S1P analog and a derivative of the natural immunosuppressant myriocin that has been recently described to cause peripheral lymphopenia by inhibiting cellular egress from lymphoid tissues (164). We demonstrated FTY to induce delayed endothelial barrier enhancement through a Gi-coupled receptor and to protect against murine inflammatory lung injury (153). Thus, targeting S1PR1 activation, either directly or via S1PR1 trans-activation by agonists such as activated protein C (57,165) and high molecular weight hyaluronan (58,166) (both robustly barrier protective), or antagonism of S1PR3 as with methylnaltrexone (167) appears to be promising strategies for attenuating the vascular leak associated with ALI.

C. Hepatocyte Growth Factor (HGF)

The stabilization of the EC barrier within newly formed capillaries is perhaps the critical feature of angiogenesis because newly formed capillaries are extremely leaky and not entirely functional. Important angiogenic factors that regulate this complex process are HGF, VEGF, and ANG-1 and -2. HGF is a heparin-binding protein with diverse func-tions including mitogenesis, organogenesis, cell survival, and angiogenesis (168,169). It stimulates EC motility, proliferation, protease production, and cytoskeletal reorganization through ligation of its tyrosine kinase domains and resultant recruitment of downstream signaling molecules. We previously demonstrated that HGF enhances barrier permeability by increasing cortical actin rearrangement and stabilizing AJs (11,168). Inhibitor studies found that phosphorylation of a glycogen synthase kinase 3β (GSK-3β) led to attenuation of the above responses. It appears as though stimulation of GSK-3β leads to enhanced endothelial junction integrity by increasing the amount of β-catenin, which link the AJ to the actin cytoskeleton, and therefore strengthen cell–cell tethering and cell adhesion forces.

Similar to protein C and hyaluronan, further evidence of the importance of S1PR1 as the primary vascular EC barrier-regulatory receptor, is transactivation of S1PR1 by other EC barrier-regulatory receptors relevant to angiogenesis and inflammatory regulation (57,58,64) including HGF. Ligation of c-Met, the receptor for HGF (64) results in prompt transactivation of S1PR1, which is essential for the HGF-mediated EC Akt kinase activation, EC cytoskeletal rearrangement, and barrier protection (14,82,83).

D. Simvastatin and ATP

Simvastatin, an HMG-CoA reductase inhibitor that lowers serum cholesterol levels, has been demonstrated to improve endothelial barrier function through activation of a Rac1-dependent cytoskeleton mechanism that is independent of its cholesterol lowering effects (170). Aside from their well-known cholesterol lowering effects, statins inhibit prenylation, a covalent addition of farnesyl (15-carbon) or geranylgeranyl (20-carbon) side chains. The activation of Rac is also dependent on this modification. Cultured ECs treated with simvastatin demonstrate cytoskeletal rearrangement, increased cortical actin, and reduced stress fibers. This same study demonstrated that cortactin is mediated to some degree by Rac, since it also appears in the periphery of these cultured cells. This study may provide future direction for the use of simvastatin in ALI therapies (171,172).

Through a mechanism that does not involve adenosine receptors, ATP induces barrier enhancement via phospholipase C- and Rac1-dependent cytoskeleton reorganization (173,174). Injection of nonhydrolyzable ATP in mice confers protection from endotoxin-induced lung injuries (175). ECs treated with ATP also demonstrate peripheral cortactin movement and reductions in paracellular gaps. These barrier-protective effects are due to Rac activation and the translocation of cortactin. The effects of ATP on the endothelium are of interest since ATP is released by activated platelets in response to shear stress and inflammation (173).

X. Conclusion

Newer and deeper insights into the regulation of lung vascular barrier properties and lung fluid balance continue to evolve. As evidenced by the specific features of thrombin-induced EC barrier disruption and S1P-mediated EC barrier enhancement, cytoskeletal components contribute greatly to the initiation and restoration of altered barrier properties. Over the past decade, a number of promising therapeutic strategies have been identified that offer hope that vascular leak can be addressed in the clinical setting. Agents such as oxidized phospholipids confer barrier enhancement by inducing unique Rac1-dependent actin rearrangement to limit VILI (176,177). FTY720 in Phase III trials and the statins, activated protein C and methylnaltrexone, are all currently approved by the FDA albeit for other medical conditions. These agents and others like them that target the EC cytoskeleton offer the prospect for rapid translation of lung vascular barrier-protective strategies to clinical practice (11,78,149,171,178,179). Further mechanistic investigation of barrier-regulatory agonists will identify novel biomarkers and novel molecular targets that may aid in development of new, more effective strategies to alleviate the dysregulated vascular leak seen in many inflammatory lung disorders. Future studiers that rely on thoughtful experimental design and powerful high-throughput tools such as cDNA microarray analysis and proteomic approaches will ultimately allow us to optimally match therapies to specific patients who suffer from aberrant EC barrier function and the resultant organ dysfunction and offer promise for the management of the critically ill.

References

1. Ware LB. Pathophysiology of acute lung injury and the acute respiratory distress syndrome. Semin Respir Crit Care Med 2006; 27(4):337–349.
2. Ware LB, Matthay MA. The acute respiratory distress syndrome. N Engl J Med 2000; 342(18):1334–1349.
3. O'Day-Bowman MB, Mavrogianis PA, Minshall RD, et al. In vivo versus in vitro oviductal glycoprotein (OGP) association with the zona pellucida (ZP) in the hamster and baboon. Mol Reprod Dev 2002; 62(2):248–256.
4. Majno G, Palade GE. Studies on inflammation. 1. The effect of histamine and serotonin on vascular permeability: an electron microscopic study. J Biophys Biochem Cytol 1961; 11:571–605.
5. Majno G, Palade GE, Schoefl GI. Studies on inflammation. II. The site of action of histamine and serotonin along the vascular tree: a topographic study. J Biophys Biochem Cytol 1961; 11:607–626.
6. Garcia JG, Schaphorst KL. Regulation of endothelial cell gap formation and paracellular permeability. J Investig Med 1995; 43(2):117–126.
7. Lum H, Malik AB. Regulation of vascular endothelial barrier function. Am J Physiol 1994; 267 (3, pt 1):L223–L241.
8. Lum H, Malik AB. Mechanisms of increased endothelial permeability. Can J Physiol Pharmacol 1996; 74(7):787–800.
9. Dudek SM, Jacobson JR, Chiang ET, et al. Pulmonary endothelial cell barrier enhancement by sphingosine 1-phosphate: roles for cortactin and myosin light chain kinase. J Biol Chem 2004; 279(23):24692–24700.
10. Birukov KG, Birukova AA, Dudek SM, et al. Shear stress-mediated cytoskeletal remodeling and cortactin translocation in pulmonary endothelial cells. Am J Respir Cell Mol Biol 2002; 26(4):453–464.
11. Liu F, Schaphorst KL, Verin AD, et al. Hepatocyte growth factor enhances endothelial cell barrier function and cortical cytoskeletal rearrangement: potential role of glycogen synthase kinase-3beta. FASEB J 2002; 16(9):950–962.
12. Petrache I, Verin AD, Crow MT, et al. Differential effect of MLC kinase in TNF-alpha-induced endothelial cell apoptosis and barrier dysfunction. Am J Physiol Lung Cell Mol Physiol 2001; 280(6):L1168–L1178.
13. Verin AD, Cooke C, Herenyiova M, et al. Role of Ca2+/calmodulin-dependent phosphatase 2B in thrombin-induced endothelial cell contractile responses. Am J Physiol 1998; 275 (4, pt 1):L788–L799.
14. Stasek JE Jr, Garcia JG. The role of protein kinase C in alpha-thrombin-mediated endothelial cell activation. Semin Thromb Hemost 1992; 18(1):117–125.
15. Nieminen M, Henttinen T, Merinen M, et al. Vimentin function in lymphocyte adhesion and transcellular migration. Nat Cell Biol 2006; 8(2):156–162.
16. Dudek SM, Garcia JG. Cytoskeletal regulation of pulmonary vascular permeability. J Appl Physiol 2001; 91(4):1487–1500.
17. Shasby DM, Shasby SS, Sullivan JM, et al. Role of endothelial cell cytoskeleton in control of endothelial permeability. Circ Res 1982; 51(5):657–661.

18. Garcia JG, Siflinger-Birnboim A, Bizios R, et al. Thrombin-induced increase in albumin permeability across the endothelium. J Cell Physiol 1986; 128(1):96–104.
19. Thomas GH. Spectrin: the ghost in the machine. Bioessays 2001; 23(2):152–160.
20. Broderick MJ, Winder SJ. Spectrin, alpha-actinin, and dystrophin. Adv Protein Chem 2005; 70:203–246.
21. Bogatcheva NV, Verin AD. The role of cytoskeleton in the regulation of vascular endothelial barrier function. Microvasc Res 2008; 76(3):202–207.
22. Kreis T, Vale R. eds. Guidebook to the Cytoskeletal and Motor Proteins. New York: Oxford Press Incorporated, 1993.
23. Dubreuil RR. Structure and evolution of the actin crosslinking proteins. Bioessays 1991; 13(5):219–226.
24. Garcia JG, Verin AD, Schaphorst K, et al. Regulation of endothelial cell myosin light chain kinase by Rho, cortactin, and p60(src). Am J Physiol 1999; 276(6, pt 1):L989–L998.
25. Dudek SM, Birukov KG, Zhan X, et al. Novel interaction of cortactin with endothelial cell myosin light chain kinase. Biochem Biophys Res Commun 2002; 298(4):511–519.
26. Lua BL, Low BC. Cortactin phosphorylation as a switch for actin cytoskeletal network and cell dynamics control. FEBS Lett 2005; 579(3):577–585.
27. Garcia JG, Patterson C, Bahler C, et al. Thrombin receptor activating peptides induce Ca2+ mobilization, barrier dysfunction, prostaglandin synthesis, and platelet-derived growth factor mRNA expression in cultured endothelium. J Cell Physiol 1993; 156(3):541–549.
28. Borbiev T, Verin AD, Shi S, et al. Regulation of endothelial cell barrier function by calcium/calmodulin-dependent protein kinase II. Am J Physiol Lung Cell Mol Physiol 2001; 280(5):L983–L990.
29. Garcia JG. Molecular mechanisms of thrombin-induced human and bovine endothelial cell activation. J Lab Clin Med 1992; 120(4):513–519.
30. Garcia JG, Fenton JW II, Natarajan V. Thrombin stimulation of human endothelial cell phospholipase D activity. Regulation by phospholipase C, protein kinase C, and cyclic adenosine 3'5'-monophosphate. Blood 1992; 79(8):2056–2067.
31. Ono S. Mechanism of depolymerization and severing of actin filaments and its significance in cytoskeletal dynamics. Int Rev Cytol 2007; 258:1–82.
32. Moriyama K, Yahara I. Two activities of cofilin, severing and accelerating directional depolymerization of actin filaments, are affected differentially by mutations around the actin-binding helix. EMBO J 1999; 18(23):6752–6761.
33. Roland J, Berro J, Michelot A, et al. Stochastic severing of actin filaments by actin depolymerizing factor/cofilin controls the emergence of a steady dynamical regime. Biophys J 2008; 94(6):2082–2094.
34. Rousseau S, Houle F, Landry J, et al. p38 MAP kinase activation by vascular endothelial growth factor mediates actin reorganization and cell migration in human endothelial cells. Oncogene 1997; 15(18):2169–2177.
35. Schneider GB, Hamano H, Cooper LF. In vivo evaluation of hsp27 as an inhibitor of actin polymerization: hsp27 limits actin stress fiber and focal adhesion formation after heat shock. J Cell Physiol 1998; 177(4):575–584.
36. Rentsendorj O, Mirzapoiazova T, Adyshev D, et al. Role of vasodilator-stimulated phosphoprotein in cGMP-mediated protection of human pulmonary artery endothelial barrier function. Am J Physiol Lung Cell Mol Physiol 2008;294(4):L686–L697.
37. Furman C, Sieminski AL, Kwiatkowski AV, et al. Ena/VASP is required for endothelial barrier function in vivo. J Cell Biol 2007;179(4):761–775.
38. Jockusch BM, Murk K, Rothkegel M. The profile of profilins. Rev Physiol Biochem Pharmacol 2007; 159:131–149.
39. Gunst SJ. Actions by actin: reciprocal regulation of cortactin activity by tyrosine kinases and F-actin. Biochem J 2004; 380(pt 2):e7–e8.

40. DeMali KA, Barlow CA, Burridge K. Recruitment of the Arp2/3 complex to vinculin: coupling membrane protrusion to matrix adhesion. J Cell Biol 2002; 159(5):881–891.

41. Fujita H, Allen PG, Janmey PA, et al. Characterization of gelsolin truncates that inhibit actin depolymerization by severing activity of gelsolin and cofilin. Eur J Biochem 1997; 248(3):834–839.

42. Spinardi L, Witke W. Gelsolin and diseases. Subcell Biochem 2007; 45:55–69.

43. Garcia JG, Lazar V, Gilbert-McClain LI, et al. Myosin light chain kinase in endothelium: molecular cloning and regulation. Am J Respir Cell Mol Biol 1997; 16(5):489–494.

44. Garcia JG, Davis HW, Patterson CE. Regulation of endothelial cell gap formation and barrier dysfunction: role of myosin light chain phosphorylation. J Cell Physiol 1995; 163(3):510–522.

45. Bogatcheva NV, Birukova A, Borbiev T, et al. Caldesmon is a cytoskeletal target for PKC in endothelium. J Cell Biochem 2006; 99(6):1593–1605.

46. Mirzapoiazova T, Kolosova IA, Romer L, et al. The role of caldesmon in the regulation of endothelial cytoskeleton and migration. J Cell Physiol 2005; 203(3):520–528.

47. Ziegler WH, Gingras AR, Critchley DR, et al. Integrin connections to the cytoskeleton through talin and vinculin. Biochem Soc Trans 2008; 36(pt 2):235–239.

48. Ziegler WH, Liddington RC, Critchley DR. The structure and regulation of vinculin. Trends Cell Biol 2006; 16(9):453–460.

49. Rudiger M. Vinculin and alpha-catenin: shared and unique functions in adherens junctions. Bioessays 1998; 20(9):733–740.

50. Birukova AA, Fu P, Chatchavalvanich S, et al. Polar head groups are important for barrier-protective effects of oxidized phospholipids on pulmonary endothelium. Am J Physiol Lung Cell Mol Physiol 2007; 292(4):L924–L935.

51. Taveau JC, Dubois M, Le Bihan O, et al. Structure of artificial and natural VE-cadherin-based adherens junctions. Biochem Soc Trans 2008; 36(pt 2):189–193.

52. Uetrecht AC, Bear JE. Coronins: the return of the crown. Trends Cell Biol 2006; 16(8):421–426.

53. Shikata Y, Birukov KG, Garcia JG. S1P induces FA remodeling in human pulmonary endothelial cells: role of Rac, GIT1, FAK, and paxillin. J Appl Physiol 2003; 94(3):1193–1203.

54. Becker PM, Verin AD, Booth MA, et al. Differential regulation of diverse physiological responses to VEGF in pulmonary endothelial cells. Am J Physiol Lung Cell Mol Physiol 2001; 281(6):L1500–L1511.

55. Mirzapoiazova T, Moitra J, Sammani S, et al. Critical role for non-muscle MLCK in ventilator-induced lung injury (VILI). Am J Respir Crit Care Med 2009; 179:A3822.

56. Gao L, Grant A, Halder I, et al. Novel polymorphisms in the myosin light chain kinase gene confer risk for acute lung injury. Am J Respir Cell Mol Biol 2006; 34(4):487–495.

57. Flores C, Ma SF, Maresso K, et al. A variant of the myosin light chain kinase gene is associated with severe asthma in African Americans. Genet Epidemiol 2007; 31(4):296–305.

58. Carbajal JM, Schaeffer RC Jr. H2O2 and genistein differentially modulate protein tyrosine phosphorylation, endothelial morphology, and monolayer barrier function. Biochem Biophys Res Commun 1998; 249(2):461–466.

59. Garcia JG, Schaphorst KL, Verin AD, et al. Diperoxovanadate alters endothelial cell focal contacts and barrier function: role of tyrosine phosphorylation. J Appl Physiol 2000; 89(6):2333–2343.

60. Pries AR, Secomb TW, Gaehtgens P. The endothelial surface layer. Pflugers Arch 2000; 440(5):653–666.

61. Maekawa M, Ishizaki T, Boku S, et al. Signaling from Rho to the actin cytoskeleton through protein kinases ROCK and LIM-kinase. Science 1999; 285(5429):895–898.

62. Huot J, Houle F, Spitz DR, et al. HSP27 phosphorylation-mediated resistance against actin fragmentation and cell death induced by oxidative stress. Cancer Res 1996; 56(2):273–279.

63. Landry J, Huot J. Regulation of actin dynamics by stress-activated protein kinase 2 (SAPK2)-dependent phosphorylation of heat-shock protein of 27 kDa (Hsp27). Biochem Soc Symp 1999; 64:79–89.

64. Nwariaku FE, Chang J, Zhu X, et al. The role of p38 map kinase in tumor necrosis factor-induced redistribution of vascular endothelial cadherin and increased endothelial permeability. Shock 2002; 18(1):82–85.

65. Bogatcheva NV, Dudek SM, Garcia JG, et al. Mitogen-activated protein kinases in endothelial pathophysiology. J Investig Med 2003; 51(6):341–352.

66. Borbiev T, Birukova A, Liu F, et al. p38 MAP kinase-dependent regulation of endothelial cell permeability. Am J Physiol Lung Cell Mol Physiol 2004; 287(5):L911–L918.

67. Borbiev T, Verin AD, Birukova A, et al. Role of CaM kinase II and ERK activation in thrombin-induced endothelial cell barrier dysfunction. Am J Physiol Lung Cell Mol Physiol 2003; 285(1):L43–L54.

68. van Nieuw Amerongen GP, Draijer R, Vermeer MA, et al. Transient and prolonged increase in endothelial permeability induced by histamine and thrombin: Role of protein kinases, calcium, and RhoA. Circ Res 1998; 83(11):1115–1123.

69. McKenzie JA, Ridley AJ. Roles of Rho/ROCK and MLCK in TNF-alpha-induced changes in endothelial morphology and permeability. J Cell Physiol 2007; 213(1):221–228.

70. Birukova AA, Smurova K, Birukov KG, et al. Role of Rho GTPases in thrombin-induced lung vascular endothelial cells barrier dysfunction. Microvasc Res 2004; 67(1):64–77.

71. Goode BL, Drubin DG, Barnes G. Functional cooperation between the microtubule and actin cytoskeletons. Curr Opin Cell Biol 2000; 12(1):63–71.

72. Klymkowsky MW. Weaving a tangled web: the interconnected cytoskeleton. Nat Cell Biol 1999; 1(5):E121–E123.

73. Birukova AA, Smurova K, Birukov KG, et al. Microtubule disassembly induces cytoskeletal remodeling and lung vascular barrier dysfunction: role of Rho-dependent mechanisms. J Cell Physiol 2004; 201(1):55–70.

74. Petrache I, Birukova A, Ramirez SI, et al. The role of the microtubules in tumor necrosis factor-alpha-induced endothelial cell permeability. Am J Respir Cell Mol Biol 2003; 28(5):574–581.

75. Bershadsky A, Chausovsky A, Becker E, et al. Involvement of microtubules in the control of adhesion-dependent signal transduction. Curr Biol 1996; 6(10):1279–1289.

76. Danowski BA. Fibroblast contractility and actin organization are stimulated by microtubule inhibitors. J Cell Sci 1989; 93(pt 2):255–266.

77. Birukova AA, Birukov KG, Smurova K, et al. Novel role of microtubules in thrombin-induced endothelial barrier dysfunction. FASEB J 2004; 18(15):1879–1890.

78. Birukov KG, Leitinger N, Bochkov VN, et al. Signal transduction pathways activated in human pulmonary endothelial cells by OxPAPC, a bioactive component of oxidized lipoproteins. Microvasc Res 2004; 67(1):18–28.

79. Helfand BT, Chang L, Goldman RD. The dynamic and motile properties of intermediate filaments. Annu Rev Cell Dev Biol 2003; 19:445–467.

80. Helfand BT, Chang L, Goldman RD. Intermediate filaments are dynamic and motile elements of cellular architecture. J Cell Sci 2004; 117(pt 2):133–141.

81. Stasek JE Jr, Patterson CE, Garcia JG. Protein kinase C phosphorylates caldesmon77 and vimentin and enhances albumin permeability across cultured bovine pulmonary artery endothelial cell monolayers. J Cell Physiol 1992; 153(1):62–75.

82. Tsuruta D, Jones JC. The vimentin cytoskeleton regulates focal contact size and adhesion of endothelial cells subjected to shear stress. J Cell Sci 2003; 116(pt 24):4977–4984.

83. Birukov KG, Jacobson JR, Flores AA, et al. Magnitude-dependent regulation of pulmonary endothelial cell barrier function by cyclic stretch. Am J Physiol Lung Cell Mol Physiol 2003; 285(4):L785–L797.

84. Siegel G, Walter A, Kauschmann A, et al. Anionic biopolymers as blood flow sensors. Biosens Bioelectron 1996; 11(3):281–294.
85. Dull RO, Dinavahi R, Schwartz L, et al. Lung endothelial heparan sulfates mediate cationic peptide-induced barrier dysfunction: a new role for the glycocalyx. Am J Physiol Lung Cell Mol Physiol 2003; 285(5):L986–L995.
86. Echtermeyer F, Baciu PC, Saoncella S, et al. Syndecan-4 core protein is sufficient for the assembly of focal adhesions and actin stress fibers. J Cell Sci 1999; 112(pt 20):3433–3441.
87. Takeda T, Go WY, Orlando RA, et al. Expression of podocalyxin inhibits cell-cell adhesion and modifies junctional properties in Madin-Darby canine kidney cells. Mol Biol Cell 2000; 11(9):3219–3232.
88. Dull RO, Garcia JG. Leukocyte-induced microvascular permeability: how contractile tweaks lead to leaks. Circ Res 2002; 90(11):1143–1144.
89. Gautam N, Olofsson AM, Herwald H, et al. Heparin-binding protein (HBP/CAP37): a missing link in neutrophil-evoked alteration of vascular permeability. Nat Med 2001; 7(10):1123–1127.
90. Laffey JG, Kavanagh BP. Ventilation with lower tidal volumes as compared with traditional tidal volumes for acute lung injury. N Engl J Med 2000; 343(11):812.
91. Birukov KG, Csortos C, Marzilli L, et al. Differential regulation of alternatively spliced endothelial cell myosin light chain kinase isoforms by p60(Src). J Biol Chem 2001;276(11):8567–8573.
92. Parker JC. Inhibitors of myosin light chain kinase and phosphodiesterase reduce ventilator-induced lung injury. J Appl Physiol 2000; 89(6):2241–2248.
93. Shikata Y, Rios A, Kawkitinarong K, et al. Differential effects of shear stress and cyclic stretch on focal adhesion remodeling, site-specific FAK phosphorylation, and small GTPases in human lung endothelial cells. Exp Cell Res 2005; 304(1):40–49.
94. Nonas SA, Finigan JH, Gao L, et al. Functional genomic insights into acute lung injury: role of ventilators and mechanical stress. Proc Am Thorac Soc 2005; 2(3):188–194.
95. Rubenfeld GD, Caldwell E, Peabody E, et al. Incidence and outcomes of acute lung injury. N Engl J Med 2005; 353(16):1685–1693.
96. Mura M, dos Santos CC, Stewart D, et al. Vascular endothelial growth factor and related molecules in acute lung injury. J Appl Physiol 2004; 97(5):1605–1617.
97. Yuan SY. Protein kinase signaling in the modulation of microvascular permeability. Vascul Pharmacol 2002; 39(4–5):213–223.
98. Ozawa M. Beta-catenin: its discovery as a cadherin-associated protein and its function as a transcription activator. Tanpakushitsu Kakusan Koso 2001; 46(3):197–207.
99. Ozawa M, Kemler R. Altered cell adhesion activity by pervanadate due to the dissociation of alpha-catenin from the E-cadherin.catenin complex. J Biol Chem 1998; 273(11):6166–6170.
100. Ukropec JA, Hollinger MK, Salva SM, et al. SHP2 association with VE-cadherin complexes in human endothelial cells is regulated by thrombin. J Biol Chem 2000; 275(8):5983–5986.
101. Vandenbroucke E, Mehta D, Minshall R, et al. Regulation of endothelial junctional permeability. Ann N Y Acad Sci 2008; 1123:134–145.
102. Pries AR, Kuebler WM. Normal endothelium. Handb Exp Pharmacol 2006; 176(pt 1):1–40.
103. Mitic LL, Anderson JM. Molecular architecture of tight junctions. Annu Rev Physiol 1998; 60:121–142.
104. Kevil CG, Payne DK, Mire E, et al. Vascular permeability factor/vascular endothelial cell growth factor-mediated permeability occurs through disorganization of endothelial junctional proteins. J Biol Chem 1998; 273(24):15099–15103.
105. Mehta D, Malik AB. Signaling mechanisms regulating endothelial permeability. Physiol Rev 2006; 86(1):279–367.
106. Rotundo RF, Curtis TM, Shah MD, et al. TNF-alpha disruption of lung endothelial integrity: reduced integrin mediated adhesion to fibronectin. Am J Physiol Lung Cell Mol Physiol 2002; 282(2):L316–L329.

107. Burridge K, Molony L, Kelly T. Adhesion plaques: sites of transmembrane interaction between the extracellular matrix and the actin cytoskeleton. J Cell Sci Suppl 1987; 8:211–229.
108. Romer LH, Burridge K, Turner CE. Signaling between the extracellular matrix and the cytoskeleton: tyrosine phosphorylation and focal adhesion assembly. Cold Spring Harb Symp Quant Biol 1992; 57:193–202.
109. Bhattacharya S, Fu C, Bhattacharya J, et al. Soluble ligands of the alpha v beta 3 integrin mediate enhanced tyrosine phosphorylation of multiple proteins in adherent bovine pulmonary artery endothelial cells. J Biol Chem 1995; 270(28):16781–16787.
110. Bhattacharya S, Ying X, Fu C, et al. Alpha(v)beta(3) integrin induces tyrosine phosphorylation-dependent Ca(2+) influx in pulmonary endothelial cells. Circ Res 2000; 86(4):456–462.
111. Moore TM, Chetham PM, Kelly JJ, et al. Signal transduction and regulation of lung endothelial cell permeability. Interaction between calcium and cAMP. Am J Physiol 1998; 275(2, pt 1):L203–L222.
112. Lollar P, Owen WG. Clearance of thrombin from circulation in rabbits by high-affinity binding sites on endothelium. Possible role in the inactivation of thrombin by antithrombin III. J Clin Invest 1980; 66(6):1222–1230.
113. Vu TK, Hung DT, Wheaton VI, et al. Molecular cloning of a functional thrombin receptor reveals a novel proteolytic mechanism of receptor activation. Cell 1991; 64(6):1057–1068.
114. Vogel SM, Gao X, Mehta D, et al. Abrogation of thrombin-induced increase in pulmonary microvascular permeability in PAR-1 knockout mice. Physiol Genomics 2000; 4(2):137–145.
115. Minnear FL, DeMichele MA, Moon DG, et al. Isoproterenol reduces thrombin-induced pulmonary endothelial permeability in vitro. Am J Physiol 1989; 257(5, pt 2):H1613–H1623.
116. Aschner JL, Lennon JM, Fenton JW II, et al. Enzymatic activity is necessary for thrombin-mediated increase in endothelial permeability. Am J Physiol 1990; 259(4, pt 1):L270–L275.
117. Mantovani A, Bussolino F, Introna M. Cytokine regulation of endothelial cell function: from molecular level to the bedside. Immunol Today 1997; 18(5):231–240.
118. Angelini DJ, Hyun SW, Grigoryev DN, et al. TNF-alpha increases tyrosine phosphorylation of vascular endothelial cadherin and opens the paracellular pathway through fyn activation in human lung endothelia. Am J Physiol Lung Cell Mol Physiol 2006; 291(6):L1232–L1245.
119. Orfanos SE, Armaganidis A, Glynos C, et al. Pulmonary capillary endothelium-bound angiotensin-converting enzyme activity in acute lung injury. Circulation 2000; 102(16):2011–2018.
120. Ye SQ, Simon BA, Maloney JP, et al. Pre-B-cell colony-enhancing factor as a potential novel biomarker in acute lung injury. Am J Respir Crit Care Med 2005; 171(4):361–370.
121. Ye SQ, Zhang LQ, Adyshev D, et al. Pre-B-cell-colony-enhancing factor is critically involved in thrombin-induced lung endothelial cell barrier dysregulation. Microvasc Res 2005; 70(3):142–151.
122. McGlothlin JR, Gao L, Lavoie T, et al. Molecular cloning and characterization of canine pre-B-cell colony-enhancing factor. Biochem Genet 2005; 43(3–4):127–141.
123. Hong SB, Huang Y, Moreno-Vinasco L, et al. Essential role of pre-B-cell colony enhancing factor in ventilator-induced lung injury. Am J Respir Crit Care Med 2008; 178(6):605–617.
124. Maniatis NA, Orfanos SE. The endothelium in acute lung injury/acute respiratory distress syndrome. Curr Opin Crit Care 2008; 14(1):22–30.
125. Penninger J, Imai Y, Kuba K. The discovery of ACE2 and its role in acute lung injury. Exp Physiol 2008; 93(5):543–548.
126. Chen CM, Chou HC, Wang LF, et al. Captopril decreases plasminogen activator inhibitor-1 in rats with ventilator-induced lung injury. Crit Care Med 2008; 36(6):1880–1885.
127. Jerng JS, Hsu YC, Wu HD, et al. Role of the renin-angiotensin system in ventilator-induced lung injury: an in vivo study in a rat model. Thorax 2007; 62(6):527–535.
128. Jiang JS, Wang LF, Chou HC, et al. Angiotensin-converting enzyme inhibitor captopril attenuates ventilator-induced lung injury in rats. J Appl Physiol 2007; 102(6):2098–2103.

129. Patan S, Haenni B, Burri PH. Implementation of intussusceptive microvascular growth in the chicken chorioallantoic membrane (CAM): 1. Pillar formation by folding of the capillary wall. Microvasc Res 1996; 51(1):80–98.

130. Pardanaud L, Yassine F, Dieterlen-Lievre F. Relationship between vasculogenesis, angiogenesis and haemopoiesis during avian ontogeny. Development 1989; 105(3):473–485.

131. Hynes RO. A reevaluation of integrins as regulators of angiogenesis. Nat Med 2002; 8(9):918–921.

132. Fong GH, Rossant J, Gertsenstein M, et al. Role of the Flt-1 receptor tyrosine kinase in regulating the assembly of vascular endothelium. Nature 1995; 376(6535):66–70.

133. Ellis LM, Hicklin DJ. VEGF-targeted therapy: Mechanisms of anti-tumour activity. Nat Rev Cancer 2008; 8(8):579–591.

134. Voelkel NF, Cool C, Taraceviene-Stewart L, et al. Janus face of vascular endothelial growth factor: the obligatory survival factor for lung vascular endothelium controls precapillary artery remodeling in severe pulmonary hypertension. Crit Care Med 2002; 30(Suppl. 5):S251–S256.

135. Moreno-Vinasco L, Gomberg-Maitland M, Maitland ML, et al. Genomic assessment of a multikinase inhibitor, sorafenib, in a rodent model of pulmonary hypertension. Physiol Genomics 2008; 33(2):278–291.

136. Mirzapoiazova T, Kolosova I, Usatyuk PV, et al. Diverse effects of vascular endothelial growth factor on human pulmonary endothelial barrier and migration. Am J Physiol Lung Cell Mol Physiol 2006; 291(4):L718–L724.

137. Thickett DR, Armstrong L, Christie SJ, et al. Vascular endothelial growth factor may contribute to increased vascular permeability in acute respiratory distress syndrome. Am J Respir Crit Care Med 2001; 164(9):1601–1605.

138. Li X, Stankovic M, Bonder CS, et al. Basal and angiopoietin-1-mediated endothelial permeability is regulated by sphingosine kinase-1. Blood 2008; 111(7):3489–3497.

139. Gallagher DC, Parikh SM, Balonov K, et al. Circulating angiopoietin 2 correlates with mortality in a surgical population with acute lung injury/adult respiratory distress syndrome. Shock 2008; 29(6):656–661.

140. Patterson CE, Lum H, Schaphorst KL, et al. Regulation of endothelial barrier function by the cAMP-dependent protein kinase. Endothelium 2000; 7(4):287–308.

141. Stelzner TJ, Weil JV, O'Brien RF. Role of cyclic adenosine monophosphate in the induction of endothelial barrier properties. J Cell Physiol 1989; 139(1):157–166.

142. Stevens T, Creighton J, Thompson WJ. Control of cAMP in lung endothelial cell phenotypes. Implications for control of barrier function. Am J Physiol 1999; 277(1, pt 1):L119–L126.

143. Liu F, Verin AD, Wang P, et al. Differential regulation of sphingosine-1-phosphate- and VEGF-induced endothelial cell chemotaxis. Involvement of G(ialpha2)-linked Rho kinase activity. Am J Respir Cell Mol Biol 2001; 24(6):711–719.

144. English D, Kovala AT, Welch Z, et al. Induction of endothelial cell chemotaxis by sphingosine 1-phosphate and stabilization of endothelial monolayer barrier function by lysophosphatidic acid, potential mediators of hematopoietic angiogenesis. J Hematother Stem Cell Res 1999; 8(6):627–634.

145. English D, Welch Z, Kovala AT, et al. Sphingosine 1-phosphate released from platelets during clotting accounts for the potent endothelial cell chemotactic activity of blood serum and provides a novel link between hemostasis and angiogenesis. FASEB J 2000; 14(14):2255–2265.

146. Kovala AT, Harvey KA, McGlynn P, et al. High-efficiency transient transfection of endothelial cells for functional analysis. FASEB J 2000; 14(15):2486–2494.

147. Lee MJ, Thangada S, Claffey KP, et al. Vascular endothelial cell adherens junction assembly and morphogenesis induced by sphingosine-1-phosphate. Cell 1999; 99(3):301–312.

148. Pyne S, Pyne NJ. Sphingosine 1-phosphate signalling in mammalian cells. Biochem J 2000; 349(pt 2):385–402.

149. Garcia JG, Liu F, Verin AD, et al. Sphingosine 1-phosphate promotes endothelial cell barrier integrity by Edg-dependent cytoskeletal rearrangement. J Clin Invest 2001; 108(5):689–701.
150. English D, Garcia JG, Brindley DN. Platelet-released phospholipids link haemostasis and angiogenesis. Cardiovasc Res 2001; 49(3):588–599.
151. Wang F, Van Brocklyn JR, Hobson JP, et al. Sphingosine 1-phosphate stimulates cell migration through a G(i)-coupled cell surface receptor. Potential involvement in angiogenesis. J Biol Chem 1999; 274(50):35343–35350.
152. Liu F, Verin AD, Borbiev T, et al. Role of cAMP-dependent protein kinase A activity in endothelial cell cytoskeleton rearrangement. Am J Physiol Lung Cell Mol Physiol 2001; 280(6):L1309–L1317.
153. Peng X, Hassoun PM, Sammani S, et al. Protective effects of sphingosine 1-phosphate in murine endotoxin-induced inflammatory lung injury. Am J Respir Crit Care Med 2004;169(11):1245–1251.
154. McVerry BJ, Peng X, Hassoun PM, et al. Sphingosine 1-phosphate reduces vascular leak in murine and canine models of acute lung injury. Am J Respir Crit Care Med 2004;170(9):987–93.
155. Edwards DC, Sanders LC, Bokoch GM, et al. Activation of LIM-kinase by Pak1 couples Rac/Cdc42 GTPase signalling to actin cytoskeletal dynamics. Nat Cell Biol 1999; 1(5):253–259.
156. Lee MJ, Van Brocklyn JR, Thangada S, et al. Sphingosine-1-phosphate as a ligand for the G protein-coupled receptor EDG-1. Science 1998; 279(5356):1552–1555.
157. Zondag GC, Postma FR, Etten IV, et al. Sphingosine 1-phosphate signalling through the G-protein-coupled receptor Edg-1. Biochem J 1998; 330(pt 2):605–609.
158. Schaphorst KL, Chiang E, Jacobs KN, et al. Role of sphingosine-1 phosphate in the enhancement of endothelial barrier integrity by platelet-released products. Am J Physiol Lung Cell Mol Physiol 2003; 285(1):L258–L267.
159. English D, Brindley DN, Spiegel S, et al. Lipid mediators of angiogenesis and the signalling pathways they initiate. Biochim Biophys Acta 2002; 1582(1–3):228–239.
160. McVerry BJ, Garcia JG. In vitro and in vivo modulation of vascular barrier integrity by sphingosine 1-phosphate: mechanistic insights. Cell Signal 2005; 17(2):131–139.
161. McVerry BJ, Garcia JG. Endothelial cell barrier regulation by sphingosine 1-phosphate. J Cell Biochem 2004; 92(6):1075–1085.
162. Yang N, Higuchi O, Ohashi K, et al. Cofilin phosphorylation by LIM-kinase 1 and its role in Rac-mediated actin reorganization. Nature 1998; 393(6687):809–812.
163. Singleton PA, Dudek SM, Chiang ET, et al. Regulation of sphingosine 1-phosphate-induced endothelial cytoskeletal rearrangement and barrier enhancement by S1P1 receptor, PI3 kinase, Tiam1/Rac1, and alpha-actinin. FASEB J 2005; 19(12):1646–1656.
164. Matloubian M, Lo CG, Cinamon G, et al. Lymphocyte egress from thymus and peripheral lymphoid organs is dependent on S1P receptor 1. Nature 2004; 427(6972):355–360.
165. Finigan JH, Dudek SM, Singleton PA, et al. Activated protein C mediates novel lung endothelial barrier enhancement: role of sphingosine 1-phosphate receptor transactivation. J Biol Chem 2005; 280(17):17286–17293.
166. Singleton PA, Dudek SM, Ma SF, et al. Transactivation of sphingosine 1-phosphate receptors is essential for vascular barrier regulation. Novel role for hyaluronan and CD44 receptor family. J Biol Chem 2006; 281(45):34381–34393.
167. Singleton PA, Moreno-Vinasco L, Sammani S, et al. Attenuation of vascular permeability by methylnaltrexone: role of mOP-R and S1P3 transactivation. Am J Respir Cell Mol Biol 2007; 37(2):222–231.
168. Singleton PA, Salgia R, Moreno-Vinasco L, et al. CD44 regulates hepatocyte growth factor-mediated vascular integrity. Role of c-Met, Tiam1/Rac1, dynamin 2, and cortactin. J Biol Chem 2007; 282(42):30643–30657.

169. Birukova AA, Alekseeva E, Mikaelyan A, et al. HGF attenuates thrombin-induced endothelial permeability by Tiam1-mediated activation of the Rac pathway and by Tiam1/Rac-dependent inhibition of the Rho pathway. FASEB J 2007; 21(11):2776–2786.

170. Chen W, Pendyala S, Natarajan V, et al. Endothelial cell barrier protection by simvastatin: GTPase regulation and NADPH oxidase inhibition. Am J Physiol Lung Cell Mol Physiol 2008; 295(4):L575–L583.

171. Jacobson JR, Dudek SM, Birukov KG, et al. Cytoskeletal activation and altered gene expression in endothelial barrier regulation by simvastatin. Am J Respir Cell Mol Biol 2004; 30(5):662–670.

172. Jacobson JR, Barnard JW, Grigoryev DN, et al. Simvastatin attenuates vascular leak and inflammation in murine inflammatory lung injury. Am J Physiol Lung Cell Mol Physiol 2005; 288(6):L1026–L1032.

173. Jacobson JR, Dudek SM, Singleton PA, et al. Endothelial cell barrier enhancement by ATP is mediated by the small GTPase Rac and cortactin. Am J Physiol Lung Cell Mol Physiol 2006; 291(2):L289–L295.

174. Kolosova IA, Mirzapoiazova T, Adyshev D, et al. Signaling pathways involved in adenosine triphosphate-induced endothelial cell barrier enhancement. Cir Res 2005; 97(2):115–124.

175. Kolosova IA, Mirzapoiazova T, Moreno-Vinasco L, et al. Protective effect of purinergic agonist ATPgammaS against acute lung injury. Am J Physiol Lung Cell Mol Physiol 2008; 294(2):L319–L324.

176. Birukov KG, Bochkov VN, Birukova AA, et al. Epoxycyclopentenone-containing oxidized phospholipids restore endothelial barrier function via Cdc42 and Rac. Circ Res 2004; 95(9):892–901.

177. Nonas S, Birukova AA, Fu P, et al. Oxidized phospholipids reduce ventilator-induced vascular leak and inflammation in vivo. Crit Care 2008; 12(1):R27.

178. Thurston G, Rudge JS, Ioffe E, et al. Angiopoietin-1 protects the adult vasculature against plasma leakage. Nat Med 2000; 6(4):460–463.

179. Wolfson RK, Lang GD, Jacobson JR, et al. The Pulmonary Endothelium: Function in Health and Disease. Hoboken, NJ: John Wiley & Sons, Ltd, 2009; 21:337–354.

16
Surfactant Therapy in the Acute Respiratory Distress Syndrome

ROGER G. SPRAGG
University of California, San Diego, and Medicine Service, San Diego VA Medical Center, San Diego, California, U.S.A.

JAMES F. LEWIS
University of Western Ontario and St. Joseph's Health Center, Ontario, Canada

I. Introduction

In the first medical description of the acute respiratory distress syndrome (ARDS) provided in 1967 by Ashbaugh and coworkers (1), the authors postulated that surfactant function might be diminished in patients with ARDS, with resultant alveolar collapse, edema, increased shunt, and hypoxemia. Indeed, using tools available at the time, a loss of surface-tension lowering capacity in fluid from the lungs of ARDS patients was demonstrated (2). Subsequent investigations have firmly established that there is diminished surfactant mass and function in the lungs of patients with ARDS, and have also provided excellent rationale for surfactant replacement in those patients. Although clinical trials have shown modest improvement in gas exchange after surfactant replacement, none has yet to show improved survival. Nevertheless, because of the strong rationale for this intervention and because of the lack of efficacy of any other pharmacologic intervention, efforts to establish a role for the application of exogenous surfactant in the treatment of patients with ARDS continue.

A description of the abnormalities of function and lipid composition of surfactant recovered in lavage fluid from ARDS patients was provided by Hallman and coworkers in 1982 (3), and subsequent investigations have provided more detailed descriptions of these abnormalities and of changes in the quantity of surfactant-associated proteins recoverable in both lavage fluid and serum (4–8). To determine the clinical relevance of these surfactant changes, it is critical to understand the normal functions of the surfactant system and how loss of these functions may affect patients with ARDS. This knowledge, together with results from preclinical investigations, continues to provide strong rationale for experimental treatment of ARDS patients using exogenous surfactant. Although the value of this treatment is yet to be convincingly demonstrated, further insights into the various factors that may influence patient responses to this therapy have been gained.

II. The Surfactant System of the Mature Lung

The surfactant system of the mature lung is a complex mixture of lipids and proteins that has both biophysical and nonbiophysical functions (9). The former include prevention of alveolar collapse at low lung volume, maintenance of patency of small airways, and prevention of alveolar edema. Possible nonbiophysical functions include protection from bacterial and viral infection and modulation of the activity of alveolar macrophages, polymorphonuclear leukocytes (pmn), and immunocompetent cells present in the airway. Surfactant is produced in the alveolar type II epithelial cell where the mature complex is found in lamellar bodies, secreted into the alveolar hypophase in the form of tubular myelin, and adsorbed in a thin film to the alveolar air–liquid interface. Compression and expansion of this film during ventilation is believed to result in removal of proteins and nonsaturated lipid components, resulting in a purified film able to reduce surface tension to close to 0 mN/m. Surfactant is cleared from the alveolar space by movement to the central airways, by macrophages, and by reuptake by alveolar type II cells for either degradation or resynthesis into functional components.

A. Composition and Biophysical Function of Lung Surfactant

The composition and biophysical function of lung surfactant are described operationally through investigation of material recovered from lung bronchoalveolar lavage fluid (BAL), minced lung, or type II pneumocyte fractions that contain lamellar bodies. Most commonly, crude surfactant preparations are made from cell-free BAL that is subjected to high-speed (approximately $40,000 \times g$) centrifugation. The resultant pellet, which may be further purified by differential density gradient centrifugation, is defined as the large-aggregate lung surfactant fraction, which is composed of large lamella-like structures and tubular myelin. In a normal individual, this fraction represents 80–90% of extracellular surfactant and has excellent surface-tension lowering properties. It is from this pellet that surfactant lipids and proteins are frequently isolated and studies of biophysical function are performed. Small surfactant aggregates are found in the supernatant of the high-speed centrifugation and comprise the remaining 10–20% of extracellular surfactant. These small vesicular forms have limited biophysical function when tested either in vitro or in vivo. The ratio of large to small aggregates (frequently expressed in terms of phosphorus content) is decreased in certain pathological states, including pneumonia and ARDS (6,7). Of note, surfactant may also be purified directly from BAL by equilibrium buoyant density gradient centrifugation, and the resulting material, while qualitatively similar to that obtained by differential centrifugation, has somewhat different composition (10). The techniques for acquiring surfactant by lavage and for isolating it from BAL are not standardized, and therefore comparisons between reports from different laboratories must be made carefully.

The biophysical function of lung surfactant may be assessed quantitatively in several ways. Measurements with the bubble surfactometer, which has commonly been used to study the function of surfactant recovered from BAL, require small amounts of material, may be performed rapidly, and are quite reproducible in the hands of experienced investigators (11). This device has been criticized, however, for being an open system from which minute amounts of surfactant may escape, thereby impairing accurate studies of very small amounts of surfactant. This objection is overcome by the captive bubble surfactometer (12). However measurements with this device, which requires only very small quantities of material for analysis, are technically demanding, and it has not been used for analysis of large numbers of clinical samples. Measurements made with a Langmuir–Wilhelmy balance have been used for decades, but require greater amounts of surfactant and are also technically demanding. Improvement in oxygenation and/or compliance of the lungs of the premature rabbit pup or of the lavaged rat after intratracheal injection of surfactant have also been used to test the biophysical properties of surfactant preparations (13,14).

Despite the differences in techniques for recovering, preparing, and analyzing lung surfactant, results are quite similar. Surfactant from normal subjects is composed of approximately 80% phospholipids, 5–10% neutral lipids (predominately cholesterol), and 8–10% proteins, predominately the specific surfactant proteins (Table 1). The most abundant phospholipid is phosphatidylcholine (PC), which comprises approximately 70% of the phospholipids present. Unlike the PC of cell membranes, which is approximately 10% saturated, over 60% of the PC of lung surfactant is disaturated PC, predominately dipalmitoylphosphatidylcholine (DPPC), and this component is believed to be of critical importance in providing surfactant's biophysical function. Indeed, DPPC is an integral component of all exogenous surfactant preparations currently in clinical use. In addition, lung surfactant contains an abundance of phosphatidylglycerol (PG), which may also contribute to surface-tension lowering properties.

Surfactant contains four recognized surfactant associate proteins, all of which have been extensively characterized at the molecular and gene level. In addition, the contributions of these proteins to the structure of the surfactant film, including specific protein–lipid interactions, have been extensively investigated (19). SP-A and SP-D are relatively hydrophilic, whereas SP-B and SP-C are markedly hydrophobic. SP-A, the most abundant surfactant protein, is a 32 kDa glycoprotein member of the collectin family with structure that includes a collagen-like domain and a calcium-dependent lectin domain also known as a carbohydrate recognition domain (CRD). The CRD is able to bind to type II cells, lipids, and surfaces of microorganisms. Alveolar SP-A has a "bouquet" structure that is an octadecamer composed of 18 SP-A monomers.

SP-A facilitates the formation of tubular myelin, enhances the adsorption of surfactant phospholipids at the air–liquid interface, modulates the secretion and uptake of surfactant by type II cells, and participates in innate defense against infection. Despite lacking in tubular myelin, SP-A knockout mice have close to normal lung structure and function, but increased susceptibility to a variety of infections (20–22).

SP-D (43 kDa) is also a collectin and in mature form in the alveolus is a dodecamer with regions that may bind to bacterial lipopolysaccharide, macrophages, and various lipids (23). SP-D shares many of the antimicrobial properties of SP-A (24), but clearly has additional effects, as mice deficient in SP-D develop emphysema-like changes, pulmonary inflammation, and fibrosis, and have hypertrophic alveolar macrophages, increased production by macrophages of hydrogen peroxide and metalloproteinases, and increased amounts of saturated PC (25).

SP-B, an 8 kDa molecule present as a dimer in the alveolar space, serves to increase markedly the adsorption of surfactant lipids to the air–liquid interface. SP-C, a 4 kDa intensely hydrophobic molecule, is dipalmitoylated and is intimately associated with the surfactant lipid film. SP-B knockout mice, which die of respiratory failure soon after birth, also have abnormal processing of SP-C precursor, and thus have deficient alveolar levels of both proteins (26). On the other hand, SP-C deficient mice have normal lung morphology, surfactant synthesis, tubular myelin and PC pool sizes, and have only subtle biophysical abnormalities at low lung volume that suggest a role for SP-C in stabilization of the surfactant film (27).

The extracellular metabolism of alveolar surfactant, specifically the conversion within the airspace of the surface-active large aggregates into small aggregates, has been

Table 1 Composition and Function of Surfactant from Normal Subjects and from Patients with ARDS

Author	Griese 1999 (15)	Hallman et al. 1982 (3)		Pison et al. 1989 (16)		Gregory et al. 1991 (4)		Günther et al. 1996 (6)		Nakos et al. 1998 (17)		Bersten et al. 1998 (18)		Greene et al. 1999 (5)		Schmidt et al. 2007 (8)	
Sampling technique	Meta-analysis	Lavage (1 × 20 mL)		Lavage (5 × 20 mL)		Lavage (3 × 50 mL)		Lavage (10 × 20 mL)		Lavage (6 × 20 mL)		Lavage (4 × 20 mL)	Airway aspirate	Lavage (5 × 30 mL)		Lavage (10 × 20 mL)	
Patients	Normal	Normal	ARDS	Normal	ARDS	Normal	ARDS	Normal	ARDS	Normal	ARDS	Normal	ARDS	Normal	ARDS day 1	Normal (ug/mL)	ARDS % day 1
Number of subjects	7	13		10	17	16–29	34–64	13		6	6	16	15	15–35	41	15	15
Component																	
PL concentration (or % normal)	0.04 mg/mL				78%		31%		96%		45%					35.9 ug/mL	31.9 ug/mL %
PL composition																	
PC (% total)	68.7	73.0	59.5	62.8	52.8	76.2	63.1	83.1	81.9	68.3	43.0	68.1	57.5			73.3	81.3
PG (% total)	12.6	12.4	0.3	10.0	1.7	10.7	4.0	8.6	3.5	8.4	6.8	8.3	9.3			3.6	11.6
PI (% total)	4.1	2.7	3.1	8.3	13.7	2.7	6.8	3.2	6.5	3.9	7.2	13.5	6.0			5.3	2.5
PE (% total)	5.3	2.6	4.3	4.8	15.8	2.8	5.7	1.7	1.9	3.4	11.0	4.0	12.1			4.8	1.4
PS (% total)	2.3	3.3	13.0	4.5	ND	1.8	2.2	1.2	1.8	4.5	9.2	5.7	7.1			6.5	1.8
Sph. (% total)	3.3	3.7	17.5	7.4	13.1	1.1	4.0	0.8	3.5	4.9	11.0	2.6	7.7			5	0.6
LysoPC (% total)	1	0.4	1.5	1.3	1.4	0.0	0.0	0.1	0.3			0.8	1.1				
Surfactant proteins						In pellet										Estimated	
SP-A (ug/mL)	4.5					118.0	6.2	1.5	0.8				759	4.8	1.2	1.5	0.8
SP-B (ug/mL)	4.9					0.7	0.1	0.9	0.8				7174	0.11	0.04	1.3	0.7
SP-C (ug/mL)																0.8	0.4
SP-D (ug/mL)	1.1													1.03	1.08	0.01	0.01
Function																	
γ_{min} (mN/m)	0–23	13.9	21			4.1	24.0	0–1	15–20							2	27

In pellet = measurement in resuspended pellet.

Estimated = estimated by multiplying values reported as group mean% PL × PL concentration.

Abbreviations: PL, phospholipid; PI, phosphatidylinositol; PE, phosphatidylethanolamine; PS, phosphatidylserine; Sph., sphingomyelin.

investigated using both in vitro and in vivo approaches. In vitro studies involve the end-over-end cycling of test tubes partially filled with a suspension of large surfactant aggregates. This cycling causes expansion and contraction of the surface film, which is believed to mimic changes at the alveolar air–liquid interface including formation of nonfunctional, small vesicles that are presumed to result from the preferential removal of surfactant components from the film. In vivo studies, in which trace doses of radio-labeled large aggregates are delivered to animals' lungs, show a direct relationship between tidal volume size and the rate of conversion of instilled large aggregates into small aggregates. In normal animals, conversion has no impact on aggregate pool sizes, presumably due to compensatory responses (i.e., uptake of small aggregates), while in animals with pre-existing acute lung injury, the increased conversion results in a decreased ratio of large to small aggregates thereby decreasing the pool of functional surfactant within the airspace. These findings are consistent with clinical observations in patients with ARDS (6,7). Aggregate conversion, at least in some species, appears to be mediated by serine protease activity. An enzyme identified as a carboxylesterase and termed "convertase" has been isolated from mouse BAL, purified and shown to have a target other than dipalmitoylphosphatidylcholine (DPPC), perhaps SP-B (28–31). Porcine liver carboxylesterase does cleave SP-B during cycling, yielding cleavage products of the same molecular weight as found in native lavage fluid after in vitro conversion mediated by the endogenous convertase. Thus, SP-B may represent a target of endogenous convertase and play a pivotal role during aggregate conversion (32).

B. Host Defense Properties of Lung Surfactant

Given the continuous exposure of the respiratory system, and in particular, pulmonary surfactant, to the external environment, it is not unexpected that surfactant plays an important role in host defense. Not only does it provide a physical barrier between the atmosphere and the pulmonary tissues, but surfactant also directly interacts with particles deposited in the distal lung, including various microorganisms such as fungi, viruses, *Pneumocystis carinii*, and a variety of bacteria. As collectins, SP-A and SP-D have a relatively high affinity for oligosaccharides on the surface of these organisms and by opsonizing and aggregating them enhance clearance by phagocytes of the innate immune system. The critical roles of SP-A and SP-D are emphasized by experiments in which SP-A$^{(-/-)}$ or SP-D$^{(-/-)}$ mice are shown to be more susceptible to bacterial and viral infections and to inflammation mediated by lipopolysaccharide (33).

These collectins indirectly influence inflammatory mediator release, in part, by modulating macrophage function (24). For example, SP-A is reported to inhibit production of cytokines by stimulated macrophages through mechanisms that include inhibition of NF-κB activation (34), and SP-A-deficient mice, relative to wild-type mice, have increased BAL levels of TNFα and MIP-2 after exposure to lipopolysaccharide (35). In the presence of SP-A, production of proinflammatory cytokines by stimulated macrophages and peripheral blood monocytes is increased (36).

Interpretation of studies investigating similar host defense properties for the collectin SP-D is more difficult due to the phenotypic abnormalities of SP-D$^{(-/-)}$ animals, as noted previously. Nevertheless, alveolar macrophages of SP-D$^{(-/-)}$ mice ingest fewer microbes and exhibit significantly greater levels of proinflammatory cytokines compared to wild-type animals when challenged with bacteria or viruses. Perhaps more important from a clinical perspective, exogenous replacement with SP-D corrects these abnormalities (37).

The roles of the hydrophobic components of surfactant in host defense are felt to be primarily indirect, through their biophysical properties in forming the surface layer as well as in particle removal via enhancement of mucociliary movement. SP-B in the absence of surfactant phospholipids, however, has been shown to kill bacteria in vitro (38), and SP-C directly binds to the lipid A component of LPS and reduces LPS-induced effects in macrophages (39).

Mice partially deficient in SP-B [SP-B$^{(+/-)}$] and fully or partially deficient in SP-C have been used to help elucidate the roles of these two proteins in host defense (40). SP-B$^{(+/-)}$ mice, when stressed with hyperoxia, develop a pulmonary injury characterized by increased BAL levels of total protein, IL-6, IL-1β, and MIP-2, fall in BAL saturated PC, and decreased compliance. These responses are maximal in the absence of SP-C and markedly attenuated in the presence of that protein. Thus, SP-C may have a physiologic role in maintenance of lung function during periods of stress when SP-B levels are diminished. Indeed, mice in which conditional regulation of SP-B expression is used to modestly reduce total levels of that protein have increased amounts of pro-SP-C in areas where SP-B is focally deficient (41) and develop lung inflammation that is reversed by restoration of SP-B expression (42). Whether SP-C can fully substitute for SP-B is unknown.

While the host defense properties of surfactant function are to maintain normal pulmonary health throughout life, specific components of surfactant are intimately involved in the pathophysiology of various lung pathologies such as acute lung injury.

III. Surfactant Alterations Associated with Acute Lung Injury

Over the past several decades, investigators have compared the amount, composition, and function of surfactant in BAL obtained from ARDS patients to values in BAL from patients with normal lungs (Table 1). Because of variability in lavage and analytic technique, comparison among studies can be risky. However, overall, the results are relatively uniform and indicate a loss of total phospholipid and alteration in the composition and function of the remaining phospholipids. Specifically, the fractional contents of PC and PG, the most surface-active lipid components, are reduced significantly, while the fractional contents of other phospholipids show a compensatory increase. Increases in the fractional content of sphingomyelin, however, are likely to be due, in part, to contributions from membranes of necrotic cells in the airway. Using ^{13}C-PC as a tracer, Cogo and coworkers estimate alveolar pool sizes and de novo synthesis rates of DPPC to be reduced by 80% or more in patients with ARDS (43). Detailed examination of the fatty acid profiles of surfactant phospholipids shows that the fatty acids of PC isolated from surfactant of normal individuals are 88% saturated (and composed 80% of palmitate), whereas those from ARDS patients are only 74% saturated (and composed 66% of palmitate) (44). Schmidt and coworkers found that the phospholipid profile tended to normalize during the initial five days of ARDS, with significant increases in the fractional content of PG and the degree of dipalmitoylation of PC. In patients who subsequently survived, the fraction of large-aggregate subtypes increased significantly (8).

In addition to changes in surfactant lipids, observations on the levels in lavage fluid of surfactant proteins document marked changes (Table 1). There is a significant decrement in the level of SP-A, and most investigators also report decrements in the BAL level of SP-B (4–6,45). BAL SP-A levels correlate inversely with disease progression, and in the study of Greene and coworkers, no patients with BAL SP-A concentrations greater than 1.2 ug/mL progressed to meet the criteria for ARDS. In addition, SP-A levels increased subsequent to the insult in patients who ultimately survived (8).

SP-D BAL concentrations, while in the normal range in surviving patients, are very low early in the course of ARDS in those patients who eventually die (5). Reasons for the loss of surfactant components are not well studied, but are likely to be due to injury to type II cells, with decreased production, rather than to increased clearance.

Alterations in plasma levels of surfactant proteins are found in patients developing acute lung injury, and in some cases may help predict disease progression. Increases in plasma levels of surfactant proteins are believed to be due to leakage of the protein across the damaged alveolar-capillary membrane into blood. In a study of 54 patients with hypoxemic respiratory failure, plasma samples were collected daily and analyzed by ELISA for SP-A and for SP-B antigen (46). Plasma SP-A circulates as a complex with IgG, while the precise nature of SP-B antigen detected in plasma is uncertain. Initial plasma SP-A and SP-B levels were higher in patients with direct (as opposed to indirect) lung injury, and plasma SP-B was significantly greater in patients who developed ARDS. Plasma values for both SP-B and SP-B/SP-A have been reported to be inversely related to blood oxygenation (47). In a study of 22 patients with respiratory failure and at risk for ARDS, and 41 patients with established ARDS, serum SP-A and SP-D levels increased significantly above normal with onset of the syndrome and two days later were maximal, with a median values approximately 20 and 3 times, respectively, higher than control. Despite the reported correlations with gas exchange, neither serum SP-A nor serum SP-D levels were predictive of survival (5).

Few studies have addressed the possibility that genetic abnormalities of surfactant proteins may result in phenotypes that are at increased risk for the development of ARDS. Two single nucleotide polymorphisms in the surfactant protein B (SFTPB) gene have been found to be associated with ARDS. A potentially important allelic polymorphism (C/T) at nucleotide 1580 within codon 131 (Thr131Ile) of the SP-B gene has the possibility of determining the presence or absence of a potential N-linked glycosylation site. Lin and coworkers have reported that the C/C genotype is found with significantly increased frequency in the subset of patients with ARDS who have predominately direct pulmonary injuries (48). In two small studies, the variant allele in the insertion/deletion polymorphism in intron 4 was associated with susceptibility to ARDS (49,50).

Surfactant biophysical function is also markedly altered in patients with ARDS. Minimum surface-tension measurements in the bubble surfactometer show, for normal surfactant, a value that is close to 0 mN/m. Values for surfactant from ARDS patients are most commonly in the range of 20 mN/m—a loss of function that is felt to be consistent with, and contribute to, the impaired physiologic function. This loss of activity is most likely the result of multiple factors, one of which is the altered fatty acid composition of PC. In analyses of surfactants from normal and ARDS patients, Günther and coworkers found that the minimum surface tension of the surfactant from normal subjects was near zero, while that from ARDS patients was markedly increased and correlated inversely with the palmitate content of PC. In reconstitution experiments, addition of DPPC to surfactant resulted in significant reduction of minimum surface tension. These results underscore the physiologic significance of alteration in the biochemical composition of surfactant lipids.

Both in vitro and in vivo experiments demonstrate that inhibition of surfactant function by plasma proteins present in alveolar edema fluid of patients with established ARDS may contribute to impaired surfactant biophysical function. Albumin, hemoglobin, fibrinogen, and fibrin monomers are all capable of inhibiting biophysical function of surfactant at low concentrations (e.g., <2 mg/mL), perhaps through competition for sites at the air–liquid interface (51–53). Surfactants lacking the hydrophobic proteins B and C are particularly sensitive to fibrinogen inhibition (53), and SP-A also contributes to resistance to protein inhibition (54).

Although several components of serum leaking into the airspace can inhibit surfactant function, not all have the same potency or significance. For example the inhibition associated with fibrinogen products may be of particular importance in patients with ARDS, as active fibrin polymerization is likely to occur in the alveoli of these patients as hyaline membranes are formed. In addition, the surfactant-inhibitory capacity of polymerizing fibrin surpasses that of soluble fibrin monomers or fibrinogen by several orders of magnitude, making it the most powerful surfactant inhibitor described (55). Seeger and coworkers have proposed that surfactant phospholipids (PL) and hydrophobic surfactant proteins are incorporated into the fibrin matrix and thus are effectively removed from the air–liquid interface and unable to form a surfactant film. They have also demonstrated that incorporated surfactant components are released by application of fibrinolytic agents, with restoration of surface activity (56,57). This finding may have future therapeutic application in treatment of patients with ARDS.

Fortunately, several in vitro and in vivo studies have shown that protein inhibition of surfactant function can be overcome in the presence of sufficient quantities of added surfactant, a concept that is of critical importance in developing strategies for surfactant replacement therapy. These observations have provided rationale for the utilization of relatively high doses of exogenous surfactant in clinical trials (58,59). At these higher concentrations, inhibition by proteins is transient, and may occur via direct interference with the structure of the surfactant film itself rather than through competition for sites at the air–liquid interface.

In addition to plasma proteins, neutral lipids may also modify surfactant function. Although physiologic levels of cholesterol are essential for organizing the surfactant surface film (60), elevated levels may result in a marked and sustained inhibition of function (61). The neutral lipid fraction of surfactant from patients with ARDS is increased, relative to controls, with fractional increase in the amounts of cholesterol, diglycerides, and triglycerides. Exposure of functional surfactant to this neutral lipid profile results in sustained loss of function, with diglycerides exerting a marked effect (62).

Another important mechanism that contributes to loss of surfactant function in ARDS patients is the increased conversion of surfactant from large to small aggregate forms, with a consequent decrease in the functional pool of large surfactant aggregates. Since most patients with ARDS are mechanically ventilated, and most if not all have significant quantities of proteases present within their airspaces, it is quite likely that increased conversion of large to small aggregate forms does occur in these patients. Indeed, animal studies specifically evaluating surfactant aggregate conversion in injured lungs show that modes of ventilation that use lower tidal volumes (5 mL/kg) and higher PEEP levels (9 cm H_2O) result in less conversion of large aggregates, greater large aggregate pool sizes and better lung function than found in similar animals ventilated with higher tidal volumes (10 mL/kg) and lower PEEP levels (5 cm H_2O) (63,64). Recently, strategies involving ventilation of animals with high-frequency oscillation (HFO) involving extremely low tidal volumes (e.g., <1 mL/kg) and adequate lung recruitment resulted in minimal large-aggregate conversion and superior outcomes, even when compared to the low tidal volume/high PEEP strategies (65).

Reactive nitrogen and oxygen radicals are present in the airways of ARDS patients, and are able to react with surfactant lipids and proteins (13,66,67). In vitro experiments demonstrate that oxidation of lipid components results in loss of biophysical function (13,68), and that pmn are able to accomplish such oxidation (69). In addition, nitric oxide metabolites, particularly peroxynitrite that is released from stimulated phagocytes, can modify tyrosine residues present in the CRD of SP-A and impair interaction of that molecule with surfactant lipids and with at least one microorganism—*Pneumocystis carinii* (67,70).

Active proteases, including elastase and collagenase, are present as well in the airways of patients with ARDS (71,72), and are capable of degrading surfactant apoproteins (69,73). BAL fluid from ARDS patients shows evidence of proteolytic cleavage of SP-A that is consistent with cleavage by neutrophil elastase (74). Phospholipase A_2 activity is present in the lungs of ARDS patients (3), and group I secretory phospholipase A_2 is able to hydrolyze PC, thereby producing free fatty acids and lysophosphatidylcholine, depleting phospholipid stores, and also impairing biophysical surfactant function (75). This loss of function is due predominately to the release of lysophospholipids (76).

In summary, diverse mechanisms may contribute to loss of surfactant function during the course of ARDS. Understanding specifically how and when these changes occur in different types of lung injury may lead to more effective treatment strategies.

IV. Preclinical Observations

Animal models of acute lung injury have been investigated to determine whether administration of exogenous surfactant may be of benefit and what factors may influence efficacy of this therapy. The variety of injury models utilized for these studies is exemplified in Table 2. The most commonly used model is one in which sequential whole lung lavages are performed. This approach not only removes airway surfactant but also results in an intense inflammatory response, with influx of pmn into the lung interstitium and airways, especially when followed by mechanical ventilation. Almost all experiments using animal models of acute lung injury have been acute, usually not more then eight hours in duration, and thus long-term outcomes such as mortality have not been investigated. Rather, measures of gas exchange and lung mechanics have served as surrogates to evaluate the presumed beneficial effects of surfactant administration. However, given the ARDS Network clinical trial, which showed decreased mortality in patients with ALI ventilated with lower tidal volumes compared to higher tidal volumes, the relevance of these surrogate markers for clinical outcomes has been questioned (77). Indeed, in that trial use of lower tidal volumes was associated with lower oxygenation values, lower serum levels of inflammatory cytokines, and less organ failure compared to patients in the higher tidal volume group. These findings suggest that future preclinical study of any lung-targeted therapy should include alternative outcomes, and these are likely to include detection of molecules reflecting the generation of mediators of inflammation.

Preclinical evaluation of surfactant replacement has revealed some additional unexpected results. For example, it has been demonstrated that delivery of a relatively low dose of surfactant by aerosol can be as effective as delivery of higher doses by intratracheal instillation. An important factor to consider when interpreting these results however, is

Table 2 Examples of Mature Lung Injury Models in Which Surfactant Application is Effective

Model	Species	Surfactant preparation	Delivery method	Improvements	References
Lavage					
Saline	Guinea pig	Porcine	Bolus	ABG, morphology	(78)
Saline	Sheep	Survanta, BLES	Bolus, aerosol	ABG, mechanics	(79)
Saline	Pig	Venticute	Bolus	ABG, mechanics, morphology	(80)
Ventilator-induced					
	Rat	Porcine	Bolus	ABG, mechanics, morphology	(81)
Aspiration					
HCl	Rat	Rabbit	Bolus ± lavage	ABG	(82)
HCl	Rabbit	Synthetic lipids, natural proteins	Bolus	ABG, mechanics, morphology	(83)
Pneumonia					
Influenza A	Mice	Bovine	Bolus	Mechanics	(84)
Sendai virus	Rats	Bovine	Bolus	ABG, mechanics, morphology	(85)
P. carinii	Rats	Bovine	Bolus	ABG, histology	(86)
Neurogenic					
Cervical vagotomy	Rabbit	Bovine	Bolus	ABG, mechanics, morphology	(87)
Toxic					
NNNMU	Rat	Survanta	Bolus	ABG	(88)
NNNMU	Rat	Survanta	Bolus	Survival	(89)
Paraquat	Rat	Survanta	Bolus	ABG, mechanics, morphology	(90)
Hyperoxia	Baboon	Exosurf	Aerosol	ABG, mechanics, morphology	(91)
Hyperoxia	Rabbit	CLSE	Bolus	Shunt, morphology	(92)
Xanthine oxidase	Guinea pig	Bovine	Bolus	Mechanics	(93)

that these studies utilized the saline lavage model described above, which is characterized primarily by surfactant deficiency and involves a relatively uniform pattern of injury
factors that may not adequately represent the more complex situation within the lungs of
ARDS patients (94).

    These types of preclinical studies have also shown that not all surfactants have
equivalent effects on gas exchange when delivered in a similar fashion. For example,
when a bovine lipid extract surfactant (BLES) was compared with a minced lung extract

(Survanta) in saline-lavaged sheep model of ARDS, instilled BLES improved gas exchange to a greater extent than instilled Survanta. However, when these surfactants were administered as aerosols, the opposite response was observed (79). Interactions between the exogenous surfactant and endogenous surfactant proteins may affect the physiologic response. Thus, these puzzling observations might be explained if these interactions vary with different delivery modalities and different exogenous preparations. Added to the complexity of specific patient responses to exogenous surfactant in the clinical setting is the observation from recent clinical trials that some subsets of patients with ALI (i.e., those with direct lung injuries) may respond better to exogenous surfactant than others (i.e., indirect injuries) (95). Future preclinical studies involving exogenous surfactant should therefore take this factor into account when interpreting potential efficacy.

Finally, the effect of mechanical ventilation on endogenous surfactant aggregate conversion has been well demonstrated in studies of preclinical models, and the same effects have been shown for exogenously administered surfactants. Higher tidal volumes convert the predominantly large-aggregate exogenous surfactant preparations into poorly functioning small aggregates to a greater extent than ventilation strategies using smaller tidal volumes. Thus, the duration of clinical improvement observed after a particular dose of exogenous surfactant is likely to be influenced by the ventilation strategy that is employed.

V. Clinical Trials of Surfactant Replacement

Rational for proceeding to clinical trials of surfactant replacement includes the observations listed in Table 3. First, a variety of mechanisms may result in loss of surfactant function, and it is reasonable to assume that this loss of function contributes to the alveolar collapse, edema, increased resistance to airflow in small airways, shunt, and hypoxemia that are seen in patients with ARDS. Second, loss of the anti-inflammatory and antibacterial functions of lung surfactant might contribute to the inflammation and high risk of infection that are features of ARDS. Third, surfactant administration markedly improves gas exchange in multiple animal models of acute lung injury. Finally, infants with established respiratory distress syndrome (RDS) have markedly improved survival when treated with exogenous surfactant. The cause of surfactant deficiency in these infants is due to prematurity, while in ARDS patients it is due both to impaired production and to a variety of mechanisms that inhibit function. Nevertheless, in both settings surfactant function is critically lacking and intense pulmonary inflammation is present. That exogenous

Table 3 Rationale for Clinical Trials of Surfactant Treatment of Acute Lung Injury

---

Quantitative and qualitative surfactant abnormalities are found in patients with ALI, including loss of surfactant function.
In animal models, loss of surfactant function results in ALI.
Surfactant deficiency may promote inflammation.
Treatment of (many) animal models of ALI with surfactant improves gas exchange.
Surfactant treatment of patients with ALI/ARDS reduces lung inflammation, improves gas exchange, and may reduce mortality.
Neonates with deficient surfactant function and RDS are rescued with exogenous surfactant.

---

surfactant is clearly efficacious in the setting of RDS provides substantial hope that it may also be effective in treating patients with ARDS.

A.   Critical Variables Affecting Studies of Surfactant Treatment of ARDS Patients

A number of important variables must be dealt with when planning studies of surfactant treatment of patients with ARDS. These include the choice of surfactant preparation, mode of administration, amount of surfactant to deliver, volume in which to deliver it, frequency and duration of retreatments, and, finally, the ventilation strategy during and after treatment.

Surfactant Preparations

Surfactants that have seen clinical use may be divided into protein-containing and nonprotein-containing preparations and are summarized in Table 4. The former are either of natural origin (e.g., derived from porcine or bovine lungs or from human amniotic fluid), or are based either on a surfactant protein produced in *Escherichia coli* by recombinant gene expression or on synthetic peptides. Surfactants of animal origin are usually subjected to organic solvent extraction and chromatographic purification, and thus contain neither SP-A not SP-D. Nonprotein-containing preparations contain lipid (i.e., DPPC and/or PG) and may contain additional constituents such as cetyl alcohol or tyloxapol.

There are certain advantages and disadvantages inherent in each class of surfactant. Protein-containing preparations appear to have superior function either when analyzed in vitro or in vivo. In addition, protein-containing preparations are more resistant to inhibition by plasma proteins. However, protein-containing preparations of animal origin have limited availability, are frequently inconsistent in composition, and have the theoretical possibility of transmitting infectious agents and nonsurfactant lipid-soluble molecules of animal origin such as platelet-activating factor (109). Preparations containing synthetic peptides or recombinant proteins appear to have excellent biophysical function and have the advantage of consistent and defined composition. Their production is, however, technically demanding and expensive. Two nonprotein-containing preparations that contain DPPC and PG have been tested in adults with ARDS. Such compounds have inferior biophysical properties and resistance to protein inhibition when compared to protein-containing preparations and therefore are unlikely to benefit patients with ARDS (110,111).

As reviewed recently (112), surfactant preparations vary significantly in their ability to affect bacterial growth. In the future, synthetic surfactants may include novel protein components designed to address this and other properties. One such component is "Mini-B," a 34-residue peptide that incorporates residues 8–25 and 63–78 of native human SP-B. This peptide joins the critical N- and C-terminal portions of SP-B that are largely responsible for the interaction of SP-B with surfactant lipids (113). Another possible component is SP-C33, a synthetic poly-Leu analog of SP-C that can substitute for isolated SP-C when used (in conjunction with SP-B) in treatment of a premature rabbit lung model of surfactant deficiency (114). Other possibilities include peptoids that mimic the structure and function of SP-B and/or SP-C, but are resistant to degradation (115), or the use of phospholipase-resistant diether phosphonolipids that exhibit resistance to inhibition by phospholipase A_2 or lysophosphatidylcholine (116).

Table 4 Surfactants That Have Been Used clinically

Generic name	Brand name	Constituents	Natural source	Manufacturer
Protein-containing				
Natural origin				
Amniotic fluid surfactant (96)		Natural lipids, SP-A, SP-B, SP-C, SP-D	Human amniotic fluid	(Not available)
Beractant (97)	Survanta	Natural lipids, SP-B, SP-C	Minced bovine lung	Abbott Laboratories (USA)
Bovine lipid extract surfactant (98)	BLES	Natural lipids, SP-B, SP-C	Bovine lavage	BLES Biochem (Canada)
Calfactant (99)	Infasurf	Natural lipids, SP-B, SP-C	Bovine calf lavage	Forest Laboratories (USA)
HL-10 (100)		Natural lipids, SP-B, SP-C	Minced porcine lung	Leo Pharmaceuticals (Denmark)
Poractant alfa (101)	Curosurf	Natural lipids, SP-B, SP-C	Minced porcine lung	Chiesi Pharmaceuticals (Italy)
SF-RI 1 (102)	Alveofact	Natural lipids, SP-B, SP-C	Bovine lavage	Boehringer Ingelheim (Germany)
Surfactant-TA (103)	Surfacten	Natural lipids, SP-B, SP-C	Minced bovine lung	Mitsubishi Pharma Corp (Japan)
Surfactant-BL (104)		Natural lipids, SP-B, SP-C	Bovine minced lung	Biosurf (Russia)
Synthetic origin				
Lucinactant (105)	Surfaxin	DPPC, POPG, PA, KL4 peptide		Discovery Laboratories (USA)
Lusupultide (106)	Venticute	DPPC, POPG, PA, rhSP-C		BYK Pharm (Germany)
Nonprotein containing				
Pumactant (107)	ALEC	DPPC, PG		Britannia Pharm (UK)
Colfosceril palmitate (108)	Exosurf Neonatal	DPPC, hexadecanol, tyloxepol		Glaxo Wellcome (USA)

Abbreviations: DPPC, dipalmitoylphosphatidylcholine; PA, palmitic acid; PG, phosphatidylglycerol; POPG, palmitoyloleoylphosphatidylglycerol; rhSP-C, recombinant human SP-C; SP-A, surfactant protein A; SP-B, surfactant protein B; SP-C, surfactant protein C; SP-D, surfactant protein C.

Mode of Administration

Surfactant may be delivered to the airway in a variety of ways. These include intratracheal instillation by bolus or infusion, bronchoscopic delivery to each lobar or segmental bronchus, delivery during lung lavage, or aerosolization.

Intratracheal bolus instillation has been used in the majority of clinical trials, and is usually accomplished through a catheter that is passed via the endotracheal tube to a point just caudal to the carina. Patients may be placed in various positions during instillation of serial surfactant aliquots to facilitate homogeneous distribution. Instillation of aliquots up to 50 mL has been done safely with the ventilator paused and positive end-expiratory pressure maintained. Slow continuous intratracheal instillation appears, in preclinical studies, to have inferior effects on gas exchange relative to bolus instillation (117). Advantages of bolus instillation include the rapidity of treatment and the ability to give large amounts over a short period of time. In one study, a dose of 100 mg/kg delivered in 25 mL aliquots could be given in as little as 10 to 15 minutes (118). Distribution may be affected adversely by gravitational forces, with preferential delivery of the instillate to dependent lung zones. However, both aerated and nonaerated lung zones are likely to receive surfactant if the rapid bolus technique is used and the patient is repositioned during administration. Treatment is limited to intubated patients, preventing study with this technique of patients supported by noninvasive ventilation.

Bronchoscopic instillation of surfactant has also been used clinically, and is both technically feasible and accompanied by apparent improvement in gas exchange (119). However, despite the theoretical possibility that distribution might be more homogeneous than with bolus instillation, preclinical studies have not demonstrated this advantage (120). In addition, it is somewhat time-consuming as administration of a single dose of 100 mg/kg may take one to two hours. Lavage fluid containing suspended surfactant may be tidally administered via a wedged bronchoscope and this lavage technique has the theoretic advantage of removing cell products and serum proteins that may promote inflammation and surfactant inhibition. Preclinical evaluation supports the concept that surfactant delivery by lavage may be an effective delivery technique (121).

Aerosolization of surfactant has been the subject of several preclinical and clinical studies. This modality has the advantages of delivering surfactant continuously, not requiring the presence of a bronchoscopist, avoiding airway obstruction, and, theoretically, providing homogeneous delivery. However, preclinical studies suggest that nonventilated lung units receive little surfactant relative to more compliant ventilated lung units (122). Perhaps the major drawback to current aerosol delivery techniques is limitation of the amount of surfactant that can be delivered in a 24-hour period.

Surfactant Dose and Dose Volume

The dose of surfactant necessary to treat patients with ARDS is undefined, as clinical studies have not yet shown convincing evidence of benefit. Furthermore, the optimal dose of surfactant for a particular patient will likely depend on factors such as the severity of the injury at the time of treatment, the specific type of surfactant used and the method used for delivery. Nevertheless, preclinical studies suggest that doses (given by bolus instillation) in the range of 50 to 100 mg of phospholipids/kg may be required. This amount of surfactant is approximately 25 times that existing in the healthy adult human airway, but such large doses may be required to overcome the inhibition of surfactant biophysical function by components of alveolar edema fluid and to assure treatment of most lung areas despite lack of fully homogeneous delivery (123).

The dose and dose volume of administered surfactant should be considered to be independent variables, with concentration a dependent variable. Dose volume is likely to be of considerable importance when delivery is as a bolus into the airway. Investigators have shown that relatively large dose volumes may result in more homogeneous distribution (124). However, as shown in Figure 1, delivery to pigs of 50 or 100 mg rSP-C surfactant/kg in 1 or 2 mL/kg resulted in a greater improvement in gas exchange than was

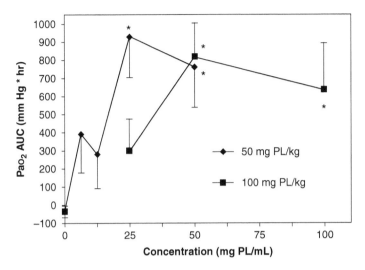

Figure 1 Pigs with acute lung injury induced by repetitive saline lavage received either 50 or 100 mg rSP-C surfactant phospholipids (PL) in volumes that varied from 1 to 6 mL/kg. The area under the Pao_2 versus time curve for four hours after treatment ($Pao_2 \cdot AUC$) is displayed as a function of the concentration of the surfactant delivered for each dose. Control animals received saline only (0 mg PL/mL). Values significantly different from control are indicated with an asterisk and indicate that animals receiving either 1 or 2 mL/kg, containing either 50 or 100 mg PL/mL had a significant improvement in gas exchange (80). *Source*: Courtesy of American Physiological Society.

achieved with the same dose delivered in 4 or 6 mL/kg, despite similar lobar distribution of the instilled surfactant (80). This result may reflect over-dilution of the exogenous surfactant.

Timing of Surfactant Administration

The timing of surfactant administration may also impact efficacy. Prophylactic treatment of premature neonates is effective in preventing lung injury (125), and prophylactic treatment of donor canine lungs prevents postimplantation injury (126). While study of the prophylactic treatment of patients at risk of developing ARDS would be attractive, the current power of predicting development of the syndrome is insufficient to support such clinical application or even investigation.

Treatment of lung injury early in the course of disease is supported by preclinical studies and by observations that patients who have significant respiratory failure but who have not yet met criteria for ARDS also have impaired surfactant function (4). There is little information that addresses the question of how frequently retreatment should occur. In trials of rSP-C surfactant, increased levels of SP-C, relative to untreated patients, could be detected in the lower airway 24 hours but not 96 hours after administration of the last dose, suggesting the possibility that treatments might rationally be spaced less frequently than every six hours, and extend over more than 24 hours (62,127). In addition, there are no data that address the question of how late in the course of ARDS surfactant treatment might be of benefit. Further clinical investigation of treatment schedules is required.

Finally, choice of the correct ventilation strategy may be critical in achieving successful treatment of ARDS patients with lung surfactant. Fortunately, the rational choice for ventilating these patients is a low-volume strategy (77), and as noted previously, it is likely that this strategy is also likely to minimize conversion of large functional surfactant aggregates to small poorly functional forms. Thus, one would theorize that use of low ventilating volumes should help preserve exogenous surfactant in the large aggregate form. Preclinical studies evaluating the efficacy of exogenous surfactant in the setting of novel modes of mechanical ventilation such as HFO are currently being conducted.

B. Results of Individual Investigations of Surfactant Treatment of ARDS Patients

The first suggestion that exogenous surfactant might be of value in treating ARDS patients was offered by Lachmann, who treated a morbidly ill patient with a natural surfactant (93). In the first small trial in nonterminal patients, in which those patients served as their own controls, Curosurf®, a natural surfactant of porcine origin, was delivered bronchoscopically to each lobar bronchus (128). Patients had a small but significant increase in gas exchange, and in several patients the minimum surface tension of surfactant recovered in BAL several hours after treatment was significantly lower than the pretreatment values.

Subsequently, additional small studies were performed using Exosurf (129). These provided rationale for a large prospective randomized multicenter Phase III trial in which 364 patients received aerosolized Exosurf and 361 received aerosolized 0.45% saline (130). The aerosolized drug contained 13.5 mg DPPC/mL, and approximately 112 mg/kg/day was aerosolized for up to five days. Results of this study were conclusively negative. Thirty-day mortality in both the treated and placebo group was 41%, and no differences were seen when groups were stratified by APACHE III score or etiology. The placebo and treated groups had similar numbers of days of mechanical ventilation and length of ICU stay, and no differences in gas exchange were detected. There are several reasons that the hypothesis that exogenous surfactant might benefit patients with ARDS was not adequately tested in this study. First, the nonprotein containing Exosurf has inferior biophysical activity and is quite susceptible to protein inhibition. Second, it is highly likely that inadequate amounts were able to be delivered by aerosolization. Finally, distribution of the aerosolized material is likely to have been predominately to well aerated lung units, with resultant failure to recruit poorly ventilated or nonventilated units. In addition to this trial, a small study of the efficacy of a second nonprotein-containing surfactant has had results consistent with the findings of the Exosurf study. Four patients with late-stage ARDS received a single dose of ALEC, a preparation containing only DPPC and palmitoyloleoylphosphatidylglycerol (POPG), without evidence of therapeutic effect (131).

A more promising phase II trial of a natural surfactant, Survanta®, was reported in 1997. In this prospective, randomized, multicenter study, patients received either standard treatment or standard treatment plus instillation of surfactant. Three surfactant-treated groups were studied. Patients received up to eight doses of 50 mg PL/kg, up to eight doses of 100 mg PL/kg, or up to four doses of 100 mg PL/kg. The inspired oxygen concentration (Fio_2) was significantly decreased at 120 hours only in the group receiving up to four doses of 100 mg PL/kg. Mortality in that same group was 18.8% as compared to 43.8% mortality in the group receiving standard treatment. Patients were lavaged prior to treatment and 120 hours after initiation of treatment to assess effects of treatment. Significant increases in lavage PL and disaturated PC concentrations were seen in the groups receiving the higher concentrations of surfactant, and biophysical function of surfactant recovered from lavage fluid at 120 hours was significantly (although minimally) decreased in the group receiving eight doses of 100 mg PL/kg. No significant adverse events were reported.

Similar findings resulted from a pilot study and subsequent randomized study of bovine surfactant (Alveofact) treatment of infants with ARDS. In the randomized study, children aged 0 to 13 years with pneumonia or sepsis and severe hypoxemia received 100 mg/kg surfactant intratracheally, and then were retreated, if necessary, 48 hours later ($n = 20$) or received standard care ($n = 15$). Significant improvement in oxygenation occurred in the treated group two hours after the initial treatment. Trends toward sustained oxygenation improvement and decreased survival were observed (132).

This study was followed by two phase II investigations of the safety and efficacy of Venticute®, a preparation containing 1 mg rSP-C/mL and 50 mg PL/mL. Based on information from preclinical studies, Venticute was delivered intratracheally in a dose volume of 1 mL/kg. In the study performed in North America, patients were prospectively randomized to receive rSP-C surfactant plus standard therapy or standard therapy alone ($n = 13$). Patients received either 100 ($n = 12$) or 200 ($n = 15$) mg PL/kg ideal body weight given in four divided doses over 24 hours. No safety concerns were identified, and the higher dose of rSP-C surfactant was associated with the most ventilator-free days to day 28 (VFDs), greatest improvement in gas exchange, and least mortality (127). In the second study, conducted in Europe and South Africa, patients were randomized to standard therapy ($n = 12$) or to receive 200 ($n = 14$) or 500 mg PL/kg. As in the former study, the group receiving 200 mg PL/kg had the greatest number of VFDs, greatest improvement in gas exchange, and least mortality (133), and surfactant treatment restored surface-tension lowering function of the large aggregate fraction recovered from BAL for up to five days (62).

These promising results were followed by two prospective, randomized, double-blind, multicenter trials designed to examine the efficacy of the 200 mg PL/kg dose of rSP-C surfactant in the treatment of ARDS patients. Parallel trials in North American and in Europe/South Africa included 221 and 227 patients, respectively (134). The most prevalent predisposing events for ARDS in both studies were sepsis, pneumonia and trauma, or surgery. The median increases in PaO_2/FiO_2 in treated versus control patients were 34 versus 15 mm Hg ($p < 0.01$) and 23 versus 11 mm Hg ($p = 0.04$) in the North American and European/South African studies, respectively (Fig. 2). No differences in survival were detected between groups treated with or without rSP-C surfactant. In a subsequent pooled analysis of all five multicenter studies in which patients with ARDS due to various predisposing events were treated with rSP-C surfactant ($n = 266$) or received usual care ($n = 266$), treatment with rSP-C surfactant significantly improved oxygenation but had no effect on mortality (32.6%). In the subgroup of patients with severe ARDS due to pneumonia or aspiration, surfactant treatment was associated with markedly improved oxygenation and improved survival (95). These observations led to a phase III trial of Venticute for patients with severe lung injury due to aspiration or pneumonia. This trial was stopped in 2008 due to lack of efficacy, and preliminary evidence suggests that

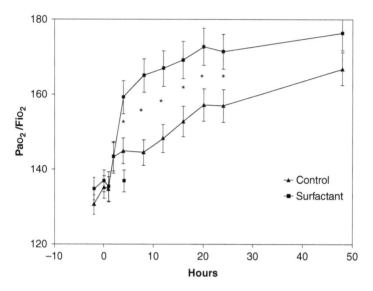

Figure 2   The average Pao_2/Fio_2 values for patients receiving usual care ($n = 224$, triangles) or treated with up to four doses in 24 hours of rSP-C surfactant ($n = 224$, squares). Between 2 and 24 hours after the first treatment, values were significantly greater in the surfactant treated group (134). *Source*: Courtesy of Massachusetts Medical Society.

an agitation maneuver designed to resuspend the powdered Venticute led to significant inactivation of the material such that not even the expected improvement in oxygenation was detected.

Although a preliminary report of a prospective randomized multicenter open-label phase II trial of HL 10, a surfactant derived from minced porcine lung, in the treatment of ARDS patients suggested that treatment with up to four doses of 100 to 200 mg PL/kg was associated with significant improvement in gas exchange and survival (100), a subsequent phase III trial in patients with ARDS associated with direct or indirect causes was stopped for lack of efficacy (135).

Calfactant, a surfactant derived from calf lung lavage, has been evaluated in the treatment of ARDS. In a pilot study, this surfactant was administered to pediatric patients, 11 of whom were between 5 and 16 years of age. The investigators concluded that surfactant administration rapidly improved oxygenation and allowed moderation of ventilator support in the majority of children studied (136). A second small prospective randomized controlled study showed that patients (age 0–16 years) who received intratracheal instillation of 80 mL/m^2 of Infasurf within 24 hours of initiation of mechanical ventilation, with retreatment if indicated, had significant immediate improvement in oxygenation and decreased requirement for mechanical ventilation (137).

In a subsequent multicenter, randomized, blinded phase III trial of calfactant compared with placebo, 153 infants, children, and adolescents with acute lung injury were enrolled within 48 hours of intubation. Patients received up to two intratracheal instillations of 80 mL/m^2 calfactant or an equal volume of air as placebo. Treated patients had a significant improvement in oxygenation and lessened mortality (19.5% vs. 36%), although the primary outcome, VFDs, was not different between groups. The improvement in survival was due entirely to improved survival in the group of patients with direct lung injury (138). This study is being followed up by a prospective randomized double-blind study that plans to enroll 480 patients aged one month to 85 years with direct ARDS who have been intubated less than 48 hours.

In addition to these 11 randomized controlled trials, several uncontrolled trials also suggest the possible efficacy of exogenous protein-containing surfactants in the treatment of patients with ARDS. In a study involving pediatric patients, BLES, a bovine lung surfactant similar to Infasurf, was administered to 13 children with severe ARDS. Results suggested benefit to those children treated within two days of ARDS diagnosis (139).

The safety and possible efficacy of surfactant delivered by bolus instillation through a bronchoscope into each segmental bronchus has been reported by several investigators. Walmrath and coworkers have administered Alveofac to patients with ARDS secondary to sepsis and observed improvement in oxygenation (119). Surfactant treatment of patients who develop ARDS after cardiac surgery has been evaluated by Bautin and coworkers who instilled surfactant-BL bronchoscopically into 78 patients who developed ARDS within 72 hours after surgery. Treatment was associated with a trend toward improvement in oxygenation and survival relative to an historical control group (104). Finally, bronchoscopic lavage has been used to deliver Surfaxin (KL$_4$-surfactant) in an uncontrolled open-label trial in which 12 adults with ARDS were studied. This study also reported modest improvement in gas exchange, with no serious adverse events associated with the procedure (140).

These trials, taken together, show that despite the strong rational for surfactant therapy of ARDS (Table 3) and the promise of uncontrolled and phase II trials, that promise has not been realized in the larger phase III trials that have used adequate amounts of highly active surfactants. The reasons for this are unclear. One possibility is that, despite similar inclusion and exclusion criteria, the patients enrolled in these studies are qualitatively different with respect to their disease, and that these differences result in substantially different responses to surfactant administration, obscuring any benefit that might be derived from surfactant treatment. A second possibility is that only an ARDS patient subset, perhaps those with direct lung injury, will benefit from surfactant treatment. Most studies performed to date have included a broad spectrum of patients with ARDS, and the signal from a responding subgroup may not yet be apparent. Finally, although surfactant replacement therapy in ARDS is both a biologically plausible hypothesis and a therapeutic possibility, it may have an insignificant role in the treatment of patients with ARDS.

VI. Summary

Since the first medical description of the ARDS, investigators have postulated that loss of lung surfactant function may be of pathophysiologic importance. This belief has deepened as multiple studies have confirmed that surfactant function is impaired in patients with ARDS. The hope that restoration of surfactant function may benefit patients with ARDS has been fostered by studies of individual patients and by a limited number of clinical trials. However, phase III studies, though often showing modest improvement in oxygenation, have failed to demonstrate improved survival. Hopefully, further study will identify effective treatment strategies and patient subgroups that this promising treatment may benefit.

References

1. Ashbaugh DG, Bigelow DB, Petty TL, et al. Acute respiratory distress in adults. Lancet 1967; 2:319–323.
2. Petty TL, Reiss OK, Paul GW, et al. Characteristics of pulmonary surfactant in adult respiratory distress syndrome associated with trauma and shock. Am Rev Respir Dis 1977; 115:531–536.
3. Hallman M, Spragg RG, Harrell JH, et al. Evidence of lung surfactant abnormality in respiratory failure: study of bronchoalveolar lavage phospholipids, surface activity, phospholipase activity, and plasma myoinositol. J Clin Invest 1982; 70:673–683.
4. Gregory TJ, Longmore WJ, Moxley MA, et al. Surfactant chemical composition and biophysical activity in acute respiratory distress syndrome. J Clin Invest 1991; 88:1976–1981.
5. Greene KE, Wright JR, Steinberg KP, et al. Serial changes in surfactant-associated proteins in lung and serum before and after onset of ARDS. Am J Respir Crit Care Med 1999;160:1843–1850.
6. Günther A, Siebert C, Schmidt R, et al. Surfactant alterations in severe pneumonia, acute respiratory distress syndrome, and cardiogenic lung edema. Am J Respir Crit Care Med 1996; 153:176–184.
7. Veldhuizen RA, McCaig LA, Akino T, et al. Pulmonary surfactant subfractions in patients with the acute respiratory distress syndrome. Am J Respir Crit Care Med 1995; 152:1867–1871.
8. Schmidt R, Markart P, Ruppert C, et al. Time-dependent changes in pulmonary surfactant function and composition in acute respiratory distress syndrome due to pneumonia or aspiration. Respir Res 2007; 8:55.
9. Robertson B, Van Golde LMJ, Battenberg JJ, eds. Pulmonary Surfactant: From Molecular Biology to Clinical Practice. New York: Elsevier, 1992.
10. Gross NJ, Kellam M, Young J, et al. Separation of alveolar surfactant into subtypes. A comparison of methods. Am J Respir Crit Care Med 2000; 162:617–622.
11. Enhorning G. A pulsating bubble technique for evaluating pulmonary surfactant. J Appl Physiol 1977; 43:198–201.
12. Schurch S, Bachofen H, Possmayer F. Surface activity in situ, in vivo, and in the captive bubble surfactometer. Comp Biochem Physiol A Mol Integr Physiol 2001: 129:195–207.
13. Gilliard N, Heldt GP, Loredo J, et al. Exposure of the hydrophobic components of porcine lung surfactant to oxidant stress alters surface tension properties. J Clin Invest 1994; 93:2608–2615.
14. Gupta M, Hernandez-Juviel JM, Waring AJ, et al. Comparison of functional efficacy of surfactant protein B analogues in lavaged rats. Eur Respir J 2000; 16:1129–1133.
15. Griese M. Pulmonary surfactant in health and human lung diseases: state of the art. Eur Respir J 1999; 13:1455–1476.
16. Pison U, Seeger W, Buchhorn R, et al. Surfactant abnormalities in patients with respiratory failure after multiple trauma. Am Rev Respir Dis 1989; 140:1033–1039.
17. Nakos G, Kitsiouli EI, Tsangaris I, et al. Bronchoalveolar lavage fluid characteristics of early intermediate and late phases of ARDS. Alterations in leukocytes, proteins, PAF and surfactant components. Intensive Care Med 1998; 24:296–303.
18. Bersten AD, Doyle IR, Davidson KG, et al. Surfactant composition reflects lung overinflation and arterial oxygenation in patients with acute lung injury. Eur Respir J 1998; 12:301–308.

19. Perez-Gil J. Structure of pulmonary surfactant membranes and films: the role of proteins and lipid-protein interactions. Biochim Biophys Acta 2008; 1778:1676–1695.
20. Korfhagen TR, LeVine AM, Whitsett JA. Surfactant protein A (SP-A) gene targeted mice. Biochim Biophys Acta 1998; 1408:296–302.
21. LeVine AM, Hartshorn K, Elliott J, et al. Absence of SP-A modulates innate and adaptive defense responses to pulmonary influenza infection. Am J Physiol Lung Cell Mol Physiol 2002; 282:L563–L572.
22. Linke MJ, Harris CE, Korfhagen TR, et al. Immunosuppressed surfactant protein A-deficient mice have increased susceptibility to Pneumocystis carinii infection. J Infect Dis 2001; 183:943–952.
23. Hawgood S, Poulain FR. The pulmonary collectins and surfactant metabolism. Annu Rev Physiol 2001; 63:495–519.
24. Crouch E, Wright JR. Surfactant proteins A and D and pulmonary host defense. Annu Rev Physiol 2001; 63:521–554.
25. Wert SE, Yoshida M, LeVine AM, et al. Increased metalloproteinase activity, oxidant production, and emphysema in surfactant protein D gene-inactivated mice. Proc Natl Acad Sci USA 2000; 97:5972–5977.
26. Clark JC, Wert SE, Bachurski CJ, et al. Targeted disruption of the surfactant protein B gene disrupts surfactant homeostasis, causing respiratory failure in newborn mice. Proc Natl Acad Sci USA 1995; 92:7794–7798.
27. Glasser SW, Burhans MS, Korfhagen TR, et al. Altered stability of pulmonary surfactant in SP-C-deficient mice. Proc Natl Acad Sci USA 2001; 98:6366–6371.
28. Krishnasamy S, Gross NJ, Teng AL, et al. Lung "surfactant convertase" is a member of the carboxylesterase family. Biochem Biophys Res Commun 1997; 235:180–184.
29. Krishnasamy S, Teng AL, Dhand R, et al. Molecular cloning, characterization, and differential expression pattern of mouse lung surfactant convertase. Am J Physiol 1998; 275: L969–L975.
30. Dhand R, Young J, Teng A, et al. Is dipalmitoylphosphatidylcholine a substrate for convertase? Am J Physiol Lung Cell Mol Physiol 2000; 278:L19–L24.
31. Veldhuizen RA, Inchley K, Hearn SA, et al. Degradation of surfactant-associated protein B (SP-B) during in vitro conversion of large to small surfactant aggregates. Biochem J 1993; 295:141–147.
32. Ruppert C, Bagheri A, Markart P, et al. Liver carboxylesterase cleaves surfactant protein (SP-) B and promotes surfactant subtype conversion. Biochem Biophys Res Commun 2006; 348:1449–1454.
33. Wright JR. Immunoregulatory functions of surfactant proteins. Nat Rev Immunol 2005; 5:58–68.
34. Moulakakis C, Adam S, Seitzer U, et al. Surfactant protein A activation of atypical protein kinase C zeta in IkappaB-alpha-dependent anti-inflammatory immune regulation. J Immunol 2007; 179:4480–4491.
35. Borron P, McIntosh JC, Korfhagen TR, et al. Surfactant-associated protein A inhibits LPS-induced cytokine and nitric oxide production in vivo. Am J Physiol Lung Cell Mol Physiol 2000; 278:L840–L847.
36. Kremlev SG, Phelps DS. Surfactant protein A stimulation of inflammatory cytokine and immunoglobulin production. Am J Physiol 1994; 267:L712–L719.
37. Ikegami M, Scoville EA, Grant S, et al. Surfactant protein-D and surfactant inhibit endotoxin-induced pulmonary inflammation. Chest 2007; 132:1447–1454.
38. Ryan MA, Akinbi HT, Serrano AG, et al. Antimicrobial activity of native and synthetic surfactant protein B peptides. J Immunol 2006; 176;416–425.
39. Chaby R, Garcia-Verdugo I, Espinassous Q, et al. Interactions between LPS and lung surfactant proteins. J Endotoxin Res 2005; 11:181–185.

40. Ikegami M, Weaver TE, Conkright JJ, et al. Deficiency of SP-B reveals protective role of SP-C during oxygen lung injury. J Appl Physiol 2002; 92:519–526.

41. Nesslein LL, Melton KR, Ikegami M, et al. Partial SP-B deficiency perturbs lung function and causes air space abnormalities. Am J Physiol Lung Cell Mol Physiol 2005; 288:L1154–L1161.

42. Ikegami M, Whitsett JA, Martis PC, et al. Reversibility of lung inflammation caused by SP-B deficiency. Am J Physiol Lung Cell Mol Physiol 2005; 289:L962–L970.

43. Cogo PE, Toffolo GM, Ori C, et al. Surfactant disaturated-phosphatidylcholine kinetics in acute respiratory distress syndrome by stable isotopes and a two compartment model. Respir Res 2007; 8:13.

44. Schmidt R, Meier U, Yabut-Perez M, et al. Alteration of fatty acid profiles in different pulmonary surfactant phospholipids in acute respiratory distress syndrome and severe pneumonia. Am J Respir Crit Care Med 2001; 163:95–100.

45. Raymondos K, Leuwer M, Haslam PL, et al. Compositional, structural, and functional alterations in pulmonary surfactant in surgical patients after the early onset of systemic inflammatory response syndrome or sepsis. Crit Care Med 1999; 27:82–89.

46. Bersten AD, Hunt T, Nicholas TE, et al. Elevated plasma surfactant protein-B predicts development of acute respiratory distress syndrome in patients with acute respiratory failure. Am J Respir Crit Care Med 1998; 164:648–652.

47. Doyle IR, Bersten AD, Nicholas TE. Surfactant proteins-A and -B are elevated in plasma of patients with acute respiratory failure. Am J Respir Crit Care Med 1997; 156:1217–1229.

48. Lin Z, Pearson C, Chinchilli V, et al. Polymorphisms of human SP-A, SP-B, and SP-D genes: association of SP-B Thr131Ile with ARDS. Clin Genet 2000; 58:181–191.

49. Gong MN, Wei Z, Xu LL, et al. Polymorphism in the surfactant protein-B gene, gender, and the risk of direct pulmonary injury and ARDS. Chest 2004; 125:203–211.

50. Max MP, Pison U, Floros J. Frequency of SP-B and SP-A1 gene polymorphisms in acute respiratory distress syndrome (ARDS). Appl Cardiopulm Pathophysiol 1996; 6:111–118.

51. Seeger W, Stöhr G, Wolf HRD, et al. Alteration of surfactant function due to protein leakage: special interaction with fibrin monomer. J Appl Physiol 1985; 56:326–338.

52. Holm BA, Notter RH. Effects of hemoglobin and cell membrane lipids on pulmonary surfactant activity. J Appl Physiol 1987; 63:1434–1442.

53. Seeger W, Günther A, Thede C. Differential sensitivity to fibrinogen inhibition of SP-C- vs. SP-B-based surfactants. Am J Physiol 1992; 261:L286–L291.

54. Cockshutt AM, Weitz J, Possmayer F. Pulmonary surfactant-associated protein A enhances the surface activity of lipid extract surfactant and reverses inhibition by blood proteins in vitro. Biochemistry 1990; 29:8424–8429.

55. Seeger W, Elssner A, Günther A, et al. Lung surfactant phospholipids associate with polymerizing fibrin: loss of surface activity. Am J Respir Cell Mol Biol 1993; 9:213–220.

56. Günther A, Markart P, Kalinowski M, et al. Cleavage of surfactant-incorporating fibrin by different fibrinolytic agents. Kinetics of lysis and rescue of surface activity. Am J Respir Cell Mol Biol 1999; 21:738–745.

57. Schermuly RT, Gunther A, Ermert M, et al. Conebulization of surfactant and urokinase restores gas exchange in perfused lungs with alveolar fibrin formation. Am J Physiol Lung Cell Mol Physiol 2001; 280:L792–L800.

58. Holm BA, Wang Z, Notter RH. Multiple mechanisms of lung surfactant inhibition. Pediatr Res 1999; 46:85–93.

59. Lachmann B, Eijking EP, So KL, et al. In vivo evaluation of the inhibitory capacity of human plasma on exogenous surfactant function. Intensive Care Med 1994; 20:6–11.

60. Bernardino de la Serna J, Perez-Gil J, Simonsen AC, et al. Cholesterol rules: direct observation of the coexistence of two fluid phases in native pulmonary surfactant membranes at physiological temperatures. J Biol Chem 2004; 279:40715–40722.

61. Gunasekara L, Schoel WM, Schurch S, et al. A comparative study of mechanisms of surfactant inhibition. Biochim Biophys Acta 2008; 1778:433–444.
62. Markart P, Ruppert C, Wygrecka M, et al. Patients with ARDS show improvement but not normalisation of alveolar surface activity with surfactant treatment: putative role of neutral lipids. Thorax 2007; 62:588–594.
63. Veldhuizen RA, Marcou J, Yao LJ, et al. Alveolar surfactant aggregate conversion in ventilated normal and injured rabbits. Am J Physiol 1996; 270:L152–L158.
64. Ito Y, Veldhuizen RA, Yao LJ, et al. Ventilation strategies affect surfactant aggregate conversion in acute lung injury. Am J Respir Crit Care Med 1997; 155:493–499.
65. Kerr CL, Veldhuizen RA, Lewis JF. Effects of high-frequency oscillation on endogenous surfactant in an acute lung injury model. Am J Respir Crit Care Med 2001; 164:237–242.
66. Haddad IY, Ischiropoulos H, Holm BA, et al. Mechanisms of peroxynitrite-induced injury to pulmonary surfactants. Am J Physiol 1993; 265:L555–L564.
67. Haddad IY, Crow JP, Hu P, et al. Concurrent generation of nitric oxide and superoxide damages surfactant protein A. Am J Physiol 1994; 267:L242–L249.
68. Seeger W, Lepper H, Hellmut RD, et al. Alteration of alveolar surfactant function after exposure to oxidative stress and to oxygenated and native arachidonic acid in vitro. Biochim Biophys Acta 1985; 835:58–67.
69. Liau DF, Yin NX, Huang J, et al. Effects of human polymorphonuclear leukocyte elastase upon surfactant proteins in vitro. Biochim Biophys Acta 1996; 1302:117–128.
70. Zhu S, Kachel DL, Martin WJ, et al. Nitrated SP-A does not enhance adherence of Pneumocystis carinii to alveolar macrophages. Am J Physiol 1998; 275:L1031–L1039.
71. McGuire WW, Spragg RG, Cohen AB, et al. Studies on the pathogenesis of the adult respiratory distress syndrome. J Clin Invest 1982; 69:543–553.
72. Christner P, Fein A, Goldberg S, et al. Collagenase in the lower respiratory tract of patients with adult respiratory distress syndrome. Am Rev Respir Dis 1985; 131:690–695.
73. Pison U, Tam EK, Caughey GH, et al. Proteolytic inactivation of dog lung surfactant-associated proteins by neutrophil elastase. Biochim Biophys Acta 1989; 992:251–257.
74. Baker CS, Evans TW, Randle BJ, et al. Damage to surfactant-specific protein in acute respiratory distress syndrome. Lancet 1999; 353:1232–1237.
75. Hite RD, Seeds MC, Jacinto RB, et al. Hydrolysis of surfactant-associated phosphatidyl-choline by mammalian secretory phospholipases A_2. Am J Physiol 1998; 275:L740–L747.
76. Hite RD, Seeds MC, Jacinto RB, et al. Lysophospholipid and fatty acid inhibition of pulmonary surfactant: non-enzymatic models of phospholipase A_2 surfactant hydrolysis. Biochim Biophys Acta 2005; 1720:14–21.
77. The Acute Respiratory Distress Syndrome Network. Ventilation with lower tidal volumes as compared with traditional tidal volumes for acute lung injury and the acute respiratory distress syndrome. N Engl J Med 2000; 342:1301–1308.
78. Berggren P, Lachmann B, Curstedt T, et al. Gas exchange and lung morphology after surfactant replacement in experimental adult respiratory distress syndrome induced by repeated lung lavage. Acta Anaesthesiol Scand 1986; 30:321–328.
79. Lewis JF, Goffin J, Yue P, et al. Evaluation of exogenous surfactant treatment strategies in an adult model of acute lung injury. J Appl Physiol 1996; 80:1156–1164.
80. Spragg RG, Smith RM, Harris K, et al. Effect of recombinant SP-C surfactant in a porcine lavage model of acute lung injury. J Appl Physiol 2000; 88:674–681.
81. Vazquez dAG, Lachmann RA, Gommers D, et al. Treatment of ventilation-induced lung injury with exogenous surfactant. Intensive Care Med 2001; 27:559–565.
82. Eijking EP, Gommers D, So KL, et al. Surfactant treatment of respiratory failure induced by hydrochloric acid aspiration in rats. Anesthesiology 1993; 78:1145–1151.
83. Strohmaier W, Redl H, Schlag G. Studies of the potential role of a semisynthetic surfactant preparation in an experimental aspiration trauma in rabbits. Exp Lung Res 1990; 16:101–110.

84. van Daal GJ, Bos JA, Eijking EP, et al. Surfactant replacement therapy improves pulmonary mechanics in end-stage influenza A pneumonia in mice. Am Rev Respir Dis 1992; 145:859–863.
85. van Daal GJ, So KL, Gommers D, et al. Intratracheal surfactant administration restores gas exchange in experimental adult respiratory distress syndrome associated with viral pneumonia. Anesth Analg 1991; 72:589–595.
86. Eijking EP, van Daal GJ, Tenbrinck R, et al. Improvement of pulmonary gas exchange after surfactant replacement in rats with Pneumocystis carinii pneumonia. Adv Exp Med Biol 1992; 316:293–298.
87. Berry D, Ikegami M, Jobe A. Respiratory distress and surfactant inhibition following vagotomy in rabbits. Am J Physiol 1986; 61:1741–1748.
88. Harris JD, Jackson FJ, Moxley MA, et al. Effect of exogenous surfactant instillation on experimental acute lung injury. J Appl Physiol 1989; 66:1846–1851.
89. Anderson BM, Jackson FJ, Moxley MA, et al. Effects on experimental acute lung injury 24 hours after exogenous surfactant instillation. Exp Lung Res 1992; 18:191–204.
90. Chen CM, Fang CL, Chang CH. Surfactant and corticosteroid effects on lung function in a rat model of acute lung injury. Crit Care Med 2001; 29:2169–2175.
91. Huang YC, Sane AC, Simonson SG, et al. Artificial surfactant attenuates hyperoxic lung injury in primates. I. Physiology and biochemistry. J Appl Physiol 1995; 78:1816–1822.
92. Loewen GM, Holm BA, Milanowski L, et al. Alveolar hyperoxic injury in rabbits receiving exogenous surfactant. J Appl Physiol 1989; 66:1087–1092.
93. Lachmann B. Surfactant replacement in acute respiratory failure: animal studies and first clinical trials. In: Lachmann B, ed. Surfactant Replacement Therapy. New York: Springer, 1987:212–223.
94. Lewis JF, Tabor B, Ikegami M, et al. Lung function and surfactant distribution in saline-lavaged sheep given instilled vs. nebulized surfactant. J Appl Physiol 1993; 74:1256–1264.
95. Taut FJH, Rippin G, Schenk DB, et al. A search for subgroups of patients with the acute respiratory distress syndrome who may benefit from surfactant replacement therapy: a pooled analysis of five studies with rSP-C surfactant (Venticute®). Chest 2008; 134(4):724–732.
96. Hallman M, Merritt TA, Schneider H, et al. Isolation of human surfactant from amniotic fluid and a pilot study of its efficacy in respiratory distress syndrome. Pediatrics 1983; 71:473–482.
97. Taeusch HW, Keough KM, Williams M, et al. Characterization of bovine surfactant for infants with respiratory distress syndrome. Pediatrics 1986; 77:572–581.
98. Enhorning G, Shennan A, Possmayer F, et al. Prevention of neonatal respiratory distress syndrome by tracheal instillation of surfactant: a randomized clinical trial. Pediatrics 1985; 76:145–153.
99. Onrust SV, Dooley M, Goa KL. Calfactant: a review of its use in neonatal respiratory distress syndrome. Paediatr Drugs 1999; 1:219–243.
100. Kesecioglu J, Schultz MJ, Lundberg D, et al. Treatment of acute lung injury (ALI/ARDS) with surfactant. Am J Respir Crit Care Med 2001; 165:A819.
101. Robertson B, Curstedt T, Johansson J, et al. Structural and functional characterization of porcine surfactant isolated by liquid-gel chromatography. In: von Wichert P, Muller B, eds. Basic Research on Lung Surfactant. Progress in Respiration Research. Basel: Karger, 1990:237–246.
102. Disse B, Gortner L, Weller E, et al. Efficacy and standardization of SF-RI 1: a preparation from bovine lung surfactant. In: Lachmann B, ed. Surfactant Replacement Therapy in Neonatal and Adult Respiratory Distress Syndrome. Berlin: Springer, 1999:37–41.
103. Fujiwara T, Chida S, Watabe Y, et al. Artificial surfactant therapy in hyaline-membrane disease. Lancet 1980; 1:55–59.
104. Bautin A, Khubulava G, Kozlov I, et al. Surfactant therapy for patients with ARDS after cardiac surgery. J Liposome Res 2006; 16:265–272.

105. Cochrane CG, Revak SD, Merritt TA, et al. The efficacy and safety of KL4-surfactant in preterm infants with respiratory distress syndrome. Am J Respir Crit Care Med 1996; 153:404–410.
106. Häfner D, Germann PG, Hauschke D. Effects of lung surfactant factor (LSF) treatment on gas exchange and histopathological changes in an animal model of adult respiratory distress syndrome (ARDS): comparison of recombinant LSF with bovine LSF. Pulm Pharmacol 1994; 7:319–332.
107. Morley CJ, Bangham AD, Miller N, et al. Dry artificial lung surfactant and its effect on very premature babies. Lancet 1981; 1:64–68.
108. Durand DJ, Clyman RI, Heymann MA, et al. Effects of a protein-free, synthetic surfactant on survival and pulmonary function in preterm lambs. J Pediatr 1985; 107:775–780.
109. Moya FR, Hoffman DR, Zhao B, et al. Platelet-activating factor in surfactant preparations. Lancet 1993; 341:858–860.
110. Häfner D, Beume R, Kilian U, et al. Dose-response comparisons of five lung surfactant factor (LSF) preparations in an animal model of adult respiratory distress syndrome (ARDS). Br J Pharmacol 1995; 115:451–458.
111. Amirkhanian JD, Bruni R, Waring AJ, et al. Inhibition of mixtures of surfactant lipids and synthetic sequences of surfactant proteins SP-B and SP-C. Biochim Biophys Acta 1991; 1096:355–360.
112. Blanco O, Perez-Gil J. Biochemical and pharmacological differences between preparations of exogenous natural surfactant used to treat Respiratory Distress Syndrome: role of the different components in an efficient pulmonary surfactant. Eur J Pharmacol 2007; 568:1–15.
113. Walther FJ, Waring AJ, Sherman MA, et al. Hydrophobic surfactant proteins and their analogues. Neonatology 2007; 91:303–310.
114. Almlen A, Stichtenoth G, Linderholm B, et al. Surfactant proteins B and C are both necessary for alveolar stability at end expiration in premature rabbits with respiratory distress syndrome. J Appl Physiol 2008; 104:1101–1108.
115. Seurynck-Servoss SL, Brown NJ, Dohm MT, et al. Lipid composition greatly affects the in vitro surface activity of lung surfactant protein mimics. Colloids Surf B Biointerfaces 2007; 57:37–55.
116. Wang Z, Chang Y, Schwan AL, et al. Activity and inhibition resistance of a phospholipase-resistant synthetic surfactant in rat lungs. Am J Respir Cell Mol Biol 2007; 37:387–394.
117. Segerer H, van Gelder W, Angenent FW, et al. Pulmonary distribution and efficacy of exogenous surfactant in lung-lavaged rabbits are influenced by the instillation technique. Pediatr Res 1993; 34:490–494.
118. Gregory TJ, Steinberg KP, Spragg R, et al. Bovine surfactant therapy for patients with acute respiratory distress syndrome. Am J Respir Crit Care Med 1997; 155:1309–1315.
119. Walmrath D, Günther A, Ghofrani HA, et al. Bronchoscopic surfactant administration in patients with severe adult respiratory distress syndrome and sepsis. Am J Respir Crit Care Med 1996; 154:57–62.
120. Lewis J, McCaig L, Hafner D, et al. Dosing and delivery of a recombinant surfactant in lung-injured adult sheep. Am J Respir Crit Care Med 1999; 159:741–747.
121. Schlosser RL, Veldman A, Fischer D, et al. Comparison of effects of perflubron and surfactant lung lavage on pulmonary gas exchange in a piglet model of meconium aspiration. Biol Neonate 2002; 81:126–131.
122. Lewis JF, McCaig L. Aerosolized versus instilled exogenous surfactant in a nonuniform pattern of lung injury. Am Rev Respir Dis 1993; 148:1187–1193.
123. Rebello CM, Jobe AH, Eisele JW, et al. Alveolar and tissue surfactant pool sizes in humans. Am J Respir Crit Care Med 1996; 154:625–628.
124. Gilliard N, Richman PM, Merritt TA, et al. Effect of volume and dose on the pulmonary distribution of exogenous surfactant administered to normal rabbits or to rabbits with oleic acid lung injury. Am Rev Respir Dis 1990; 141:743–747.

125. Soll RF, Morley CJ. Prophylactic versus selective use of surfactant in preventing morbidity and mortality in preterm infants. Cochrane Database Syst Rev 2001; CD000510.

126. Novick RJ, MacDonald J, Veldhuizen RA, et al. Evaluation of surfactant treatment strategies after prolonged graft storage in lung transplantation. Am J Respir Crit Care Med 1996; 154:98–104.

127. Spragg RG, Lewis JF, Wurst W, et al. Treatment of acute respiratory distress syndrome with recombinant surfactant protein C surfactant. Am J Respir Crit Care Med 2003; 167:1562–1566.

128. Spragg RG, Gilliard N, Richman P, et al. Acute effects of a single dose of porcine surfactant on patients with the adult respiratory distress syndrome. Chest 1994; 105:195–202.

129. Weg JG, Balk RA, Tharratt RS, et al. Safety and potential efficacy of an aerosolized surfactant in human sepsis-induced adult respiratory distress syndrome. JAMA 1994; 272:1433–1438.

130. Anzueto A, Baughman R, Guntupalli KK, et al. Aerosolized surfactants in adults with sepsis-induced acute respiratory distress syndrome. N Engl J Med 1996; 334:1417–1421.

131. Haslam PL, Hughes DA, MacNaughton PD, et al. Surfactant replacement therapy in late-stage adult respiratory distress syndrome. Lancet 1994; 343:1009–1011.

132. Moller JC, Schaible T, Roll C, et al. Treatment with bovine surfactant in severe acute respiratory distress syndrome in children: a randomized multicenter study. Intensive Care Med 2003; 29:437–446.

133. Günther A, Ruppert C, Schmidt R, et al. Surfactant alteration and replacement in acute respiratory distress syndrome. Respir Res 2001; 2:353–364.

134. Spragg RG, Lewis JF, Walmrath H-D, et al. Effect of recombinant surfactant protein-C based surfactant on the acute respiratory distress syndrome. N Engl J Med 2004; 351:884–892.

135. http://www.leo-pharma.com/41256A84002BE7FC/0/59400A0E93DD0652C1256EAD007 340E5?OpenDocument. Accessed August 23, 2009.

136. Willson DF, Jiao JH, Bauman LA, et al. Calf's lung surfactant extract in acute hypoxemic respiratory failure in children. Crit Care Med 1996; 24:1316–1322.

137. Willson DF, Zaritsky A, Bauman LA, et al. Instillation of calf lung surfactant extract (calfactant) is beneficial in pediatric acute hypoxemic respiratory failure. Members of the Mid-Atlantic Pediatric Critical Care Network. Crit Care Med 1999; 27:188–195.

138. Willson DF, Thomas NJ, Markovitz BP, et al. Effect of exogenous surfactant (calfactant) in pediatric acute lung injury: a randomized controlled trial. JAMA 2005; 293:470–476.

139. Lewis JF, Dhillon JS, Singh RN, et al. Exogenous surfactant therapy for pediatric patients with the acute respiratory distress syndrome. Can Respir J 1997; 4:21–26.

140. Wiswell TE, Smith RM, Katz LB, et al. Bronchopulmonary segmental lavage with Surfaxin (KL(4)-surfactant) for acute respiratory distress syndrome. Am J Respir Crit Care Med 1999; 160:1188–1195.

17
Prone Position in ARDS

ANTONIO ANZUETO
South Texas Veterans Health Care System, Audie L. Murphy Division, and The University of Texas Health Science Center at San Antonio, San Antonio, Texas, U.S.A.

LUCIANO GATTINONI
Ospedale Maggiore Policlinico, Milan, Italy

I. Introduction

Since the description of acute respiratory distress syndrome (ARDS) in 1967 (1), mechanical ventilation has been the mainstay therapy of support to these patients. Furthermore, mechanical ventilation has been shown to result in lung injury, thus therapeutic strategies focused on preventing this injury have been shown to significantly decrease mortality (2). It was almost 10 years after the clinical description of ARDS that Piehl and Brown (3) first described the benefit of positional changes to improve arterial oxygenation in five patients with acute respiratory failure. Douglas and coworkers (4) confirmed these data in a more extensive study, and also described significant improvement in arterial oxygenation in most, but not all, patients who were placed in prone position. Possible mechanisms to explain the improvement of gas exchange during prone position included a redistribution of blood flow and/or ventilation, an increase in lung functional and residual capacities, and changes in intrapulmonary pressure gradients. These two studies were based on the theoretical work by Bryan (5), who advocated prone position in mechanically ventilated patients in order to improve regional inflation of dorsal portions of the lung. Over the last 20 years, there have been extensive reports on the pathophysiology of prone ventilation as well as the clinical application in acute lung injury (ALI) and ARDS.

This chapter reviews the factors related to improvement of oxygenation due to prone ventilation; the effect on ventilation and perfusion; then uses this information to demonstrate how changes in body position affect gas exchange; and provides an update on the potential effect of the mediastinum weight over the lung parenchyma. Finally, there is a summary of clinical data available, including a recently published multicenter, randomized trial on the use of prone ventilation in patients with ALI/ARDS and other forms of ALI.

A. Pathophysiology in ARDS

ARDS is characterized by pulmonary infiltrates, which were previously considered to be rather homogenously distributed throughout the lung, as evidenced by conventional chest radiographs (6,7). Considering the complexity of the anatomical changes occurring in ARDS lung structure, regional chest tomography analysis allows the assessment of these parenchyma abnormalities. Chest tomography technology shows that in the ARDS lung, the lung abnormalities are primarily located in the dependent regions, that is, the dorsal regions (lower) in supine position (8–10). In contrast, the nondependent regions, that is, the sternal regions (upper) in supine position, seem, at least to visual inspection, quite normal. These findings have challenged the commonly held opinion that ALI/ARDS are a generalized lung disease and suggest that the lung parenchyma is not affected in a uniform way.

In ALI/ARDS patients, infiltrates in lung parenchyma are seen by chest radiographs in up to 70–80% of the lung fields, depending on the severity of respiratory failure. The proportion of lung that can be ventilated, is consequently being reduced to almost 20–30% of a normal lung, and therefore, may have the dimensions of a baby lung (11). Thus, the ARDS lung has three compartments: one substantially normal (healthy zone); one fully diseased without any possibility of recruitment (diseased zone); and finally one composed of collapsed alveolar, potentially recruitable with maneuvers (recruitable zone) (12). Thus, the overall thorax volume is not substantially different between ARDS and normal patients, suggesting that in ARDS, the decrease in lung volume does not indicate a decrease in total thoracic volume, but a simple replacement of gas with tissue volume (13).

The reduction of respiratory compliance, a typical finding in ARDS, was previously attributed to the severity of the disease and/or to intrinsic mechanical alterations of the lung tissue. Using chest tomography, Gattinoni and coworkers (12) demonstrated that, contrary to commonly accepted notion, respiratory compliance was not related to the amount of "disease" tissue, but to the amount of residual inflated lung, indicating that the smaller the portion of lung open to gas, the lower the compliance. Whereas respiratory compliance was correlated with a normally inflated part of the lung, the gas exchange impairment was strongly related to the amount of noninflated tissue mass, that is, to the extent of the disease (12). These data suggest that the main cause of severe hypoxemia is the perfusion of the noninflated lung tissue. Moreover, these investigators hypothesized that the dependent lung regions, where the majority of noninflated tissue is present, may be underperfused, as evidenced by the discrepancy between the shunt fraction and the noninflated tissue fraction (i.e., 30% of shunt with 60% of noninflated tissue). The underperfusion of this lung region resulted in mechanical compression of the blood vessels and worsening hypoxic pulmonary constriction (13).

Further studies using regional computer tomography analysis of the lung, Brismar and coworkers (14) found that in the supine position, the disease homogenously affected all lung parenchyma with no part of the lung being healthy, and interstitial edema did not exhibit gravity-dependent distribution along the vertical gradient (Fig. 1). These findings were in accordance with previous reports obtained in a number of animal experiments of respiratory failure (15,16) and in cardiogenic pulmonary edema (17). It appears that the primary mechanism leading to edema, at least in ARDS, acts equally in each part of the lung. Thus, edema cannot move freely through the interstitial space, but the reason for this distribution is not completely understood. As a consequence, whatever the role of the thoracic or lung shape, in ARDS the increased regional superimposed pressure is the major factor explaining the increased regional inflation gradients, since it causes lung deflation and collapse along the vertical gradient due to increased weight (18).

Understanding the regional perfusion and ventilation factors is important in order to determine the effect of body position on these variables. In the upright position, perfusion increases from the nondependent to the dependent lung regions, approximately three

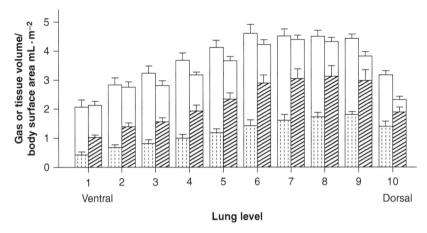

Figure 1 Tissue and gas volumes in supine lung levels 1 (ventral) to 10 (dorsal) in normal subjects (first bar in each pair) and in patients with ARDS (second bar in each pair). The total lung volumes were similar in the two groups. In patients with ARDS, the gas volume was lower and tissue volume higher in each level. *Source*: From Ref. 14.

quarters of the way down the lung and below (19–21). The increase in perfusion gradients has classically been explained by the relationship between the intravascular hydrostatic pressure and the alveolar pressure at various gravitational levels (lung zone 1 and 2) together with distensibility to the pulmonary circulation (zone 3) (19). The decrease in perfusion occurring in more dependent regions (i.e., zone 4) has been attributed to several factors including extra-alveolar vessel narrowing resulting from low volumes; interstitial edema present in the area (21,22); and hypoxic vasoconstriction (23). At the same time, the gravitational gradient described in the upright position has also been observed in the supine and lateral decubitus positions.

Several investigators have shown that there is a gravitational gradient of regional alveolar volume in the different body positions. In upright and supine position, the nonde-pendent alveoli are more expanded than those in the dependent lung regions at functionally residual capacity (FRC) and at all lung volumes above FRC until the lung reaches total lung capacity (20,24,25). Accordingly, under normal conditions, during tidal breathing from FRC to end expiration, alveolar volume ventilation increases along the gravitational gradients (26). When ventilation is below FRC, small airways in the dependent lung regions are closed and the early part of inhalation is directed to less dependent regions. In summary, in patients with ALI/ARDS the changes in perfusion and ventilation to the lung parenchyma are reduced by placing these patients in a supine position, and as a consequence, there is an improvement in oxygenation.

B. Effects of Prone Position
The gravitational gradients of perfusion described in upright lungs have also been observed at the head-down, supine, and right and left lateral decubitus positions (27,28). Although some investigators have observed an increased gravitational gradient of perfusion in prone

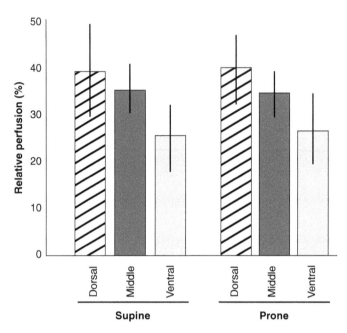

Figure 2 Effect of position on regional distribution of perfusion after oleic acid-induced acute lung injury. Note that prone position has no effect on regional perfusion distribution. *Source*: From Ref. 30.

position, this gradient is markedly reduced compared with that found in the other positions (28,29). In animal studies, Wiener and coworkers (30) described strong gravitational gradient of perfusion in the supine position before and after ALI was produced with oleic acid, but when the animals were turned to prone position, these perfusion gradients changed very little. These observations confirm that the "gravitational" gradient in perfusion does exist, but the role played by gravity in determining the gradient is minimal (Fig. 2).

Several mechanisms have been suggested to explain the more uniform lung perfusion seen in prone positions. Reed and Wood (28) suggested that there might be regional differences in pulmonary vascular resistance resulting from changes in interstitial pressure due to variable regional lung expansion in the two positions. More recently, Beck and Lai-Fook (31) suggested that this explanation is unlikely, particularly over the range of lung volume at which tidal breathing occurs and changes in pulmonary vascular resistance that occur with tidal breathing are extremely small. Other mechanisms may be that caudal movement of the ventral portion of the diaphragm might be reduced in a prone position (29), but this hypothesis has not been supported by recent reports (32). Other investigators suggest that the improvement in oxygenation seen with changes in body position is secondary to improvement of ventilation to dependent lung regions. This explanation is supported by both clinical data and animal experiments demonstrating that prone position reduces arterio-venous shunt. Lung perfusion is preferentially directed to dorsal lung regions regardless of position, such that prone position causes minimum, if any, alteration in regional perfusion. Thus, if there is no change in perfusion, turning a

Table 1 Differences in Transpulmonary Pressure (Ppl cm of water) in Prone and Supine Positions Before and After Volume Infusion

	Before volume infusion		After volume infusion	
	Supine	Prone	Supine	Prone
Nondependent	-3 ± 0.6	-1.3 ± 0.2^a	-2.3 ± 0.2	-0.9 ± 0.2^a
Dependent	7 ± 0.3	-0.1 ± 0.2^a	3 ± 0.5^b	0.9 ± 0.3^b

[a] $p < 0.05$ supine versus prone position, before and after volume infusion.
[b] $p < 0.05$ before versus after volume infusion, supine or prone position.

patient to the prone position mostly improved regional ventilation. Several investigators have studied the effect of the gravitational pleural gradient. The gravitational pleural pressure gradient is more uniform in the prone position compared with the supine position, but the pleural pressure in the dependent regions become positive in the setting of lung edema when measured in the supine position, and turning the patient prone reduces the pleural pressure in the dependent regions (Table 1). Lamm and coworkers (33) directly measured the regional ventilation/perfusion (VE/Q) ratios with SPECT scanning. In the supine position, the VE/Q ratio in normal lungs was distributed in the skewed fashion with the median VE/Q shifted toward values approximating 0.8 (Fig. 3). The VE/Q ratios increased from the dorsal (dependent) to the ventral (nondependent) regions. On turning the animals to prone position, the VE/Q was distributed in a more "gaussian fashion." The median VE/Q was improved and no gravitational gradient were observed. These investigators found that in injured lungs, the VE/Q distribution was markedly altered, and after turning the animal into prone position, the VE/Q distribution shifted considerably. These observations confirm the premise that the pleural pressure gradient did not simply reverse on turning prone such that pleural pressure in these ventral regions was not sufficiently positive because of airspace collapse or failure of airspace opening (Fig. 4).

C. Effect of Mediastinal Weight on Lung Parenchyma

Above, we have discussed that reversible airspace closure occurs in the dorsal lung regions when patients with ALI/ARDS are placed in supine positions, and that turning patients into prone position will alter dorsal lung transpulmonary pressures and reverse airway closure. A number of factors would contribute to the ability of prone position to alter dorsal lung transpulmonary pressures, including among others compressive effects of consolidated lung (34); direct transmission of the weight of abdominal content to the caudal regions of the dorsal lung (5,35); and direct transmission of the heart weight to the lung regions located beneath it (36,37). The idea that the heart can have an impact on the regional lung distention and that the lung can be affected by heart transmural pressures dates back to 1947 when Brookhart and Boyd (36) noted that "the dog's heart produces deformation of the adjacent lung, raising pressure on the external surface of the heart above the pressure existing between the lung and the wall of the thorax." These observations were confirmed by other investigators who suggested that the weight of the heart accounts for regional differences in pleural pressures and compression of lung parenchyma (38–41). The heart–lung interaction and its effect on ventilation were noted by oscillation in expired gas flow (measured at the mouth with a body plethysmograph) that corresponded to the heartbeat

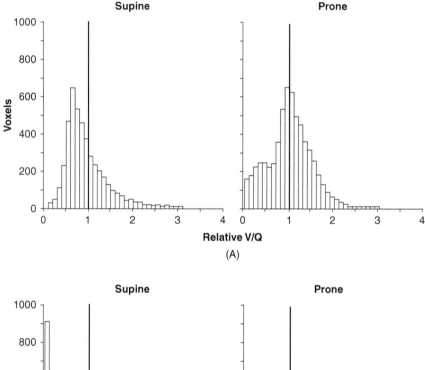

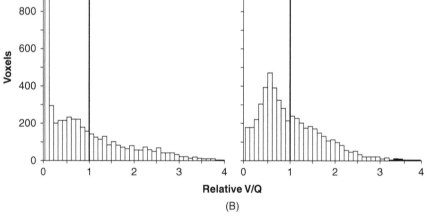

Figure 3 Distribution of regional ventilation and perfusion in (**A**) normal dog, supine and prone. (**B**) Injured dogs after oleic acid-induced acute lung injury, supine and prone. *Source*: From Ref. 33.

(42). These effects are due to a direct local mechanical distortion of the lungs. Other investigators described differences in a single breath oxygen test, which is attributed in part to the weight of the heart (43). Wiener and coworkers (44) described that left lower lobe ventilation is impaired when patients with cardiomegaly were positioned supine, but not when they were positioned prone. All these observations were later confirmed by

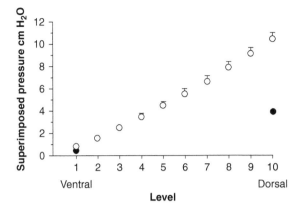

Figure 4 Superimposed pressure in patients with ARDS (open circles) and reference normals (close circles). The superimposed pressure overlying each lung level from nondependent to dependent regions is markedly increased as compared with normals. *Source*: From Ref. 14.

Ball and coworkers (45), who studied the effects of posture on thoracic anatomy using chest tomography and by spatial reconstruction. Hoffman observed marked supine-to-prone differences in the regional air content of the lung, and found that these differences correlated with shift in the position of the mediastinal content, including the heart (46).

Albert and Hubmayr (47) measured the relative lung volume that is located directly under the heart both in supine and prone position. The study population consisted of normal subjects (four male and three females), mean age of 49 ± 18 years (range 28–73). None of the patients had a history of cardiac disease. Four exhaled tomography sections between the carina and the diaphragm were analyzed (sections 1 through 4). When supine, the percent of the total lung volume located under the heart increased from $7 \pm 4\%$ to $42 \pm 8\%$ and from $11 \pm 4\%$ to $16 \pm 40\%$ in sections 1 through 4, in the left and right lungs, respectively. When patients were studied in prone position, the percent of lung volume located under the heart was less than 1% and 4%, left and right lung respectively, in all four sections ($p < 0.05$ for each section, supine vs. prone) (Fig. 5). The main finding of this study was that in the supine position, considerable fraction of both lungs is located underneath the heart and, as such, would be subjected to compressive forces resulting from weight of the heart and the blood contained therein. In the prone position, only a very small fraction of either lung was similarly affected. The investigators suggested that the clinical implications of these findings are that these changes will lower the inspiratory and end-expiratory pressures required to obtain maximum airspace recruitment (i.e., alveolar recruitment and/or airway opening), and reduce cyclical airspace opening and closing. If ventilator-induced lung injuries are related to any or all of these factors, then routine use of prone position could translate into reduction of morbidity and mortality in patients with ALI/ARDS.

A major limitation of this study is that it was done on normal subjects and we do not know if the same changes are going to happen in patients with underlying lung disease. The isolated effect of heart weight will be difficult to estimate in patients with ARDS.

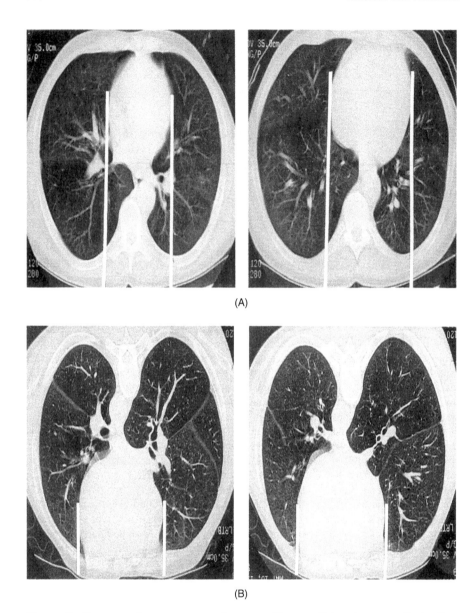

(A)

(B)

Figure 5 Computer chest tomograms, the areas of lung medial to the perpendicular lines were quantified as being under the heart. (**A**) supine position (**B**) prone position. *Source*: From Ref. 47.

In this disease state, there are markedly regional variations in lung volume; the alveolar space is fluid filled to variable degrees; there is soft tissue edema that alters thoracic and abdominal compliance; there are variable abdominal wall edema, ascites, and increased abdominal pressure; and patients may or may not have cardiomegaly. All these parameters may explain the variability in gas exchange improvement that is seen when patients with ARDS are turned from supine to prone position.

D. Can Prone Position Have an Impact in Ventilator-Induced Injury?

Numerous reports have indicated that ventilating the lungs with excessive volume is deleterious and ventilator-induced lung injury can occur (48,49). Furthermore, we now understand that the lung injury is not homogenous and as previously described, mechanical ventilation is limited to a small portion of the lung parenchyma ("baby lung") (11,15). So, consensus has emerged that tidal volume should be kept at or below the static inflation pressure of 35 cm of H_2O; and PEEP should be titrated to exceed airway-opening pressure (50). The initial studies by Webb and Tierney (51) demonstrated that although high inflation pressure and large volume ventilation produce lung injury and edema, the adverse effects were markedly reduced by adding PEEP. The working hypothesis is that lung injury results from the sheer force associated with repeat airspace opening and closing, and lung injury is not uniform (52). If volutrauma were caused by lung overdistention, this effect will be distributed preferentially to the lung ventral regions where lung distention is greater. The fact that they were not, is consistent with the idea that sheer forces associated with airspace opening and closing are responsible for the injury (53). These data suggest that our attention should be directed more toward preventing airspace closure than on avoiding lung overdistention. Accordingly, various ventilatory strategies have been proposed to counter this effect. Amato and coworkers (54), first demonstrated that such an approach could reduce the mortality of patients with ARDS. This work was confirmed by the study completed by the ARDS Network, which found that using a tidal volume of 6 mL/kg as opposed to 12 mL/kg ideal body weight decreased mortality by 25% (from 40% to 30%) (2). Accordingly, strong arguments can be made today that ventilator-induced injuries are clinical important entities that adversely affect clinical outcome. These studies also confirmed a decrease in the number of multiple organ failure, confirming the prior hypothesis that how mechanical ventilation is applied will have an impact on patient survival, not only by improving oxygenation, but also by decreasing other organ damage (2).

It has been suggested by animal experiments that the severity and distribution of ventilator-induced lung injury is altered by the combination of PEEP, prone position, and respiratory frequency (55). The ability of prone ventilator position to generate more uniform lung distention and to reduce the compressive effect of the dorsal lung in the setting of ALI would seem to be major theoretical benefit and may account for the improvement of oxygenation seen in most patients. Broccard and coworkers (56) have expanded this theory by confirming that supine ventilation can cause lung injury and by demonstrating that ventilating animals in prone position can reduce the extent of lung injury. Albert and Lamm (57) showed in an oleic acid injured dog model that early prone position could markedly reduce the lung inflammatory response. In this study, after the animals were injured, they were immediately randomized to either supine or prone position, and then ventilated for six hours on 100% oxygen. Thirty minutes after the start of mechanical ventilation, there were significant differences in oxygenation between groups. Furthermore, there were also differences in lung weight to dry ratio; whole lung lavage cell counts and protein content. The percentage of polymorphic nucleated white blood cells (WBC) was lower in animals ventilated in prone position than in supine, 49 ± 21 versus 77 ± 24 ($p = 0.06$) respectively. These data suggested that early use of prone ventilation in dogs, not only improved oxygenation, but also limited the inflammatory burden. These data have not been confirmed in humans.

E. Impact of Prone Ventilation on the Heart

Patients with ARDS develop acute cor-pulmonale and this condition may worsen by ventilator settings such as pressure-limited ventilation and the development of hypercarbia. Prone ventilation has been shown to reduce airway pressure and improved alveolar ventilation. The effect of prone ventilation on right ventricle (RV) overload in ARDS patients was reported by Vieillard-Baron and coworkers (80). These investigators studied 42 ARDS patients treated with prone position with PaO_2/FiO_2 ratio of <100 mm Hg. RV function was evaluated by bedside transesophageal echocardiography before and after prone positioning. The investigators found that before prone positioning 50% patients had acute cor-pulmonale, defined by RV enlargement associated with septal dyskinesia. In these patients, prone ventilation produced a significant decrease in mean RV enlargement and significant reduction in mean septal dyskinesia. These data demonstrate that prone ventilation may have significant impact in RV pressure overload and function in patients with severe ARDS.

F. The Use of Prone Ventilation in ARDS

The importance of body position changes during mechanical ventilation was first demonstrated by Ray and coworkers (58) in three groups of anesthetized dogs with experimentally induced ALI. A control group was left immobile; a second group was turned from side to side every hour; and a third group was turned every half hour. The PaO_2 values fell sharply in the control group, and there was significant arterial-venous shunting. The second group had some improvement in PaO_2 values and decreased shunting, but the PaO_2 values returned to normal in only the third group. The first use of changes in body position in humans was reported by Piehl and Brown (3) in five patients with ARDS. Their data suggest that $180°$ changes in position resulted in a significant increase in PaO_2 (47 torr), presumably by reduction of alveolar-arterial oxygen gradients and improvement in ventilation-perfusion ratios. These data were later confirmed by Douglas and coworkers (4) who studied the benefit of prone positioning in six patients; five on the ventilator and one with a nonrebreather oxygen mask. These patients had variable periods of prone ventilation, but overall there was a significant increase in PaO_2 by a mean of 69 mm Hg [range 2–178 mm Hg using the same tidal volume, fraction of inspired oxygen (FiO_2), and level of PEEP]. The prone position made it possible to reduce the FiO_2 in four of the five patients who required mechanical ventilation. The investigators did not notice any significant change in other parameters, including $PaCO_2$, respiratory frequency, or static compliance. These studies were done based on the theoretical work postulated by Bryan (5) who advocated a trial of prone position for patients who required mechanical ventilation, suggesting that position changes may enhance the patient's lung expansion and ventilation of the dorsal areas. Despite these encouraging clinical results, prone ventilation has not become an integral part of the treatment of respiratory failure. Langer and

Table 2 Ventilation/Perfusion Effect of Prone Position in ARDS

1. Reduction in shunt.
2. Perfusion is preferentially directed to dorsal lung regions regardless of position.
3. The gravitational pleural pressure gradient is more uniform.
4. Pleural pressure is reduced in dependent regions.
5. The regional ventilation/perfusion ratio is more uniform and better matched.

coworkers (59) demonstrated that prone position resulted in a disappearance of infiltrates in the dorsal regions of the lung visualized by computed tomography scan, and at the same time there was an increase in arterial oxygenation in some, but not all patients. Since then, a large number of research studies have been focused on trying to understand the pathophysiology and the reason for improvement in oxygenation previously discussed with prone ventilation in ALI/ARDS, the potential mechanisms are summarized in Table 2.

While most of the clinical studies focused on the short-term physiological effect and the mechanism why prone position improved oxygenation, Fridrich and coworkers (60) demonstrated a significant long-term benefit on gas exchange in a group of patients with trauma-induced ARDS. These investigators studied 20 patients with ARDS and severe hypoxemia despite the fact they were ventilated using inversed ratio ventilation and high PEEP. These patients were periodically placed in prone position up to 20 hours per day over several days without any major complications. Patients were reassessed every morning in a supine position, and if the patient's hypoxemia persisted, they were again placed in the prone position. The oxygen variables improved significantly each time the patient was placed in the prone position. Immediately after the first turn from the supine to prone position, the investigators observed that the Pao_2 increased from a mean of 97 ± 4 to 152 ± 15 mm Hg ($p \leq 0.05$) with a significant decrease in intrapulmonary shunt. Most of these improvements were lost when the patients were turned supine, but could be reproduced when prone position was repeated after a short period (four hours) in the supine position. Investigators placed patients in supine position in order to allow nursing care, medical evaluation, and intervention such as placement of central lines. No position-dependent changes in systemic hemodynamics were observed. The overall mortality of the study group was 10%. The homogeneity of the patient group in terms of etiology, prestudy ventilation time, early onset of positioned therapy may be all important factors for the positive response of prone position seen in these patients.

Chatte and coworkers (61) reported the pattern of Pao_2 and Fio_2 response when patients with severe acute respiratory failure (Pao_2/Fio_2 ratio of less than 150) were turned from a supine to prone position. Thirty-two consecutive patients with heterogenous causes of ARDS including sepsis, aspiration, pneumonia, etc., were studied one hour before, one and four hours during, and one hour after being placed in prone position. The Pao_2/Fio_2 was 103 ± 28, 158 ± 62, 159 ± 59, and 128 ± 52, respectively (ANOVA, $p < 0.01$). Seven patients in the study (22%) did not show an improvement in oxygenation; they are referred as nonresponders. Twenty-three patients (78%) had a significant improvement and they are referred as responders. Among the seven nonresponders, two did not tolerate the prone position and were returned to preprone position before the end of the four-hour trial. In the other five patients, the Pao_2/Fio_2 ratio remained below 90. In 10 of the 23 responders (43%), the Pao_2/Fio_2 ratio returned to their preprone value when

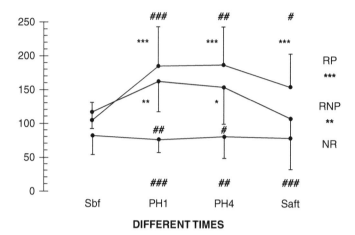

Figure 6 Evolution of Pao_2/Fio_2 before, during, and after the first four hours of prone trial. *Abbreviations*: RP, responders persistent; RNP, responders nonpersistent; NR, no responders; Sbf, one hour before prone; PH1, first hour during prone; PH4, fourth hour during prone; Saft, one hour after supine. $*, **, *** = p < 0.05$ vs. NR; $\#, \#\#, \#\#\# = p < 0.05$ vs. RNP. *Source*: From Ref. 61.

patients were repositioned—these patients are called partial responders. In 13 of the other 23 patients (57%), improvement in oxygenation persisted in the supine position. These patients did not require repositioning from supine to prone (Fig. 6). The investigators collected safety data during 994 episodes of prone positioning. Superficial cutaneous and mucosa damage was frequently seen, mainly affecting the anterior chest wall, lips, tongue, or forehead. Subcutaneous edema was seen in all the patients. Two patients had severe decrease in their oxygen saturation when placed in the prone position. Overall, excluding cutaneous and mucosa damage, these investigators reported, a low number of side effects in 6/32 (19%) of all patients, but only 6/294 during prone position (2%). The overall mortality of the study group was 56% (18/32) and none were related to prone position. It is important to point out that in this study, the investigators stated that four attendants helped turning the patients from supine to prone position. The tolerance to prone position was systematically monitored during this trial; hemodynamic measures did not show any significant changes in cardiac output, mean arterial pressure, capillary wedge pressure, and pulmonary and/or systemic vascular resistance. This was the first study to identify that there are three different types of response when patients with ARDS are placed from supine to prone position: nonresponders, partial responders, and responders. Furthermore, this study identified that patients with the lower Pao_2/Fio_2 ratio and the highest PEEP are the less likely to improve during prone position.

Studies by Jolliet and coworkers (62) reported a lower percentage of patients responding to prone position (57%). These investigators described that if a patient improved during prone, when returned to supine position were more likely to respond to additional prone positioning (71% of the time), but if the patients were initially nonresponders, they were less likely to respond (25%). Furthermore, these investigators described the absence of response to prone position was not accompanied by worsening hypoxemia or hemodynamic instability. They concluded that repeated daily trials of prone position should be considered in the management of ARDS patients with severe hypoxemia.

The application of ventilator-protective strategies such as low-volume, pressure-limited ventilation in combination with prone position was first reported by Stocker and coworkers (63). These investigators studied 25 patients with a mean age of 38 years who had trauma or postoperative-induced ARDS. Based on the APACHE II score of 24, the predicted mortality rate of the study groups was 35.4%. Seventeen of the 25 patients were treated employing prone position. Patients were not placed in the prone position if they had severe head injury with elevated intracranial pressure, spine fractures that could not be stabilized, and the presence of focal neurologic deficits. The median time interval between ICU admission and first prone position was 10 days (1–26 days). The prone protocol consisted of turning the patients to prone position and keeping them as long as Pao_2/Fio_2 ratio improved and/or remained stable. These investigators reported that all the patients had an improvement in their Pao_2/Fio_2 ratio when they were placed in prone position. Prone/supine position periods varied considerably from patient to patient (range 2–66 hours). The number of prone positions and maneuvers varied noticeably as well (range 1–9 times). These investigators reported two serious complications during prone positions. In one, the patient became septic after turned to prone, and another suffered an infectious corneal ulceration and needed immediate surgery. The mortality of the overall group was 12%, significantly lower than the predicted mortality. The major contribution of the work of Stocker and coworkers was that these investigators kept their patients in the prone position as long as gas exchange improved or least did not deteriorate (up to 48 hours). However, the response in terms of required number and duration of positional maneuvers differ significantly among the patients. Furthermore, they also reported that the clinical response was independent for the patient's initial Fio_2, lung injury score, and days of ventilator support prior to position changes. Whereas some of the patients showed an immediate improvement, other started to improve after variable time intervals, up to 24 hours. The investigators hypothesized that the improvement in oxygenation was due to a more homogenous regional inflation distribution, and therefore a redistribution of ventilation from dorsal areas, the nondependent lung regions. For the delayed response, the investigators do not have any explanation and they speculate that edema redistribution, reabsorption, and/or that the increase of ventilated lung volume may augment PEEP effects in the nonventilated lung areas. The data suggest that low-volume, pressure-limited ventilation combined with permissive hypercapnia and prone positioning lowers mortality of ARDS.

Nakos and coworkers (64) examined the effect of prone positioning in mechanically ventilated patients with hydrostatic pulmonary edema (HPE), patients with ARDS (early and late disease), and patients with pulmonary fibrosis. All the patients were ventilated with volume-control ventilation, the tidal volume was set at 6 to 8 mL/kg body weight, frequency set 15 to 25 per minute, PEEP was set just above the value of lower inflation point of the pressure volume curve, or 10 cm H_2O if they were not able to determine this value. Plateau pressure was kept lower than 35 cm of H_2O in all the patients. Patients with HPE were turned to the prone position after being mechanically ventilated for at least six hours, needed an Fio_2 of more than 60% to achieve an oxygen saturation of 90% or more, and did not respond to recruiting maneuvers. All patients with HPE had a significant improvement in oxygenation when they were placed in the prone position. The Pao_2/Fio_2 ratio increased from 72 ± 16 in the supine position to 208 ± 61 after six hours in prone position ($p < 0.001$). This increase in oxygenation was persistent and was not associated with any detrimental effect on hemodynamics. Fifteen of 20 patients with ARDS (75%) improved oxygenation in the prone position. The Pao_2/Fio_2 ratio increased form 83 ± 14 in the supine position to 189 ± 34 after six hours of prone position ($p < 0.01$). In contrast, five of 20 patients with ARDS (25%) and none of the patients with pulmonary fibrosis showed any improvement in oxygenation during prone position. In this study, not all the patients with ARDS had a significant response. These investigators were able to identify that patients with "early ARDS" (less than 36 hours elapsed from the onset of the precipitating factor and diagnosis of ARDS) responded better to prone position that patients with "late ARDS" (more than 36 hours elapsed from the onset to the diagnosis of ARDS). It is worth to point out that in all the "late ARDS" the precipitating factor was related to direct insult to the lung. This study showed an improvement in the mortality rate for both patients with HPE and ARDS who were turned prone, compared with their predicted mortality. However, the small number of patients made this comparison powerless to draw definitive conclusions about the influence of position on outcome. In patients with HPE, the oxygenation improvement could be partially due to the relief of the compressive effect of an enlarged heart to the dorsal lung regions. The persistent improvement after turning the patient back to the supine position may be due to a substantial decrease in pulmonary edema, and the relative decrease in heart size, because of treatment. Most of these patients had significant improvement in hemodynamics, mainly manifested by an increase in cardiac index. The increase in cardiac index will improve the V/Q relationship and could be related to the reduction in pulmonary vascular resistance, and improved performance of both right and left ventricle. The reduction in pulmonary vascular resistance in both HPE and ARDS patients probably is related to decreased hypoxic pulmonary vasoconstriction or recruitment of atelectatic areas (65). Apart from prone position, factors such as low tidal volume and PEEP could have contributed to the favorable outcomes seen in this study. The major contributions of this study are that the clinical utility of prone ventilation has been shown in other conditions, such as HPE. On one side, the existence of pulmonary edema, in both early ARDS and HPE, can be considered as predictors of beneficial effect of prone positioning on gas exchange. On the other side, the presence of lung fibrosis, such as in late ARDS or pulmonary fibrosis, results in no effect to prone positioning.

In order to assess the effect of prone ventilation on survival in ARDS, several large, randomized, international clinical studies have been conducted. Gattinoni and coworkers (66) reported the results of an international multicenter, randomized trial of patients with ALI and/or ARDS that compared treatment in the supine position with a predefined strategy of placing patients in a prone position for six or more hours daily for up to 10 days. These investigators enrolled 304 patients, 152 patients in each group. Patients were assessed each morning while in supine position and were changed to prone if the Pao_2/Fio_2 ratio was 200 or less, with a PEEP of at least 6 cm of H_2O; or a Pao_2/Fio_2 ratio of 300 or less with a PEEP of at least 10 cm of H_2O. In two patients assigned to the supine group, the prone position was used due to persistent hypoxemia. In the prone group, logistic problems, mainly staffing limitations, resulted in noncompliance in 41 patients, a total of 91 missing periods of prone positioning over a 10-day period. The mortality rate was 23% during the 10-day study period, 49.3% at the time of discharge from the intensive care unit, and 60.5% at six months. The relative rate of death in the prone group as compared with the supine group was 0.84 at the end of the study period

(95% confidence interval; 0.56–1.27), 1.05 at the time of discharge from the intensive care unit (95% confidence interval, 0.84–1.32); and 1.06 at six months (95% confidence interval, 0.88–1.28). Patients randomized to the prone position remained in this position for an average of 7.0 ± 1.8 hours per day. For all 721 maneuvers, the median change in the Pao_2/Fio_2 ratio was 28 at one hour (range 128–303) and 44 (range 101–319) at the end of the period of pronation. In 73.2% of the pronation procedures, the Pao_2/Fio_2 ratio increased more than 10, with 69.9% of the total response observed during the first hour (Fig. 7). A posthoc analysis showed a significant lower 10-day mortality rate in the prone group compared to the supine group in the patients with the lowest quartile Pao_2/Fio_2 ratio <88%; 23.1% versus 47.2% (relative risk of death 0.49, 95% confidence interval, 0.25–0.95). Other parameters identified in posthoc analysis that were associated with decreased mortality associated with prone ventilation included the highest Simplified Acute Physiological Score II (>49), and the quartile with the highest tidal volume, >12 mL/kg predicted body weight. The number of new or worsening pressure sores per patient was significantly higher in the prone than in the supine group during the 10-day study period, whereas the number of total days with pressure sores per patient was similar in both groups. As expected, the patients' weight bearing areas, thorax, cheekbone, iliac crest, breast, and neck were significantly more likely to be affected in the prone group. There were no differences in other adverse events including accidental displacement of tracheal or thoracotomy tube, or loss of venous access. The investigators concluded that despite the limitations related to having a smaller number of patients than the originally estimated sample size, the data suggested that prone ventilation of patients with ALI/ARDS did not improve survival. However, these investigators found that prone position improved oxygenation in more than 70% of time in which it was used, with

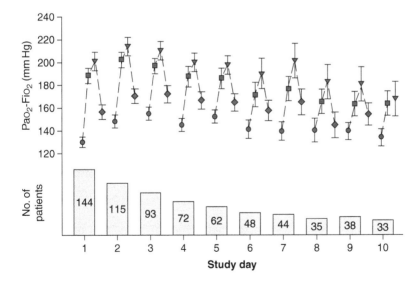

Figure 7 Changes in Pao_2/Fio_2 over 10 days. Data shown are daily measures before prone positioning (circles), after one hour (squares), at the end period of pronation (triangles), and on the morning following day (diamonds). *Source*: From Ref. 71.

about 30% of the effect occurring during the first hour of pronation. Thus, the Pao_2/Fio_2 ratio increased significantly in the prone patients. These data suggest that prone position alters the underlying conditions in the respiratory system that leads to worsening of gas exchange in ALI/ARDS. Furthermore, the effect persists in part beyond the period of pronation. Safety has been one of the major concerns with use of prone ventilation; this study found that in a multicenter trial, there was no increase in complications. It is important to point out that the percentages of patients with new or worsening pressure sores or with displacement of endotracheal tubes, vascular catheters, or thoracotomy tubes were similar in the two groups.

Guerin and coworkers (67) reported the results of a French multicenter, randomized trial of patients with ALI and/or ARDS randomly assigned to prone position for at least eight hours per day on standard beds, or supine position placement. These investigators enrolled 791 patients, 413 patients in the prone position group and 378 patients in the supine group. The primary end point was 28-day mortality, secondary end points were 90-day mortality, duration of mechanical ventilation, incidence of ventilator-associated pneumonia (VAP), and oxygenation. The study protocol mandated that patients received prone ventilation for at least eight hours a day. The two groups had comparable baseline demographic characteristics. Prone position was applied a mean of 8.6 (6.6) hours/day for 4.1 (4.7) days. Prone position was not adequately placed in 25% of patients. The 28-day mortality rate was 32.4% for the prone position group, and 31.5% for the supine group [relative risk (RR), 0.97; 95% confidence interval (CI), 0.79–1.19; $p = 0.77$]. Ninety-day mortality for the prone group was 43.3% versus 42.2 for the supine group (RR, 0.98; 95% CI, 0.84–1.13; $p = 0.75$). The mean duration of mechanical ventilation was 13.7 (7.8) days for the prone group versus 14.1 (8.6) days for the supine group ($p = 0.93$); and the VAP incidence was 1.66 versus 2.14 episodes per 100 patients days of intubation, respectively ($p = 0.045$). The median change in the Pao_2/Fio_2 ratio was higher in patients in the prone position during the first 28 days of mechanical ventilation. The number of new or worsening pressure sores per patient was significantly higher in the prone than in the supine group. There were also increased incidence of accidental displacement of endotracheal tube, and tube obstruction in the prone ventilation group. This study demonstrated no benefit of prone ventilation on patients' outcomes, including mortality, and duration of ventilator support. The investigators reported reduction in complications such as VAP. This study has important limitation that we need to point out. First, several patients with severe hypoxemia that were randomized to the supine group, were allowed to be place in a prone position. Second, in this study the investigators did not mandate a ventilator and/or weaning management protocol. Thus, patients did not receive current standard of care of protective ventilation strategist. This study showed similar improvement of oxygenation as Gattinoni and coworkers (66), but also demonstrate that oxygenation can not accurately predict mortality in these patients.

More recent, Mancebo and coworkers (68) and Fernandez and coworkers (69) reported the results of two multicenter, randomized trial of patients with ALI and/or ARDS that were already been treated with protective ventilation strategies and randomly assigned to prone position continuous for >20 hours per day on standard beds, or supine position placement. Both trials were prematurely stopped due to a low patient recruitment rate. These studies verified prior observations, that the oxygenation was significant improved in the prone group. Fernandez and coworkers (69) reported that the Pao_2/Fio_2 tended to be higher in prone patient after six hours; on day 3 was 234 ± 85 versus 159 ± 78

prone and supine groups, respectively ($p < 0.05$). The intensive care unit mortality in the Mancebo and coworkers study (68) was 43% (33/76) in patients ventilated prone; and 58% (35/60) in patients ventilated supine, but this difference did not reach statistical significance. Multivariate analysis showed that simplified acute physiology score II at inclusion (OR 1.07; $p < 0.001$); number of days elapsed between ARDS diagnosis and inclusion (OR 2.83; $p < 0.001$); and randomized to supine position (OR 2.53; $p < 0.003$) were independent risks factors for mortality. These investigators demonstrated that prone ventilation is feasible, safe, and may reduce mortality.

More recently, Abroug and coworkers (70) published a meta-analysis of five trials that included 1372 patients that met a predefined criteria for mortality analysis. Using a fixed-effects model, the investigators did not find a significant effect of prone position on mortality. Clinical parameters including Pao_2/Fio_2 increased significantly with proning, but there was no significant reduction of mechanical ventilation such as VAP, airway complications, length of intensive care unit. The investigators concluded that in order to draw definitive conclusions on the value of prone ventilation in ALI/ARDS, the appropriate clinical trial needs to be designed with a patient sample, adequately sized and optimizing the duration of proning and ventilation strategy. Thus, the number of patients who are required in order to demonstrate the difference in survival will make it necessary to have a heterogeneous patient population with ARDS (e.g., trauma, sepsis, aspiration, pneumonia, etc.) (71). Gattinoni and coworkers (66) have suggested that this study is the beginning of further research collaboration that will address these limitations and evaluate the value of longer periods of prone position and the need for standardization of mechanical ventilation in both prone and supine groups according to predefined lung-protective strategies. A clear message of these data is that prone ventilation protects the lung against ventilator-induced injury.

All these studies have shown that patient selection, studying patients with ARDS caused by primary pulmonary disease, or secondary to extrapulmonary conditions have an impact on outcome. Several investigators have suggested that based on the etiology of ARDS, there may be two separate syndromes (72–75). Differences in respiratory mechanics and response to mechanical ventilation and PEEP are consistent with the presence of consolidation in the lung parenchyma as opposed to edema and alveolar collapse (34,74). Furthermore, patients with ARDS as their main cause of mechanical ventilation may have different disease than ARDS that develops during the course of mechanical ventilation (76). The latter syndrome is associated with increased multiple organ failure and increased mortality (76). Therefore, due to the heterogenicity of this syndrome, both precipitating factors and onset of presentation will have to be taken into consideration when designing clinical trials in ARDS.

In order to improve patient's long-term outcomes and survival in ARDS, it may be necessary to use a combination of several adjunctive therapies. Papazian and coworkers (77) evaluated the hemodynamic and respiratory effect of the combination of inhaled nitric oxide and prone position in patients with ARDS. These investigators studied supine and prone position with and without nitric oxide. Inhaled nitric oxide resulted in an increase in Pao_2/Fio_2 ratio that was comparable to the changes seen with prone position alone. The association of nitric oxide and prone position resulted in a further improvement in Pao_2/Fio_2 ratio when compared with baseline, or prone position alone, and/or supine position with nitric oxide. Analysis of variance showed a significant additive effect of nitric oxide to prone position in both Pao_2/Fio_2 ratio ($p < 0.0001$) and shunt fraction

($p < 0.01$). This study showed that there is an additive effect in oxygenation by using these two therapies. This study suggested a decrease in mortality when these two therapies are used, but it is important to point out that this was not the main endpoint, and it was not statistically powered to show a difference or decreased mortality. These observations have been confirmed by Johannigman and coworkers (78) in 16 patients with ARDS who were ventilated in the supine position with nitric oxide (one part per million) or prone position with nitric oxide. The Pao_2/Fio_2 increased by 14% with nitric oxide in 62% of patients (10/16 patients) in the supine position, and by 33% in 87% of the patients (14/16) in the prone position. The combination of nitric oxide and prone position resulted in an improvement in 94% of patients (15/16) with a mean increase in Pao_2/Fio_2 of 59%. The investigators also noted that there was a significant reduction in pulmonary vascular resistance during the use of nitric oxide in both supine and prone position. There were no significant hemodynamic effects of either therapy. The investigators conclude that there may be synergistic effect of these two therapies. Other combinations of therapies that have been used included the report by Varkul and coworkers (79) of high frequency oscillatory ventilation, prone positioning, and inhaled nitric oxide in patients with severe hypoxemia. Due to the fact that patients with ARDS clearly have many complex and dynamic physiological derangements, it may be necessary to consider the combination of multiple therapies for patients with severe disease or persistent hypoxemia.

II. Conclusion

Clinical studies have clearly demonstrated in ALI/ARDS patients, prone position results in significant and clinical relevant improvement in oxygenation, and these changes occur within the first hours. We also know that the degree of oxygenation improvement is not related to the extent to which gas exchange was impaired; improvement can persist in patients when they are returned to supine position; and beneficial response is not limited to patients who are turned early in the course of the disease, although the data suggest that early use may be more beneficial. Patients who fail to respond initially may improve during subsequent attempts of turning. The incidence of complications associated with the use of prone ventilation is small. Animal research and clinical experience suggest that prone ventilation may protect the lung from the potential detrimental effects of mechanical ventilation. Further studies are needed to further characterize these findings.

References

1. Ashbaugh DG, Bigelow DB, Petty TL, et al. Acute respiratory distress in adults. Lancet 1967; ii:319–323.
2. The Acute Respiratory Distress Syndrome Network. Ventilation with lower tidal volumes as compared with traditional tidal volumes for acute lung injury and the acute respiratory distress syndrome. N Engl J Med 2000; 342:1301–1308.
3. Piehl MA, Brown RS. Use of extreme position changes in acute respiratory failure. Crit Care Med 1976; 4:13–14.
4. Douglas WW, Rehder K, Beynen FM, et al. Improved oxygenation in patients with acute respiratory failure: the prone position. Am Rev Respir Dis 1977; 115:559–566.
5. Bryan AC. Comments of a devil's advocate. Am Rev Respir Dis 1974; 110:43.
6. Gattinoni L, Pesenti A, Torresin A, et al. Adult respiratory distress syndrome profiles by computed tomography. J Thorac Imaging 1986; 1:25–30.

7. Rinaldo JE, Rogers RM. Adult respiratory distress syndrome: changing concepts of lung injury and repair. N Engl J Med 1982; 306:900–909.
8. Gattinoni L, Mascheroni D, Torresin A, et al. Morphological response to positive end-expiratory pressure in acute respiratory failure: computerized tomography study. Intensive Care Med 1986; 56:1091–1130.
9. Rommelscheim K, Lakner K, Westhofen P, et al. Das respiratorische distress-syndrom des erwachsenen (ARDS) im computer-tomogramn. Anasth Intensivther Notfallmed 1983; 18: 59–644.
10. Maunder RJ, Shuman WP, McHugh JW, et al. Preservation of normal lung region in adult respiratory distress syndrome: analysis by computed tomography. JAMA 1986; 255: 2463–2465.
11. Gattinoni L, Pesenti A. ARDS: the dishomogeneous lung: facts and hypothesis. Intensive Crit Care Digest 1987; 6:1–4.
12. Gattinoni L, Pesenti A, Avalli L, et al. Pressure volume curve of total respiratory system in acute respiratory failure. Am Rev Respir Dis 1987; 36:730–736.
13. Jones R, Reid L, Zapol WM, et al. Pulmonary vascular pathology: human and experimental studies. In: Zapol WM, Falke KJ, eds. Acute Respiratory Failure. New York/Basel: Marcel Dekker Inc., 1985:23–160.
14. Brismar B, Hedenstierna G, Lundquist H, et al. Pulmonary densities during anesthesia with muscular relaxation: a proposal of atelectasis. Anesthesiology 1985: 62:422–428.
15. Gattinoni L, Pelosi P, Pesenti A, et al. CT scan in ARDS: clinical and physiopathological insights. Acta Anaesthesiol Scand Suppl 1991; 95:87–96.
16. Jones T, Jones HA, Rhodes CG, et al. Distribution of extravascular fluid volumes in isolated perfused lungs measured with H_2O. J Clin Invest 1976; 57:706–713.
17. Wollmer P, Rhodes CG, Deanfield J, et al. Regional extravascular density of the lung in patients with acute pulmonary edema. J Appl Physiol 1970; 8:204–229.
18. Pelosi P, D'Andrea L, Vitale G, et al. Vertical gradient of regional lung inflation in adult respiratory distress syndrome. Am J Respir Crit Care Med 1994; 149:8–13.
19. West JB, Dollery CT. Distribution of blood flow and ventilation-perfusion ratio in the lung, measured with radioactive CO_2. J Appl Physiol 1960; 15:405–410.
20. Ball WC, Stewart PB, Newsham LG, et al. Regional pulmonary function studied with xenon. J Clin Invest 1962; 41:519–531.
21. Bryan AC, Bentivoglio LG, Beerel F, et al. Factors affecting regional distribution of ventilation and perfusion in the lung. J Appl Physiol 1964; 19:395–402.
22. Hughes JMB, Glazier JB, Maloney JE, et al. Effects of extra-alveolar vessels on distribution of blood flow in the dog lung. J Appl Physiol 1968; 25:701–712.
23. Prefaut C, Engel LA. Vertical distribution of perfusion and inspired gas in supine man. Respir Physiol 1981; 43:209–219.
24. Agostoni E, Hyatt RE. Static behavior of the respiratory system. In: Macklem PT, Mead J, eds. Handbook of Physiology. The Respiratory System. Vol 3. Mechanics of Breathing. Bethesda, MD: American Physiological Society, 1986:113–130.
25. Milic-Emili J, Henderson JAM, Dolovich MB, et al. Regional distribution of inspired gas in the lung. J Appl Physiol 1966; 21:749–759.
26. Amis TC, Jones HA, Hughes JMB. Effect of posture on inter-regional distribution of pulmonary ventilation in man. Respir Physiol 1984; 56:145–167.
27. West JB, Dollery CT, Naimark A. Distribution of blood flow in isolated lung: relation to vascular and alveolar pressures. J Appl Physiol 1964; 19:713–724.
28. Reed JH, Wood EH. Effect of body position on vertical distribution of pulmonary blood flow. J Appl Physiol 1979; 28:303–311.
29. Orphanidou D, Hughes JMB, Myers MJ, et al. Tomography of regional ventilation and perfusion using krypton 81 m in normal subjects and asthmatic patients. Thorax 1986; 41:542–551.

30. Wiener CM, Kirk W, Albert RL. Prone position reverses gravitational distribution of perfusion in dog lungs with oleic acid-induced injury. J Appl Physiol 1990; 68:1386–1392.
31. Beck KC, Lai-Fook SJ. Pulmonary blood flow vs. gas volume at various perfusion pressures in rabbit lung. J Appl Physiol 1985; 58:2004–2010.
32. Albert RK, Leasa D, Sanderson M, et al. The prone position improves arterial oxygenation and reduces shunt in oleic acid-induced acute lung injury. Am Rev Respir Dis 1987; 135: 628–635.
33. Lamm WJE, Graham MM, Albert RK. Mechanism by which the prone position improves oxygenation in acute lung injury. Am J Respir Crit Care Med 1994; 150:184–193.
34. Gattinoni LL, D'Andrea P, Pelos P, et al. Regional effects and mechanisms of positive end-expiratory pressure in early adult respiratory distress syndrome. JAMA 1993; 269:2122–2127.
35. Froese AB, Bryan AC. Effects of anesthesia and paralysis on diaphragmatic mechanics in man. Anesthesiology 1974; 41:242–255.
36. Brookhart JM, Boyd TE. Local differences in intrathoracic pressure and their relation to cardiac filling pressure in the dog. Am J Physiol 1947; 148:434–444.
37. Rutishauser WJN, Banchero AG, Tsakiris AC, et al. Pleural pressures at dorsal and ventral sites in supine and prone body positions. J Appl Physiol 1966; 21:1500–1510.
38. Wood EH. Some effects of gravitational and inertial forces on the cardiopulmonary system. Aerosp Med 1967; 38:225–233.
39. Hyatt RE, Bar-Yishay E, Abel MD. Influence on the heart on the vertical gradient of transpulmonary pressure in dogs. J Appl Physiol 1985; 58:52–57.
40. Scharf SM, Caldini P, Ingram RH. Cardiovascular effects of increasing airway pressure in the dog. Am J Physiol 1977; 232:H35–H43.
41. Culver BH, Marini JJ, Butler J. Lung volume and pleural pressure effects on ventricular function. J Appl Physiol 1981; 50:630–635.
42. Bosman AR, Lee GD. The effects of cardiac action upon lung gas volume. Clin Sci 1965; 28:311–324.
43. Cortese DA, Rodarte JR, Rehder K, et al. Effect of posture on the single-breath oxygen test in normal subjects. J Appl Physiol 1976; 41:474–479.
44. Wiener CM, McKenna WJ, Myers MJ, et al. Left lower lobe ventilation is reduced in patients with cardiomegaly in the supine but not in the prone position. Am Rev Respir Dis 1990; 141:150–155.
45. Ball WC, Wicks JD, Mettler FA. Prone-supine change in organ position: CT demonstration. AJR Am J Roentgenol 1980; 135:815–820.
46. Hoffman EA. Effect of body orientation on regional lung expansion: a computed tomographic approach. J Appl Physiol 1985; 59:468–480.
47. Albert RK, Hubmayr RD. The prone position eliminates compression of the lungs by the heart. Am J Respir Crit Care Med 2000; 161:1660–1665.
48. Dreyfuss D, Basset G, Soler P, et al. Intermittent positive-pressure hyperventilation with high inflation pressures produces pulmonary microvascular injury in rats. Am Res Respir Dis 1985; 132:880–884.
49. Dreyfuss D, Saumon G. Role of tidal volume, FRC and end-expiratory volume in the development of pulmonary edema following mechanical ventilation. Am Rev Respir Dis 1993; 148;1194–1203.
50. Slutsky AS. Mechanical ventilation. American College of Chest Physicians' Consensus Conference. Chest 1993; 104:1833–1859.
51. Webb H, Tierney D. Experimental pulmonary edema due to intermittent positive pressure ventilation with high inflation pressures: protection by positive end-expiratory pressure. Am Rev Respir Dis 1974; 110:556–565.
52. Muscedere JG, Mullen JMB, Gan K, et al. Tidal ventilation at low airway pressures can augment lung injury. Am J Respir Crit Care Med 1994; 149:1327–1334.

53. Kolobow T, Moretti MP, Fumagalli R, et al. Severe impairment in lung function induced by high peak airway pressure during mechanical ventilation: an experimental study. Am Rev Respir Dis 1987; 135:312–315.

54. Amato MB, Barbas CS, Medeiros DM, et al. Effect of a protective-ventilation strategy on mortality in the acute respiratory distress syndrome. N Engl J Med 1998; 338:347–354.

55. Sinclair SE, Souders J, Hlastala MP. Severity and distribution of ventilator-induced lung injury (VILI) is altered by PEEP, prone position, and respiratory frequency in normal rabbits. Am J Respir Dis 1998; 157:A107.

56. Broccard A, Shapiro RS, Schmitz LL, et al. Prone position attenuates and redistributes ventilator-induced lung injury in dogs. Crit Care Med 2000; 28:295–303.

57. Albert RK, Lamm WJE. Ventilator-induced augmentation of acute lung injury is limited by prone ventilation. Am J Respir Crit Care Med 1998; 157:A460.

58. Ray JF III, Yost L, Moallem S, et al. Immobility, hypoxemia, and pulmonary arteriovenous shunting. Arch Surg 1974; 109:537.

59. Langer M, Mascheroni D, Marcolin R, et al. The prone position in ARDS patients. A clinical study. Chest 1988; 94:103–107.

60. Fridrich P, Krafft P, Hochlenthner H, et al. Effects of long-term prone positioning n patients with trauma-induced adult respiratory distress syndrome. Anesth Analg 1996; 83:1206–1211.

61. Chatte G, Sab JM, Dubois JM, et al. Prone position in mechanically ventilated patients with severe acute respiratory failure. Am J Respir Crit Care Med 1997; 1555:473–478.

62. Jolliet P, Bulpa P, Chevrolet J-C. Effects of the prone position on gas exchange and hemodynamics in severe acute respiratory distress syndrome. Crit Care Med 1998; 26:1977–1985.

63. Stocker R, Neff T, Stein S, et al. Prone positioning and low-volume pressure-limited ventilation improve survival in patients with severe ARDS. Chest 1997; 111:1008–1017.

64. Nakos G, Tsangaris I, Kostamis E, et al. Effect of the prone position on patients with hydrostatic pulmonary edema compared with patients with acute respiratory distress syndrome and pulmonary fibrosis. Am J Respir Crit Care Med 2000; 161:360–368.

65. Benumof JL. Mechanism of decreased blood flow to atelectatic lung. J Appl Physiol 1979; 46:1047–1048.

66. Gattinoni L, Tognoni G, Pesenti A, et al. Effect of prone positioning on the survival of patients with acute respiratory failure. N Engl J Med 2001; 345:568–573.

67. Guerin C, Gaillard S, Lemasson S, et al. Effects of systematic prone positioning in hypoxemic acute respiratory failure. A randomized Controlled Trial. JAMA 2004; 292:2379–2387.

68. Mancebo J, Fernanandez R, Blanch L, et al. A Multicenter trial of prolonged prone ventilation in severe acute respiratory distress syndrome. Am J Respir Crit Care Med 2006; 173: 1233–1239.

69. Fernandez R, Trenchs X, Klamburg J, et al. Prone positioning in acute respiratory distress syndrome: a multicenter randomized clinical trial. Intensive Care Med 2008; 34:1487–1491.

70. Abroug F, Ouanes-Besbes L, Elantrous S, et al. The effect of prone positioning in acute respiratory distress syndrome or acute lung injury: a meta-analysis. Areas of uncertainty and recommendations for research. Intensive Care Med 2008; 34:1002–1011.

71. Slutsky AS. Prone positioning of patients with acute respiratory failure (correspondence). N Engl J Med 2002; 346(4):295–297.

72. Gattinoni L, Bombino M, Pelosi P, et al. Lung structure and function in different stages of severe adult respiratory distress syndrome. JAMA 1994; 271:1772–1779.

73. Gattinoni L, Pelosi P, Suter PM, et al. Acute respiratory distress syndrome caused by pulmonary and extrapulmonary disease. Am J Respir Crit Care Med 1998; 158:3–11.

74. Rocker GM. Acute respiratory distress syndrome: different syndromes, different therapies? Crit Care Med 2001; 29:210–211.

75. Croce MA, Fabian TC, Davis KA, et al. Early and late acute respiratory distress syndrome: two distinct clinical entities. J Trauma 1999; 46:361–368.

76. Anzueto A, Esteban A, Alia, et al. ARDS before and after start of mechanical ventilation. Am J Respir Crit Care Med 2000; 161:A-382.
77. Papazian L, Bregeon F, Gaillat F, et al. Respective and combined effects of prone position and inhaled nitric oxide in patients with acute respiratory distress syndrome. Am J Respir Crit Care Med 1998; 157:580–585.
78. Johannigman JA, Davis K Jr, Miller SL, et al. Prone positioning and inhaled nitric oxide: synergistic therapies for acute respiratory distress syndrome. J Trauma 2001; 50:589–596.
79. Varkul MD, Stewart TE, Lapinsky SE, et al. Successful use of combined high-frequency oscillatory ventilation, inhaled nitric oxide, and prone positioning in the acute respiratory distress syndrome. Anesthesiology 2001:95:797–799.
80. Vieillard-Baron A, Charron C, Caille V, et al. Prone positioning unloads the right ventricle in severe ARDS. Chest 2007; 132:1440–1446.

18

Mechanical Ventilation in the Acute Respiratory Distress Syndrome

ROY G. BROWER
Pulmonary and Critical Care Medicine, Johns Hopkins University,
Baltimore, Maryland, U.S.A.

LAURENT BROCHARD
Réanimation Médicale, INSERM U 492 and Hopital Henri Mondor,
Université Paris 12, Créteil, France

I. Introduction

Mechanical ventilation (MV) is critical for survival of many patients with acute lung injury and the acute respiratory distress syndrome (ALI/ARDS). Without MV death may occur within hours to days from acute hypoxemic and hypercarbic respiratory failure. With MV there is more time for administration of therapies specific to the cause of ALI/ARDS, such as antibiotics for pneumonia or sepsis, for the host's immune system to fight infections, and for natural healing processes to occur. However, MV can also cause additional lung injury (ventilator-induced lung injury, VILI), which may delay or prevent recovery from acute respiratory failure. Thus, clinicians are challenged to use MV in a manner that maintains acceptable gas exchange but also avoids VILI.

In the first edition of this book (1), we provided an extensive review of the historical evolution of MV in ARDS, mechanisms of injury from MV, lung-protective ventilation strategies, and use of different modes of MV and gas exchange support, including high frequency ventilation and noninvasive ventilation. In this second edition, we focus on information that has become available and ideas that have evolved since publication of the first edition.

II. VILI from High Volumes and Pressures During Inspiration

Traditional approaches to MV in ARDS utilized tidal volumes of approximately 10 to 15 mL/kg (2–4). These large tidal volumes were helpful for maintaining normal arterial PCO_2 and pH despite elevations in dead space. Large tidal volumes were also helpful for maintaining acceptable arterial PO_2 (5,6). However, large tidal volumes (with associated high inspiratory airway pressures) can cause VILI (high volume/pressure VILI). Even when there are no gross manifestations of barotrauma, overdistention of aerated lung tissue can cause inflammation, increased pulmonary vascular permeability, leak of protein-rich fluid from the vascular space into the pulmonary interstitium and alveolar airspaces, shunt, and hypoxemia (7–11). MV with lower tidal volumes and inspiratory airway pressures is associated with modest worsening of gas exchange, but in-hospital mortality is lower with this approach (12–14). Therefore, current recommendations for MV in ARDS include a tidal volume goal of approximately 6 mL/kg predicted (lean) body weight (15–17).

A. Is There a Safe Upper Limit for Inspiratory Plateau Pressure?

Inspiratory plateau pressure (Pplat) is measured in the ventilator circuit with an inspiratory hold, after a tidal volume is delivered and before exhalation (18). In the absence of respiratory muscle activity, Pplat represents the distending pressure of the respiratory system (lungs and chest wall combined). If chest wall elastance did not vary between patients, then higher Pplats in some patients could be attributed to higher distending pressures of their lungs. Some researchers have suggested that Pplats as high as 30 to 35 cm H_2O are safe, and that tidal volume reduction is unnecessary if Pplat is below this level (19,20). This is suggested by several lines of evidence, but different points of view regarding each of these have also been offered.

1. Considerations of normal physiology: In a subject with a normal respiratory system, the Pplat that would result from inflation to a normal total lung capacity is approximately 35 cm H_2O (21). This suggests that a Pplat of 35 cm H_2O is safe. Normal people may perform total lung capacity maneuvers several times in one day, but ALI/ARDS patients usually receive more than 20,000 tidal volumes in one day. Studies in large mammals with initially normal lungs demonstrated ALI after several hours of ventilation with peak lung volumes that were less than total lung capacity (8,22). Moreover, in experimental models injurious effects of overdistention were additive to those of other causes of acute lung inflammation (23,24).

2. Experimental models: VILI was not apparent in some models after MV at peak airway pressures of approximately 30 cm H_2O (9,25,26), but these experiments were of brief duration (less than one hour). VILI *was* apparent after hours-days of MV with peak pressures of 20 to 30 cm H_2O (7,8,22,27), especially when there were other causes of lung inflammation.

3. Comparisons of trials of volume-and-pressure limited MV strategies: In two randomized clinical trials in which volume-and-pressure limited strategies were associated with improved clinical outcomes, the mean Pplat in the higher tidal volume/pressure group exceeded 32 cm H_2O (12,13). In contrast, in three trials in which volume-and-pressure limited MV strategies were not associated with improved clinical outcomes, the mean Pplats in the higher tidal volume/pressure groups were lower than 32 cm H_2O (28–30). This suggested that 32 cm H_2O was the safe upper limit for Pplat (19,31). However, in the three trials that failed to demonstrate beneficial effects of volume-and-pressure limitation, the proportions of patients with Pplats that exceeded 32 cm H_2O were greater in the higher tidal volume/pressure groups than in the lower tidal volume/pressure groups. If 32 cm H_2O was a safe upper limit for Pplat, then we would expect to see trends favoring the lower tidal volume/pressure groups in these trials. Absence of such trends suggests that confounding factors affected the outcomes in these trials (32).

Three studies completed since the first edition of this book suggest that in ARDS patients, the safe upper limit for Pplat is less than 30 cm H_2O. First, in an analysis of the NIH tidal volume trial, the beneficial effects of volume-and-pressure limited MV were

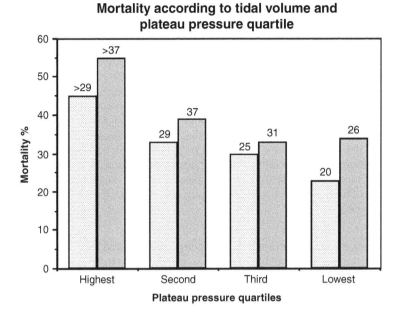

Figure 1 Patients in each of the two study groups in the NIH tidal volume trial (13) were ranked according to plateau pressure on the first day after randomization. Both study groups were then divided into quartiles according to these plateau pressures. Each quartile contained approximately 100 patients. Each vertical bars shows mortality for one of the quartiles of one study group. Lighter bars represent quartiles of the lower tidal volume group. Darker bars represent quartiles of the higher tidal volume group. Numbers above each bar represent the highest plateau pressures in the quartiles. Plateau pressures were below 32 cm H_2O in the third and fourth quartiles of the higher tidal volume study group. Mortality was lower in the lower tidal volume quartiles than in the respective higher tidal volume quartiles. The interaction between quartiles and study group was not significant ($p = 0.23$). *Source*: From Ref. 33.

not significantly different in subsets of patients whose Pplats would have been greater than or less than 32 cm H_2O had they received the higher tidal volume/pressure strategy (Fig. 1) (33). These results suggest that lowering Pplat is of value even when Pplat is already below 30 cm H_2O. It is also possible that the amplitude of the tidal swing in airway pressures affects the development of VILI, independent of Pplat. Second, in a study of ARDS patients receiving tidal volumes of 6 mL/kg predicted body weight, computed tomography in 10 patients (with Pplats of 28–30 cm H_2O) demonstrated that tidal ventilation occurred predominantly in a hyperinflated compartment. In the remaining 20 patients (with Pplats of 25–26 cm H_2O), tidal ventilation occurred predominantly in a normally aerated compartment. Inflammatory cytokine concentrations in bronchoalveolar lavage fluid were significantly greater and ventilator-free days were significantly fewer in the former group (34). Third, in a study of 15 ARDS patients with focal distribution of aeration loss and tidal volumes of 6 mL/kg predicted body weight, Pplats were less than 30 cm H_2O. An analysis of the airway pressure–time relationship suggested that overdistention occurred on these settings. When PEEPs were lowered to reduce overdistention, plasma concentrations of IL-6, IL-8, and sTNF-α RI decreased significantly (35).

These observations strongly suggest that deliberate efforts should be made in most patients to maintain Pplat (or inspiratory pressure with pressure-cycled modes) below 30 cm H_2O. Several clinical recommendations for ventilator management in ARDS suggest the use of a tidal volume goal of 6 mL/kg (15–17). In most ARDS patients, Pplats of 20 to 30 cm H_2O result from tidal volumes of 6 mL/kg. The studies cited in the preceding paragraphs suggest that outcomes could be better if tidal volumes and resulting Pplats were even lower. However, this would probably cause additional hypercapnia and acidosis, deterioration in arterial oxygenation, and increased requirements for sedative medications and, possibly, neuromuscular blockade. Depending on individual clinical circumstances, there may be additional beneficial effects from further reductions in inspiratory pressures and volumes. Effects of more aggressive volume-and-pressure limited MV strategies on clinical outcomes such as mortality and ventilator-free days have not been studied rigorously.

B. Is There a Better Approach to Adjusting Tidal Volume?

In addition to tidal volume, PEEP, and lung elastance, Pplat can also be affected by chest wall elastance and pleural disease. In patients with high chest wall elastance or large pleural effusions, a high Pplat could be associated with relatively low levels of lung stretch. In patients with low chest wall elastance, MV with tidal volumes of 6 mL/kg and with Pplats less than 30 cm H_2O may cause high volume/pressure VILI. A better method of monitoring lung stretch could allow more individualized ventilator management and possibly better clinical outcomes. Some researchers suggest measuring esophageal pressure to estimate pleural pressure and then estimating transpulmonary pressure (P_L) at end inspiration from the difference between Pplat and esophageal pressures (36,37):

$$P_L = \text{Pplat} - \text{Pesoph}$$

This is an attractive idea because P_L reflects lung stress specifically (38), and lung stress is a marker of stretch in aerated lung tissue. However, use of esophageal pressure as a surrogate for pleural pressure is confounded by artifacts in critically ill patients (39–42). To minimize the effects of these artifacts, other workers have estimated lung stress at end inspiration from the *difference* between estimations of P_L at relaxation volume (at airway pressure of zero) and at the peak of inspiration (43):

$$\Delta P_L = (\text{Pao} - \text{Pesoph})_{\text{inspiration}} - (\text{Pao} - \text{Pesoph})_{\text{relaxation}}$$

Assuming the artifacts in esophageal pressure are the same at end expiration and end inspiration, they would disappear in the calculation of the difference. Another assumption in this approach is that changes in esophageal pressure during inspiration represent changes in pleural pressure in general. Another potentially superior alternative to Pplat for monitoring lung stretch is lung strain at peak inspiration. This can be estimated from the ratio of lung volume at peak inspiration to relaxation lung volume (at airway pressure of zero) (43). These are intriguing ideas for monitoring stretching forces in the lungs specifically, and they offer the potential for customizing ventilator settings to the physiologic characteristics of individual patients. However, we need more information regarding safe upper limits for these estimations of stress and strain before we can use these techniques in usual care. Moreover, lung stress and strain at peak inspiration do not account for variations in the pathway to peak inspiration. *Changes* in lung stress and strain during inspiration may be important determinants of VILI, in addition to the peak levels (44,45). Moreover, inspiratory flow rates and waveforms may modulate VILI from high volumes and pressures during inspiration, independent of the maximum or the change in stress or strain (46,47).

C. Volume-and-Pressure Limited MV in Patients Without ALI/ARDS?

In a retrospective analysis of a clinical database (48), the odds ratio for developing ALI was significantly greater when tidal volumes prescribed for usual care exceeded 6 mL/kg predicted body weight (Odds Ratio 1.3 for each mL/kg above 6 mL/kg predicted body weight). Some patients in this study may have received higher tidal volumes because there were greater challenges to gas exchange or severe metabolic acidosis. If so, then the association of higher tidal volumes with worse outcomes might reflect severity of disease rather than effects of higher tidal volumes. In their analyses the investigators adjusted for indices of risk, such as APACHE scores and reason for admission to the intensive care unit. However, it is possible that they did not have sufficient information to adjust for severity. In a randomized trial in patients undergoing esophagectomy for cancer, patients received tidal volumes of either 9 mL/kg or 5 mL/kg during the single lung ventilation phase of the surgery (49). In the study group that received lower tidal volumes, plasma levels of IL-1, IL-6, and IL-8 were significantly lower in the postoperative period. Also, PaO_2/FiO_2s were significantly higher and extravascular lung water (measured with double indicator dilution) and the duration of MV after surgery were significantly lower in the lower tidal volume group. This study suggests that MV with lower tidal volumes is beneficial in patients at risk for developing ALI.

III. VILI from Low Volumes and Pressures During Expiration

In ARDS patients, some unstable lung units open with each inspiration and close during expiration. Mechanical forces associated with repeated opening and closing may deplete surfactant and injure small bronchioles and alveoli (50,51). Lung injury may also result from excessive stress and strain in the parenchymal connections between aerated and nonaerated lung units (52). Also, some alveoli and small bronchioles may fill with fluid and foam at low lung volumes (53), causing tidal volumes to be delivered preferentially to the remaining aerated lung units, causing injury from overdistention.

Traditional approaches to MV in ARDS utilize PEEPs of approximately 5 to 12 cm H_2O (2,54,55). With these PEEP levels, acceptable arterial oxygenation can be achieved in most ARDS patients without using very high, potentially toxic concentrations of inspired oxygen. However, PEEP may also prevent low volume/pressure VILI by reducing the proportion of atelectatic or fluid-filled lung at end expiration. This lung-protective effect of PEEP was demonstrated in several experimental models in which low volume/pressure VILI was attenuated by PEEP (7,50,56,57). In humans with ARDS, clinical outcomes improved and concentrations of inflammatory cytokines in blood and bronchoalveolar lavage fluid decreased when higher levels of PEEP were combined with lower tidal volumes and inspiratory airway pressures (12,14,58). However, it is not clear if the beneficial effects associated with higher PEEP in these clinical studies were from lung protection from low volume/pressure VILI, high volume/pressure VILI, or both. Nonetheless, some researchers and clinicians recommend the use of higher levels of PEEP than those utilized in the traditional MV approach (41,59–63).

A. Clinical Trials of MV with Higher Peep in ALI/ARDS

Three randomized trials of MV strategies with higher versus lower PEEP (64–66) levels were completed since publication of the first edition of this book (Table 1). In each of the trials, all patients received MV strategies designed to prevent high volume/pressure VILI. The primary outcome variable in each of the trials was mortality, which was not significantly different in any of the studies. Ventilator-free days were not significantly different in two of the trials, but in one of the trials higher PEEP *was* associated with more ventilator-free days (medians of 7 vs. 3, $p = 0.04$) and more organ failure-free days (6 vs. 2, $p = 0.04$).

There are several possible explanations for the generally disappointing effects of the higher PEEP strategies in these trials.

1. Higher PEEP was associated with higher Pplats. Thus, it possible that beneficial effects of higher PEEP (reduced low volume/pressure VILI) were counteracted by detrimental effects (increased high volume/pressure VILI).
2. All patients in the three clinical trials received MV with lower tidal volumes. The primary intention of this approach is to reduce high volume/pressure VILI. However, MV with lower tidal volumes may also reduce low volume/pressure VILI by reducing tidal swings in lung volume and pressure. Thus, the potential beneficial effects of higher PEEP may have been reduced by using lower tidal volumes.

Table 1 Three Clinical Trials of Mechanical Ventilation with Higher Versus Lower Levels of Positive End-Expiratory Pressure

	Mean PEEPs on days 1 and 3 (cm H_2O)		Mortality in hospital (%)		Ventilator-free days or mechanical ventilation in survivors ($^$) (median)	
	Lower PEEP groups	Higher PEEP groups	Lower PEEP groups	Higher PEEP groups	Lower PEEP groups	Higher PEEP groups
NIH ARDS Network	8.9	14.7	24.9	27.5	14.5	13.8
($n = 549$) (64)	8.5	12.9				
Canadian ($n = 983$) (66)	10.1	15.6	40.4	36.4	$10^$	$10^$
	8.8	11.8				
French ($n = 767$) (65)	7.1	14.6	39.0	35.4	3	7^a
	6.7	13.4				

[a] $p = 0.04$ for comparison of ventilator-free days in the higher versus the lower PEEP study groups.
Methods for setting higher PEEP:
ARDS Network—table of fixed combinations of PEEP and Fio_2.
Canadian—table of fixed combinations of PEEP and Fio_2.
French—PEEP raised until inspiratory plateau pressure = 28 to 30 cm H_2O.

3. In some ARDS patients, higher PEEP causes substantial recruitment of previously atelectatic or fluid-filled alveoli (PEEP-responders). In other ARDS patients, higher PEEP causes little or no recruitment (PEEP-nonresponders) (67–70). PEEP-induced increments in Pplat and in radiographic indicators of lung overdistention are greater in the nonresponders than in responders. Thus, it is possible that in responders the beneficial effects (recruitment) may exceed the detrimental effects (overdistention). In contrast, in nonresponders the detrimental effects may exceed the beneficial effects. This hypothesis is supported by a comparison of the methods used in the three trials of higher PEEP. In the two trials in which higher PEEP was not associated with improved outcomes, the higher PEEP approach utilized tables of combinations of PEEP and Fio_2 to achieve a clinically acceptable level of arterial PO_2 (64,66). With this approach, PEEP would not be raised above initial levels unless arterial PO_2 was below the acceptable range. Arterial oxygenation usually increases substantially in responders when higher PEEP is applied (68,69), so PEEP was probably not raised above initial levels in many of the responder subset. In contrast, in the trial in which higher PEEP was associated with greater ventilator-free and organ failure-free days, the higher PEEP strategy required increases in PEEP until Pplat increased to approximately 28 to 30 cm H_2O (65). With this approach, responders may have received higher PEEPs than they would have received in the other two trials, and nonresponders probably received lower levels of PEEP. Thus, beneficial effects of the higher PEEP strategy in the third trial may have been greater in the responder subset compared to the effects in the responder subsets of the trials that used PEEP-Fio_2 tables. Also because of the different methods for raising PEEP, higher PEEP nonresponders in the two studies that utilized PEEP-Fio_2 tables may have received higher PEEPs than in the third study. Thus, detrimental effects of higher PEEP in the nonresponder subsets in these two studies may have been greater than the detrimental effects in the nonresponder subset of the third trial.

B. Identifying Responders and Nonresponders

The different physiologic behaviors of responders and nonresponders stimulated the search for clinically useful methods for identifying these two subsets. Computerized tomography was used in several studies to assess recruitment versus overdistention from PEEP (63,67,68,71), but this approach is cumbersome and costly. In a study of 19 ARDS patients, recruitment from PEEP was assessed by constructing volume–pressure curves on the same volume and pressure axes during MV with lower and higher PEEP and referring volume to the elastic equilibrium volume of the respiratory system (69). In nine patients, the change from lower to higher PEEP caused substantial increases in end-expiratory volume [587 ± 158 mL (standard deviation)]. This probably represented lung recruitment because it was associated with substantial increases in Pao_2/Fio_2 (from 150 ± 36 to 396 ± 138 mm Hg) and reductions in lung elastance (23 ± 3 to 20 ± 2 cm H_2O/L). In contrast, in the remaining 10 patients the increment from lower to higher PEEP caused minimal increases in end-expiratory volume (70 ± 38 mL), and this was associated with no improvement in Pao_2/Fio_2 (from 149 ± 38 to 142 ± 36) or in lung elastance (27 ± 6 to 28 ± 6 cm H_2O/L). This study suggests that responders can be distinguished from nonresponders by monitoring arterial oxygenation and respiratory system elastance at the bedside when raising PEEP from lower to higher levels.

In a study of 68 ALI patients (49 with ARDS), recruitment responses to PEEP were assessed by computerized tomography at PEEPs of 5 and 15 cm H_2O (68). PEEP responsiveness could be predicted with moderate sensitivity and specificity by the following three physiologic variables, each of which can be assessed at the bedside: Pao_2/Fio_2 < 150 on PEEP of 5 cm H_2O, a decrease in alveolar dead space (or improved CO_2 clearance) when PEEP was raised from 5 to 15 cm H_2O, and an increase in respiratory system compliance when PEEP was raised from 5 to 15 cm H_2O. If two of these three variables were present, the sensitivity and specificity for recruitment in response to an increase in PEEP from 5 to 15 cm H_2O were 79% and 81%, respectively.

To identify patients more likely to benefit from higher PEEP, some investigators estimated pleural pressure using esophageal manometry. Transpulmonary pressure (P_L) at end expiration was then calculated by subtracting esophageal pressure from airway opening pressure. In many patients receiving traditional levels of PEEP, P_L values were negative because esophageal pressures were higher than the PEEP (36,37). In a small clinical trial (37), patients were randomized to receive a traditional PEEP strategy [as in the ARDS Network tidal volume trial (13)] or a strategy in which PEEP was adjusted to ensure a positive end-expiratory P_L. With this approach, patients with elevated esophageal pressures received higher levels of PEEP. As in the other trials of higher PEEP, this approach was associated with improved arterial oxygenation and reduced respiratory system elastance. The P_L-guided approach was also associated with a trend toward reduced mortality. However, there are several reasons why the value of using esophageal manometry for managing PEEP must be confirmed in additional studies. First, at a given airway opening pressure or lung volume, pleural pressure can vary substantially throughout the thorax (72–74). Therefore, it is not clear that a single value of P_L estimated from esophageal manometry can provide useful guidance for managing PEEP for the whole lung. A study in dogs suggests that esophageal pressure is a fair representation of average pleural pressure (72). However, in many supine, critically ill patients, pressure in the esophagus is elevated considerably by compression from the weight of the mediastinum and cephalad displacement of the left hemidiaphragm. Thus, esophageal pressure in supine subjects probably overestimates average pleural pressure. Second, with the P_L strategy as used in the recent trial, PEEP was raised to high levels in some patients (in whom esophageal pressures were high). In some patients, Pplats exceeded 35 cm H_2O (51 cm H_2O in one patient). It is not clear that the benefits of lung recruitment with higher PEEP exceed the adverse effects of overdistention with such high plateau pressures. Third, although there were trends favoring mortality in the P_L-guided study group, the study was terminated early on the basis of the primary outcome of improved arterial oxygenation. Mortality was a secondary outcome in this small, unblinded study.

C. Patients More Vulnerable to Adverse Effects of Higher PEEP

Recent studies suggest that three groups of patients may be more vulnerable to detrimental effects of high airway pressures.

1. Focal ARDS: In some ARDS patients the morphological distribution of lung injury is diffuse; in other patients the lesions are patchy or focal (75,76). Focal ARDS usually involves consolidation of lower lobes with preserved aeration in the remainder of the lungs. These focal lesions tend to be nonresponsive to PEEP. Pressure–volume

curves in these patients frequently lack an identifiable lower inflection point (77). These patients are at higher risk of overdistension from higher PEEP.

2. Acute cor pulmonale: Pulmonary hypertension is often associated with ARDS. Some patients also exhibit right ventricular dysfunction with right ventricle dilation and abnormal septal motion (78,79). This can cause circulatory depression with systemic hypotension and requirements for vasopressors. High airway pressures contribute to right ventricular failure (80) and should be avoided, if possible, in patients with severe acute cor pulmonale. Monitoring with serial cardiac echography may be useful.

3. Mild hypoxemia: Posthoc analyses of two of the large trials of higher PEEP suggested that patients with Pao_2/Fio_2 between 300 and 200 may respond poorly to higher PEEP, with non significant trends toward increased mortality (65,66). These patients generally have low potential for recruitment (68). Detrimental effects of higher PEEP may outweigh the beneficial effects in this group.

D. How Much PEEP Should Nonresponders Receive?

In a recent study, 15 patients were selected because they had focal loss of aeration on computerized tomography (35). In previous studies, focal or lobar loss of aeration predicted a lack of response to PEEP (67). All 15 patients received MV with tidal volumes of 6 mL/kg and with PEEP set initially according to the NIH ARDS Network lower PEEP table (13). With these settings, the slope of the airway pressure–time relationship (with constant inspiratory airflow) increased during each inspiration, suggesting that aerated lung had become overdistended during inspiration (35,81). When PEEP was decreased until the slope of the pressure–time relationship became constant during inspiration, plasma concentrations of interleukin-6, interleukin-8, and soluble tumor necrosis factor receptor I decreased significantly. The decreases in PEEP were not associated with significantly worse arterial oxygenation, but arterial PCO_2 decreased, suggesting that dead space had decreased when PEEP was lowered. This study suggests that PEEP nonresponders should receive lower PEEPs than those that they would receive on the NIH ARDS Network lower PEEP table.

E. Methods for Setting PEEP

Assuming that PEEP is beneficial for some ARDS patients, it is not yet clear how to set PEEP in individual patients. An earlier study suggested that PEEP should be adjusted to achieve maximal systemic oxygen delivery, and that this objective could be met by adjusting PEEP until respiratory system elastance is minimized (from lung recruitment) (82). Clinical outcomes were not assessed in this study, and subsequent studies in patients with sepsis and ALI did not demonstrate improved outcomes with hemodynamic management strategies designed to promote oxygen delivery (83,84).

Another approach to setting PEEP is to construct a static or quasi-static pressure–volume relationship of the respiratory system (12,14). In most ARDS patients this relationship has three phases (85,86). At low pressures and volumes, the slope is typically low (low compliance or high elastance) because more lung tissue is atelectatic. The slope then increases over a relatively narrow range of pressure and volume as some lung units open. In a second phase at moderate pressures and volumes, the slope is maximal and approximately rectilinear. In a third phase at higher pressures and volumes the slope decreases, as aerated lung units approach their elastic limits and become overdistended. If tidal ventilation encompasses the range of pressure and volume of the transition between the first and second phases, there may be substantial VILI from recruitment and derecruitment of lung units with each breath. The approximately rectilinear phase II portion has been interpreted to represent a range of pressure and volume in which there is neither recruitment nor overdistention. According to these interpretations of the pressure–volume curve, PEEP should be set at the lower end of the second phase, to maintain lung recruitment above the level of the transition between the first and second phases. This is an attractive physiologic concept, but several recent studies suggest that the three phases of the pressure–volume curve do not represent distinctly different physiologic behaviors of the lung. The transition from the first to the second phase represents substantial recruitment, but substantial *additional* recruitment continues through phase II and into phase III (70,87). Moreover, some lung units may become overdistended in the second phase. The approximately rectilinear shape of the second phase may be explained by the opposing effects of recruitment (which causes the slope to increase) and overdistention (which causes the slope to decrease). Thus, setting PEEP at the lower end of the second phase will not prevent the low volume/pressure VILI that occurs from MV over the ranges of pressure and volume of the second phase. Another limitation of the pressure–volume curve approach for setting PEEP is that static or quasi-static pressure–volume curves do not necessarily represent the pressure–volume relationship during tidal ventilation. When PEEP is relatively low, the pressure–volume relationship during tidal ventilation is closer to the inspiratory limb of the pressure–volume curve. However, at higher PEEPs the relationship during tidal ventilation approaches the expiratory limb of the pressure–volume loop (88,89).

Some investigators recommend an approach to setting PEEP in which airway pressure is initially raised to a high level, such as 40 to 45 cm H_2O, to achieve high levels of arterial oxygenation (62). Tidal ventilation is then resumed, and PEEP is decreased in small decrements until arterial oxygenation begins to decrease. Airway pressure is then raised back to the previous high level to restore recruitment, and PEEP is then set approximately 2 cm H_2O higher than the level at which arterial oxygenation decreased. Like the pressure–volume approach, this approach is designed to identify the individual patient-specific lowest level of PEEP necessary to maintain a high level of lung recruitment. One limitation of this approach is that in addition to lung recruitment, arterial oxygenation is affected by several other factors that vary with airway pressure, such as cardiac output and ventilation-perfusion ratios (90). Thus, the level of PEEP at which arterial oxygenation begins to decrease may not represent the level of PEEP at which lung recruitment begins to decrease. A second limitation is that this approach usually results in relatively high PEEPs, which are associated with relatively high Pplats. It is not clear if the beneficial effects of lung recruitment with this approach outweigh the detrimental effects of lung overdistention. Because of limitations such as these, this approach has not been recommended widely.

Another approach to setting PEEP uses noninvasive bedside electrical impedance tomography of the chest to monitor the distribution of ventilation (91). At low PEEPs, the tomographic images demonstrate preferential distribution of tidal volumes to some lung units, usually in ventral regions, and little-no ventilation to other lung units. At higher PEEPs, the distribution of tidal ventilation becomes more homogeneous as previously atelectatic or fluid-filled lung units become aerated. At even higher PEEP levels, some lung units (usually in ventral regions) receive less ventilation because they become overdistended. This approach avoids the limitations of using arterial oxygenation as a surrogate for lung recruitment. However, like the decremental PEEP approach described in the previous paragraph, this approach will lead to higher PEEPs than those used in traditional approaches, which may increase high volume/pressure during inspiration. The imaging techniques for this approach need further refinement, and this approach should be tested against other MV approaches in which PEEP levels are not raised to high levels.

F. Recruitment Maneuvers

RMs consist of relatively brief (30 seconds–2 minutes) exposures to airway pressures that are higher than those that result from tidal ventilation. The purpose of RMs is to open some lung units that are atelectatic or fluid-filled during tidal ventilation. Because of hysteresis in the pressure–volume relationship of the respiratory system, some of these lung units may subsequently remain open during tidal ventilation. If so, then the lungs may be ventilated more homogeneously, inspiratory airway pressures and lung overdistention may decrease, and gas exchange (arterial PO_2 and PCO_2) may improve. Several studies have demonstrated beneficial effects of RMs on pertinent physiologic characteristics such as arterial oxygenation, venous admixture, respiratory system elastance, and recruited volume. Although the results are somewhat variable, some generalizations are possible.

1. As with PEEP, some patients respond to RMs with substantial increases in arterial oxygenation and reductions in respiratory system elastance, but responses in other patients are much less (92–94).
2. RMs are more likely to be effective early in the course (days 1–2 of MV) than later in the course of ARDS (92).
3. Although some investigators showed sustained effects of RMs on gas exchange (63), in most studies these effects disappeared within 60 minutes (92–96). Some investigators suggest that the effects of RMs persist if PEEP is raised after conducting an RM (97,98). But such sustained improvements in arterial oxygenation, elastance, and related variables could be from effects of the increments in PEEP rather than effects of RMs.
4. Higher RM pressures are generally associated with a higher proportion of responders and with greater effects on lung recruitment. An RM approach that raised airway pressure to as high as 60 cm H_2O for two minutes (tidal cycling between 45 and 60 cm H_2O) reversed a high proportion of atelectatic lung in 24 of 26 patients, including some with focal or lobar distribution of the loss of aeration (63).
5. Some studies report brief episodes of hypotension, bradycardia, and tachycardia during or shortly after RMs (94,99,100). Recruitment maneuvers can cause transient but substantial dilatation of the right ventricle and collapse of the left ventricle (101). This may explain the decrease in cardiac output that frequently occurs during and immediately after RMs (92). In an experimental model of pneumonia-induced ARDS, hemodynamic alterations persisted after 15 minutes of RMs (99). These data suggest that great precautions should be taken before using RMs in patients with hemodynamic instability, especially in patients with right ventricular dysfunction before the use of RMs.

Several methods have been proposed for conducting RMs. A simple approach is to apply continuous positive airway pressure of approximately 40 cm H_2O for 30 to 60 seconds (12,92,94). Other approaches maintain a respiratory cycle during the RM and raise either the PEEP (at constant tidal volume or increment in inspiratory airway pressure) or the pressure during inspiration (at constant PEEP) for 30 seconds to 2 minutes (63,93,99,102). Maintaining the respiratory cycle during the RM may be more effective for recruitment because it involves repeated increments in airway pressure to high levels. It may also cause less circulatory depression because mean airway pressure is lower than when the high airway pressure is maintained throughout the period of the RM.

Some investigators recommend conducting RMs on a regular basis, especially when PEEP is raised because arterial oxygenation is not acceptable. Others suggest that RMs should be reserved for situations in which gas exchange deteriorates, presumably because of derecruitment. For example, a patient whose arterial oxygenation worsens after a brief disconnection of the endotracheal tube from the ventilator circuit may benefit from a RM to restore the level of recruitment before the disconnection. There are no studies that clearly define a role for RMs, and there is no consensus on the role of RMs in MV management of ALI/ARDS.

IV. High Frequency Ventilation

This approach to MV utilizes very small tidal volumes and relatively high mean airway pressures. Therefore, it is attractive for management of ARDS because of the potential to increase lung recruitment (to reduce low volume/pressure VILI) while avoiding overdistention during inspiration (to reduce high volume/pressure VILI) (103). This may be a more effective approach to prevention of VILI than lung-protective strategies that utilize conventional mechanical ventilators. However, HFV requires substantially more sedation and, sometimes, neuromuscular blockade than conventional modes of ventilation. Recent studies emphasize the clinical value of reducing sedation, to reduce time on MV and, perhaps, mortality (104). Therefore, it is not yet clear if HFV will improve clinical outcomes from ARDS.

Many randomized clinical trials of HFV versus conventional MV were conducted in neonates and small children with respiratory distress syndromes (reviewed in the first edition of this chapter). None of the trials demonstrated reduced mortality. Some studies demonstrated an association between the use of HFV and a reduction in chronic lung disease (usually defined as a requirement for supplemental oxygen approximately one month after enrollment or before hospital discharge). Since the first edition of this book at least two more trials of HFV in neonates yielded different results: one demonstrated no beneficial effects (105) and the other demonstrated a reduction in chronic lung disease (106).

A recent randomized trial of HFV in adults with ARDS did not demonstrate beneficial effects of HFV. A subset analysis suggested that there were beneficial effects in patients with more severe lung disease (107). However, the number of patients in this trial was modest, and the value of the subset analysis is very limited.

Recent physiologic studies suggest that under some circumstances, the size of the tidal volumes that result from HFV may approach the size used in lung-protective approaches that use conventional MV (108,109). Moreover, the approach that was initially recommended for use of HFV may not be as lung protective as some alternative approaches. More studies are needed to refine HFV techniques and optimize its potential for lung protection. Routine use of HFV is not currently recommended because its role has not been clearly defined in clinical studies. At least three randomized trials of HFV are currently in progress (clinicaltrials.gov NCT00399581 and NCT00474656; controlled-trials.com ISRCTN10416500).

V. Extracorporeal Gas Exchange

Controlled clinical trials of extracorporeal membrane oxygenation and extracorporeal CO_2 removal were reviewed in the first edition of this book. The earlier trials did not demonstrate improved clinical outcomes with these techniques, perhaps because beneficial effects were counteracted by detrimental effects. Despite these disappointing results, some centers have continued to refine the criteria used to select patients to receive extracorporeal support and to test newer techniques designed to reduce complications. Initial reports of a more recent controlled clinical trial were promising (http://www.cesar-trial.org, http://www.medscape.com/viewarticle/569740), but the trial design and data analysis have not yet been reported after peer review. Extracorporeal gas exchange may be a useful technique for some patients in the future, but at this time this approach can be recommended for more widespread use.

VI. Noninvasive Ventilation

With noninvasive ventilation (NIV), a face mask is used instead of an endotracheal tube to connect the patient to the ventilator. This approach may avoid many complications of endotracheal intubation, such as mechanical injury to the upper airway, aspiration, and adverse effects of sedative and analgesic medications. Many patients require only intermittent ventilator support, which can be accomplished easily by removing and replacing the NIV face mask. Some patients can eat, speak, and attend to hygiene during respites from NIV. However, it is not possible to provide the same high levels of ventilator support through the face mask interface, and several technical challenges must be overcome before sufficient support can be achieved (110–112).

NIV is well established for us in patients with acute respiratory acidosis, as in chronic obstructive lung disease (113–115). In these patients, NIV is associated with reduced mortality and use of intensive care resources. In patients with ALI and ARDS, NIV with 10 to 15 cm H_2O of pressure support reduced neuromuscular drive, respiratory muscle effort, and sensation of dyspnea (116). In an earlier randomized study in patients with hypoxemic respiratory failure but no history of chronic lung disease, beneficial effects of NIV were apparent only in a subgroup of patients with acute hypercapnia (117). Several studies subsequently showed that in some patients with hypoxemic respiratory failure, NIV can reduce the need for endotracheal intubation and improve important clinical outcomes (118–123). In one notable study, patients with hypoxemic respiratory failure but without chronic obstructive pulmonary disease, hemodynamic instability, or neurological impairment were randomized to receive NIV with pressure support and PEEP or MV with an endotracheal tube when protocol-defined criteria for intubation were identified (115). Improvements in oxygenation were similar with the noninvasive and invasive approaches, but patients treated with NIV had shorter durations of MV and intensive care unit stay and experienced fewer complications. There was a 30% failure rate of NIV, and mortality was high in patients who were intubated after failing NIV, suggesting that delayed intubation may adversely affect outcomes. Several additional clinical studies also demonstrated some beneficial effects, but NIV failure rates were substantial, and mortality among those who failed were also high (118,119,122,124–126). It is not clear if failure of NIV is a marker of severity or if delayed intubation in some patients who attempt NIV causes complications that contribute to mortality. Earlier initiation of NIV (before criteria for intubation are identified) may reduce the frequency of NIV failure and the associated risks of delayed intubation. ARDS patients who receive NIV must be monitored carefully for signs of worsening respiratory failure to prevent complications of delayed and hasty endotracheal intubation.

Avoiding endotracheal intubation substantially reduces the risk of nosocomial pneumonia and other infectious complications (127,128). Therefore, patients who are at high risk for nosocomial infections may be most likely to benefit from NIV. Several recent trials showed substantial beneficial effects of NIV when used as a preventive measure during episodes of acute hypoxemic respiratory failure in solid organ-transplant patients and in patients with severe immunosuppression, as in hematological malignancies and neutropenia (127,129,130). The rates of intubation and of infectious complications, length of stay, and mortality were significantly reduced in patients who received NIV.

Selection of ARDS patients to receive NIV must be based on clinical factors that reflect the severity of lung injury and the presence of associated organ dysfunctions. Hemodynamic instability or neurological dysfunction usually contraindicates NIV. In a study of 354 patients with acute hypoxemic respiratory failure, age greater than 40 years and a simplified acute physiologic score greater than 35 predicted NIV failure (119). Other predictors of NIV failure include an APACHE II score greater than 17, metabolic acidosis, and respiratory rate greater than 25/min before NIV (121,122,125). After one hour of NIV, failure of the respiratory rate to decrease to less than 25/min was a strong predictor of failure (122).

VII.   Spontaneous Ventilation Versus Neuromuscular Blockade

Dysynchrony between a patient's respiratory efforts and a MV respiratory cycle may lead to the administration of sedative medications to suppress spontaneous respiratory efforts. Airway pressure release ventilation (APRV) and Bilevel ventilation are timed pressure-cycling modes of MV in which the ventilator cycle is independent of a patient's respiratory efforts (131–133). Patients can initiate inspiration and expiration at any time during the cycle of the ventilator. This approach is designed to allow positive pressure ventilation and spontaneous breathing to coexist while reducing the conflict (and resulting discomfort and agitation) that frequently occurs between patients' respiratory efforts and ventilators' attempts to assist with those efforts. This may allow lower doses of sedative medications. Spontaneous respiratory efforts may reduce basilar atelectasis, improve ventilation-perfusion matching, and increase venous return and cardiac output (131,132). However, many patients have vigorous spontaneous respiratory efforts while receiving MV with other modes. More studies are needed to demonstrate improvements in clinical outcomes such as time on MV with APRV and Bilevel ventilation.

In a recent controlled clinical trial, 36 patients with ARDS were randomized to receive a neuromuscular blocking agent (NMBA, cisatracurium) or placebo within 48 hours of the onset of ARDS (134). All patients received a volume-and-pressure limited MV approach in the volume-assist-control mode. After 48 hours of study drug treatment, concentrations of inflammatory cytokines (IL-1β, IL-6, and IL-8) in bronchoalveolar lavage fluid and in blood were lower in patients who received the NMBA. Moreover, arterial oxygenation improved more during the 48 hours of NMBA treatment than placebo treatment, and improved oxygenation in the NMBA group continued for at least 72 hours after discontinuation of the study medication. Reducing oxygen consumption by skeletal muscles could have contributed to improved arterial oxygenation during the 48 hours of NMBA treatment, but this effect would be unlikely to persist after the 48-hour period of NMBA treatment. Another possible explanation for the positive effects of NMBA on lung function is that the elimination of muscular activity reduced proinflammatory cytokine release from muscles into the systemic circulation, leading to decreased inflammation in the lung. However, studies in exercising subjects suggest that the cytokines released from exercising muscles *reduce* systemic inflammation (135,136). The investigators suggested that elimination of patient-ventilator dysynchrony with NMBA allowed a more homogenous delivery of tidal volumes and reduced derecruitment of dependent lung areas. This explanation may contradict the rationale for *promoting* spontaneous breathing, as with APRV or Bilevel ventilation. A larger randomized, controlled clinical trial NMBAs in ARDS is needed to confirm the clinical findings in the recent pilot study and to define mechanisms by which NMBAs reduce inflammation (www.clinicaltrials.gov NCT00299650).

VIII.   Recommendations for Clinical Use of MV in ALI/ARDS

Interpretation of studies to draw direct recommendations for clinical practice must be made cautiously. Airway pressures and lung volumes are tightly linked. Changing PEEP frequently causes inspiratory pressures to rise, and changing pressures and volumes during inspiration can affect lung volume and recruitment at end expiration. Therefore, the respective effects of individual changes in pressures and volumes are very difficult to isolate. Pplat varies with tidal volumes, but we do not know if the beneficial effects of tidal volume reduction are due to a lowering of Pplat (reflecting decreased end-inspiratory alveolar distension) or to a lower amplitude of tidal swings in lung volume (reflecting lower tidal strain)? When PEEP is modified with constant tidal volume, the resulting effects on outcomes may be caused by changes in lung recruitment at end expiration, changes in lung distention at end inspiration, or changes in tidal swings in lung volume and pressure. Recent studies allow us to make MV safer, but many uncertainties persist. Therefore, we offer the following recommendations with these caveats in mind.

A.   NIV

NIV may be used early in the course of ARDS in patients without hemodynamic compromise, before gas exchange becomes severely compromised, and before a patient's sensorium becomes impaired. With early use of NIV, some patients may be spared from complications of endotracheal intubation, such as nosocomial pneumonia and adverse effects of heavy sedation and neuromuscular blockade. However, NIV cannot provide enough support for many, perhaps most, ALI/ARDS patients. In a large cohort study, failure of NIV was significantly associated with an increase in the risk of death even after adjustment for severity factors (137). Such an association was not found in patients treated with NIV for exacerbation of chronic obstructive pulmonary disease (COPD) or cardiogenic pulmonary edema. Therefore, we suggest that NIV can be used in ALI/ARDS patients if some component of respiratory failure can be reversed quickly. However, intubation should not be delayed if NIV does not lead to stability or improvement. Criteria that indicate failure include hypoxemia despite an elevated Fio_2, worsening respiratory acidosis, tachypnea, and excessive use of accessory muscles of breathing.

B.   Ventilator Mode

Either a volume- or pressure-control mode can be used. The same pressure and volume objectives can be achieved with either approach, and neither mode is superior to the other for achieving important clinical objectives. Therefore, the choice of mode should be made primarily on the basis of familiarity of the clinical staff. However, with all modes, it is crucial that the user understands the physiologic relationships between volume and the different pressures that can be measured on the ventilator. Regardless of mode, both inspiratory pressures and tidal volumes should be monitored and adjusted to achieve specific volume-and-pressure limited ventilation goals. This monitoring must be specific to either the volume- or pressure-based approach. When volume-control modes are used, it is important to monitor plateau pressures. When pressure-control modes are used, it is important to monitor expired tidal volumes.

When using pressure-control modes, clinicians must remember that the ventilator reports only the pressure at the airway opening. If a patient has spontaneous inspiratory efforts, transpulmonary pressure can be considerably augmented and cause substantial overdistention even when airway opening pressures are not elevated. Tidal volume monitoring is very important in this condition.

C.   Tidal Volumes and Inspiratory Pressures

If a volume-control mode is used, tidal volume should be set at approximately 6 mL/kg predicted body weight (15–17). Tidal volumes of 7 to 8 mL/kg should be considered for patients who experience severe respiratory acidosis, especially when there is elevated intracranial pressure (13). In volume-cycled modes, some severely dyspneic patients trigger second tidal volumes before exhalation of initial tidal volumes, effectively increasing the delivered tidal volume to twice the intended volume. A modest increase in tidal volume may reduce the sensation of dyspnea in these patients and prevent the double breaths. Also, in some patients work-of-breathing with small tidal volumes may be excessive. It may be prudent to allow modestly higher tidal volumes or inspiratory pressures in these patients, to avoid complications from excessive sedative or neuromuscular blocking medications. Lower tidal volumes should be considered if plateau pressures exceed 30 cm H_2O.

If a pressure-control mode is used, ventilator inspiratory pressure should be adjusted to achieve average tidal volumes of approximately 6 mL/kg. Higher or lower inspiratory pressures should be considered using the same factors suggested for modifying the volume-control tidal volume goal.

Regardless of ventilator mode, ventilator circuit dead space should be reduced as much as is practical. The internal volumes of many heat and moisture exchangers approach 100 mL (138–141). At constant tidal volume, these devices reduce alveolar ventilation of each breath, which may increase dyspnea, tachypnea, work-of-breath, and respiratory acidosis. In ALI/ARDS patients inspired gases should be conditioned with heated humidifiers, which do not contribute to dead space. Moreover, when minute ventilation is elevated, heated humidifiers are more effective for warming and humidifying inspired gases.

D. PEEP and Fio$_2$

The approach used in the NIH trial of volume-and-pressure limited ventilation (13) represented a consensus of how PEEP and Fio$_2$ were used by the NIH investigators and clinical colleagues in 1995. The consensus evolved with the knowledge that both PEEP and supplemental oxygen can support arterial oxygenation, but that both can also have adverse effects (142). The table of PEEP and Fio$_2$ pairs has been used in several subsequent trials of different lung-protective MV strategies (64–66). It is a clinically practical approach that has been adopted for usual care in many intensive care units.

However, a shortcoming of the NIH approach is that it may not adjust PEEP according to physiologic characteristics that best represent recruitment in individual patients. PEEP nonresponders recruit little (and arterial Pao$_2$ improves little) in response to higher levels of PEEP. Oxygenation can improve in these patients with the use of higher Fio$_2$, but with fixed pairings of PEEP and Fio$_2$, patients must receive higher PEEP to also receive higher Fio$_2$. Higher levels of PEEP may cause high volume/pressure VILI (35). Moreover, PEEP responders may benefit from higher levels of PEEP than they would receive on the table of fixed pairings of PEEP and Fio$_2$ because increasing PEEP levels are paired with increasing Fio$_2$s. For these reasons, we recommend an approach that attempts to distinguish PEEP responders from nonresponders, and to apply higher levels of PEEP in the responders and lower levels in nonresponders.

Three approaches to identifying responders and nonresponders were reviewed in the previous section of this chapter on setting PEEP (65,68,69). Two of the approaches are more clinically practical than the third because they can be more easily incorporated into usual care MV strategies. In the approach by Grasso and coworkers, Pao$_2$/Fio$_2$ and lung elastance were first measured during MV on the NIH lower PEEP table. These values were then compared to the Pao$_2$/Fio$_2$ on the NIH higher PEEP table. In responders Pao$_2$/Fio$_2$ increased and lung elastance decreased significantly (69); in nonresponders there was little change in Pao$_2$/Fio$_2$ and lung elastance increased. Using this approach, patients whose Pao$_2$/Fio$_2$ increases substantially in the transition from the lower to the higher PEEP table should continue on the higher PEEP table. In nonresponders, PEEP may be lowered (and overdistention reduced) while monitoring arterial oxygenation. In most nonresponders, lowering PEEP from the lower PEEP table causes little change in arterial oxygenation (35).

The approach used in the third clinical trial of higher PEEP is also clinically practical (65). After initially setting PEEP according to the NIH lower PEEP table, PEEP is raised in increments until the plateau pressure is 28 to 30 cm H$_2$O. This approach will yield higher levels of PEEP in responders than in nonresponders. If Pao$_2$/Fio$_2$ does not increase substantially when the plateau pressure limit has been reached, then PEEP should be returned to the lower PEEP table level (or even lower) to reduce unnecessary inspiratory pressures and volumes (35).

E. Recruitment Maneuvers

We suggest conducting a RM shortly after initiating conventional MV and on occasions when arterial oxygenation worsens because of an event that causes derecruitment, such as a disconnection of the endotracheal tube from the MV circuit. Some investigators also recommend conducting a RM whenever PEEP is raised because arterial oxygenation fell below acceptable limits. Clinicians should take special precautions when conducting RMs in patients with circulatory failure, especially those with cor pulmonale.

References

1. Brower R, Brochard L. Mechanical ventilation in the acute respiratory distress syndrome. In: Matthay M, Lenfant C, eds. Acute Respiratory Distress Syndrome. New York: Marcel Dekker, Inc., 2003:589–631.
2. Petty TL. Acute respiratory distress syndrome (ARDS). Dis Mon 1990; 36(1):1–58.
3. Pontoppidan H, Geffin B, Lowenstein E. Acute respiratory failure in the adult. N Engl J Med 1972; 287:799–806.
4. Brochard L, Lemaire F. Tidal volume, positive end-expiratory pressure, and mortality in acute respiratory distress syndrome. Crit Care Med 1999; 27(8):1661–1663.
5. Hedley-Whyte J, Laver MB, Benedixen HH. Effect of changes in tidal ventilation on physiologic shunting. Am J Physiol 1964; 206:891–897.
6. Benedixen HH, Hedley-Whyte J, Laver MB. Impaired oxygenation in surgical patients during general anesthesia with controlled ventilation. N Engl J Med 1963; 269:991–997.
7. Webb HH, Tierney DF. Experimental pulmonary edema due to intermittent positive pressure ventilation with high pressures. Am Rev Respir Dis 1974; 110:556.
8. Tsuno K, Prato P, Kolobow T. Acute lung injury from mechanical ventilation at moderately high airway pressures. J Appl Physiol 1990; 69(3):956–961.
9. Parker JC, Townsley MI, Rippe B, et al. Increased microvascular permeability in dog lungs due to high peak airway pressures. J Appl Physiol 1984; 57:1809–1816.
10. Dreyfuss D, Soler P, Basset G, et al. High inflation pressure pulmonary edema. Am Rev Respir Dis 1988; 137:1159–1164.
11. Dreyfuss D, Saumon G. State of the art: ventilator-induced lung injury; lessons from experimental studies. Am J Respir Crit Care Med 1998; 157:294–323.
12. Amato MBP, Barbas CSV, Medeiros DM, et al. Effect of a protective-ventilation strategy on mortality in the acute respiratory distress syndrome. N Engl J Med 1998; 338(6):347–354.
13. Acute Respiratory Distress Syndrome Network. Ventilation with lower tidal volumes as compared with traditional tidal volumes for acute lung injury and the acute respiratory distress syndrome. N Engl J Med 2000; 342:1301–1308.
14. Villar J, Kacmarek RM, Perez-Mendez L, et al. A high positive end-expiratory pressure, low tidal volume ventilatory strategy improves outcome in persistent acute respiratory distress syndrome: a randomized, controlled trial. Crit Care Med 2006; 34(5):1311–1318.
15. Malhotra A. Low-tidal-volume ventilation in the acute respiratory distress syndrome. N Engl J Med 2007; 357(11):1113–1120.
16. Wheeler AP, Bernard GR. Acute lung injury and the acute respiratory distress syndrome: a clinical review. Lancet 2007; 369(9572):1553–1564.
17. Fan E, Needham DM, Stewart TE. Ventilatory management of acute lung injury and acute respiratory distress syndrome. JAMA 2005; 294(22):2889–2896.
18. Tobin MJ, Van de Graaff WB. Monitoring of lung mechanics and work of breathing. In: Tobin MJ, ed. Principles and Practice of Mechanical Ventilation. New York: McGraw-Hill, Inc., 1994:967–1004.
19. Tobin M. Culmination of an era in research on the acute respiratory distress syndrome. N Engl J Med 2000; 342:1360–1361.
20. Eichacker PQ, Gerstenberger EP, Banks SM, et al. A metaanalysis of ALI and ARDS trials testing low tidal volumes. Am J Respir Crit Care Med 2002; 166:1510–1514.
21. Rahn H, Otis AB, Chadwick LE, et al. The pressure-volume diagram of the thorax and lung. Am J Physiol 1946; 146;161–178.
22. Mascheroni D, Kolobow T, Fumagalli R, et al. Acute respiratory failure following pharmacologically induced hyperventilation: an experimental animal study. Intensive Care Med 1988; 15(1):8–14.
23. Dreyfuss D, Soler P, Saumon G. Mechanical ventilation-induced pulmonary edema: interaction with previous lung alterations. Am J Respir Crit Care Med 1995; 151:1568–1575.

24. Whitehead TC, Zhang H, Mullen B, et al. Effect of mechanical ventilation on cytokine response to intratracheal lipopolysaccharide. Anesthesiology 2004; 101(1):52–58.
25. Parker JC, Hernandez LA, Longenecker GL, et al. Lung edema caused by high peak inspiratory pressures in dogs. Am Rev Respir Dis 1990; 142:321–328.
26. Carlton DP, Cummings JJ, Scheerer RG, et al. Lung overexpansion increases pulmonary microvascular protein permeability in young lambs. J Appl Physiol 1990; 69(2): 577–583.
27. Frank JA, Gutierrez JA, Jones KD, et al. Low tidal volume reduces epithelial and endothelial injury in acid-injured rat lungs. Am J Respir Crit Care Med 2002; 165(2):242–249.
28. Brower RG, Shanholtz CB, Fessler HE, et al. Prospective randomized, controlled clinical trial comparing traditional vs. reduced tidal volume ventilation in ARDS patients. Crit Care Med 1999; 27;1492–1498.
29. Brochard L, Roudot-Thoraval F, Roupie E, et al. Tidal volume reduction for prevention of ventilator-induced lung injury in the acute respiratory distress syndrome. Am J Respir Crit Care Med 1998; 158:1831–1838.
30. Stewart TE, Meade MO, Cook DJ, et al. Evaluation of a ventilation strategy to prevent barotrauma in patients at high risk for acute respiratory distress syndrome. N Engl J Med 1998; 338(6):355–361.
31. Eichacker PQ, Banks SM, Natanson C. Meta-analysis of tidal volumes in ARDS (letter). Am J Respir Crit Care Med 2003; 167:798–799.
32. Amato M, Brochard L, Stewart T, et al. Metaanalysis of tidal volume in ARDS. Am J Respir Crit Care Med 2003; 168(5):612–613.
33. Hager DN, Krishnan JA, Hayden DL, et al. Tidal volume reduction in patients with acute lung injury when plateau pressures are not high. Am J Respir Crit Care Med 2005; 172(10): 1241–1245.
34. Terragni PP, Rosboch G, Tealdi A, et al. Tidal hyperinflation during low tidal volume ventilation in acute respiratory distress syndrome. Am J Respir Crit Care Med 2007; 175(2): 160–166.
35. Grasso S, Stripoli T, De Michele M, et al. ARDSnet ventilatory protocol and alveolar hyperinflation: role of positive end-expiratory pressure. Am J Respir Crit Care Med 2007; 176(8): 761–767.
36. Talmor D, Sarge T, O'Donnell CR, et al. Esophageal and transpulmonary pressures in acute respiratory failure. Crit Care Med 2006; 34(5):1389–1394.
37. Talmor D, Sarge T, Malhotra A, et al. Mechanical ventilation guided by esophageal pressure in acute lung injury. N Engl J Med 2008; 359(20):2095–2104.
38. Gibson GJ, Pride NB. Lung distensibility. The static pressure-volume curve of the lungs and its use in clinical assessment. Br J Dis Chest 1976; 70(3):143–184.
39. Milic-Emili J, Mead J, Turner JM, et al. Improved technique for estimating pleural pressure from esophageal balloons. J Appl Physiol 1964; 19:207–211.
40. Marini JJ, O'Quin R, Culver BH, et al. Estimation of transmural cardiac pressures during ventilation with PEEP. J Appl Physiol 1982; 53(2):384–391.
41. Baydur A, Cha EJ, Sassoon CS. Validation of esophageal balloon technique at different lung volumes and postures. J Appl Physiol 1987; 62(1):315–321.
42. Cherniack RM, Farhi LE, Armstrong BW, et al. A comparison of esophageal and intrapleural pressure in man. J Appl Physiol 1955; 8(2):203–211.
43. Chiumello D, Carlesso E, Cadringher P, et al. Lung stress and strain during mechanical ventilation of the acute respiratory distress syndrome. Am J Respir Crit Care Med 2008; 178(4):346–355.
44. Birukov KG, Jacobson JR, Flores AA, et al. Magnitude-dependent regulation of pulmonary endothelial cell barrier function by cyclic stretch. Am J Physiol Lung Cell Mol Physiol 2003; 285(4):L785–L797.

45. Tschumperlin DJ, Oswari J, Margulies SS. Deformation-induced injury of alveolar epithelial cells: effect of frequency, duration and amplitude. Am J Respir Crit Care Med 2000; 162: 357–362.

46. Amato M, Barbas CSV, Pastore L, et al. Minimizing barotrauma in ARDS: protective effects of PEEP and the hazards of driving and plateau pressures. Am J Respir Crit Care Med 1996; 153: A375.

47. Maeda Y, Fujino Y, Uchiyama A, et al. Effects of peak inspiratory flow on development of ventilator-induced lung injury in rabbits. Anesthesiology 2004; 101(3):722–728.

48. Gajic O, Dara SI, Mendez JL, et al. Ventilator-associated lung injury in patients without acute lung injury at the onset of mechanical ventilation. Crit Care Med 2004; 32(9):1817–1824.

49. Michelet P, D'Journo XB, Roch A, et al. Protective ventilation influences systemic inflammation after esophagectomy: a randomized controlled study. Anesthesiology 2006; 105(5): 911–919.

50. Muscedere JG, Mullen JBM, Gan K, et al. Tidal ventilation at low airway pressures can augment lung injury. Am J Respir Crit Care Med 1994; 149:1327–1334.

51. Faridy EE, Permutt S, Riley RL. Effect of ventilation on surface forces in excised dogs' lungs. J Appl Physiol 1966; 21:1453–1462.

52. Mead J, Takishima T, Leith D. Stress distribution in lungs: a model of pulmonary elasticity. J Appl Physiol 1970; 28:596–608.

53. Martynowicz MA, Walters BJ, Hubmayr RD. Mechanisms of recruitment in oleic acid-injured lungs. J Appl Physiol 2001; 90(5):1744–1753.

54. Carmichael LC, Dorinsky PM, Higgins SB, et al. Diagnosis and therapy of acute respiratory distress syndrome in adults: an international survey. J Crit Care 1996; 11(1):9–18.

55. Thompson BT, Hayden D, Matthay MA, et al. Clinicians' approaches to mechanical ventilation in acute lung injury and ARDS. Chest 2001; 120:1622–1627.

56. Tremblay L, Valenza F, Ribeiro SP, et al. Injurious ventilatory strategies increase cytokines and c-fos m-RNA expression in an isolated rat lung model. J Clin Invest 1997; 99(5):944–952.

57. Corbridge TC, Wood LDH, Crawford GP, et al. Adverse effects of large tidal volume and low PEEP in canine acid aspiration. Am Rev Respir Dis 1990; 142:311–315.

58. Ranieri VM, Suter P, Tortorella C, et al. Effect of mechanical ventilation on inflammatory mediators in patients with acute respiratory distress syndrome. JAMA 1999; 282(1):54–61.

59. Lachman B. Open up the lung and keep the lung open. Intensive Care Med 1992; 18:319–321.

60. Verbrugge SJ, Lachmann B, Kesecioglu J. Lung protective ventilatory strategies in acute lung injury and acute respiratory distress syndrome: from experimental findings to clinical application. Clin Physiol Funct Imaging 2007; 27(2):67–90.

61. Haitsma JJ, Lachmann RA, Lachmann B. Lung protective ventilation in ARDS: role of mediators, PEEP and surfactant. Monaldi Arch Chest Dis 2003; 59(2):108–118.

62. Girgis K, Hamed H, Khater Y, et al. A decremental PEEP trial identifies the PEEP level that maintains oxygenation after lung recruitment. Respir Care 2006; 51(10):1132–1139.

63. Borges JB, Okamoto VN, Matos GF, et al. Reversibility of lung collapse and hypoxemia in early acute respiratory distress syndrome. Am J Respir Crit Care Med 2006; 174(3): 268–278.

64. Acute Respiratory Distress Syndorme Network. Higher versus lower positive end-expiratory pressures in patients with the acute respiratory distress syndrome. N Engl J Med 2004; 351(4):327–336.

65. Mercat A, Richard JC, Vielle B, et al. Positive end-expiratory pressure setting in adults with acute lung injury and acute respiratory distress syndrome: a randomized controlled trial. JAMA 2008; 299(6):646–655.

66. Meade MO, Cook DJ, Guyatt GH, et al. Ventilation strategy using low tidal volumes, recruitment maneuvers, and high positive end-expiratory pressure for acute lung injury and acute respiratory distress syndrome: a randomized controlled trial. JAMA 2008; 299(6):637–645.

67. Rouby JJ, Lu Q, Goldstein I. Selecting the right level of positive end-expiratory pressure in patients with acute respiratory distress syndrome. Am J Respir Crit Care Med 2002; 165(8):1182–1186.

68. Gattinoni L, Caironi P, Cressoni M, et al. Lung recruitment in patients with the acute respiratory distress syndrome. N Engl J Med 2006; 354(17):1775–1786.

69. Grasso S, Fanelli V, Cafarelli A, et al. Effects of high versus low positive end-expiratory pressures in acute respiratory distress syndrome. Am J Respir Crit Care Med 2005; 171(9): 1002–1008.

70. Richard JC, Maggiore SM, Johnson B, et al. Influence of tidal volume on alveolar recruitment: respective role of PEEP and a recruitment maneuver. Am J Respir Crit Care Med 2001; 163:1609–1613.

71. Puybasset L, Cluzel P, Chao N, et al. A computed tomography scan assessment of regional lung volume in acute lung injury. The CT Scan ARDS Study Group. Am J Respir Crit Care Med 1998; 158(5, pt 1):1644–1655.

72. Pelosi P, Goldner M, McKibben A, et al. Recruitment and derecruitment during acute respiratory failure: an experimental study. Am J Respir Crit Care Med 2001; 164(1):122–130.

73. Agostoni E, D'Angelo E, Bonanni MV. Topography of pleural surface pressure above resting volume in relaxed animals. J Appl Physiol 1970; 29(3):297–306.

74. Agostoni E, Miserocchi G. Vertical gradient of transpulmonary pressure with active and artificial lung expansion. J Appl Physiol 1970; 29(5):705–712.

75. Puybasset L, Cluzel P, Gusman P, et al. Regional distribution of gas and tissue in acute respiratory distress syndrome. I. Consequences for lung morphology. CT Scan ARDS Study Group. Intensive Care Med 2000; 26(7):857–869.

76. Puybasset L, Gusman P, Muller JC, et al. Regional distribution of gas and tissue in acute respiratory distress syndrome. III. Consequences for the effects of positive end-expiratory pressure. CT Scan ARDS Study Group. Adult Respiratory Distress Syndrome. Intensive Care Med 2000; 26(9):1215–1227.

77. Malbouisson LM, Muller J-C, Constantin J-M, et al. Computed tomography assessment of positive end-expiratory pressure-induced alveolar recruitment in patients with acute respiratory distress syndrome. Am J Respir Crit Care Med 2001; 163:1444–1450.

78. Jardin F, Dubourg O, Bourdarias JP. Echocardiographic pattern of acute cor pulmonale. Chest 1997; 111(1):209–217.

79. Vieillard-Baron A, Prin S, Chergui K, et al. Echo-Doppler demonstration of acute cor pulmonale at the bedside in the medical intensive care unit. Am J Respir Crit Care Med 2002; 166(10):1310–1319.

80. Viellard-Baron A, Schmitt J-M, Augarde R, et al. Acute cor pulmonale in acute respiratory distress syndrome submitted to protective ventilation: incidence, clinical implications, and prognosis. Crit Care Med 2001; 29:1551–1555.

81. Ranieri VM, Zhang H, Mascia L, et al. Pressure-time curve predicts minimally injurious ventilatory strategy in an isolated rat lung model. Anesthesiology 2000; 93:1320–1328.

82. Suter P, Fairley HB, Isenberg MD. Optimum end-expiratory airway pressure in patients with acute pulmonary failure. N Engl J Med 1975; 292:284–289.

83. Gattinoni L, Brazzi L, Pelosi P, et al. A trial of goal oriented hemodynamic therapy in critically ill patients. N Engl J Med 1995; 333:1025–1032.

84. Wiedemann HP, Wheeler AP, Bernard GR, et al. Comparison of two fluid-management strategies in acute lung injury. N Engl J Med 2006; 354(24):2564–2575.

85. Amato MBP, Barbas CSV, Medeiros DM, et al. Beneficial effects of the "open lung approach" with low distending pressures in acute respiratory distress syndrome. Am J Respir Crit Care Med 1995; 152:1835–1846.

86. Matamis D, Lemaire F, Hart A, et al. Total respiratory pressure-volume curves in the adult respiratory syndrome. Chest 1984; 86:58–66.

87. Jonson B, Richard JC, Straus C, et al. Pressure-volume curves and compliance in acute lung injury: evidence of recruitment above the lower inflection point. Am J Respir Crit Care Med 1999; 159;1172–1178.

88. Kolobow T, Moretti MP, Fumagalli R, et al. Severe impairment in lung function induced by high peak airway pressure during mechanical ventilation. Am Rev Respir Dis 1987; 135: 312–315.

89. Rimensberger PC, Pristine G, Mullen BM, et al. Lung recruitment during small tidal volume ventilation allows minimal positive end-expiratory pressure without augmenting lung injury. Crit Care Med 1999; 27(9):1940–1945.

90. Dantzker DR, Lynch JP, Weg JG. Depression of cardiac output is a mechanism of shunt reduction in the therapy of acute respiratory failure. Chest 1980; 77:636–642.

91. Victorino JA, Borges JB, Okamoto VN, et al. Imbalances in regional lung ventilation: a validation study on electrical impedance tomography. Am J Respir Crit Care Med 2004; 169(7):791–800.

92. Grasso S, Mascia L, Del Turco M, et al. Effects of recruiting maneuvers in patients with acute respiratory distress syndrome ventilated with protective ventilatory strategy. Anesthesiology 2002; 96(4):795–802.

93. Villagra A, Ochagavia A, Vatua S, et al. Recruitment maneuvers during lung protective ventilation in acute respiratory distress syndrome. Am J Respir Crit Care Med 2002; 165: 165–170.

94. Brower RG, Morris A, MacIntyre N, et al. Effects of recruitment maneuvers in patients with acute lung injury and acute respiratory distress syndrome ventilated with high positive end-expiratory pressure. Crit Care Med 2003; 31(11):2592–2597.

95. Oczenski W, Hormann C, Keller C, et al. Recruitment maneuvers after a positive end-expiratory pressure trial do not induce sustained effects in early adult respiratory distress syndrome. Anesthesiology 2004; 101:620–625.

96. Pelosi P, Cadringher P, Bottino N, et al. Sigh in acute respiratory distress syndrome. Am J Respir Crit Care Med 1999; 159:872–880.

97. Suh GY, Kwon OJ, Yoon JW, et al. A practical protocol for titrating "optimal" PEEP in acute lung injury: recruitment maneuver and PEEP decrement. J Korean Med Sci 2003; 18(3): 349–354.

98. Tugrul S, Akinci O, Ozcan PE, et al. Effects of sustained inflation and postinflation positive end-expiratory pressure in acute respiratory distress syndrome: focusing on pulmonary and extrapulmonary forms. Crit Care Med 2003; 31(3):738–744.

99. Lim SC, Adams AB, Simonson DA, et al. Transient hemodynamic effects of recruitment maneuvers in three experimental models of acute lung injury. Crit Care Med 2004; 32(12): 2378–2384.

100. Lapinsky SE, Aubin M, Mehta S, et al. Safety and efficacy of a sustained inflation for alveolar recruitment in adults with respiratory failure. Intensive Care Med 1999; 25(11): 1297–1301.

101. Nielsen J, Ostergaard M, Kjaergaard J, et al. Lung recruitment maneuver depresses central hemodynamics in patients following cardiac surgery. Intensive Care Med 2005; 31(9):1189–1194.

102. Foti G, Cereda M, Sparacino ME, et al. Effects of periodic lung recruitment maneuvers on gas exchange and respiratory mechanics in mechanically ventilated acute respiratory distress syndrome (ARDS) patients. Intensive Care Med 2000; 26:501–507.

103. Krishnan J, Brower R. High-frequency ventilation for acute lung injury and ARDS. Chest 2000; 118:795–807.

104. Kress JP, Pohlman AS, O'Connor MF, et al. Daily interruption of sedative infusions in critically ill patients undergoing mechanical ventilation. N Engl J Med 2000; 342: 1471–1477.

105. Johnson AH, Peacock JL, Greenough A, et al. High-frequency oscillatory ventilation for the prevention of chronic lung disease of prematurity. N Engl J Med 2002; 347(9):633–642.

106. Courtney SE, Durand DJ, Asselin JM, et al. High-frequency oscillatory ventilation versus conventional mechanical ventilation for very-low-birth-weight infants. N Engl J Med 2002; 347(9):643–652.

107. Bollen CW, van Well GT, Sherry T, et al. High frequency oscillatory ventilation compared with conventional mechanical ventilation in adult respiratory distress syndrome: a randomized controlled trial [ISRCTN24242669]. Crit Care 2005; 9(4):R430–R439.

108. Hager DN, Fessler HE, Kaczka DW, et al. Tidal volume delivery during high-frequency oscillatory ventilation in adults with acute respiratory distress syndrome. Crit Care Med 2007; 35(6):1522–1529.

109. Sedeek KA, Takeuchi M, Suchodolski K, et al. Open-lung protective ventilation with pressure control ventilation, high-frequency oscillation, and intratracheal pulmonary ventilation results in similar gas exchange, hemodynamics, and lung mechanics. Anesthesiology 2003; 99(5):1102–1111.

110. Mehta S. Noninvasive positive pressure ventilation in acute respiratory failure. Intensive Care Med 1998; 24:1113–1114.

111. Brochard L. Noninvasive ventilation in acute respiratory failure. Respir Care 1996; 41:456–465.

112. Mehta S, Hill NS. Noninvasive ventilation. Am J Respir Crit Care Med 2001; 163:540–577.

113. Hill NS. Noninvasive positive pressure ventilation for respiratory failure caused by exacerbations of chronic obstructive pulmonary disease: a standard of care? Crit Care 2003; 7(6):400–401.

114. Brochard L, Isabey D, Piquet J, et al. Reversal of acute exacerbations of chronic obstructive lung disease by inspiratory assistance with a face mask. N Engl J Med 1990; 323:1523–1530.

115. Antonelli M, Conti G, Rocco M, et al. A comparison of noninvasive positive-pressure ventilation and conventional mechanical ventilation in patients with acute respiratory failure. N Engl J Med 1998; 339:429–435.

116. L'Her E, Deye N, Lellouche F, et al. Physiologic effects of noninvasive ventilation during acute lung injury. Am J Respir Crit Care Med 2005; 172(9):1112–1118.

117. Wysocki M. Noninvasive ventilation in acute cardiogenic pulmonary edema: better than continuous positive airway pressure? Intensive Care Med 1999; 25:1–2.

118. Honrubia T, Garcia Lopez FJ, Franco N, et al. Noninvasive vs. conventional mechanical ventilation in acute respiratory failure: a multicenter, randomized controlled trial. Chest 2005; 128(6):3916–3924.

119. Antonelli M, Conti G, Moro ML, et al. Predictors of failure of noninvasive positive pressure ventilation in patients with acute hypoxemic respiratory failure: a multi-center study. Intensive Care Med 2001; 27(11):1718–1728.

120. Lellouche F. Noninvasive ventilation in patients with hypoxemic acute respiratory failure. Curr Opin Crit Care 2007; 13(1):12–19.

121. Antonelli M, Conti G, Esquinas A, et al. A multiple-center survey on the use in clinical practice of noninvasive ventilation as a first-line intervention for acute respiratory distress syndrome. Crit Care Med 2007; 35(1):18–25.

122. Yoshida Y, Takeda S, Akada S, et al. Factors predicting successful noninvasive ventilation in acute lung injury. J Anesth 2008; 22(3):201–206.

123. Guisset O, Vargas F, Gabinski C, et al. Non-invasive ventilation (NIV) in acute respiratory distress syndrome (ARDS) patients-oral presentation. Intensive Care Med 2003; 29:S124.

124. Ferrer M, Esquinas A, Leon M, et al. Noninvasive ventilation in severe hypoxemic respiratory failure: a randomized clinical trial. Am J Respir Crit Care Med 2003; 168(12):1438–1444.

125. Rana S, Jenad H, Gay PC, et al. Failure of non-invasive ventilation in patients with acute lung injury: observational cohort study. Crit Care 2006; 10(3):R79.

126. Domenighetti G, Gayer R, Gentilini R. Noninvasive pressure support ventilation in non-COPD patients with acute cardiogenic pulmonary edema and severe community-acquired pneumonia: acute effects and outcome. Intensive Care Med 2002; 28(9):1226–1232.

127. Antonelli M, Contin G, Bufi M, et al. Noninvasive ventilation for treatment of acute respiratory failure in patients undergoing solid organ transplantation. JAMA 2000; 283:235–241.

128. Girou E, Schortgen F, Delclaux C, et al. Association of noninvasive ventilation with nosocomial infections and survival in critically ill patients. JAMA 2000; 284:2361–2367.

129. Hilbert G, Gruson D, Vargas F, et al. Noninvasive ventilation in immunosuppressed patients with pulmonary infiltrates, fever, and acute respiratory failure. N Engl J Med 2001; 344(7):481.

130. Azoulay E, Alberti C, Bornstain C, et al. Improved survival in cancer patients requiring mechanical ventilatory support: impact of non-invasive mechanical ventilatory support. Crit Care Med 2001; 29:519–525.

131. Putensen C, Rasanen J, Lopez F, et al. Effect of interfacing between spontaneous breathing and mechanical cycles on the ventilation-perfusion distribution in canine lung injury. Anesthesiology 1994; 81:921–930.

132. Putensen C, Zech S, Wrigge H, et al. Long-term effects of spontaneous breathing during ventilatory support in patients with acute lung injury. Am J Respir Crit Care Med 2001; 164:43–49.

133. Downs JB, Stock MC. Airway pressure release ventilation: a new concept in ventilatory support. Crit Care Med 1987; 15:459–461.

134. Forel JM, Roch A, Marin V, et al. Neuromuscular blocking agents decrease inflammatory response in patients presenting with acute respiratory distress syndrome. Crit Care Med 2006; 34(11):2749–2757.

135. Pedersen BK, Steensberg A, Schjerling P. Muscle-derived interleukin-6: possible biological effects. J Physiol 2001; 536(pt 2):329–337.

136. Pedersen BK, Steensberg A, Fischer C, et al. Searching for the exercise factor: is IL-6 a candidate? J Muscle Res Cell Motil 2003; 24(2–3):113–119.

137. Demoule A, Girou E, Richard JC, et al. Benefits and risks of success or failure of noninvasive ventilation. Intensive Care Med 2006; 32(11):1756–1765.

138. Cook D, Ricard JD, Reeve B, et al. Ventilator circuit and secretion management strategies: a Franco-Canadian survey. Crit Care Med 2000; 28:3547–3554.

139. Le Bourdelles G, Mier L, Fiquet B, et al. Comparison of the effects of heat and moisture exchangers and heated humidifiers on ventilation and gas exchange during weaning trials from mechanical ventilation. Chest 1996; 110:1294–1298.

140. Pelosi P, Solca M, Ravagnan I, et al. Effects of heat and moisture exchangers on minute ventilation, ventilatory drive, and work of breathing during pressure-support ventilation in acute respiratory failure. Crit Care Med 1996; 24:1184–1188.

141. Moran I, Bellapart J, Vari A, et al. Heat and moisture exchangers and heated humidifiers in acute lung injury/acute respiratory distress syndrome patients. Effects on respiratory mechanics and gas exchange. Intensive Care Med 2006; 32(4):524–531.

142. Almog A, Brower R. Complications of mechanical ventilation. In: Matthay MA, Schwartz DE, eds. Complications in the Intensive Care Unit. New York: Chapman & Hall, 1997:50–61.

19
Fluid Therapy and Hemodynamic Monitoring in Acute Lung Injury

CAROLYN S. CALFEE
Pulmonary and Critical Care Medicine and Cardiovascular Research Institute,
University of California, San Francisco, California, U.S.A.

NAVEEN GUPTA
Department of Medicine, Division of Pulmonary and Critical Care, University of Pittsburgh
School of Medicine, Pittsburgh, Pennsylvania, U.S.A.

MICHAEL A. MATTHAY
Pulmonary and Critical Care Medicine and Cardiovascular Research Institute,
University of California, San Francisco, California, U.S.A.

I. Introduction

Fluid management for patients with acute lung injury (ALI) has been an area of uncertainty and controversy for approximately three decades (1–4). Several observational studies have suggested that restricting the quantity of fluid replacement might be beneficial in reducing the extent of pulmonary edema in patients with ALI. On the other hand, there has been concern that a restrictive fluid management strategy might potentiate nonpulmonary organ failure. From a physiologic perspective, although the fundamental mechanism responsible for pulmonary edema formation in ALI can be best explained by an increase in lung vascular permeability, elevation in lung vascular hydrostatic pressures also does result in a greater increase in extravascular lung water (Fig. 1). Short-term experimental studies demonstrated that lowering pulmonary vascular pressure was an effective mechanism for reducing lung edema in models of lung injury. A classic study by Prewitt and coworkers (5) published in 1981 demonstrated that lowering left atrial hydrostatic pressure reduced the quantity of lung edema in short-term studies of oleic acid-induced lung injury in dogs. Also, based on several experimental studies in 1978, Staub provided a convincing physiologic rationale for the likely value of lowering pulmonary vascular pressures in noncardiogenic pulmonary edema (6).

In an attempt to address the unresolved clinical question of the optimal fluid replacement strategy in ALI, the National Heart, Lung and Blood Institute Acute Respiratory Distress Syndrome Network recently completed a 1000-patient clinical trial entitled the Fluid and Catheter Treatment Trial (FACTT) (7). This trial compared a conservative to a liberal fluid management strategy in patients with ALI. In both arms of the trial, fluid and diuretic management were dictated by a protocolized regimen. The fluid management strategies were tested in a factorial design that also evaluated the utility of a central venous catheter versus a pulmonary artery catheter for hemodynamic monitoring (8). Because the results of this clinical trial have provided the first evidence-based guidelines for fluid management of patients with ALI, this chapter will focus on the primary results of this trial and the implications for clinical practice.

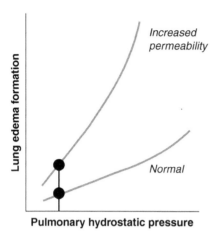

Pulmonary hydrostatic pressure

Figure 1 Relationship between pulmonary hydrostatic pressure and lung edema formation under normal conditions and increased permeability. Under normal conditions, an increase in pulmonary hydrostatic pressure results in increased lung edema formation. In the setting of increased lung epithelial permeability, this relationship is further accentuated. *Source*: From Ref. 6.

II. Design of the Trial

Patients were enrolled in the FACTT within 48 hours of the onset of lung injury. The diagnostic criteria for ALI were based on the American-European consensus conference (9) and included the acute onset of bilateral pulmonary infiltrates on chest radiograph, a $Pao_2/Fio_2 < 300$, and no clinical evidence of left atrial hypertension. Important exclusions were the presence of a pulmonary artery catheter, the need for dialysis, and chronic lung disease. All participants in the trial were ventilated with the lung-protective low tidal volume, plateau pressure-limited ventilator strategy, previously published by the ARDS Network and demonstrated to reduce mortality (10).

Patients were randomly assigned to receive either a central venous catheter or pulmonary artery catheter for hemodynamic management, with stratification by the presence of sepsis. In addition, patients were then randomized to either a fluid-conservative or fluid-liberal strategy. Importantly, the fluid management strategies were not instituted until patients had been out of shock for 12 hours. Shock was defined as a mean arterial pressure <60 mm Hg, or the requirement for vasopressors (other than dopamine at a dose less than 5 μg/kg/min). For patients in shock, fluid management was left to the judgment of the managing physicians.

Hemodynamic measurements were made every four hours, and adjustments in fluid or diuretic management were instituted according to those findings. For patients randomized to the fluid-conservative group, the primary goal of the protocol was to lower central venous pressure with fluid restriction and diuretic therapy to less than 4 mm Hg or the pulmonary artery wedge pressure to less than 8 mm Hg. For patients randomized to the fluid-liberal strategy, the protocol goal was a central venous pressure of 10 to 14 mm Hg or a pulmonary artery pressure of 14 to 18 mm Hg. Adherence to both the fluid-conservative and fluid-liberal strategies was excellent, with approximately 90% of protocol orders accepted (8).

III. Hemodynamic Monitoring

In terms of monitoring hemodynamics with either a central venous catheter or pulmonary artery catheter, the trial found no differences between the two groups in any of the major clinical outcomes, including mortality, ventilator-free days, or organ failure-free days (Fig. 2) (8). In addition, there was no difference in the requirement for hemodialysis between the two catheter groups (8). There was an increase in minor complications with the pulmonary artery catheter, but there was no mortality attributable to the insertion or presence of a pulmonary artery catheter (Table 1).

The results of this part of the trial were in agreement with several other recent clinical trials that found no significant benefit of monitoring critically ill patients with a pulmonary artery catheter versus a central venous catheter. Specifically, trials from Canada, France, and the UK respectively found no benefit of using a pulmonary artery catheter compared to a central venous catheter in the management of high-risk surgical patients (11), ALI and shock (12), or general critical illness (13). Also, a U.S.-based study of congestive heart failure found no benefit of using a pulmonary artery catheter for management of decompensated congestive heart failure (14).

Interestingly, 29% of the patients randomized to the pulmonary artery catheter arm in the FACTT had a pulmonary artery occlusion pressure of greater than 18 mm Hg; half of these patients had a pulmonary artery occlusion pressure of 19 or 20 mm Hg. However, only 3.5% of patients had both a pulmonary artery occlusion pressure of greater than 18 mm Hg and a cardiac index of less than 2.5 L per minute per square meter, indicating that few patients with purely cardiogenic pulmonary edema were enrolled in the trial. Nonetheless, the finding that more than 25% of the patients with ALI had an

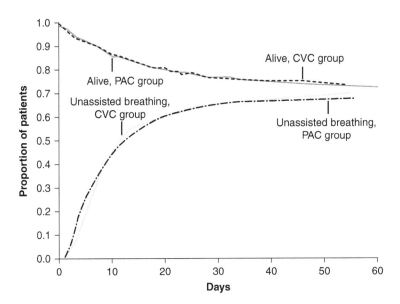

Figure 2 Kaplan–Meier estimates of the probability of survival and of survival without the need for assisted ventilation during the first 60 days after randomization. *Source*: From Ref. 8.

Table 1 Catheter-Related Complications

	Number of patients						
	PAC group				CVC group		
Complication	Sheath	PAC	CVC	Total	Sheath	CVC	Total
Technical and mechanical complications							
Difficult placement	1	8	1	10	0	2	2
Catheter malfunction	0	4	0	4	0	0	0
Pneumothorax	3	2	1	6	0	6	6
Air embolism	1	1	1	3	0	0	0
Arterial puncture	1	0	2	3	0	0	0
Arrhythmia							
Atrial	3	15	0	18	0	0	0
Ventricular	4	15	0	19	1	5	6
Conduction defect	1	4	0	5	1	0	1
Bleeding and clotting							
Hemothorax	2	1	0	3	1	0	1
Insertion-site bleeding	2	1	3	6	1	2	3
Thromboembolism	0	0	0	0	1	0	1
Local thrombosis	1	1	1	3	0	6	6
Infection							
Local	3	2	7	12	1	8	9
Bloodstream[a]	1	3	1	5	0	3	3
Other	0	2	1	3	0	3	3
Total	23	59	100	100	6	35	41

[a]Positive blood cultures were believed to be related to the presence of the catheter. Overall, 19% of patients in the PAC group and 18% of patients in the CVC group had one or more positive blood cultures ($p = 0.43$).
Abbreviations: PAC, pulmonary artery catheter; CVC, central venous catheter.
Source: From Ref. 8.

elevated pulmonary arterial wedge pressure further underscored the potential relevance of a conservative approach to fluid management by demonstrating that many patients with ALI also have concomitant volume overload.

IV. The Fluid Strategies

Patients in the conservative fluid management arm had significantly more ventilator-free days than patients in the liberal fluid management arm (14.6 ± 0.5 vs. 12.1 ± 0.5 days, respectively, mean $\pm$ SE, $p < 0.001$) (Table 2). This increase in ventilator-free days was associated with concordant improvements in pulmonary physiology; specifically the oxygenation index and the lung injury score were significantly improved in the conservative fluid group compared to the liberal fluid group (Table 3) (7). In addition, there was a nearly significant improvement in the Pao_2/Fio_2 in the conservative group ($p = 0.07$), and the plateau airway pressure was 1.5 cm H_2O lower in the conservative fluid group ($p = 0.01$). Thus, the improvement in pulmonary physiologic indices suggested that

Table 2 Main Outcome Variables[a]

Complication	Conservative strategy	Liberal strategy	p-value
Death at 60 days (%)	25.5	28.4	0.30
Ventilator-free days from days 1–28[b]	14.6 ± 0.5	12.1 ± 0.5	<0.001
ICU-free days[b]			
Days 1–7	0.9 ± 0.1	0.6 ± 0.1	<0.001
Days 1–28	13.4 ± 0.4	11.2 ± 0.4	<0.001
Organ failure-free days[b,c]			
Days 1–7			
Cardiovascular failure	3.9 ± 0.1	4.2 ± 0.1	0.04
CNS failure	3.4 ± 0.2	2.9 ± 0.2	0.02
Renal failure	5.5 ± 0.1	5.6 ± 0.1	0.45
Hepatic failure	5.7 ± 0.1	5.5 ± 0.1	0.12
Coagulation abnormalities	5.6 ± 0.1	5.4 ± 0.1	0.23
Days 1–28			
Cardiovascular failure	19.0 ± 0.5	19.1 ± 0.4	0.85
CNS failure	18.8 ± 0.5	17.2 ± 0.5	0.03
Renal failure	21.5 ± 0.5	21.2 ± 0.5	0.59
Hepatic failure	22.0 ± 0.4	21.2 ± 0.5	0.18
Coagulation abnormalities	22.0 ± 0.4	21.5 ± 0.4	0.37
Dialysis to day 60			
Patients (%)	10	14	0.06
Days	11.0 ± 1.7	10.9 ± 1.4	0.96

[a]Plus–minus values are means ± SE. CNS denotes central nervous system.
[b]This was an a priori secondary outcome.
[c]For this analysis, cardiovascular failure was defined by a systolic blood pressure of 90 mm Hg or less or the need for a vasopressor [in contrast, shock was defined by a mean arterial pressure of less than 60 mm Hg or the need for a vasopressor (except a dose of dopamine of 5 μg per kilogram per minute or less)]; a coagulation abnormality was defined by a platelet count of 80,000 per cubic millimeter or less; hepatic failure was defined by a serum bilirubin level of at least 2 mg per deciliter (34 μmol per liter); and renal failure was defined by a serum creatinine level of at least 2 mg per deciliter (177 μmol per liter). We calculated the number of days without organ or system failure by subtracting the number of days with organ failure from the lesser of 28 days or the number of days to death. Organs and systems were considered failure-free after patients were discharged from the hospital.
Source: From Ref. 7.

patients treated with the fluid-conservative protocol had reduced quantities of pulmonary edema, although there was no direct evidence for this conclusion since extravascular lung water was not measured in this trial. Patients in the conservative fluid management arm also had more intensive care unit-free days than those in the liberal fluid management arm (13.4 ± 0.4 vs. 11.2 ± 0.4 days, respectively; mean ± SE, $p < 0.001$).

In terms of the primary outcome of the study, there was a nonsignificant 2.9% reduction in 60-day mortality in the fluid-conservative management group compared with the liberal fluid management group (25.5% vs. 28.4%, respectively; $p = 0.30$; 95% confidence interval for the difference, minus 2.6–8.4%) (Table 2). In addition, there were no differences between the two fluid strategies in the incidence or prevalence of shock.

Table 3 Pulmonary Outcomes in the Fluid and Catheter Treatment Trial (FACTT)

Variable	Fluid-conservative group	Fluid-liberal group	p-value[a]
Ventilator-free days	14.6 ± 0.5	12.1 ± 0.5	<0.001
ICU-free days (1–28)	13.4 ± 0.4	11.2 ± 0.4	<0.001
Plateau pressure, cm H_2O	24.2 ± 0.6	25.7 ± 0.5	0.002
Dialysis to day 60[a]	10%	14%	0.06
Oxygenation index	10.1 ± 0.8	11.8 ± 0.7	0.003
Lung injury score	2.03 ± 0.07	2.27 ± 0.06	<0.001

All variables reported as mean $\pm$ SE. p-Values for the physiologic variables are for comparison of trends over time using repeated measures analysis of variance, though only day 7 values are shown in the table for simplicity.
Oxygenation index calculated as (mean airway pressure $\times$ Fio_2/Pao_2) $\times$ 100, with a lower number indicating better gas exchange. Lung injury score is calculated as previously described.
[a]Patients (%).

Although there was concern that a fluid-conservative strategy would have a deleterious effect on renal function, there was a trend toward a higher need for renal replacement therapy in the fluid-liberal group (10% in fluid conservative vs. 14% in fluid liberal; $p = 0.06$); the mean number of days of dialysis required did not differ between the two groups (conservative fluid group = 11.0 ± 1.7 days vs. liberal fluid management group 10.9 ± 1.4 days; $p = 0.96$). Thus, there was no evidence that the conservative fluid management strategy had a negative impact on renal function. Furthermore, there was a small but significant improvement in central nervous system status in the fluid-conservative group (Table 2).

V. Relevance of This Trial to Clinical Practice

When considering how to translate the results of this trial into clinical practice, it is important to remember that the FACTT trial was designed to address the issue of fluid management in patients with ALI who were *not* in shock. Thus, the results of the FACTT trial do not conflict with the finding that early goal-directed therapy and the concomitant fluid resuscitation improve outcomes in patients with septic shock (15). Of note, a prospective NIH-supported trial at the University of Pittsburgh is underway to test and validate the results of the Rivers trial, which at this time remains the only trial of early goal-directed therapy.

An additional consideration for clinicians wanting to implement the results of this trial in their own practice is how to translate the somewhat complex FACTT fluid management algorithm into a real-world setting. To address this issue, and to generate a template for use in ongoing and future clinical trials, the ARDS Network Investigators have provided a simplified version of the conservative fluid management protocol (Table 4). In addition, the cumulative fluid balance observed over the first seven days of the trial can provide some guidance to physicians trying to implement a fluid-conservative strategy. The average daily fluid balance for patients in the trial in the liberal fluid group was approximately 1 L positive per day. This positive fluid balance is similar to the results of prior studies from the ARDS Network in which fluid management was not protocolized, suggesting that the fluid-liberal strategy approximated typical fluid management (Fig. 3) (7). In sharp contrast, the conservative fluid management patients had a net even fluid

Table 4 Algorithm for Conservative Management of Fluids in Patients with Acute Lung Injury

CVP (mm Hg) (recommended)	PAOP (mm Hg) (optional)	MAP ≥ 60 mm Hg and off vasopressors for ≥ 12 hr	
		Average urine output <0.5 mL/kg/hr	Average urine output ≥ 0.5 mL/kg/hr
>8	>12	Furosemide*; reassess in 1 hr	Furosemide; reassess in 4 hr
4–8	8–12	Fluid bolus as fast as possible;† reassess in 1 hr	Furosemide; reassess in 4 hr
<4	<8	Fluid bolus as fast as possible;† reassess in 1 hr	No intervention; reassess in 4 hr

Patients must have had a MAP of greater than 60 mm Hg without requiring vasopressors for at least 12 hours before this protocol is initiated.
*For diuretics, the furosemide dosing begins with 20 mg bolus, 3 mg/hr infusion, or last known effective dose. Double each subsequent dose until goal achieved (oliguria reversal or intravascular pressure target), with maximal dose of 160 mg bolus or 24 mg/hr. Do not exceed 620 mg/day. If patient has heart failure, treatment with dobutamine may be considered. Diuretic therapy should be withheld for patients with renal failure, defined as dialysis dependence, oliguria with serum creatinine >2 mg/dl, or oliguria with serum creatinine <2 mg/dl but urinary indices indicative of acute renal failure.
†Fluid bolus: 15 mL/kg crystalloid (round to nearest 250 mL) or 1 unit packed red blood cells or 25 g albumin.
Abbreviations: CVP, central venous pressure; PAOP, pulmonary artery occlusion pressure; MAP, mean arterial pressure.

balance over the first seven days of the protocol (Fig. 3) (7). This finding provides a practical guideline for fluid management in critically ill patients with ALI. It is important to appreciate that aggressive diuresis needs to be accompanied by careful monitoring of the patient's serum potassium and bicarbonate and careful monitoring of overall electrolyte and metabolic balance.

Patients with ALI due to severe trauma comprised a small percentage of patients (8%); thus, extrapolation of the results of this trial to this patient group should be done with caution. Patients with trauma-induced lung injury have had a markedly improved mortality over the past two decades (16), and recent data suggest that the biologic features of trauma-related ALI may differ substantially from those of ALI due to other causes (17).

VI. Limitations of the FACTT Trial
The FACTT did not address the question of whether colloid or crystalloid should be used for management of patients with ALI. In the FACTT protocol, fluid boluses were administered in the form of normal saline, Plasmalyte, Lactated Ringers, packed red blood cells, or albumin, depending on the physician's preference. In 2004, the SAFE trial (Saline Versus Albumin Fluid Evaluation Trial) reported that saline was equivalent to an albumin solution for resuscitation of critically ill patients (18).

At the same time, previous studies have demonstrated that the subset of ALI patients with hypoproteinemia may benefit from albumin therapy. Martin and coworkers (19) randomized 37 patients with ALI and a serum protein concentration less than 5.0 g/dL to

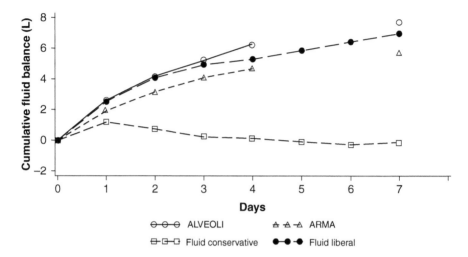

Figure 3 Cumulative fluid balance in patients enrolled in the FACTT compared to patients in prior acute respiratory distress syndrome network studies. Fluid administration in the liberal fluid management arm of the FACTT was similar to fluid administration in two prior acute respiratory distress syndrome network studies of ventilator management strategy. The fluid-liberal strategy, like the unprotocolized fluid management in prior trials, resulted in a gain of approximately 1 L/day. In contrast, fluid administration in the conservative fluid management arm results in a net even fluid balance over the first seven days of the study. *Abbreviations*: ARMA, acute respiratory distress syndrome network trial of 6 versus 12 mL/kg tidal volume ventilation; ALVEOLI, acute respiratory distress syndrome network trial of low versus high positive end-expiratory pressure. *Source*: From Ref. 7.

receive either furosemide in albumin every eight hours for five days or double placebo. The intervention group had improved oxygenation, fluid balance, and hemodynamics; although no differences in mortality were observed, this study was a phase II trial that was not powered to assess mortality as a major outcome. In a follow-up trial that compared the administration of furosemide with albumin to furosemide without albumin, the combination of both the diuretic and albumin appeared to be superior, using similar endpoints (20). Thus, further clinical trials in ALI are needed to assess the potential role of albumin therapy, perhaps in combination with diuretics and a fluid-conservative strategy.

VII. Conclusions

Although the results of a single trial must be interpreted cautiously when applied to patients with ALI, the results of the FACTT trial are sufficiently impressive so that clinical practice should change in at least two respects.

First, the pulmonary artery catheter should not be considered beneficial in the vast majority of patients with ALI, particularly those patients without shock. Monitoring the central venous pressure should be adequate. The pulmonary artery catheter may still be valuable in the management of patients with severe or persistent shock or a clinical presentation complicated by the combination of cardiac insufficiency and sepsis (21), although the FACTT did not address this issue. Furthermore, the results of the FACTT demonstrated that 29% of patients had an initial pulmonary arterial wedge pressure greater than 18 mm Hg (7), consistent with the general hypothesis that ALI is often complicated by elevated intravascular pressures that may augment the degree of pulmonary edema (6).

Second, the results of the FACTT support the value of inducing a negative fluid balance in patients with ALI who are not in shock. In order to achieve this objective, measurements and management of hemodynamics need to be done on a frequent basis (Table 4). In the FACTT trial, central venous pressure or the pulmonary arterial wedge pressure was measured every four hours, and clinical decisions were made to administer diuretics and/or to limit fluid administration in order to achieve a central venous pressure that was less than or equal to 4 mm Hg. The results of the FACTT trial also indicate that acute renal failure was not precipitated by a fluid-conservative therapy. Although there was no significant difference in mortality between the two groups ($p = 0.30$), mortality was almost 3% less in the fluid-conservative group.

In our opinion, the results of the NHLBI ARDS Network clinical FACTT trial should transform the care of patients with ALI. It is now clear that a fluid-conservative management strategy should be instituted for most patients with ALI, if they are not in shock. After so many years of opinion-based recommendations for fluid management in patients with ALI, it is gratifying to have the results of a randomized clinical trial that provides the basis for evidence-based recommendations.

Acknowledgments

We appreciate the assistance of Andrew Manies in preparing this manuscript. Dr. Matthay was supported by NHLBI HL51856 and HL51854. Dr. Gupta was supported by a Parker B. Francis Career Development Award and Dr. Calfee was supported by a FAMRI Career Award and an NHLBI K23 Award.

References

1. Hyers TM. ARDS: the therapeutic dilemma. Chest 1990; 97:1025.
2. Schuster DP. The case for and against fluid restriction and occlusion pressure reduction in adult respiratory distress syndrome. New Horiz 1993; 1:478–488.
3. Simmons RS, Berdine GG, Seidenfeld JJ, et al. Fluid balance and the adult respiratory distress syndrome. Am Rev Respir Dis 1987; 135:924–929.
4. Humphrey H, Hall J, Sznajder I, et al. Improved survival in ARDS patients associated with a reduction in pulmonary capillary wedge pressure. Chest 1990; 97:1176–1180.
5. Prewitt RM, McCarthy J, Wood LD. Treatment of acute low pressure pulmonary edema in dogs: relative effects of hydrostatic and oncotic pressure, nitroprusside, and positive end-expiratory pressure. J Clin Invest 1981; 67: 409–418.
6. Staub NC. Pulmonary edema: physiologic approaches to management. Chest 1978; 74:559–564.
7. Wiedemann HP, Wheeler AP, Bernard GR, et al. Comparison of two fluid-management strategies in acute lung injury. N Engl J Med 2006; 354:2564–2575.
8. Wheeler AP, Bernard GR, Thompson BT, et al. Pulmonary-artery versus central venous catheter to guide treatment of acute lung injury. N Engl J Med 2006; 354: 2213–2224.
9. Bernard GR, Artigas A, Brigham KL, et al. The American-European consensus conference on ARDS: Definitions, mechanisms, relevant outcomes, and clinical trial coordination. Am J Resp Crit Care Med 1994; 149:818–824.

10. The Acute Respiratory Distress Syndrome Network. Ventilation with lower tidal volumes as compared with traditional tidal volumes for acute lung injury and the acute respiratory distress syndrome. N Engl J Med 2000; 342:1301–1308.
11. Sandham JD, Hull RD, Brant RF, et al. A randomized, controlled trial of the use of pulmonary-artery catheters in high-risk surgical patients. N Engl J Med 2003; 348:5–14.
12. Richard C, Warszawski J, Anguel N, et al. Early use of the pulmonary artery catheter and outcomes in patients with shock and acute respiratory distress syndrome: a randomized controlled trial. JAMA 2003; 290:2713–2720.
13. Harvey S, Harrison DA, Singer M, et al. Assessment of the clinical effectiveness of pulmonary artery catheters in management of patients in intensive care (PAC-Man): a randomised controlled trial. Lancet 2005; 366:472–477.
14. Binanay C, Califf RM, Hasselblad V, et al. Evaluation study of congestive heart failure and pulmonary artery catheterization effectiveness: the ESCAPE trial. JAMA 2005; 294:1625–1633.
15. Rivers E, Nguyen B, Havstad S, et al. Early goal-directed therapy in the treatment of severe sepsis and septic shock. N Engl J Med 2001; 345:1368–1377.
16. Stapleton RD, Wang BM, Hudson LD, et al. Causes and timing of death in patients with ARDS. Chest 2005; 128:525–532.
17. Calfee CS, Eisner MD, Ware LB, et al. Trauma-associated acute lung injury differs clinically & biologically from acute lung injury due to other clinical disorders. Crit Care Med 2007; 35:2243–2250.
18. Myburgh J, Cooper DJ, Finfer S, et al. Saline or albumin for fluid resuscitation in patients with traumatic brain injury. N Engl J Med 2007; 357:874–884.
19. Martin GS, Mangialardi RJ, Wheeler AP, et al. Albumin and furosemide therapy in hypoproteinemic patients with acute lung injury. Crit Care Med 2002; 30:2175–2182.
20. Martin GS, Moss M, Wheeler AP, et al. A randomized, controlled trial of furosemide with or without albumin in hypoproteinemic patients with acute lung injury. Crit Care Med 2005; 33:1681–1687.
21. Ware LB, Matthay MA. Clinical practice. Acute pulmonary edema. N Engl J Med 2005; 353:2788–2796.

20

Pathogenesis of Sepsis and Sepsis-Induced Acute Lung Injury

ESTELLE S. HARRIS and MATTHEW T. RONDINA
Divisions of Respiratory and Critical Care Medicine and General Internal Medicine,
Department of Medicine, University of Utah, Salt Lake City, Utah, U.S.A.

HANSJÖRG SCHWERTZ
Division of Vascular Surgery, Department of Surgery, University of Utah, Salt Lake City,
Utah, U.S.A.

ANDREW S. WEYRICH and GUY A. ZIMMERMAN
Division of Respiratory and Critical Care Medicine, Department of Medicine, and the Program
in Human Molecular Biology and Genetics, University of Utah, Salt Lake City, Utah, U.S.A.

I. Introduction

And here comes in the great tragedy—sepsis everywhere, unavoidable sepsis!

—Sir William Osler

Sepsis, a systemic condition with several stages and degrees of severity resulting from dysregulated activation of the innate immune and hemostatic systems, is a lethal syndrome and a major cause of acute lung injury (ALI) and its progression to the acute respiratory distress syndrome (ARDS). The concept that sepsis can lead to end-organ injury and dysfunction dates to the Greek origin of the term ("*sepsios*") and to investigations of its pathogenesis that predate modern times (1). Although not reported as a cause of lung injury in the 12 patients in the seminal description of ARDS by Petty and coworkers (2), sepsis was later recognized as a major inciting factor (3). In addition, many subsequent reports demonstrated an association between sepsis and ALI, and consensus statements and recent reviews identify it as a leading condition that "triggers" the molecular and cellular cascades that culminate in ALI and ARDS (ALI/ARDS) in humans (4–8). These and related issues were discussed in a previous version of this chapter (9), which will be referred to frequently and which contains additional references that will not be cited here. A very large number of studies and reports relevant to sepsis, ALI, and ARDS have appeared since that time; we profile this literature, but do not attempt to discuss each key area in comprehensive fashion. Many of the topics discussed in the chapter are themselves the subjects of detailed reviews, which are given in the reference list.

Sepsis-induced ALI and ARDS (ALI/ARDS) (Fig. 1) can be caused by infection with gram-positive bacteria, gram-negative organisms, and/or fungi (9). Circulating bacterial lipopolysaccharide (LPS, also generally called "endotoxin") (10) has been associated

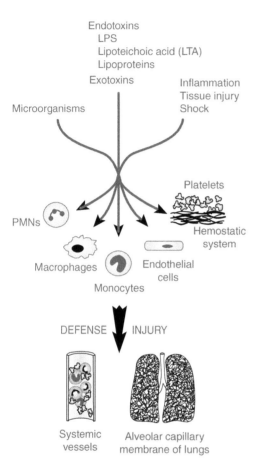

Figure 1   Cellular effectors mediate sepsis and sepsis-induced acute lung injury and ARDS (ALI/ARDS). Pathogens, microbial endotoxins and exotoxins, and endogenous host mediators generated in response to infection, inflammation, tissue injury, and/or shock trigger signaling cascades, leading to activation of myeloid leukocytes, endothelial cells, platelets, and other cellular systems. Activation of the coagulation cascade occurs in parallel. Each of these is a facet of defensive responses to microorganisms, but can be an effector of vascular dysfunction and tissue damage if it becomes dysregulated and maladaptive in septic syndromes. Systemic vessels as well as the alveolar-capillary membrane are involved in septic ALI/ARDS (see text for details).

with development of ARDS induced by diverse predisposing conditions in some, but not all, studies, indicating that it may act in an additive or synergistic fashion with trauma, hemorrhage, and other insults to induce alveolar-capillary membrane injury (11,12). Nevertheless, in this chapter we largely focus on sepsis as the principal or only inciting condition for ALI and ARDS.

The incidence of ARDS associated with septic syndromes (see below) is variable, but is in the range of 25–40% (5,9,13,14). It is estimated that between 400,000 and 750,000 episodes of severe sepsis occur annually in the United States (potentially as high as 3.0 cases per 1000 population) and that this may increase to as many as 1,100,000 cases by the year 2020 (9). In that event the number of sepsis-induced cases of ALI and ARDS might approach or exceed 440,000/yr, resulting in mortality of devastating proportion based on past and current outcomes and management (5,9,15–17). To this would be added the morbidity and mortality of sepsis-induced ALI and ARDS elsewhere in the world (9,17). Sepsis is a particularly lethal triggering condition for ALI/ARDS. In a recent study of recombinant human-activated protein C (rAPC) therapy in ALI (see below) in which subjects with severe sepsis were excluded, overall mortality was 13% compared to approximately 25% in large clinical trials that enrolled patients with ALI triggered by severe sepsis (18). In studies of low-dose glucocorticoids administered for refractory septic shock, the mortality of control patients with ALI was 67% (19).

Sepsis occurs in all phases of life. The incidence of neonatal sepsis is estimated to be one to five cases per 1000 live births, and to occur with higher frequencies after very low birth weight premature deliveries (16,20). The impact of sepsis on neonatal lung disease has not been clearly defined. Sepsis is also a triggering condition for ALI in older children (21,22), although the overall incidence of sepsis falls dramatically in children older than one year and in young adults (16). In adults, advanced age is an independent risk factor for development and negative outcomes in sepsis, and may heighten pulmonary inflammatory responses induced by LPS (23,24).

II. Definitions

Sepsis is a clinical syndrome resulting from systemic responses to intravascular or extravascular infection (9). Recent reviews and re-examinations of sepsis and its pathobiology emphasize this concept, and underscore that it is a dysregulated, maladaptive host response (17,25–30). Intravascular and extravascular bacterial infection may each have unique biologic features that will ultimately dictate different approaches to prevention and treatment (29). Septic syndromes are variable in severity, and include uncomplicated *sepsis*, *severe sepsis* with lung or other end-organ dysfunction that often culminates in the multiple organ dysfunction syndrome (MODS), and *septic shock* (17,31). Although often considered a continuum in which there is progression from one stage to the next (32), septic syndromes may be distinct in their molecular etiology (33). Severe pulmonary infection is a common triggering cause of severe sepsis (34,35) and septic shock (36). In parallel, the lung is the organ most commonly involved in severe sepsis and MODS (37).

Clinical identification of patients with septic syndromes in recent years has largely been based on consensus definitions (17,38) as is clinical identification of ALI/ARDS (5,6). The consensus definitions for sepsis also provide criteria for a systemic inflammatory response syndrome (SIRS) in the absence of documented infection, a condition that can be triggered by other insults and injuries. One potential mechanism for SIRS is entry of LPS and other bacterial toxins into the circulation because of disruption of intestinal or other barrier integrity (9,11,17). Consensus definitions for sepsis and its variable presentations are generally felt to be imperfect and have been re-evaluated and refined with the aim of establishing additional precision (17,39,40).

One of the reasons that current definitions may not be sufficiently precise is that human sepsis is extremely heterogeneous (9,17,41). This makes it difficult to define and rigorously characterize specific phenotypes within the spectrum of sepsis, and consequently to identify genetic traits that influence sepsis and its complications and to sort out interaction of these traits with environmental variables (1,42–44) (see chap. 12). Heterogeneity is likely one of the chief features of sepsis that has contributed to disappointing and confusing negative outcomes of interventional trials (9,17,45,46). Other factors that contribute to imprecision in clinical definitions of septic syndromes include the complexity of pathophysiological responses, gaps in fundamental knowledge regarding the cellular, molecular, and "systems biology" responses to infection, deficits in insight regarding variables in microbial virulence, and incomplete understanding of mechanisms that contribute to compartmentalization of molecular events triggered by microbes under some conditions yet incite dramatic systemic responses in others (9,28,29,47,48) (Fig. 2).

III. Pathophysiology of Sepsis: An Overview

Current and earlier concepts of sepsis identify dysregulated or unregulated activation of the innate immune system—leading to a systemic inflammatory response—as a central feature of the pathogenesis of sepsis and sepsis-associated ALI/ARDS; dysregulated activation of the hemostatic cascade is a second critical mechanism that goes hand-in-hand with pathologic systemic inflammation (9,25,28,29,37,49–52) (Figs. 1 and 2). Microvascular dysfunction, increased permeability, and loss of barrier function of systemic and pulmonary vessels are key pathophysiologic events (5,6,9,53,54). Additional features, including activation of nitric oxide syntheses and cyclooxygenases, altered adrenergic receptor reactivity, altered vascular reactivity, and myocardial depression mediate hemodynamic sequellae of severe sepsis and septic shock (9,17,30,31,53). There is evidence that hemodynamic responses are influenced by inflammatory and thrombotic effector systems (9), although this will not be discussed in detail.

Extracellular, cellular, and metabolic alterations add to the vascular pathophysiology of sepsis, contributing to the systemic nature of the dysregulated inflammatory state (17,31). Experimental models indicate that disrupted mitochondrial oxidative phosphorylation may be a critical feature of brain dysfunction in sepsis (55,56). A variety of additional facets of intermediary metabolism and altered glucose utilization contribute to the pathophysiology of septic syndromes (17,30,31,57).

The cellular and molecular mechanisms that drive innate immune responses in sepsis and influence its interactions with the hemostatic system (Figs. 1 and 2) are complex. Furthermore, new components continue to be discovered, and a comprehensive understanding of dysregulation of these pathways in sepsis and septic ALI remains elusive. The following sections outline some of the cellular and molecular systems that are currently thought to be critical in the dysregulated inflammatory and hemostatic responses in sepsis and septic ALI/ARDS.

A. Leukocytes in Sepsis: An Overview

Several lines of evidence indicate an essential role for host hematopoietic cells in sepsis, including experiments in which lethal effects of LPS were restored in C3H/HeJ mice—which are resistant to LPS because of a mutation in the gene for Toll-like

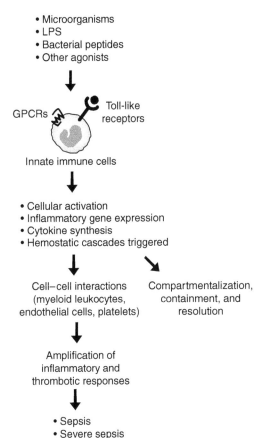

• Microorganisms
• LPS
• Bacterial peptides
• Other agonists

GPCRs   Toll-like receptors

Innate immune cells

• Cellular activation
• Inflammatory gene expression
• Cytokine synthesis
• Hemostatic cascades triggered

Cell–cell interactions
(myeloid leukocytes,
endothelial cells, platelets)

Compartmentalization,
containment, and
resolution

Amplification of
inflammatory and
thrombotic responses

• Sepsis
• Severe sepsis
• Septic shock

Figure 2 A simplified outline of pathogenetic events in sepsis. Microorganisms and/or their products activate innate immune effector cells (Fig. 1). Toll-like receptors are central to host recognition of microbial PAMPs and other components, and trigger cellular responses. Host cells also generate signaling molecules that can be recognized by TLRs or by G-protein-coupled receptors (GPCRs), providing additional avenues for cellular activation. Changes in responding cell phenotype and function occur, including inflammatory gene expression and cytokine and chemokine synthesis. In parallel, hemostatic cascades are triggered, including platelet activation and tissue factor-dependent thrombin generation and fibrin deposition (Fig. 1). If defense against the invading microbes is successful, the pathogens are compartmentalized, contained, and killed by the linked inflammatory and hemostatic events, host responses remain regulated and localized, and the infection and tissue inflammation resolve. Alternately, however, microbial inoculum and virulence and/or host genetic predispositions lead to dysregulated and maladaptive amplification of inflammation and hemostasis. Cell–cell interactions mediated by immune, neural, and metabolic pathways contribute to systemic, rather than localized, inflammation and clinically defined septic syndromes. Vascular and end organ dysfunction, including lung dysfunction culminating in ALI/ARDS, occur depending on the specific syndrome.

receptor 4 (*Tlr* 4)—by irradiation and subsequent reconstitution with hematopoietic precursors from an LPS-sensitive mouse strain (1,58). Myeloid leukocytes are key innate immune/inflammatory effector cells in sepsis (Fig. 1). These effector cells are nonclonally derived and capable of responding to pathogens without conditioning by prior exposure or antigenic specificity (1,59). Genetic defects in myeloid cell function cause leukocyte adhesion deficiency syndromes and other conditions that predispose to recurrent infections, many of which are life-threatening and involve the lungs (60,61). These genetic disorders dramatically illustrate the requisite functions of myeloid leukocytes and their molecular systems in host defense and the adaptive acute inflammatory response (51,62). The acquired syndromes of sepsis and septic ALI provide equally dramatic examples of dysregulated, maladaptive innate immune effector responses, and the balance, precision, and control that must be achieved in order to successfully defend the mammalian host when it is challenged by infection or tissue injury (9,51). Molecular mechanisms that compartmentalize and localize inflammatory responses, together with humoral and neural pathways that reduce or modulate systemic inflammation, may be critical in achieving control of myeloid and other cellular activities in acute infection and in preventing systemic injury (29,47,48) (Fig. 2).

Myeloid cells with critical roles in sepsis and sepsis-induced ALI include macrophages, neutrophils (polymorphonuclear leukocytes, PMNs), and monocytes. Macrophages recognize bacteria and bacterial products including LPS, provide "points of control" that modulate local and systemic pro- and anti-inflammatory responses to infection, and can be effectors of tissue injury as well as tissue repair (10,51,63–65). Targeted deletion ("knockout") of $\alpha_D\beta_2$, a leukocyte integrin highly expressed on subsets of splenic and other macrophages in humans and mice, dramatically altered survival in a murine model of *Salmonella* sepsis at early time points postinfection, illustrating the potential for macrophage effector mechanisms to orchestrate host responses to systemic challenge by invasive pathogens (66).

Monocytes and neutrophils are required for recognition and elimination of bacteria and other pathogens (51,59–61). In addition, however, PMNs and monocytes are mediators of injury in sepsis and septic ALI and—by virtue of mechanisms such as granular enzyme release, oxygen radical generation, and inflammatory gene expression—induce vascular leakage and tissue damage (9,67,68). Interactions of leukocytes with the pulmonary endothelium, which occurs continuously under normal conditions, are dysregulated by LPS and other factors that mediate cellular activation in bacteremia and sepsis (69). The phenotypes and functional characteristics of monocytes and neutrophils change in response to mediators generated at specific stages in sepsis, but the mechanisms involved are largely undefined (48,70–73). A subset of monocytes (CD14$^+$/CD16$^+$) is expanded in sepsis and is a major source of tumor necrosis factor (TNF-α) (74,75). Caspase 1 and other components of the "inflammasome" of circulating monocytes are altered in patients with septic shock, potentially influencing processing of key cytokines (73). Triggering receptor expressed on myeloid cells (Trem-1), a recently identified member of the immunoglobin superfamily, contributes to altered myeloid leukocyte function and may induce pathways that interface with Toll-like receptor (TLR) signaling (see below) in sepsis (9,76).

Human and rodent neutrophils and monocytes use integrins of both the β_1 and β_2 classes (61,77) for adhesion, trafficking, and signaling in localized infection and in pathologic conditions such as sepsis and sepsis-induced ALI (67,70,78,79). Neutrophil β_2 integrins, which are also called "leukocyte integrins" (61,66), modulate apoptotic cell death (80) in addition to other functions (61). PMN apoptosis is a marker of severity of sepsis and septic ARDS (81), indicating that β_2 integrin signaling may be an important component of dysregulated inflammation in septic syndromes.

Although myeloid leukocytes have been studied for over a century, new functions of PMNs and monocytes continue to be discovered. Generation of "neutrophil extracellular traps" (NETs) by human PMNs appears to be a mechanism of extracellular capture and killing of bacteria and fungi (82,83). Extrusion of NETs may also contribute to vascular injury in sepsis (84,85). Neutrophil-derived catecholamines were reported to be mediators of LPS-induced ALI in mice, identifying a new cellular pathway that may operate in sepsis (86). PMNs have important roles in immune responses and tissue repair that have not been widely recognized (51). Monocytes not only perform acute effector functions in infection and inflammation but also have incompletely—characterized activities as precursors of macrophages and dendritic cells (65).

Dendritic cells, natural killer cells, and specific populations of gamma delta T cells have activities in sepsis that are not yet completely characterized. These leukocyte subclasses add complexity to contributions by myeloid leukocytes, and are involved in critical interactions between the innate and adaptive immune systems in responses to infectious challenge (51,87–91). There is frequently a phase of relative immune refractoriness in later stages after a septic challenge that may be mediated by CD4$^+$ T lymphocytes polarized to the Th2 phenotype and that may predispose to secondary fungal or bacterial infection if the patient survives the initial septic episode (92). This could potentially reflect dysregulated signaling to, or by, dendritic cells (91). Dendritic cells mediated linked inflammation and coagulation via protease-activated receptor 1 (PAR1) signaling and the sphingosine-1-phosphate axis in a mouse model of sepsis (93), suggesting that these cells contribute to dysregulated host responses to microbial challenge in septic syndromes.

B.   Endothelial Function Is Altered in Sepsis

Endothelial cells (ECs) are critical in host defense, repair, and physiologic inflammation (9,69,94). In addition, the endothelium is an important interface between inflammatory and thrombotic pathways in sepsis and ALI induced by sepsis and other causes (9,54,95,96). Activities of systemic and pulmonary endothelium in sepsis and ALI (Figs. 1 and 3) have been reviewed (9,54,95–98). Dysregulated interactions between activated or injured ECs and myeloid leukocytes may be particularly important in experimental and clinical sepsis, and contribute to intravascular leukocyte sequestration in the lung as well as trafficking to alveolar compartments (9,67,79,99) (also see below). Recent studies in murine models suggest that leukocyte sequestration in the lungs induced by LPS is largely due to endothelial activation (48), although this contrasts with earlier work in humans and other rodent species indicating that leukocyte activation is the critical event (67,69). ECs are released into the circulation in septic patients (100), potentially as a result of injury mediated by locally activated PMNs or monocytes.

ECs express TLRs (see below) and recognize LPS and other bacterial products (9,102). In response to stimulation with LPS human ECs in culture express new gene products, including inducible adhesion molecules and chemokines that mediate interactions with leukocytes, and undergo phenotypic and functional alterations (101,103,104). Similar changes have been documented in vessels of septic patients, indicating the validity of the model (105–107). Some of the newly expressed EC chemokines, adhesion molecules, and inflammatory factors are synthesized under transcriptional control by nuclear factor Kappa B (NF-κB) (9,98). Selective genetic disruption of NF-κB in endothelium resulted

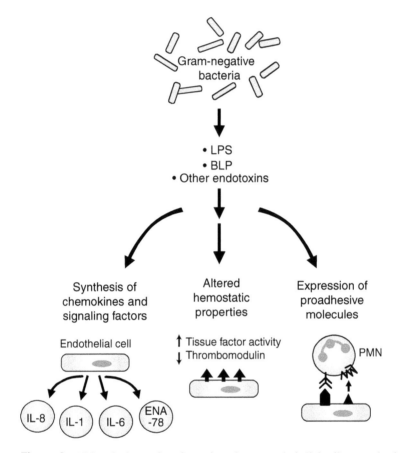

Figure 3 LPS and other endotoxins activate human endothelial cells: a mechanism of sepsis vascular dysfunction and inflammatory injury. LPS and other components of gram-negative bacteria bind to TLRs on human ECs, inducing new gene expression and other functional responses. In addition, ECs respond to components of gram-positive bacteria, such as the Braun lipoprotein (BLP), using TLRs different from those that recognize LPS; thus, ECs activation is also a fundamental mechanism in gram-positive sepsis [see (9,98,101) for details].

in improved survival in mice challenged with LPS or subjected to cecal ligation and puncture (CLP) (108). Thus, altered expression of endothelial genes and synthesis of the corresponding protein products in response to LPS may be a central feature of gram-negative bacterial infection and sepsis (Fig. 3). In addition, the pattern of messenger (mRNAs) RNAs, including transcripts that code for gene products relevant to systemic inflammatory responses and injury, is also robustly altered when human ECs are challenged with bacterial lipoproteins (101). This illustrates that "endotoxic" responses can be induced by a variety of microbial products in addition to the classic endotoxin, LPS (9,10). Expression of new gene products by ECs activated by a variety of microbial products may be one of the factors that accounts for failure of antibodies with specificity for LPS to consistently prevent septic complications in clinical trials (9,25,27,46).

Vascular endothelial growth factor (VEGF) induces endothelial permeability and promotes ECs proliferation, migration, and survival (98). Circulating VEGF levels are increased in mice and humans in experimental and clinical sepsis, and blocking VEGF protected animals against the toxic effects of LPS; furthermore, ECs treated with VEGF were sensitized to stimulation by low concentrations of TNF-α (109). This study suggested that VEGF contributes to the vascular pathophysiology of sepsis and that its inhibition may be a therapeutic strategy in sepsis (109). In addition, in illustrates complex activities of endogenous factors that are recognized by endothelium in inflammation and sepsis.

C. Platelets: Hemostatic and Inflammatory Cells That May Be Ubiquitously Activated in Sepsis

Platelets are the central effector cells of rapid hemostasis, but also have key inflammatory and immune functions that were likely retained as they evolved from ancient multifunctional innate defensive cells (110,111). Thus, platelets have the potential to mediate both hemostasis and inflammation, and to link thrombosis and inflammatory responses in sepsis and a variety of other disorders (Fig. 4). Alterations and activities of platelets in sepsis have only recently been emphasized (95,96,112–114), however, and will be summarized in overview form here. Newly recognized activities of platelets and megakaryocytes that may contribute to septic ALI/ARDS have been reviewed in detail (115).

Platelets are activated frequently, and perhaps ubiquitously, in sepsis (95,96), and alterations in their number and distribution are common (114). Sepsis is a leading risk factor for thrombocytopenia in critically ill patients (112,113). There is an inverse relationship between circulating platelet number and severity of sepsis (113). Furthermore, thrombocytopenia is a negative prognostic variable in sepsis and other critical illnesses (112). Sepsis-associated thrombocytopenia is thought to be a marker for host responses to pathogen challenge (113), although its relationship to other biomarkers of the systemic inflammatory response is not clear (114).

Disseminated intravascular coagulation (DIC) is commonly invoked as a mechanism of sepsis-induced thrombocytopenia, and is a predictor of mortality in sepsis (116–118). Nevertheless, altered platelet number in sepsis is multifactorial in origin and appears to include impaired thrombopoiesis and trapping of platelets in peripheral vascular beds ("sequestration") [Fig. 4(B)], in addition to increased peripheral destruction and consumption as a manifestation of DIC (114). Sequestration in peripheral vascular beds may involve homotypic aggregation, formation of platelet–leukocyte and platelet–fibrin complexes (see below), and interactions with ECs and/or exposed subendothelial matrix [Fig. 4(B)] (114). Sequestration may vary in different organs in sepsis (113), and circulating platelets and those that are sequestered in microvasclar beds may have different functional characteristics in clinical and experimental sepsis (114). Mechanisms independent of platelet activation by thrombin may contribute to thrombocytopenia in sepsis based on studies in surrogate animal experiments (119,120). For example, sialidase activities of microbes modify glycoproteins on the surface of murine platelets, causing them to be recognized and cleared by an asialoglycoprotein receptor on hepatocytes (120).

Alterations in platelet function in sepsis are less well characterized than alterations in number, and in some cases the results of clinical studies are conflicting (114,121).

(A)

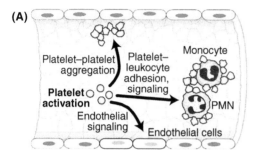

(B)

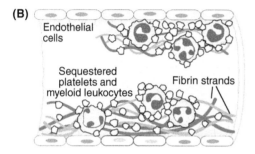

Figure 4 Platelet activation, interaction with leukocytes and ECs, and sequestration in microvessels are key events in experimental and clinical sepsis. (**A**) Activation of platelets by thrombin, PAF, or other agonists generated in sepsis induces homotypic platelet–platelet aggregation, formation of heterotypic aggregates with myeloid leukocytes, and interaction with ECs. There is evidence for each interaction in sepsis and septic ALI/ARDS based on experimental models and/or clinical observations. Intercellular signaling, functional responses, and new gene expression can result (see text and Fig. 5). LPS and other bacterial toxins can also directly activate platelets in experimental models relevant to sepsis. (**B**) Platelet sequestration in microvascular beds has the potential to mediate prolonged intercellular signaling, in addition to amplifying deposition of fibrin and contributing to microvascular obstruction (see text for details). *Source*: From Ref. 114.

Apparent differences may be due to time-dependent changes in platelet function at specific stages of septic syndromes, heterogeneous populations of juvenile and mature platelets in the blood, and other factors (114). Platelet aggregation and adhesion are reported to be variably altered, potentially in response to plasma factors in part (112,121–124). Platelets are known to release multiple inflammatory proteins and lipids into the local milieu, and other signaling factors are displayed on their surfaces (111). In sepsis, these factors include VEGF, PDGF, and thrombospondin based on clinical studies to date (121,124). Other mediators, which have not yet been identified in samples from patients, are also almost certainly released or presented at the surfaces of activated platelets in human septic syndromes as well (114).

Traditional dogma holds that hemostatic and inflammatory factors in the proteome of activated platelets are preformed; circulating platelets are not generally thought to synthesize new proteins because they are anucleate and are incapable of nuclear transcription. In contrast to this traditional view, recent discoveries demonstrate that mature circulating platelets from human subjects have a transcriptome of mRNAs and pre-mRNAs that are expressed at the megakaryocyte stage. In some cases, platelet mRNAs can be translated to their protein products in response to activating signals, a process termed "signal-dependent translation" (114,125). One mechanism involves regulated translation of stable, mature mRNAs that are "silenced," or transcriptionally repressed, in the resting state (125). Bcl-3, a protein that was recently shown to regulate clot retraction and fibrin remodeling by activated human platelets, was the first example (125–127). A second mechanism involves signal-dependent splicing of pre-mRNAs, which generates mature transcripts that are then translated. This was first reported as a mechanism of synthesis of interleukin-1β (IL-1β) in response to activation by thrombin and β_3 integrin engagement (128). Subsequently, tissue factor (TF) was shown to be synthesized in this fashion by activated platelets (129). IL-1β and TF each have major activities in clinical and experimental sepsis (9,33,50,52,114,130,131). A recent report demonstrates that splicing of the pre-mRNA for IL-1β and synthesis of the protein occur in human platelets activated with LPS, and provides evidence that splicing of the pre-mRNA for cyclooxygenase II is also triggered (132). In addition, studies of samples from patients indicate that splicing of the TF pre-mRNA, expression of mature TF mRNA, and a procoagulant surface are characteristics of platelets circulating in the intravascular milieu of human sepsis (133). Post-transcriptional expression of mRNAs and proteins by activated platelets is now also being examined in patients with ALI/ARDS, including subjects in whom lung injury is triggered by sepsis (Rondina M, Weyrich AS, Zimmerman GA, et al., unpublished studies).

Functional responses of platelets such as adhesion, aggregation, secretion, signal-dependent translation, and new protein synthesis require cellular activation and do not occur, or in some cases occur only minimally, in the basal state (114,125). Agonists with the potential to activate platelets are generated via multiple pathways in experimental and clinical sepsis, including thrombin, platelet-activating factor (PAF), and others (9,114,131,134,135). In addition, platelets interact with gram-negative and gram-positive bacteria; in many cases these interactions induce platelet activation (114,133). Furthermore, recent observations from several laboratories demonstrate that LPS directly activates murine and human platelets, inducing functional responses that include altered adhesiveness, interactions with leukocytes, splicing of pre-mRNAs, and signal-dependent translation (85,114,132,133). Consistent with this, a number of studies now indicate that mouse and human platelets express toll-like receptor 4 (TLR4) (85,114,132), the primary receptor for LPS (see below). LPS challenge and other in vivo models of experimental sepsis cause thrombocytopenia, altered thrombopoiesis, platelet activation, and deposition of platelets in the lungs and liver in experimental animals and/or humans (136–142). Factors and toxins from gram-positive bacteria also alter platelet functional responses (112,133). The ability of platelets to recognize and respond to microbial factors—in addition to endogenous agonists such as thrombin and PAF that are generated by the host—in infection may have been conserved from the repertoires of ancient multifunctional defensive cells that could directly interact and neutralize invading pathogens as well as seal wounds, and that ultimately gave rise to modern specialized mammalian platelets (110).

LPS and other bacterial products also likely alter megakaryocyte function in sepsis (137; Foulks J, Weyrich AS, Zimmerman GA, et al., unpublished studies).

D. Cell–Cell Interactions in Sepsis and Septic ALI

Myeloid leukocytes, platelets, and ECs interact in complex fashions in inflammatory syndromes, including sepsis (Figs. 1, 3, 4, and 5). As previously outlined, interactions of myeloid leukocytes with activated systemic and pulmonary endothelium [Figs. 3 and 4(A)] are critical pathogenetic mechanisms in sepsis and ALI/ARDS that have been extensively reviewed (61,97,98,114,143,144). Platelet interactions with endothelium and the vessel wall in inflammation, ALI, and sepsis have also been reviewed recently (114,115,145) [Figs. 4 and 5(C)]. In addition, activated platelets also interact directly with myeloid leukocytes and lymphocytes (9,111,145) [Figs. 4 and 5(B)].

Platelet–leukocyte interactions provide a prototype example of cellular and molecular links between hemostasis and inflammation in sepsis. Furthermore, interactions of platelets, myeloid leukocytes, fibrinogen, and fibrin in vessels of septic patients establish a milieu for complex signaling (Fig. 4), and may be therapeutic targets (114). When platelets are activated they become adhesive for PMNs and monocytes in addition to undergoing "homotypic" platelet–platelet aggregation (9,114) (Figs. 4 and 5). Formation of "heterotypic" platelet–monocyte aggregates is a sensitive marker of platelet activation in the circulating blood that links thrombosis and inflammation in atherosclerosis and its acute complications (146–149). In addition, platelet–leukocyte aggregates form in the blood in other inflammatory disorders, including sepsis (9,114). Clinical observations indicate that platelet–monocyte and platelet–neutrophil aggregates are induced in patients with septic syndromes, potentially resulting from activation of either the platelet or the leukocyte; these cellular complexes may be biomarkers of disease (150–155). Because interactions of platelets with myeloid leukocytes can induce new gene expression, these heterotypic aggregates may also be accessible "barometers" of the patterns of inflammatory genes

---

$\longrightarrow$

Figure 5   Signaling via PAR1 and 4 and PAFR pathways induces diverse cellular responses linking inflammation and thrombosis. (**A**) Thrombin induces display of P-selectin and synthesis and surface expression of PAF by engaging PAR1 on human ECs; signaling mediated by PAF, acting via the PAFR on neutrophils, mediates juxtacrine activation of PMNs tethered to the ECs surface by binding of P-selectin to PSGL-1 on the leukocyte. The activated PMNs undergo functional changes that can contribute to inflammation and thrombosis in sepsis and other pathologic syndromes. (**B**) Thrombin activates human platelets via PAR1 and PAR4, resulting in platelet–platelet aggregation mediated by integrin $\alpha_{IIb}\beta_3$ and display of P-selectin, leading to formation of platelet–monocyte aggregates. Thrombin-induced activation of platelets also mediates their adhesion to PMNs. Outside-in signaling in cellular aggregates can induce transcriptional and post-transcriptional pathways and expression of new genes, including genes that code for chemokines, cytokines, and inflammatory enzymes. PAF, like thrombin, induces platelet activation, cellular aggregation, interaction with myeloid leukocytes, and intercellular signaling. (**C**) Thrombin- and PAF-stimulated platelets synthesize and release IL-1β, which signals new gene expression in ECs. The mechanism involves signal-dependent splicing of IL-1β pre-mRNA and subsequent translation of IL-1β transcripts by activated platelets. Preformed C-X-C and CC chemokines are also released from aggregated, degranulating platelets and can directly activate PMNs and monocytes.

(A)

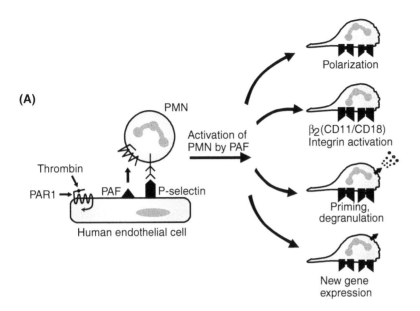

(B)

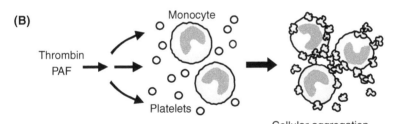

(C)

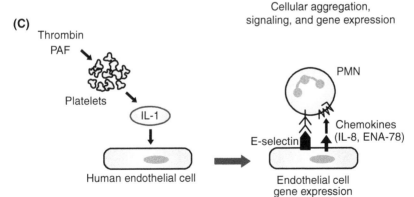

that are expressed in septic syndromes (114). Complexes of platelets and myeloid leuko-cytes are found in the blood of patients with sepsis caused by both gram-negative and gram-positive organisms (152,154,156) and in the circulation of experimental animals challenged with bacterial toxins (157–159). Platelet–leukocyte aggregates may impair microvascular blood flow in sepsis (151). Nevertheless, intercellular signaling, functional responses of the interacting cells, and new inflammatory gene expression may be as important as—or more important than—mechanical obstruction (114). Mechanistic stud-ies demonstrate that adhesive and signaling interactions between activated platelets and myeloid leukocytes involve P-selectin on the platelets binding to P-selectin glycoprotein ligand 1 on the leukocytes, other adhesion molecules including β_2 integrins, and soluble and plasma membrane-bound signaling factors (115,145).

Platelet–leukocyte interactions may contribute to end-organ complications of sepsis, including ALI/ARDS (9,114,124,160,161), although this issue has not been completely explored. In unpublished preliminary studies, we found greater numbers of aggregates consisting of platelets adherent to $CD14^+/CD16^+$ monocytes compared to aggregates consisting of platelets and $CD14^+/CD16^-$ monocytes in blood samples from patients with ALI/ARDS, some of whom had underlying sepsis (Harris E, Weyrich AS, Zimmerman GA, et al., unpublished studies; 114). This may have pathogenetic signifi-cance if intracellular signaling between the adherent platelets and monocytes occurs in the blood of septic patients and induces synthesis of TNF-α, IL-Iβ and/or other mediators, as it does in in vitro models (74,162–164). In recent experimental studies, platelet–PMN aggregates were identified as critical cellular effectors of ALI in mouse models of aspira-tion and sepsis (165), providing experimental evidence that platelet–leukocyte interactions contribute to ALI.

E. TLRs: Sensors That Recognize LPS and Other Microbial and Endogenous Ligands and Trigger Host Responses, Inflammation, and Injury

TLRs are a family of cell surface and intracellular receptors expressed by immune effector cells and other cell types. Specific TLRs recognize LPS and other microbial molecules—including bacterial lipoproteins, peptidoglycans, and lipoteichoic acid (LTA)—and trans-mit signals to intracellular transduction cascades (1,9,166,167) (Figs. 2 and 6). The first ligands for TLRs to be identified were microbial products that display pathogen-associated molecular patterns (PAMPs), which are conserved structural motifs that are critical for microbial survival. Recognition of bacterial, mycobacterial, fungal, and viral PAMPs by TLRs was originally thought to allow the mammalian host to distinguish the invading pathogen from "self" (167,168). It is now known, however, that TLRs also recognize endogenous molecules of a variety of classes that may serve as "danger signals" and trig-ger inflammatory responses and repair (166,169–172). Thus, TLRs can transmit signals and induce alterations in cellular function in response to host factors, in addition to micro-bial PAMPs. A voluminous literature involving TLRs and their functions has evolved since the first version of this chapter was published; some of these observations are out-lined in this section, together with previous background information. We cite reviews in the field heavily in this summary.

Mammalian TLRs are related to the Toll receptors in *Drosophila*, which signal responses to infection and, in addition, are critically involved in development (1,174,175).

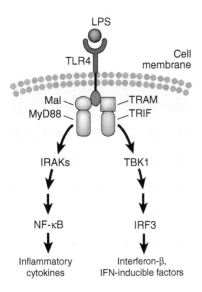

Figure 6 TLR signaling cascades lead to activation of transcriptional pathways and expression of cytokines, chemokines, and inflammatory mediators. A highly simplified outline of TLR4 signaling is illustrated [see text and (166,173) for details].

Discovery of TLRs in humans provided new molecular insight into host defense and pathological dysregulation of the innate immune system that is immediately relevant to infectious and inflammatory diseases, including sepsis (63,64,166,172,175–178). Expression of mammalian and human TLRs is differentially altered in cells challenged with microbial products or stimulated with certain cytokines (166,179), and their activity may also be regulated by other mechanisms (169). Thus, TLRs are not static components in the inflammatory response.

Characterization of strains of mice that are unresponsive to endotoxic effects of administration of LPS led to identification of the gene for TLR4 (1,10,48). Multiple additional murine and human TLRs that recognize distinct microbial components have now been discovered (166,178). TLR4 and TLR2 are particularly relevant to sepsis and septic ALI, although other TLRs are likely involved in septic syndromes (9,180,181). In humans, as in mice, TLR4 recognizes LPS, although there are species-specific differences in the recognition of partial LPS structures (1,10,48). A variety of strategies aimed at interrupting binding and recognition of LPS by TLR4 inhibit signaling in vivo; some have been evaluated as novel therapeutic approaches in clinical sepsis (46,178,182). Polymorphisms in the human *TLR4* gene are associated with altered responses to LPS and increased susceptibility to gram-negative infection in humans (43,176,183). *TLR 2* is the principal receptor for lipopeptides, which include molecules common to gram-negative and gram-positive organisms, and for peptidoglycans and LTA of gram-positive bacteria (166). A polymorphism in the human *TLR2* gene is associated with reduced responses to bacterial lipoproteins and altered frequency of septic shock in staphylococcal and other gram-positive infections (176).

TLRs act cooperatively to mediate signaling, depending on the bacterial factors and cellular systems involved (166,184–186). For example, recent experiments using genetically modified mice indicate that LTA-induced lung inflammation depends on TLR2 and combinatorial signals delivered via TLR4 and the receptor for PAF (187). PAF is also a mediator of inflammation and sepsis (134) (also see below). As a second example, TLR4-induced synthesis of interferon gamma, altered TLR2 activity, and influenced outcome in a murine model of gram-negative sepsis (185). In addition to functional interactions, there are physical associations. As an example, TLR2 associates with TLR6, providing a mechanism for discrimination of differences in the lipid components of bacterial lipopeptides (166).

TLRs interact with other key molecules and coreceptors in a cell- and tissue-specific fashion. In mammalian myeloid leukocytes and other effector cells, presentation of LPS to TLR4 involves binding of LPS to LPS-binding protein (LBP), which is present in soluble form in plasma and other fluids, and binding of the LPS–LBP complex to CD14, a protein that exists in soluble and glycophosphatidylinositol-anchored forms (9,102,188). CD14 then transfers LPS to soluble or TLR-4-associated MD-2, which binds noncovalently to the extracellular domain of TLR4 leading to activation, signal transduction, and altered trafficking of the receptor (166). CD14 presents LPS to other proteins besides TLR4 (189), and recognizes lipopeptides and peptidoglycans and presents them to TLR2 (190). Signaling via the TLR2/TLR6 heterodimer depends in part on CD14, and is further influenced by CD36 (178). Thus, CD14 influences signaling in response to a variety of bacteria (179). Stress-induced increases in soluble CD14 in plasma lead to binding and transfer of LPS to plasma lipoproteins, potentially reducing responses of monocytes to LPS in vivo (189). Polymorphisms in the *CD14* locus are associated with altered susceptibility and outcome in septic shock (43).

Recognition mechanisms for LPS and LTA mediated by TLR4 and TLR2 have been defined in the lungs of experimental animals and in humans subjected to experimental challenge with endotoxins (191–199). Pulmonary responses are diminished when C3H/HEJ mice are given LPS by systemic administration (200). Chimeric mice deficient in endothelial but not leukocyte TLR4 had dramatically decreased accumulation of PMNs in the lungs in response to systemic LPS challenge, indicating that pulmonary endothelial TLR4 is critical for this sequestration (201). Responses of mice to inhaled LPS are altered by *TLR*4 gene dosage (202), and are mediated by TLR4, LBP, and CD14 (197,198,203). TLR4 signaling was recently reported to also be central in a pathway to ALI induced by viral pathogens in mice, and to link lung injury mediated by innate immune responses and oxidative stress (204). If these studies are applicable to clinical ALI, TLR4 signaling may be pivotal in lung injury triggered by a variety of noninfectious and infectious challenges in addition to ALI/ARDS induced by gram-negative bacteria. In studies of wild type and knockout mice, TLR2 and CD14 were observed to mediate pulmonary inflammatory responses to intranasal LTA, and linked signaling via TLR4 and the PAF receptor-mediated lung cytokine and cellular responses (187). Thus, TLR4 and TLR2 have complex roles in the lungs of experimental animals characterized by bacterial products that trigger pulmonary inflammatory responses and sepsis. TLR signaling in the murine lung in response to LPS was attenuated for prolonged periods after experimental viral infection, suggesting a mechanism for secondary bacterial pneumonia in viral syndromes (205).

In human volunteers given low doses of LPS, lung inflammation occurs. In these "human models" there are differences in pulmonary inflammatory responses when the challenge is via the airway versus the systemic route (192,193,195). Similarly, there are differences in pulmonary responses in mice given LPS via the intraperitoneal and intra-tracheal routes (196). Localized alveolar instillation of LPS or LTA in human volunteers triggered different patterns of mediators and PMN activation, indicating that stimulation of TLR4 and TLR2 results in differential pulmonary inflammation in humans (199). Thus, TLR4 and TLR2 mediate lung responses to endotoxins in humans as well as in mice. It is unknown how these responses in human subjects are compared to those that are induced by multiple bacterial products that activate several TLR pathways simultaneously, and/or by bacterial products in the context of endogenous chemokines, cytokines, and other inflammatory mediators. These are conditions that occur in clinical sepsis. In addition, the patterns of TLRs and their cellular localizations in the normal, inflamed, and injured human lung are yet to be completely characterized. Furthermore, there is evidence that the LBP/CD14 components of the LPS recognition system are altered in lung injury (9,23,191). Finally, alveolar surfactant lipids and proteins bind LPS and modify its activity, providing a lung-specific component of recognition that may vary in inflammation and injury (191).

Microbial sensors in addition to TLRs have recently been identified (166,167,206). These include the NOD receptors, dectin 1, and helicase domain-containing antiviral proteins. One of the members of the latter family, RIG-I, was cloned from human ECs activated with LPS (207).

F. TLRs in Intracellular Signaling, Gene Expression Pathways, and Synthesis of Inflammatory Mediators

TLRs signal to intracellular pathways that induce altered gene expression, leading to changes in cellular phenotype, functions, and synthesis of proteins and other factors that modify the inflammatory milieu. The signaling cascades include elements shared with those activated via the interleukin-1 (IL-1) receptor family. TLRs have a motif in their cytoplasmic tails homologous to a domain in the IL-1 receptor—the toll/interleukin-1 receptor motif (TIR)—that is critical for signal transduction and triggers multiple intracellular events (166,178).

After engagement by ligands, TLRs dimerize and undergo conformational rearrangements, including alterations in the cytoplasmic tail TIR domain, that allow recruitment of intracellular adaptor molecules that contain TIR motifs (166). For TLR4, these adaptors include MyD88; MAL (MyD88-adaptor-like), also called TIR-associated protein (TIRAP); TRIF (TIR-domain-containing adaptor protein-inducing IFN-β), also called TIR-domain-containing molecule 1 (TICAM1); and TRAM (TRIF-related adaptor molecule) (166) (Fig. 6). Selective partnering of specific adaptor molecules with TLRs and with downstream signaling pathways after binding of specific ligands leads to differential cellular responses (173). Parallel signaling by engagement of other surface molecules, such as β_2 integrins or scavenger receptors, can interface with TLR signaling pathways (9,65).

MyD88 and TRIF activate signaling cascades that mediate production of proinflammatory cytokines and type I interferons, respectively (166,173). Engagement of TLR4 or TLR2 induces NF-κB activation and synthesis of NF-κB-dependent inflammatory and immune genes (9,190) via a signaling cascade that involves MyD88, MAL, IL-1R-associated kinases (IRAK) 1 and 4, and additional intermediary components (166,178) (Fig. 6). Transcriptional pathways that regulate responses to oxidant stress influence MyD88-dependent and independent signaling in mice challenged with LPS or subjected to CLP (208). This could be important in sepsis-induced ALI/ARDS, where oxidant injury and signaling play key roles (5,6). A functional variant of MAL in humans is associated with protection against bacteremia and a variety of other infectious syndromes (209). Deficiency of MyD88 in children is associated with recurrent bacterial infections, including invasive pneumococcal disease; similarly, children with IRAK-4 deficiency have increased susceptibility to pneumococcal infection and other bacterial pathogens (210). Thus, this pathway is essential for innate immunity against certain pyogenic bacteria, although there is age-related redundancy in host defense to these microbial infections and differences in humans and in mice (210). IRAK-mediated steps are points of control in TLR-triggered inflammatory signaling in humans and mice (210,211). Signaling to NF-κB-dependent transcription pathways by TLRs (Fig. 6) is not restricted to macrophages and myeloid leukocytes and occurs in ECs (101,212) and other cell types, although it is robust in myeloid cells (64,65).

Engagement of TLR3, TLR4, TLR7, and TR9 activates a TRIF-dependent pathway that leads to production of type 1 interferons as well as other proinflammatory molecules; this can be demonstrated in MyD88-deficient cells (166). TRIF transmits activating signals to a transcriptional pathway regulated by IFN regulatory factor 3 (IRF3) (213), providing a mechanism for induction of IFN-β and IFN-inducible genes (166). Endogenous inhibition of IRAK1 can mediate differential control, reducing synthesis of NF-κB-dependent inflammatory cytokines via the MyD88/MAL pathway while enhancing production of interferons (214). In addition, individual ligands can apparently induce TRIF-dependent activation of the IRF3 pathway—or, instead, the MyD88-dependent expression of NF-κB-regulated genes (Fig. 6)—by binding to MD-2 and differentially modifying association of the cytoplasmic domain of TLR4 with specific adaptor proteins (173). Specific signaling via TRIF induced by binding of oxidized phospholipids (see below) to TLR4 was reported to mediate ALI in a mouse model of influenza lung infection (215).

G. Cytokines and Chemokines: Prototype Mediators in Sepsis

As outlined, signaling to NF-κB and other transcriptional pathways, and consequent expression of inflammatory gene products, are key features of TLR biology and pathology. As an example, transcripts for NF-κB-dependent chemokines and cytokines are among the major mRNAs induced when human monocytes or ECs are stimulated with LPS or gram-positive bacterial products (101,216,217). Cytokine synthesis was critical in establishing the biologic consequences and cellular bases for signaling by TLR4 (1,9,10). Key cytokines and chemokines involved in experimental and clinical sepsis are induced by TLR engagement, including TNF-α, the α and β isoforms of IL-1, IL-6, IL-8, IFN-γ, high mobility group box 1 (HMGB1), and macrophage inhibitory factor (MIF-1) (9,33,184,217).

Proinflammatory chemokines and cytokines are also among the factors expressed in human and mouse lungs challenged with LPS or LTA (194,199). In addition to transcriptional regulation, TLR signaling influences post-transcription control and other features that regulate availability of key cytokines. As an example, post-transcriptional processing and secretion of IL-1β and other IL-1 family members are regulated by caspases and pathways controlled by a complex of proteins termed the "inflammasome" that can be altered by signaling (73,167,219). Caspase 1-deficient mice are protected in sepsis models and a polymorphism for caspase 12, which may regulate caspase 1, is associated with altered susceptibility to sepsis in humans (130,220–223).

Anti-inflammatory cytokines and factors that modulate host response are also induced by TLR signaling, and cytokine "imbalance" has been proposed as a central feature of dysregulated inflammation and tissue injury in sepsis, based on experimental models and analysis of patient samples (9,28,211,224,225) [Fig. 7(A)]. More recent observations question the concept of cytokine imbalance in septic syndromes, however (35). Alternatively, cytokine "profiles"—which are patterns of specific cytokines—are proposed to provide "codes" for distinct septic syndromes [Fig. 7(B)]. In this analysis, TNF-α is identified as a prototype mediator of septic shock, and HMGB1 as a prototype cytokine for severe sepsis; severe sepsis and septic shock are further proposed to be distinct clinical syndromes rather than stages in a continuum of severity (33). TNF-α is a classic mediator of systemic inflammation and immune response (226) that is secreted within minutes after infectious challenge or experimental bacteremia. Plasma levels are transient, however, and return to near baseline within a few hours (33). TNF-α is present in the blood of patients with septic shock, and levels are higher than those in patients with severe sepsis (33,218). Administration of exogenous TNF-α induces the manifestations of septic shock in experimental models (33).

HMGB1 was more recently discovered and assigned the role of a late and sustained mediator sepsis (9,33). HMGB1 is a nuclear DNA-binding protein that can be released by stimulated or necrotic macrophages and that functions as a proinflammatory cytokine in the extracellular milieu (9,33,227). Consistent with intricate activities in sepsis, HMGB1 binds to TLR2 and TLR4 and induces functional cellular responses (33,228). HMGB1 is also recognized by the receptor for advanced glycation end products (RAGE) (33), and lung inflammation and cytokine synthesis are retained when HMGB1 is given intratracheally to C3H/HeJ mice deficient in TLR4 (39). RAGE is induced in type 1 alveolar cells in rodents challenged with LPS and is present in edema fluid of patients with ALI (229) and BAL samples from mice given intratracheal LPS. Thus, this component of the HMGB1 recognition system is altered in ALI, as are TLRs. HMGB1 is released from hypoxic hepatocytes (230) and was interpreted to be "downstream" of apoptosis in a pathway to organ damage based on studies in an in vivo model (231). HMGB1, therefore, has the potential to contribute to end-organ injury and multiple organ dysfunction in severe sepsis (33). HMGB1 levels are increased in serum at late time points in clinical and experimental sepsis (9,33,232) and in lung and plasma samples in experimental and clinical ALI (233). Antagonist and inhibitors of HMGB1 ameliorated ALI and reduced mortality in experimental models of severe sepsis (33,233,234). Binding of HMGB1 by thrombomodulin may provide protection from its proinflammatory effects (235,236). Thus, changes in levels of thrombomodulin in sepsis and septic ALI may alter bioavailability and activity of HMGB1.

Based on these and other observations, TNF-α (together with IL-1α and IL-1β) and HMGB1 were proposed as central components in the "codes" for septic shock and severe sepsis, respectively [Fig. 7(B)] (33). It was also observed, however, that neither cytokine is absolutely specific for sepsis and that additional cytokines and inflammatory mediators also are likely to contribute to specific septic syndromes (33). It seems clear that there must indeed be additional modifying factors. For example, high levels of TNF-α have been detected in human malarial syndromes and in mice with experimental malaria, but pathophysiology similar to septic shock is uncommon (237). Nevertheless, time-dependent expression of specific cytokines—and, therefore, time-dependent therapeutic windows—may be central determinants of specific septic syndromes. This is a potential

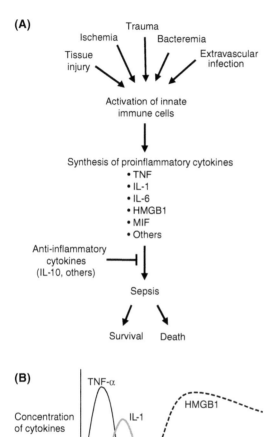

Figure 7 Cytokines are synthesized in septic syndromes and are mediators and biomarkers of inflammation, thrombosis, and tissue injury. (**A**) Multiple proinflammatory cytokines are synthesized in the systemic response to bacteremia or extravascular infection without bloodstream invasion. Host-delivered agonists can also drive proinflammatory cytokine synthesis in SIRS induced by trauma, ischemia, and other forms of tissue injury. Anti-inflammatory cytokines that can modify or blunt proinflammatory responses are also synthesized and released, leading to the concept of cytokine imbalance in sepsis. (**B**) Temporal patterns of specific cytokines ("codes") may mediate unique septic syndromes. TNF-α, acting together with IL-1 and other cytokines, is proposed to be a necessary mediator of septic shock and is sufficient to induce shock in mice. TNF-α and IL-1α and β are rapidly released in response to microbial or endotoxin challenge but are transiently present in the blood. HMGB1 is proposed to be a delayed and sustained mediator of inflammation that is requisite for organ dysfunction in severe sepsis. In this analysis, severe sepsis and septic shock are proposed to be unique syndromes and not stages in a continuum of severity [see text and (33) for details]. Panel B was redrawn from Ref. 33.

reason for failure of selective anticytokine agents in previous clinical trials of biologic intervention in sepsis (9,17,46).

Macrophage migration inhibitory factor (MIF) is a pleiotropic cytokine with activities in innate and acquired immunity that was first identified several decades ago but more recently was characterized, together with HMGB1, as a new molecular effector in septic syndromes (9). Targeted disruption of the *MIF* gene in mice conferred resistance to LPS and reduced inflammatory responses in the lungs of animals challenged with *Pseudomonas aeruginosa* (238). Among other interesting features, MIF is an antagonist of the anti-inflammatory and immunosuppressive effects of glucocorticoids and thus may enhance inflammatory injury in sepsis by this mechanism in addition to direct and proinflammatory actions (9,239). MIF is present in plasma of patients with sepsis (240) and lavage fluids from patients with ARDS (241). Plasma MIF concentrations were elevated in septic subjects both with and without shock, and elevated levels discriminated between survivors and nonsurvivors (240). Thus, additional contributors to the cytokine profiles of specific septic syndromes (33,218)—such as MIF—may influence the natural histories of these conditions and the frequency and outcome of complications such as ALI/ARDS.

H.   It Is More Than TLRs: Other Receptor Systems Signal and Modify Inflammatory and Thrombotic Responses in Sepsis

In addition to TLRs, other signaling systems are involved in complex inflammatory responses to microbial and endotoxic challenge (9,65,204). While each of these pathways cannot be comprehensively reviewed in this chapter, signaling mechanisms involving G-protein-coupled receptors (GPCRs) are important to consider. GPCRs have evolved for many biological tasks including host responses to infection (9) (Fig. 2). They are important in experimental and clinical sepsis, and are attractive therapeutic targets (25). GPCRs that have significant roles in regulated and dysregulated inflammation and activities in experimental and/or clinical sepsis include the receptor for formulated bacterial peptides, protease-activated receptors (PARs) that recognize thrombin and other ligands, chemokine receptors, the receptor for the activated 5th component of complement (C5a), the G2A receptor that recognizes lysophosphatidylcholine, eicosanoid and leukotriene receptors, histamine receptors, β-adrenergic receptors, angiotensin receptors, and the PAF receptor (9,31,41,204,242,243). PAF receptor signaling will be considered here as a prototype example because studies of its contributions to sepsis and ALI span the spectrum from basic science to clinical trials. Observations related to the PAR family and thrombin signaling (131,135,244,245) are discussed throughout this chapter.

The PAF receptor (PAFR) is constitutively expressed on human PMNs, monocytes, and other cells, and transmits outside-in signals that induce multiple functional responses when it is specifically ligated by PAF or by structurally related ligands (called "PAF-like lipids") that are generated by oxidant attack on membrane phospholipids in pathological conditions (246–248). The PAFR is also expressed on human platelets, where its engagement triggers aggregation, granule exocytosis, signal-dependent translation of IL-1β, and other responses (9). Expression on both myeloid leukocytes and platelets is an unusual pattern for a GPCR that confers the ability to rapidly induce both acute inflammatory and thrombotic events when its ligands are generated (134). In addition to displaying the PAFR and responding to PAF, myeloid leukocytes and platelets synthesize PAF when stimulated. LPS and lipopeptides induce synthesis and release of PAF by adherent human PMNs, an example of a mechanism by which PAF may be produced in septic syndromes

(249). Similarly, human ECs rapidly synthesize PAF in response to stimulation with a variety of thrombotic and proinflammatory agonists, and use it in endothelial-dependant targeting and activation of myeloid leukocytes (134) (Fig. 5).

A group of precise mechanisms has evolved to regulate cellular activation via the PAF/PAFR signaling system (9). They include tightly controlled enzymatic synthesis of PAF, expression of the PAFR on specific target cells, receptor desensitization after engagement, spatially regulated signaling by PAF localized to the surfaces of ECs and certain other cells that produce it (juxtacrine signaling), and rapid degradation of PAF by a group of endogenous enzymes termed PAF acetylhydrolases. Breakdown or dysregulation of one or more of these control mechanisms and/or unregulated nonenzymatic production of PAF-like lipids (see below) may contribute to pathological inflammation in a number of syndromes and diseases, including sepsis (9,134).

In addition to enzymatic synthesis of PAF, ligands for the PAFR can be generated in an unregulated, nonenzymatic fashion. Oxidatively modified phospholipids (OX-PLs) of a variety of structures are generated by oxidative attack on cell membranes or oxidation of synthetic substrates such as 1-palmitoyl-2-arachidonoyl-*sn*-glycero-3-phosphocholine (134,247). OX-PLs with very short *sn*-2 side chains, generated by oxidative fragmentation of native long chain fatty acids at the *SN*-2 position, are recognized by the PAFR on target cells and activate it (9,134). Thus, PAF-like OX-PLs can potentially be generated and mediate inflammatory events in pathologic conditions independently from, or together with, PAF produced by cellular synthesis (134). Interestingly, OX-PLs were recently reported to activate TLR4 (215), although specific structures of the OX-PLs species were not determined. OX-PLs derived from precursors that can yield PAF-like lipids are also reported to negatively modify TLR signaling and functional responses in vitro and in vivo (250–252). To add further complexity, the PAFR is reported to mediate a component of the pulmonary inflammatory response to LTA in mice (187), and LTA is reported to be a ligand for the PAFR on respiratory epithelium in vitro (253,254). Thus, PAFR signaling can have complex combinational features when PAF and/or PAF-like OX-PLs are produced, other OX-PLs molecular species are generated, bacterial ligands are present, and TLRs are engaged, a possibility that has sometimes not been considered in studies of OX-PLs in models relevant to sepsis and ALI.

There is extensive preclinical and clinical evidence that the PAF signaling system is involved in sepsis and its complications (9,134,255,256). Furthermore, new responses of effector cells that are mediated by PAF/PAFR signaling and are relevant to sepsis continue to be discovered. As examples, PAF activates previously unrecognized mechanisms of transcriptional and post-transcriptional gene expression in human PMNs (257), in addition to inducing post-transcriptional pathways in platelets (see above). PAF also triggers formation of extracellular NETs—which are implicated in sepsis (84)—by human neutrophils (258).

Innate immune cells from a number of other species also bear the PAFR and are activated, undergo phenotypic changes, and synthesize cytokines such as TNF-α when it is engaged (9,134,255). Administration of PAF to experimental animals and blockade of PAFR signaling in surrogate disease models indicate roles in sepsis and related syndromes (9). As an example, overexpression of the PAFR increased mortality in response to LPS challenge in a genetically altered mouse strain (259). In a second study, LPS, TNF-α, and PAF itself increased expression of the endogenous PAFR mRNA in rats with intestinal injury (260). Observations in additional in vivo models provide evidence for dysregulated signaling via the PAFR as a mechanism of septic ALI and for linked activities of LPS, PAF, and TNF-α in pathologic inflammation (9,255,261–263). In recent studies, LTA-induced lung inflammation in mice was mediated by TLR2, TLR4, and the PAFR (187). These and other models (9) identify activities of PAFR in experimental sepsis, and in responses of key end organs that are injured in septic syndromes. Animal models also suggest that signaling via the PAFR contributes to complications that may accompany sepsis and shock, including ischemia/reperfusion damage and transfusion-related lung injury (264–266). In vivo and whole lung systems further suggest new mechanisms by which the PAFR pathway mediates pulmonary edema. In murine models of LPS challenge and aspiration, PAFR signaling resulted in sphingomyelin hydrolysis, ceramide generation, synthesis of eicosanoids, and alveolar flooding (267,268).

Clinical observations parallel findings in studies of PAFR signaling in experimental models of sepsis (9). There is evidence for receptor occupancy on circulating platelets from subjects with sepsis, and activity consistent with PAF or PAF-like OX-PLs has been found in blood and/or tissue in some, but not all, samples from patients with sepsis that have been examined (9,133,255). A complicating feature of analysis of plasma or bronchoalveolar lavage (BAL) samples is that PAF can act in a juxtacrine fashion at cell surfaces, without being released into the plasma or interstitial fluids; levels measured in solution may, therefore, have little relationship to biological effects in mediating cell–cell interactions and activating target cells (9). There are a number of other technically challenging aspects of measuring PAF and PAF-like OX-PLs that can complicate assays of clinical samples (134,247).

Clinical trials of PAFR antagonists in sepsis suggested positive effects, but did not clearly establish therapeutic benefit (9,46,133,269–272). A number of variables in addition to heterogeneity of the patient populations and timing of administration of the drug may account for this. They include inefficient blockade of the PAFR and short half-lives and other pharmacological characteristics of receptor antagonists that were studied (9,134). These outcomes suggested that an alternative approach to utilizing a noncompetitive strategy might be useful (9). Recombinant plasma PAF acetylhydrolase (rPAF AH), which terminates signaling "upstream" from the PAFR by selectively hydrolyzing PAF and PAF-like OX-PLs, provided such a therapeutic option (134,248). rPAF AH improves survival in LPS challenge and CLP models of sepsis (273), consistent with previous studies in which it inactivated PAF and PAF-like OX-PLs in vitro and in vivo (9). Administration of rPAF AH to 127 patients with severe sepsis in a randomized, double blind multicenter phase IIb trial resulted in reduced 28-day all-cause mortality and a trend toward reduced multiple organ dysfunction (274). A subsequent phase III trial in subjects with severe sepsis was, however, terminated after partial enrollment because of apparent lack of efficacy (275).

Several variables may have accounted for the different outcomes in the phase II and phase III trials, including differences in the severity of illness in the study populations (276). Another key variable may be dynamic, time-dependent changes in levels of endogenous plasma PAF AH in inflammation and injury, which potentially creates a "moving therapeutic target" that was not evaluated in either clinical trial. The activity of endogenous plasma PAF AH is decreased in some—but not all—subjects with sepsis or SIRS (9,134,273) [Fig. 8(A)]. This establishes the potential for pathological imbalance resulting from enhanced generation of agonists recognized by the PAFR (PAF, PAF-like OX-PLs) and parallel depression of a key enzyme that degrades them and terminates their signals (endogenous PAF AH). Mechanisms of decreased activity of endogenous PAF AH include

LPS-mediated inhibition of its synthesis by macrophages and oxidative inactivation of the endogenous anti-inflammatory enzyme in the inflammatory milieu (9). Septic patients with depressed levels of endogenous plasma PAF AH might be expected to respond to administration of rPAF AH, whereas those with normal or increased plasma activity [Fig. 8(A)] might have lesser or no benefit (277). Endogenous levels of plasma PAF AH are, however, dynamic and change over time in inflammatory conditions. Dynamic variation in plasma PAF AH activity occurs in experimental sepsis in mice (273) [Fig. 8(B)] and in critically ill patients (278), likely reflecting new synthesis by macrophages in response to inflammatory stimuli (134). Endogenous PAF AH activity in the alveolar compartment also varies in a time-dependent fashion in patients and experimental animals with ALI, potentially due to local synthesis as well as leak from the blood (279,280) [Fig. 8(C)]. Individual variation in the duration of depressed endogenous PAF AH activity may establish subsets of patients who may respond to rPAF AH and specific temporal windows for successful therapy, in addition to partially accounting for the broad range of values in plasma and BAL PAF AH in patient samples collected in the acute phase of sepsis and ALI/ARDS (273,279). These and other unknown issues (276,277,281) suggest that the PAF/PAFR system remains a potential target for therapeutic intervention in some patients with sepsis and septic ALI.

I. The Interface Between Inflammation, Coagulation, and Thrombosis in Sepsis and Its Complications

Sepsis is perhaps the most dramatic and compelling example of the intimate relationship between the innate immune and hemostatic systems in inflammatory disease. Evolutionary and phylogenetic perspectives trace this association (52,110,282,283). In *Limulus, Drosophila*, and other invertebrates, serial activation of serine protease zymogens or release of intracellular proteases from multifunctional defensive cells generates a coagulum that walls off invading microbes (52,284,285). These invertebrate proteolytic pathways, which have similarity to mammalian clotting and complement cascades, can

--→

Figure 8   Plasma PAF AH is variably depressed in patients with sepsis and septic shock and is dynamically regulated in mice with experimental sepsis and humans with septic ALI/ARDS. (**A**) Plasma PAF AH activity was determined in samples from subjects with severe sepsis or septic shock within 48 hours of diagnosis, and in a group of controls. Both depressed and elevated activity levels were detected in septic patients (273). Depressed plasma PAF AH activity in sepsis has also been reported in other studies (9,134). (**B**) Mice were subjected to CLP and plasma PAF AH activity was determined in surviving animals over a four-day period. At 48 hours there was a mean depression of enzymatic activity, but with a broad range of values in individual animals. The activity levels then returned toward baseline over the next 48 hours. Depression of plasma PAF AH activity was more marked and prolonged in a group of animals given intrapentoneal LPS (not shown). *Source*: From Ref. 271. (**C**) Plasma PAF AH activity was measured in serial blood samples from a subject with sepsis and ARDS as described in (279). The activity assay used was different from the commercial assay employed in the studies in Panel A. Activity levels were initially moderately depressed and gradually increased over 10 days in the ICU in this subject (unpublished data).

(A)

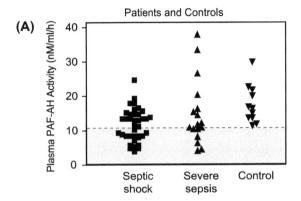

(B)

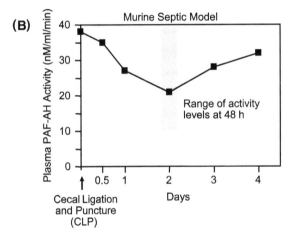

(C)

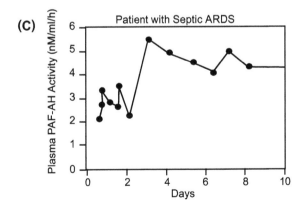

be triggered by LPS and other PAMPs (282), suggesting that the primitive coagulation response was part of a common host defense mechanism that subsequently evolved for specialized hemostatic and innate immune functions but with continued molecular links between the two parallel systems.

There is extensive evidence from experimental and clinical studies that dysregulated hemostasis influences the natural history of sepsis and its end-organ complications, including ALI (9,37,52,54,95,96,117,224,286,287). These observations spawned recent clinical trials of novel anticoagulants (25,95,96,286). The molecular basis for coagulation, including the generation of thrombin and conversion of fibrinogen to fibrin, has been extensively reviewed (52) and will not be recapitulated in detail here. Current evidence indicates that the TF pathway is the primary mechanism for thrombin generation in patients with sepsis (52,131,286). TF is synthesized by human monocytes and macrophages in response to LPS, proinflammatory cytokines, and other stimuli in vivo and in vitro and is deposited on cell surfaces or released into the flowing blood in microparticles that are shed by monocytes and other cell types (288). Recent evidence indicates that human platelets can also synthesize TF (129,288,289) (see earlier section). Thrombin generated by sequential protease-dependent steps in the TF pathway cleaves fibrinogen to yield fibrin, the ultimate end product in coagulation and the central component of the fibrin clot (52). Dysregulated fibrin deposition and fibrinolysis are key features in the pathophysiology of sepsis and septic ALI (37,52,113,224). Consistent with clinical observations and in vitro studies, TF expression mediates intravascular coagulation in endotoxemia and knockout of the *TF* gene reduces LPS-induced thrombosis in mice (131,288).

Together with its cleavage of fibrinogen, thrombin activates platelets and induces their aggregation and interaction with leukocytes and, in addition, induces inflammatory responses by ECs and certain other cell types that express the appropriate PARs (244,245) (Fig. 5). Thus, generation of thrombin and signaling via PARs on target cells are potent mechanisms that link the hemostatic and inflammatory systems. Several examples illustrate this point (Fig. 5). Activation of human ECs by thrombin induces translocation of P-selectin to their surfaces and coincident synthesis of PAF, which results in ECs-dependent adhesion and local activation of PMNs (9,290) [Fig. 5(A)]. A similar mechanism is induced when immobilized platelets are stimulated to display P-selectin and PAF on their surfaces (134). In addition, P-selectin displayed on the surfaces of platelets activated by thrombin binds to P-selectin glycoprotein ligand 1 (PSGL-1) on monocytes, resulting in transcellular signaling to transcriptional and translational control pathways that induces new expression of gene products including TNF-α, IL-8, MCP-1, cyclooxygenase 2, and other factors (9,164) [Figs. 4(A) and 5(B)]. As a third example, human platelets stimulated by thrombin synthesize and release IL-1β, which can then activate new gene expression in ECs, providing a novel mechanism with the potential to both link and amplify thrombosis and inflammation (291) [Fig. 5(C)].

In addition to these examples, thrombin induces other inflammatory response by direct and indirect actions on cells of the innate immune and vascular systems (244,245). Furthermore, additional proteases and molecular complexes generated by the coagulation cascade have proinflammatory properties (52). The mechanisms are in some cases less well characterized than are those activated by thrombin, but are nevertheless relevant to sepsis and other pathological conditions (9).

At the same time that the coagulation cascade is triggered and cellular thrombotic systems are activated, endogenous anticoagulant proteins are depleted and the fibrinolytic response is attenuated in dysregulated hemostasis induced by sepsis and tissue injury (9,18,37,52,224). The major endogenous anticoagulant systems in humans are regulated by protein C, antithrombin, and tissue factor pathway inhibitor (TFPI) (52). Recent observations indicate that disruption of the protein C/protein S/thrombomodulin pathway is a pivotal event in patients with sepsis (52,54,117,292). Current evidence demonstrates that it has a major role in preventing thrombosis in the microcirculation and, because it also has anti-inflammatory effects (see below), that its actions are not limited to controlling thrombin generation and modulating fibrinolysis (9,52,236). The ability to modulate proinflammatory as well as procoagulant pathways may be a major feature that contributes to the efficacy of endogenous APC as a control factor and rAPC as a therapeutic agent in severe sepsis (9) (see below).

Protein C circulates as an inactive precursor that is rapidly converted to a serine protease, activated protein C (APC), by a complex of thrombin and thrombomodulin (TM). TM is present on the plasma membranes of ECs under basal conditions and binds thrombin when it is generated. This inhibits the procoagulant actions of thrombin while facilitating its ability to cleave protein C to APC (52). TM not only converts thrombin from a prothrombotic factor to an anticoagulant molecule but was also recently reported to bind HMGB1 and prevent its activation of RAGE (235,236). Protein C activation is additionally enhanced by the endothelial cell protein C receptor (EPCR) (52,293). When APC is produced it associates with a plasma factor, protein S. This complex inactivates factors Va and VIIIa, inhibiting thrombin generation (9,52).

In addition to providing an endogenous anticoagulant "brake" on thrombin production that is proportional to the thrombotic stimulus under physiological conditions, APC modulates inflammatory responses (52). Blocking APC or cofactors of the pathway in primates infused with sublethal concentrations of LPS resulted not only in enhanced thrombosis and mortality but also in enhanced inflammation, as indicated by circulating levels of TNF-α, IL-6, and IL-8 (294). In additional early studies, APC also reduced blood and tissue levels of TNF-α in rodent models of sepsis and was reported to inhibit LPS-stimulated translocation of NF-κB to the nucleus and other responses in human monocytic cell lines (9,294).

More recent studies also support the idea that APC has complex anti-inflammatory functions as well as anticoagulant activities. In addition to modulating mononuclear cell function and survival, APC inhibited LPS-induced leukocyte adhesion and attenuated reduction in capillary perfusion in rodents in vivo; rAPC also reduced PMN accumulation in a human model of LPS-induced lung inflammation (295–297). Acute inflammation was worsened when mice with genetically impaired expression of endogenous protein C levels were challenged with LPS, as were intravascular coagulation, thrombocytopenia, and organ damage (298). Consistent with these observations, recombinant APC with only 10% of the anticoagulant activity of wild-type APC was as effective as the wild-type protein in reducing mortality after LPS challenge, and enhanced survival in other models (299). Additional activities may contribute to improved mortality in these experimental systems (300). APC has antiapoptotic and cytoprotective activities, and protects endothelial barrier function (300,301). Cytoprotective actions were thought to be important in the survival benefit at nonanticoagulant APC (299). Antiapoptotic, antinflammatory, and barrier protective activities appear to be mediated by EPCR and PAR2, indicating unexpected interplay between these two signaling systems (300–302). Thrombin, in low concentrations, and APC may enhance endothelial barrier function by interfacing with a pathway activated by sphingosine-1-phosphate (S1P) (300,301,303,304). Part of the mechanism appears to involve transactivation of the S1P receptor, S1P1 (303,304). Thus, there are complex interactions between APC and the EPCR, PAR1, and S1P1 signaling pathways in regulation of endothelial barrier function (300).

Plasma levels of protein C and protein S rapidly decrease in septic patients and in subjects with ALI caused by other insults, based on clinical studies (9,224,305). Consistent with these observations, in recent experimental studies protein C levels were depressed in a rat CLP model of polymicrobial sepsis and this was associated with lung inflammation: that was ameliorated by administration of APC (306). Furthermore, TM is reduced on the human endothelial surface in both in vitro models of LPS challenge and in histological analysis of biopsies from patients with clinical meningococcal sepsis, although this has not been seen in all animal models (9,236,307). In addition, levels of soluble TM—which has lower activity than cell surface TM—increase in the plasma of patients with sepsis and many other systemic inflammatory diseases (9). Reduction of TM on the endothelial surface and shedding into the plasma may result from its proteolytic cleavage by elastase and other proteases locally released by degranulating neutrophils (52) (Figs. 3 and 5). LPS-stimulated human ECs synthesize several degranulating factors that trigger the release of elastase and other granular proteases by PMNs (9), and, thrombin-stimulated human ECs "prime" neutrophils for enhanced degranulation by a mechanism involving surface display of P-selectin and PAF and engagement of the PAFR [Fig. 5(A)]. Thus, inflammatory signaling of ECs may contribute to dysregulated coagulation and subsequent thrombosis by PMN-dependent decreases in surface TM and impaired local activation of protein C. Furthermore, neutrophil-derived oxygen radicals can attack a methionine residue that is important for its activation (9,52).

There is experimental evidence that dysregulated coagulation and thrombosis are involved in septic lung injury, in addition to systemic manifestations of sepsis (9,224,308,309). Infusions of LPS in experimental animals cause intravascular fibrin deposition in the lungs, as well as in other organs involved in sepsis-induced multiple organ failure (310). In a primate model in which animals were primed with killed *Escherichia coli* and then challenged 12 hours later with live bacteria, TF generation, pulmonary fibrin deposition, and alveolar neutrophil accumulation occurred and were associated with hypoxemia, decreased lung compliance, lung edema, pulmonary hypertension, and evidence for concomitant renal failure. These pathological responses were improved by administration of a competitive inhibitor of TF, site-inactivated factor VIIa, and by administration of TFPI (311). In a similar model, an antibody against TF attenuated pulmonary dysfunction, inflammation, and fibrinogen depletion induced by challenge with gram-negative bacteria (312). In a rodent "two-hit" model, animals were subjected to hemorrhagic shock, resuscitated, and then challenged with intratracheal LPS to simulate infection after trauma, a common clinical scenario (313). Hemorrhagic shock potentiated the injury triggered by subsequent administration of low doses of LPS, and sequential challenge resulted in increased lung TF and plasminogen activator levels, and a net procoagulant state that may have involved augmented TLR4 signaling (313,314). This model may mimic some of the features of challenge by bacterial products delivered via the airway (intubation, airway colonization and/or infection, etc.) after an initial "hit" by systemic trauma and hemorrhage, a situation that commonly occurs in the intensive care unit. Two "hit" models may be particularly useful in investigation of ALI, including studies related to septic ALI/ARDS (315).

IV. Features of Septic ALI/ARDS in Critically III Patients

The systemic features of septic syndromes have been reviewed (30,31,90). This section focuses specifically on the lung in clinical sepsis. The pathobiologic basis and translational correlates of septic ALI/ARDS in human subjects have been outlined in previous sections and will be referred to again in places. Lung injury in sepsis is not a static condition but instead involves stages that have been defined by clinical and pathologic studies, and that may ultimately provide specific windows of opportunity for unique preventative and therapeutic measures (Fig. 9).

The incidence, natural history, and prognosis of ALI/ARDS precipitated by sepsis were reported in early studies, further described in subsequent clinical series, and have been reviewed (5,6,9,14,318). In general, physiological features of ALI and ARDS induced by sepsis have been reported to be similar to those in patients with ALI caused by other precipitating factors (trauma, aspiration, etc.) (5,6,224). Nevertheless, it is possible that sepsis and septic shock alter the "physiological phenotype" of individual patients (9). The mortality of ALI and ARDS associated with sepsis and septic shock is higher than that in other subsets of ALI, a feature identified in most early and more recent clinical reports (5,18,19,319–321). The mechanisms that account for the lethal nature of septis-induced ARDS remain incompletely defined, although comorbid conditions and the complicated

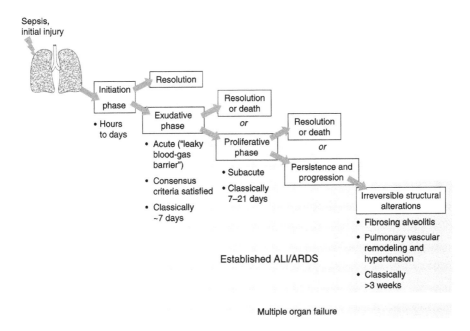

Figure 9 The natural history of septic ALI/ARDS: time-dependent phases, pathophysiologic events, and therapeutic targets. Histopathologic and clinical observation demonstrate that septic ALI and ARDS have time-dependent physiologic manifestations, phases, and outcomes (9,316,317). A key challenge in reducing morbidity in patients with ALI/ARDS associated with sepsis is to identify features that determine persistence and progression of alveolar and systemic injury versus resolution and repair (6).

molecular events, concurrent systemic injury, and frequent multiple organ failure induced by sepsis must surely contribute (9).

PMNs and monocytes accumulate in the lungs of patients with septic ALI and ARDS. This can be demonstrated using imaging with radiolabeled leukocytes, histological analysis, and BAL (9,322–325) (Fig. 10). Acute accumulation of myeloid leukocytes in the lungs has similarly been documented in virtually all animal models of sepsis, including those in rodents, ungulates, and primates. Experimental and clinical studies indicate that molecular imaging may be useful as a noninvasive approach to identifying early inflammatory events in ALI (326), potentially providing a much needed tool that narrows the gap between preclinical and clinical observations. Recent studies indicate that 18 fluorodeoxyglucose position emission tomography scanning can detect early diffuse lung inflammation in humans with ALI initiated by pulmonary contusion (327), but this has not yet been examined extensively in ALI secondary to sepsis.

Histological evaluation of lung tissue from human subjects with bacteremia or sepsis-induced ALI/ARDS has in many cases demonstrated intravascular accumulation, or "sequestration," of PMNs and monocytes in vessels of various sizes (316,317,323,328,330) (Fig. 10). Intravascular cellular aggregates may contribute to the

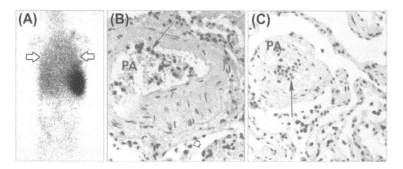

Figure 10 Neutrophils and monocytes accumulate in the lungs of patients with sepsis-induced ARDS. (**A**) Autologous radiolabeled leukocyte scanning in a patient with gram-negative sepsis 24 hours after meeting criteria for ARDS revealed diffuse accumulation of myeloid leukocytes in the lungs (arrows) (325). Consistent with imaging results, biopsy of the lungs in patients with septic ALI also demonstrates sequestration of myeloid leukocytes in microvessels (9). (**B**) PMNs and monocytes in a heterotypic cellular aggregate in a small pulmonary artery of a patient dying with ALI secondary to sepsis. Immunocytochemical analysis demonstrated that some of the myeloid leukocytes in intravascular aggregates expressed IL-8 (long arrow), whereas circulating PMNs and monocytes from control subjects do not express this chemokine. PMNs and mononuclear leukocytes in alveoli were also positive for IL-8 (short arrow) (328). (**C**) PMNs and monocytes in a heterotypic cellular aggregate (arrow) in a small pulmonary arteriole in the lung of a patient dying with ALI precipitated by sepsis. Immunostaining demonstrating expression of IL-8 by myeloid leukocytes in intravascular aggregates, and also by PMNs and monocytes in alveolar spaces. PMNs and monocytes in intravascular aggregates in lung sections from patients with sepsis also stain positively for ENA-78 (329), a second chemokine associated with ALI/ARDS (not shown).

increased pulmonary dead space fraction reported in ARDS associated with sepsis and other triggering conditions (321). Intravascular leukocyte aggregation has been thought to be an early pathological event resulting from formation of homotypic and heterotypic adhesive clusters of myeloid leukocytes in the flowing blood in response to circulating inflammatory mediators (Figs. 4 and 5), and to result in endothelial injury secondary to local release of oxygen radicals, elastase, and other proteases from leukocytes trapped in the lung microcirculation (6,9). Clinical and experimental studies provide evidence for degranulation and for cytolytic fragmentation of intravascular PMNs that could cause massive local release of granular enzymes (103,208). Monocytes or neutrophils in mixed cell aggregates in the pulmonary microvasculature may be a source of TF that induces and propagates thrombosis (9,288). In addition, intravascular neutrophils and monocytes in the lungs of septic patients express new gene products, including chemokines (328,329) (Fig. 10). The relative contributions of circulating factors versus juxtacrine signaling molecules (cell-associated chemokines, PAF, etc.) that are locally expressed by pulmonary ECs or entrapped platelets (see below) in causing intravascular leukocyte accumulation in sepsis are unknown. Direct effects of LPS or other endotoxins on both leukocytes and ECs may mediate intravascular leukocyte sequestration in sepsis based on clinical and experimental studies (48,67,69).

Morphometric analysis in classic reports documented expansion of the pulmonary intravascular leukocyte population in humans with sepsis, consistent with studies outlined above, and indicated that there were also increased numbers of platelets (316,317). Increased accumulation of platelets in the pulmonary microvasculature of septic platelets may result from platelet–platelet aggregates, local deposition of platelets in platelet–fibrin thrombi, interaction of platelets with sequestered leukocytes, and/or by formation of platelet–monocyte and platelet–PMN aggregates in the systemic blood and their deposition in the pulmonary microvasculature (Fig. 4) (see previous section) (115,323). Administration of LPS to human volunteers demonstrated that platelet–leukocyte aggregates form in the blood in response to this bacterial agonist (150). Complex interactions between platelets, myeloid leukocytes, and ECs in areas of intravascular sequestration [Figs. 4(B), 5, and 10)] may be stable over many hours, and provide a potential mechanism for intercellular signaling and new inflammatory gene expression (Fig. 5). Megakaryocytes may also be present, although this feature has not been characterized in human septic ALI/ARDS (115).

The relative contributions of intravascular, transiting, and intra-alveolar leukocytes (69,79,316,331) to alveolar-capillary membrane injury in patients with septic ALI/ARDS are not defined. Analysis of histological samples in studies in the Utah ARDS SCOR indicated that new gene products are expressed by neutrophils and monocytes in each compartment (9,328,329) (Fig. 10). New expression of inflammatory proteins and enzymes may amplify lung injury mediated by release of granular enzymes and generation of oxygen radicals by innate biochemical mechanisms (see above). Evidence for activation and degranulation of neutrophils in human ALI/ARDS secondary to sepsis and other causes has been reviewed (9,67,68). While it is possible that PMNs that are most responsive to direct stimulation with LPS or other agonists are sequestered in the lungs (332), the accumulation of PMNs in systemic vessels (Fig. 1) and formation of platelet–leukocyte aggregates in circulating blood (Figs. 4 and 5) indicate that they are also activated outside of the pulmonary circulation.

    The route(s) of neutrophil migration to interstitial and alveolar sites in human septic ALI are not definitively established. Although in mice subjected to shot-term inflammatory challenge the pulmonary capillary is the dominant site of PMN emigration (79,333), adhesion and emigration in pulmonary venules and arterioles may also occur (69). Histological observations suggest that venules and arterioles are routes of myeloid leukocyte trafficking in the inflamed or injured human lung (329; Albertine K, Zimmerman GA, unpublished observations). By whatever route, the accumulation of PMNs in the alveoli of patients with sepsis-induced ALI appears to influence outcome (9). PMN numbers in BAL samples tended to be higher in the first two weeks after onset of septic ALI in subjects that died compared to the subgroup that survived, whereas in trauma patients with ALI the BAL neutrophil counts progressively diminished over time and did not distinguish patients that died from the survivors (334). This suggests that persistence of the initial neutrophil "alveolitis" (Fig. 10) contributes to sustained injury and progression rather than resolution of ALI in patients with sepsis (Fig. 9), and thereby influences mortality. Nevertheless, this cannot necessarily be generalized to all patients with ALI and ARDS regardless of the inciting condition (12,334).

    In addition to neutrophils, monocytes accumulate in the alveolar space and are recovered in BAL samples early in the course of ALI/ARDS triggered by sepsis and other causes (9). Patterns of diminishing and sustained monocytic recruitment and differentiation have been observed in BAL samples from patients with ARDS, most of whom had sepsis and/or bacteria pneumonia (335). Identification of monocyte subsets with different functional characteristics in humans and mice (65) indicates that it will be important to examine specific contributions of unique monocytic populations to septic ALI. In a series of patients with sepsis-induced ALI/ARDS an increase in alveolar macrophages in serial lavage samples was associated with survival (334), suggesting that monocyte-to-macrophage differentiation may influence the natural history. We found evidence that the gene coding for plasma PAF AH (Fig. 8), which is induced as monocytes differentiate to macrophages (134), is expressed by alveolar macrophages in patients with ALI (279). This may be one aspect by which macrophage expansion limits inflammatory injury in subsets of patients with ALI, but the factors that influence differentiation of monocytes into pulmonary macrophages or dendritic cells and determine the expression of specific gene products by these cells in sepsis are largely unknown (9).

    The histological features of alveolar-capillary units in patients dying with ARDS caused by sepsis were described in pioneering studies of Bachofen and Weibel and later pathological investigation by others (316,317,331). In the acute or "exudative" phase (Fig. 9), they include interstitial and alveolar edema, intra-alveolar hemorrhage, relative preservation of endothelial morphology and continuity, local destruction of alveolar epithelium with denuded areas covered by fibrin-containing hyaline membranes, and intravascular and extravascular deposition of myeloid leukocytes, platelets, and fibrin (6,316). This is the key constellation of findings in the pathological diagnosis of "diffuse alveolar damage," the anatomic equivalent of the clinical condition of ARDS (316,328,331,336). These features were largely reproduced when primates were infused with LPS or live E. coli bacteria in early studies (337,338), although septic models in the mouse and other animals do not always demonstrate each of these features. While changes in the alveolar-capillary membrane in humans with septic ALI/ARDS and in animal models have been characterized based on cellular appearance, we know little about the "molecular phenotypes" of these cells: that is, the patterns of intracellular, surface, and locally released molecules that have been induced and, in parallel, the molecules that have been "downregulated" (9,339). It is likely that we will not completely understand key features of septic ALI/ARDS without this information. Histological, genomic, and proteomic studies correlated with in vitro cell models, measurement of factors in blood and BAL, and molecular imaging approaches may address this important gap in our clinical knowledge (315,326).

As with the acute phase, the histological features of the subacute proliferative and fibrotic phases of ALI/ARDS caused by documented sepsis (Fig. 9) appear to be similar to those in subjects with ALI/ARDS incited by other triggering conditions (316,317,331). We again know little about the molecular phenotypes of the lung and inflammatory cells at these later stages or how they compare to those in the earlier acute phase or in subsets of patients with different outcomes, such as alveolar fibrosis or obliterative vasculopathy with pulmonary hypertension (Fig. 9) (9). Similarly, there are gaps in our clinical knowledge regarding key repair mechanisms in the exudative and proliferative phase of septic ALI/ARDS (6,315), and it is unknown new approaches such as mesenchymal stem cell administration (340) will be of benefit. Mechanical stress and biologic signaling imposed by different patterns of mechanical ventilation may alter histologic patterns as well as clinical outcomes in septic ALI/ARDS (336).

Pathologic fibrin deposition occurs in macro and micro vessels of the lungs of patients with ALI/ARDS induced by sepsis, as it does in patients of ALI caused by other inciting conditions (37,316,317,331,341,342). This is part of a generalized dysregulation of fibrin generation and fibrinolysis in intravascular and extravascular compartments in ALI, and is consistent with findings in preclinical models as outlined in previous sections (37,224,300,308). Alveolar fluid and plasma samples from subjects with ALI/ARDS indicate that TF is a key mediator of fibrin deposition in the acutely injured human lung (300). Recent studies demonstrate that the alveolar epithelium is a source of TF, indicating that it is one of the sites of extrinsic pathway coagulation in ALI (37,343). The protein C system is also involved in human inflammatory lung injury. Circulating and alveolar protein C levels are reduced in septic ALI/ARDS and also in ALI triggered by other causes, and TM levels are increased in these compartments (344). In studies in the ARDS Network, low plasma concentrations of protein C and elevated levels of plaminogen activator inhibitor 1 were independent predictors of mortality and surrogate endpoints in patients with ALI/ARDS, including those with sepsis as an underlying cause (300). It is unclear if the deranged fibrin deposition in the lungs of septic patients is quantitatively or qualitatively different from that induced by other mechanisms of injury, or to what extent fibrin generation is required for healing and repair for the acutely injured lung (9,309). Protective modes of mechanical ventilation, which are indicated and appear to be efficacious in patients with septic ALI/ARDS (30), may reduce dysregulated pulmonary fibrin deposition (300).

The therapeutic role of rAPC in septic ALI is not yet clear. Based on the original trial (PROWESS) of patients with severe sepsis (292), rAPC is approved for use in septic patients with a high risk of death and Apache II scores ≥25 (30). Subsequent studies have not provided evidence that rAPC has efficacy in septic patients with less severe pathophysiology, or in pediatric patients (21,345). Furthermore, treatment with rAPC is associated with increased risk of bleeding so that the risk/benefit balance must be carefully considered in all subjects (27,300). Analysis of subgroups of patients in the PROWESS trial indicated that the lungs were the major source of infection and that patients with pulmonary infection had the greatest benefit from rAPC, suggesting that it may be therapeutically useful in septic ALI/ARDS (34,300). In addition, rAPC has ameliorated lung inflammation in studies employing the "human model" of LPS administration (195) and in some, but not all animal models of ALI (300). In summary, because the specific issue of septic ALI/ARDS was not explicitly evaluated in the original PROWESS trial, the therapeutic role of or rAPC in human ALI/ARDS associated with sepsis is yet to be clearly defined. Furthermore, in a recent phase II clinical study of subjects with ALI in which patients with severe sepsis and Apache II scores ≥25 were excluded, there was no survival benefit in the group treated with rAPC (18).

A variety of soluble biomarkers have been measured in samples of plasma and alveolar fluid from patients with sepsis, sepsis-induced ALI/ARDS, and ALI/ARDS associated with other triggering conditions (9,34,76,218,240,346–353). No single marker or combination of markers has emerged as specific for the etiology of ALI/ARDS or as predictive of occurrence, natural history, or outcome of these syndromes of lung injury (9,327). Approaches that may include pattern analysis using proteomic strategies together with genomic interrogation and parallel biological analysis may increase the yield from clinical samples in the future (9,315). In addition, imaging modalities that give molecular and functional information may complement current biomarkers and other surrogate end points in the study and clinical management of septic ALI/ARDS (326).

V. Research in Sepsis and Septic ALI/ARDS: Mechanisms, Models, and Challenges

Sepsis and its complications, including ALI/ARDS, are defined by clinical criteria. Basic and translational research in sepsis is focused on identifying cellular and molecular mechanisms that are tractable to specific manipulation, thus, potentially yielding new approaches to therapy and prevention of septic syndromes. Many surrogate animal models have been developed for the study of sepsis; some of these have been employed to examine mechanisms of ALI/ARDS resulting from systemic microbial challenge or direct pulmonary infection (9,25,315). Nevertheless, no animal model has yet been identified that reproduces the clinical condition of human sepsis or the end-organ complications that occur in its various syndromes, stages, and severities. In some cases, investigators in the field do not uniformly agree on the utility of an individual model, or how data generated with the model should be interpreted (25). Murine models are extremely popular because of the option of targeted genetic alteration, and many studies using mice are cited in this review. There are many differences between the immune systems and inflammatory responses of mice and humans (91,354–356), however, and as we emphasize here sepsis and septic ALI/ARDS are syndromes of immune and inflammatory dysregulation (Figs. 1 and 2). Differences between mice and humans may account for a part of the gap that currently exists between preclinical observations and clinical application in the field. Murine and other animal models will continue to be used as discovery and proof-of-principal systems (315), however, and can be very useful in combination with clinical analysis for generating mechanistic insights (Fig. 8).

Isolated human cell models continue to yield new mechanisms that are relevant to clinical sepsis (82,83,125,128,129,257), and offer the potential advantage of reducing the staggering complexity that characterizes the pathobiology of sepsis. Experimental systems utilizing isolated cells, examined individually or in studies of cell–cell interactions, are likely to provide additional mechanistic insights in the future, and are important tools for dissection of findings in in vivo models. They are insufficient to alone unlock the riddles of sepsis and septic ALI/ARDS, however. The "human models" of LPS or other microbial components administered to volunteers via the systemic circulation or delivered locally to the alveoli provide important translational insights that, like human cell models, are directly relevant to clinical sepsis, but these experimental systems, too, have limitation (17,357). A challenge for the future is to use each of these surrogate experimental systems to their greatest advantage and, in parallel, to identify new tools that bridge the gap between preclinical observations and their clinical validation, thereby accelerating mechanistic insight and consequent development of new therapies and preventative measures that have efficacy and consistent utility in the management of sepsis and septic ALI/ARDS.

Acknowledgements
The authors thank Sharren Brewer for diligent preparation of the manuscript and Diana Lim for expert preparation of the figures. We also thank our colleagues for their invaluable contributions to collaborative work that is cited and for many useful discussions, and Michael Matthay for sending preprints of unpublished articles. Projects mentioned in this review were, or are, supported by the National Institutes of Health (R37 HL44525, HL066277, HL091754, HL090870, P50 HL50153); a Western Affiliate American Heart Association Post-Doctoral Fellowship and grant-in-aid (09BGIA2250381) (H-JS); and K12 (C06-RR11234 from the National Center for Research Resources) and K23 (HL092161) (MTR).

References
1. Beutler B. Toll-like receptors: how they work and what they do. Curr Opin Hematol 2002; 9(1):2–10.
2. Ashbaugh, DG, Bigelow DB, et al. Acute respiratory distress in adults. Lancet 1967; 2(7511):319–323.
3. Kaplan RL, Sahn SA, et al. Incidence and outcome of the respiratory distress syndrome in gram-negative sepsis. Arch Intern Med 1979; 139(8):867–869.
4. Bernard GR, Artigas A, et al. The American-European Consensus Conference on ARDS. Definitions, mechanisms, relevant outcomes, and clinical trial coordination. Am J Respir Crit Care Med 1994; 149(3, pt 1):818–824.
5. Ware LB, Matthay MA. The acute respiratory distress syndrome. N Engl J Med 2000; 342(18):1334–1349.
6. Matthay MA, Zimmerman GA. Acute lung injury and the acute respiratory distress syndrome: four decades of inquiry into pathogenesis and rational management. Am J Respir Cell Mol Biol 2005; 33(4):319–327.
7. Ware LB. Pathophysiology of acute lung injury and the acute respiratory distress syndrome. Semin Respir Crit Care Med 2006; 27(4):337–349.
8. Leaver SK, Evans TW. Acute respiratory distress syndrome. BMJ 2007; 335(7616):389–394.
9. Zimmerman GA, Albertine KH, et al. Pathogenesis of sepsis and septic-induced lung injury. In: Matthay MA, ed. Acute Respiratory Distress Syndrome, vol. 179. New York/Basel: Marcel Dekker, Inc., 2003:245–287.
10. Beutler B, Rietschel ET. Innate immune sensing and its roots: the story of endotoxin. Nat Rev Immunol 2003; 3(2):169–176.

11. Parsons PE, Worthen GS, et al. The association of circulating endotoxin with the development of the adult respiratory distress syndrome. Am Rev Respir Dis 1989; 140(2):294–301.
12. Pittet JF, Mackersie RC, et al. Biological markers of acute lung injury: prognostic and pathogenetic significance. Am J Respir Crit Care Med 1997; 155(4):1187–1205.
13. Pepe PE, Potkin RT, et al. Clinical predictors of the adult respiratory distress syndrome. Am J Surg 1982; 144(1):124–130.
14. Hudson LD, Milberg JA, et al. Clinical risks for development of the acute respiratory distress syndrome. Am J Respir Crit Care Med 1995; 151(2, pt 1):293–301.
15. Rangel-Frausto MS. The epidemiology of bacterial sepsis. Infect Dis Clin North Am 1999; 13(2):299–312, vii.
16. Angus DC, Linde-Zwirble WT, Lidicker J, et al. Epidemiology of severe sepsis in the United States: analysis of incidence, outcome, and associated costs of care. Crit Care Med 2001; 29(7):1303–1310.
17. Vincent JL, Abraham E. The last 100 years of sepsis. Am J Respir Crit Care Med 2006; 173(3):256–263.
18. Liu KD, Levitt J, et al. Randomized clinical trial of activated protein C for the treatment of acute lung injury. Am J Respir Crit Care Med 2008; 178(6): 618–623.
19. Annane D, Sebille V, et al. Effect of low doses of corticosteroids in septic shock patients with or without early acute respiratory distress syndrome. Crit Care Med 2006; 34(1): 22–30.
20. Stoll BJ, Hansen RD, et al. Very low birth weight preterm infants with early onset neonatal sepsis: the predominance of gram-negative infections continues in the National Institute of Child Health and Human Development Neonatal Research Network, 2002–2003. Pediatr Infect Dis J 2005; 24:635–639.
21. Nadel S, Goldstein B, et al. Drotrecogin alfa (activated) in children with severe sepsis: a multicentre phase III randomised controlled trial. Lancet 2007; 369(9564):836–843.
22. Wong HR, Cvijanovich N, et al. Interleukin-8 as a stratification tool for interventional trials involving pediatric septic shock. Am J Respir Crit Care Med 2008; 178(3):276–282.
23. Martin GS, Mannino DM, et al. The effect of age on the development and outcome of adult sepsis. Crit Care Med 2006; 34(1):15–21.
24. Gomez CR, Hirano S, Cutro BT, et al. Advanced age exacerbates the pulmonary inflammatory response after lipopolysaccharide exposure. Crit Care Med 2007; 35(1):246–251.
25. Riedemann NC, Guo RF, et al. Novel strategies for the treatment of sepsis. Nat Med 2003; 9(5):517–524.
26. Bucala R. Series introduction: molecular and cellular basis of septic shock. J Leukoc Biol 2004; 75(3):398–399.
27. Rice TW, Bernard GR. Therapeutic intervention and targets for sepsis. Annu Rev Med 2005; 56:225–248.
28. Baron RM, Baron MJ, et al. Pathobiology of sepsis: are we still asking the same questions? Am J Respir Cell Mol Biol 2006; 34(2):129–134.
29. Munford RS. Severe sepsis and septic shock: the role of gram-negative bacteremia. Annu Rev Pathol 2006; 1:467–496.
30. Russell JA. Management of sepsis. N Engl J Med 2006; 355(16):1699–1713.
31. Annane D, Bellissant E, et al. Septic shock. Lancet 2005; 365(9453):63–78.
32. Alberti C, Brun-Buisson C, Chevret S, et al. Systemic inflammatory response and progression to severe sepsis in critically ill infected patients. Am J Respir Crit Care Med 2005; 171:461–468.
33. Ulloa L, Tracey KJ. The cytokine profile: a code for sepsis. Trends Mol Med 2005; 11(2):56–63.
34. Laterre PF, Garber G, et al. Severe community-acquired pneumonia as a cause of severe sepsis: data from the PROWESS study. Crit Care Med 2005; 33(5):952–961.

35. Kellum JA, Kong L, et al. Understanding the inflammatory cytokine response in pneumonia and sepsis: results of the Genetic and Inflammatory Markers of Sepsis (GenIMS) Study. Arch Intern Med 2007; 167(15):1655–1663.
36. Annane D, Aegerter P, et al. Current epidemiology of septic shock: the CUB-Rea Network. Am J Respir Crit Care Med 2003; 168(2):165–172.
37. Bastarache JA, Ware LB, et al. The role of the coagulation cascade in the continuum of sepsis and acute lung injury and acute respiratory distress syndrome. Semin Respir Crit Care Med 2006; 27(4):365–376.
38. Members of the American College of Chest Physicians/Society of Critical Care Medicine Consensus Conference Committee. American College of Chest Physicians/Society of Critical Care Medicine Consensus Conference: definitions for sepsis and organ failure and guidelines for the use of innovative therapies in sepsis. Crit Care Med 1992; 20(6):864–874.
39. Abraham E. Matthay MA, et al. Consensus conference definitions for sepsis, septic shock, acute lung injury, and acute respiratory distress syndrome: time for a reevaluation. Crit Care Med 2000; 28(1):232–235.
40. Levy MM, Fink MP, et al. 2001 SCCM/ESICM/ACCP/ATS/SIS International Sepsis Definitions Conference. Crit Care Med 2003; 31(4):1250–1256.
41. Wang H, Czura CJ, et al. Lipid unites disparate syndromes of sepsis. Nat Med 2004; 10(2):124–125.
42. Stüber F. Human responses to endotoxin: role of the genetic background. In: Brade H, Opal SM, Vogel SN, et al., eds. Endotoxin in Health and Disease. New York: Marcel Dekker, Inc., 1999:877–885.
43. Cariou A, Chiche JD, et al. The era of genomics: impact on sepsis clinical trial design. Crit Care Med 2002; 30(Suppl. 5):S341–S348.
44. Barnes KC. Genetic determinants and ethnic disparities in sepsis-associated acute lung injury. Proc Am Thorac Soc 2005; 2(3):195–201.
45. Opal SM, Cross AS. Clinical trials for severe sepsis. Past failures, and future hopes. Infect Dis Clin North Am 1999; 13(2):285–297, vii.
46. Marshall JC. Such stuff as dreams are made on: mediator-directed therapy in sepsis. Nat Rev Drug Discov 2003; 2(5):391–405.
47. Huston JM, Ochani M, Rosas-Ballina M, et al. Splenectomy inactivates the cholinergic antiinflammatory pathway during lethal endotoxemia and polymicrobial sepsis. J Exp Med 2006; 203(7):1623–1628.
48. Kerfoot SM, Kubes P. Local coordination verses systemic disregulation: complexities in leukocyte recruitment revealed by local and systemic activation of TLR4 in vivo. J Leukoc Biol 2005; 77(6):862–867.
49. Esmon CT. Sepsis. A myriad of responses. Lancet 2001; 358(Suppl.):S61.
50. Cohen J. The immunopathogenesis of sepsis. Nature 2002; 420(6917):885–891.
51. Nathan C. Points of control in inflammation. Nature 2002; 420(6917):846–852.
52. Opal SM, Esmon CT. Bench-to-bedside review: functional relationships between coagulation and the innate immune response and their respective roles in the pathogenesis of sepsis. Crit Care 2003; 7(1):23–38.
53. Bateman RM, Sharpe MD, et al. Bench-to-bedside review: microvascular dysfunction in sepsis–hemodynamics, oxygen transport, and nitric oxide. Crit Care 2003; 7(5):359–373.
54. Schouten M, Wiersinga WJ, et al. Inflammation, endothelium, and coagulation in sepsis. J Leukoc Biol 2008; 83(3):536–545.
55. Haden DW, Suliman HB, Carraway MS, et al. Mitochondrial biogenesis restores oxidative metabolism during *Staphylococcus aureus* sepsis. Am J Respir Crit Care Med 2007; 176:762–777.
56. d'Avila JC, Santiago AP, Amancio RT, et al. Sepsis induces brain mitochondrial dysfunction. Crit Care Med 2008; 36(6):1925–1932.

57. Singer G, Stokes KY, et al. Sepsis-induced intestinal microvascular and inflammatory responses in obese mice. Shock 2008; 31(3):275–279.

58. Michalek SM, Moore RN, et al. The primary role of lymphoreticular cells in the mediation of host responses to bacterial endotoxim. J Infect Dis 1980; 141(1):55–63.

59. Nathan C. Neutrophils and immunity: challenges and opportunities. Nat Rev Immunol 2006; 6(3):173–182.

60. Lekstrom-Himes JA, Gallin JI. Immunodeficiency diseases caused by defects in phagocytes. N Engl J Med 2000; 343(23):1703–1714.

61. Bunting M, Harris ES, et al. Leukocyte adhesion deficiency syndromes: adhesion and tethering defects involving beta 2 integrins and selectin ligands. Curr Opin Hematol 2002; 9(1):30–35.

62. Levin BR, Antia R. Why we don't get sick: the within-host population dynamics of bacterial infections. Science 2001; 292(5519):1112–1115.

63. Beutler B, Poltorak A. Sepsis and evolution of the innate immune response. Crit Care Med 2001; 29(7 Suppl):S2-6; discussion S6-7.

64. Aderem A. Role of Toll-like receptors in inflammatory response in macrophages. Crit Care Med 2001; 29(Suppl. 7):S16–S18.

65. Gordon S. The macrophage: past, present and future. Eur J Immunol 2007; 37(Suppl. 1):S9–S17.

66. Miyazaki Y, Bunting M, Stafforini DM, et al. Integrin alphaDbeta2 is dynamically expressed by inflamed macrophages and alters the natural history of lethal systemic infections. J Immunol 2008; 180(1):590–600.

67. Lee WL, Downey GP. Neutrophil activation and acute lung injury. Curr Opin Crit Care 2001; 7(1):1–7.

68. Abraham E. Neutrophils and acute lung injury. Crit Care Med 2003; 31(Suppl. 4):S195–S199.

69. Rodrigues RS, Zimmerman GA. Pulmonary endothelial interactions with leukocytes and platelets. In: Rounds A, Voelkel N, eds. The Pulmonary Endothelium. London, UK: John Wiley and Sons, Ltd, 2008.

70. Ibbotson GC, Doig C, Kaur J, et al. Functional alpha4-integrin: a newly identified pathway of neutrophil recruitment in critically ill septic patients. Nat Med 2001; 7(4):465–470.

71. Docke WD, Randow F, et al. Monocyte deactivation in septic patients: restoration by IFN-gamma treatment. Nat Med 1997; 3(6):678–681.

72. Adib-Conquy M, Adrie C, Moine P, et al. NF-kappaB expression in mononuclear cells of patients with sepsis resembles that observed in lipopolysaccharide tolerance. Am J Respir Crit Care Med 2000; 162(5):1877–1883.

73. Fahy RJ, Exline MC, Gavrilin MA, et al. Inflammasome mRNA expression in human monocytes during early septic shock. Am J Respir Crit Care Med 2008; 177(9):983–988.

74. Fingerle G, Pforte A, et al. The novel subset of CD14+/CD16+ blood monocytes is expanded in sepsis patients. Blood 1993; 82(10):3170–3176.

75. Belge KU, Dayyani F, Horelt A, et al. The proinflammatory CD14+CD16+DR++monocytes are a major source of TNF. J Immunol 2002; 168(7):3536–3542.

76. Gibot S, Kolopp-Sarda MN, et al. Plasma level of a triggering receptor expressed on myeloid cells-1: its diagnostic accuracy in patients with suspected sepsis. Ann Intern Med 2004; 141(1):9–15.

77. Bohnsack JF, Akiyama SK, et al. Human neutrophil adherence to laminin in vitro. Evidence for a distinct neutrophil integrin receptor for laminin. J Exp Med 1990; 171(4):1221–1237.

78. Guo RF, Riedemann NC, Laudes IJ, et al. Altered neutrophil trafficking during sepsis. J Immunol 2002; 169(1):307–314.

79. Reutershan J, Ley K. Bench-to-bedside review: acute respiratory distress syndrome—how neutrophils migrate into the lung. Crit Care 2004; 8(6):453–461.

80. Mayadas TN, Cullere X. Neutrophil beta2 integrins: moderators of life or death decisions. Trends Immunol 2005; 26(7):388–395.

81. Fialkow L, Filho LF, Bozzetti MC, et al. Neutrophil apoptosis: a marker of disease severity in sepsis and sepsis-induced acute respiratory distress syndrome. Crit Care 2006; 10(6):R155.

82. Brinkmann V, Reichard U, et al. Neutrophil extracellular traps kill bacteria. Science 2004; 303(5663):1532–1535.

83. Fuchs TA, Abed U, Goosmann C, et al. Novel cell death program leads to neutrophil extracellular traps. J Cell Biol 2007; 176(2):231–241.

84. Clark SR, Ma AC, Tavener SA, et al. Platelet TLR4 activates neutrophil extracellular traps to ensnare bacteria in septic blood. Nat Med 2007; 13(4):463–469.

85. Ma AC, Kubes P. Platelets, neutrophils, and neutrophil extracellular traps (NETs) in sepsis. J Thromb Haemost 2008; 6(3):415–420.

86. Flierl MA, Rittirsch D, Nadeau BA, et al. Phagocyte-derived catecholamines enhance acute inflammatory injury. Nature 2007; 449(7163):721–725.

87. Wang L, Kamath A, Das H, et al. Antibacterial effect of human V gamma 2V delta 2 T cells in vivo. J Clin Invest 2001; 108(9):1349–1357.

88. Hotchkiss RS, Tinsley KW, Swanson PE, et al. Depletion of dendritic cells, but not macrophages, in patients with sepsis. J Immunol 2002; 168(5):2493–2500.

89. Oberholzer A, Oberholzer C, Bahjat KS, et al. Increased survival in sepsis by in vivo adenovirus-induced expression of IL-10 in dendritic cells. J Immunol 2002; 168(7):3412–3418.

90. Hotchkiss RS, Karl IE. The pathophysiology and treatment of sepsis. N Engl J Med 2003; 348(2):138–150.

91. Steinman RM, Banchereau J. Taking dendritic cells into medicine. Nature 2007; 449(7161): 419–426.

92. Opal SM, Huber CE. SEPSIS. Sci Am Med 2001; 30:1–17.

93. Niessen F, Schaffner F, Furlan-Freguia C, et al. Dendritic cell PAR1-S1P3 signalling couples coagulation and inflammation. Nature 2008; 452(7187):654–658.

94. Cines DB, Pollak ES, Buck CA, et al. Endothelial cells in physiology and in the pathophysiology of vascular disorders. Blood 1998; 91(10):3527–3561

95. Aird WC. The hematologic system as a marker of organ dysfunction in sepsis. Mayo Clin Proc 2003a; 78(7):869–881.

96. Aird WC. The role of the endothelium in severe sepsis and multiple organ dysfunction syndrome. Blood 2003b; 101(10):3765–3777.

97. Hack CE, Zeerleder S. The endothelium in sepsis: source of and a target for inflammation. Crit Care Med 2001; 29(Suppl. 7):S21–S27.

98. Martinez ML, Zimmerman GA. Endothelial biomedicine. In: Aird WC, ed. Endothelium Biomedicine. Cambridge: Cambridge University Press, 2007:1178–1192.

99. Reutershan J, Morris MA, Burcin TL, et al. Critical role of endothelial CXCR2 in LPS-induced neutrophil migration into the lung. J Clin Invest 2006; 116(3):695–702.

100. Mutunga M, Fulton B, et al. Circulating endothelial cells in patients with septic shock. Am J Respir Crit Care Med 2001; 163(1):195–200.

101. Neilsen PO, Zimmerman GA, et al. Escherichia coli Braun lipoprotein induces a lipopolysaccharide-like endotoxic response from primary human endothelial cells. J Immunol 2001; 167(9):5231–5239.

102. Henneke P, Golenbock DT. Innate immune recognition of lipopolysaccharide by endothelial cells. Crit Care Med 2002; 30(Suppl. 5):S207–S213.

103. Gill EA, Imaizumi T, et al. Bacterial lipopolysaccharide induces endothelial cells to synthesize a degranulating factor for neutrophils. FASEB J 1998; 12(9):673–684.

104. Zhao B, Bowden RA, et al. Human endothelial cell response to gram-negative lipopolysaccharide assessed with cDNA microarrays. Am J Physiol Cell Physiol 2001; 281(5):C1587–C1595.

105. Turner GD, Ly VC, et al. Systemic endothelial activation occurs in both mild and severe malaria. Correlating dermal microvascular endothelial cell phenotype and soluble cell adhesion molecules with disease severity. Am J Pathol 1998; 152(6):1477–1487.

106. Leone M, Boutiere B, Camoin-Jau L, et al. Systemic endothelial activation is greater in septic than in traumatic-hemorrhagic shock but does not correlate with endothelial activation in skin biopsies. Crit Care Med 2002; 30(4):808–814.

107. Müller AM, Cronen C, Müller KM, et al. Heterogeneous expression of cell adhesion molecules by endothelial cells in ARDS. J Pathol 2002; 198(2):270–275.

108. Ye X, Ding J, Zhou X, et al. Divergent roles of endothelial NF-kappaB in multiple organ injury and bacterial clearance in mouse models of sepsis. J Exp Med 2008; 205(6):1303–1315.

109. Yano K, Liaw PC, Mullington JM, et al. Vascular endothelial growth factor is an important determinant of sepsis morbidity and mortality. J Exp Med 2006; 203(6): 1447–1458.

110. Weyrich AS, Lindemann S, et al. The evolving role of platelets in inflammation. J Thromb Haemost 2003; 1(9):1897–1905.

111. Weyrich AS, Zimmerman GA. Platelets: signaling cells in the immune continuum. Trends Immunol 2004; 25(9):489–495.

112. Vincent JL, Yagushi A, et al. Platelet function in sepsis. Crit Care Med 2002; 30(Suppl. 5):S313–S317.

113. Warkentin TE, Aird WC, et al. Platelet-endothelial interactions: sepsis, HIT, and antiphospholipid syndrome. Hematology Am Soc Hematol Educ Program 2003; 2003(1):497–519.

114. Schwertz H, Weyrich AS, et al. Interacoes entre plaquetas, leucocitos e endothelia na resposta inflamatoria sistemica e na sepse (Cellular interactions of platelets, leukocytes and endothelium in systemic inflammatory responses and sepsis). In: Caire de Castro FNH, Marcus David C, eds. Sepse: Da Bancada a Beira Do Leto. Rio de Janerio: Revinter Press, 2007:107–120.

115. Bozza FA, Shah AM, Weyrich AS, et al. Amicus or adversary: platelets in lung biology, acute injury, and inflammation. Am J Respir Cell Mol Biol 2008; 40(2):123–134.

116. Dempfle CE. Coagulopathy of sepsis. Thromb Haemost 2004; 91(2):213–224.

117. Levi M. Platelets at a crossroad of pathogenic pathways in sepsis. J Thromb Haemost 2004; 2(12): 2094–2095.

118. Zeerleder S, Hack CE, et al. Disseminated intravascular coagulation in sepsis. Chest 2005; 128(4):2864–2875.

119. Croner RS, Hoerer E, et al. Hepatic platelet and leukocyte adherence during endotoxemia. Crit Care 2006; 10(1):R15.

120. Grewal PK, Uchiyama S, Ditto D, et al. The Ashwell receptor mitigates the lethal coagulopathy of sepsis. Nat Med 2008; 14(6):648–655.

121. Yaguchi A, Lobo FL, et al. Platelet function in sepsis. J Thromb Haemost 2004; 2(12):2096–2102.

122. Evans G, Lewis AF, et al. The role of platelet aggregation in the development of endotoxin shock. Br J Surg 1969; 56(8):624.

123. Cowan DH, Bowman LS, et al. Platelet aggregation as a sign of septicemia in thermal injury. A prospective study. JAMA 1976; 235(12):1230–1234.

124. Gawaz M, Dickfeld T, Bogner C, et al. Platelet function in septic multiple organ dysfunction syndrome. Intensive Care Med 1997; 23(4):379–385.

125. Zimmerman GA, Weyrich AS. Signal-dependent protein synthesis by activated platelets: new pathways to altered phenotype and function. Arterioscler Thromb Vasc Biol 2008; 28(3):s17–24.

126. Weyrich AS, Dixon DA, Pabla R, et al. Signal-dependent translation of a regulatory protein, Bcl-3, in activated human platelets. Proc Natl Acad Sci USA 1998; 95(10):5556–5561.

127. Weyrich AS, Schwertz H, Kraiss LW, et al. Protein synthesis by platelets: historical and new perspectives. J Thromb Haemost 2009; 7(2):241–246.

128. Denis MM, Tolley ND, et al. Escaping the nuclear confines: signal-dependent pre-mRNA splicing in anucleate platelets. Cell 2005; 122(3):379–391.

129. Schwertz H, Tolley ND, et al. Signal-dependent splicing of tissue factor pre-mRNA modulates the thrombogenicity of human platelets. J Exp Med 2006; 203(11):2433–2440.

130. Ohlsson K, Björk P, Bergenfeldt M, et al. Interleukin-1 receptor antagonist reduces mortality from endotoxin shock. Nature 1990; 348(6301):550–552.

131. Pawlinski R, Mackman N. Tissue factor, coagulation proteases, and protease-activated receptors in endotoxemia and sepsis. Crit Care Med 2004; 32(Suppl. 5):S293–S297.

132. Shashkin PN, Brown GT, et al. Lipopolysaccharide is a direct agonist for platelet RNA splicing. J Immunol 2008; 181(5):3495–3502.

133. Rondina M, Schwertz H, Harris E, et al. Manuscript submitted.

134. Zimmerman GA, McIntyre TM, et al. The platelet-activating factor signaling system and its regulators in syndromes of inflammation and thrombosis. Crit Care Med 2002; 30(Suppl. 5):S294–S301.

135. Ruf W. Protease-activated receptor signaling in the regulation of inflammation. Crit Care Med 2004; 32(Suppl. 5):S287–S292.

136. Andonegui G, Kerfoot S, McNagny K, et al. Platelets express functional Toll-like receptor-4 (TLR4). Blood 2005; 106(7):2417–2423.

137. Stohlawertz P, Folman CC, et al. Effects of endotoxemia on thrombopoiesis in men. Thromb Haemost 1999; 81:613–617.

138. Zhao L, Ohtaki Y, Yamaguchi K, et al. LPS-induced platelet response and rapid shock in mice: contribution of O-antigen region of LPS and involvement of the lectin pathway of the complement system. Blood 2002; 100(9):3233–3239.

139. Aslam R, Speck ER, Kim M, et al. Platelet Toll-like receptor expression modulates lipopolysaccharide-induced thrombocytopenia and tumor necrosis factor-α production in vivo. Blood 2006; 107(2):637–641.

140. Kiefmann R, Heckel K, et al. Role of p-selectin in platelet sequestration in pulmonary capillaries during endotoxemia. J Vasc Res 2006; 43(5):473–481.

141. Rumbaut RE, Bellera RV, Randhawa JK, et al. Endotoxin enhances microvascular thrombosis in mouse cremaster venules via a TLR4-dependent, neutrophil-independent mechanism. Am J Physiol Heart Circ Physiol 2006; 290(4):H1671–H1679.

142. Kälsch T, Elmas E, Nguyen XD, et al. Endotoxin-induced effects on platelets and monocytes in an in vivo model of inflammation. Basic Res Cardiol 2007; 102(5):460–466.

143. Harlan JM, Winn RK. Leukocyte-endothelial interactions: clinical trials of anti-adhesion therapy. Crit Care Med 2002; 30(Suppl. 5):S214–S219.

144. McIntyre TM, Prescott SM, et al. Cell-cell interactions: leukocyte-endothelial interactions. Curr Opin Hematol 2003; 10(2):150–158.

145. Bergmeier W, Wagner DD. Inflammation. In: Michaelson AD, ed. Platelets. Boston, MA: Academic Press, 2007:713–726.

146. Michaelson M. A model of extraordinary social engagement, or "moral giftedness. New Dir Child Adolesc Dev 2001; (93):19–32.

147. Ma N, Hunt NH, et al. Correlation between enhanced vascular permeability, up-regulation of cellular adhesion molecules and monocyte adhesion to the endothelium in the retina during the development of fatal murine cerebral malaria. Am J Pathol 1996; 149(5):1745–1762.

148. Freedman JE, Loscalzo J. Platelet-monocyte aggregates: bridging thrombosis and inflammation. Circulation 2002; 105(18):2130–2132.

149. Brambilla M, Camera M, Colnago D, et al. Tissue factor in patients with acute coronary syndromes: expression in platelets, leukocytes, and platelet-leukocyte aggregates. Aterioscler Thromb Vasc Biol 2008; 28(5):947–953.

150. Li N, Soop A, et al. Multi-cellular activation in vivo by endotoxin in humans—limited protection by adenosine infusion. Thromb Haemost 2000; 84(3):381–387.

151. Kirschenbaum LA, Aziz M, et al. Influence of rheologic changes and platelet-neutrophil interactions on cell filtration in sepsis. Am J Respir Crit Care Med 2000; 161(5):1602–1607.

152. Ogura H, Kawasaki T, et al. Activated platelets enhance microparticle formation and platelet-leukocyte interaction in severe trauma and sepsis. J Trauma 2001; 50(5):801–809.

153. Russwurm S, Vickers J, et al. Platelet and leukocyte activation correlate with the severity of septic organ dysfunction. Shock 2002; 17(4):263–268.

154. Peters MJ, Heyderman RS, Faust S, et al. Severe meningococcal disease is characterized by early neutrophil but not platelet activation and increased formation and consumption of platelet-neutrophil complexes. J Leukoc Biol 2003; 73(6):722–730.

155. Soriano AO, Jy W, et al. Levels of endothelial and platelet microparticles and their interactions with leukocytes negatively correlate with organ dysfunction and predict mortality in severe sepsis. Crit Care Med 2005; 33(11):2540–2546.

156. Mirlashari MR, Hagberg IA, et al. Platelet-platelet and platelet-leukocyte interactions induced by outer membrane vesicles from N. meningitidis. Platelets 2002; 13(2):91–99.

157. Bryant AE, Chen RY, et al. Clostridial gas gangrene. I. Cellular and molecular mechanisms of microvascular dysfunction induced by exotoxins of Clostridium perfringens. J Infect Dis 2000; 182(3):799–807.

158. Bryant AE, Bayer CR, Chen RY, et al. Vascular dysfunction and ischemic destruction of tissue in Streptococcus pyogenes infection: the role of streptolysin O-induced platelet/neutrophil complexes. J Infect Dis 2005; 192(6):1014–1022.

159. Bryant AE, Bayer CR, Aldape MJ, et al. Clostridium perfringens phospholipase C-induced platelet/leukocyte interactions impede neutrophil diapedesis. J Med Microbiol 2006; 55(Pt 5): 495–504.

160. Gawaz M, Fateh-Moghadam S, Pilz G, et al. Platelet activation and interaction with leucocytes in patients with sepsis or multiple organ failure. Eur J Clin Invest 1995; 25(11):843–851.

161. Heffner JE. Platelet-neutrophil interactions in sepsis—platelet guilt by association? Intensive Care Med 1997; 23(4):366–368.

162. Weyrich AS, McIntyre TM, McEver RP, et al. Monocyte tethering by P-selectin regulates monocyte chemotactic protein-1 and tumor necrosis factor-alpha secretion. Signal integration and NF-kappa B translocation. J Clin Invest 1995; 95(5):2297–2303.

163. Weyrich AS, Elstad MR, McEver RP, et al. Activated platelets signal chemokine synthesis by human monocytes. J Clin Invest 1996; 97(6):1525–1534.

164. Dixon DA, Tolley ND, Bemis-Standoli K, et al. Expression of COX-2 in platelet-monocyte interactions occurs via combinatorial regulation involving adhesion and cytokine signaling. J Clin Invest 2006; 116(10):2727–2738.

165. Zarbock A, Singbartl K, Ley K. Complete reversal of acid-induced acute lung injury by blocking of platelet-neutrophil aggregation. J Clin Invest 2006; 116(12):3211–3219.

166. Akira S, Uematsu S, Takeuchi O. Pathogen recognition and innate immunity. Cell 2006; 124(4):783–801.

167. Medzhitov R. Recognition of microorganisms and activation of the immune response. Nature 2007; 449(7164):819–826.

168. Medzhitov R, Janeway CA Jr. Decoding the patterns of self and nonself by the innate immune system. Science 2002; 296(5566):298–300.

169. Brunn GJ, Platt JL. The etiology of sepsis: turned inside out. Trends Mol Med 2006; 12(1):10–16.

170. Bianchi ME. DAMPs, PAMPs and alarmins: all we need to know about danger. J Leukoc Biol 2007; 81(1):1–5.

171. Miyake K. Innate immune sensing of pathogens and danger signals by cell surface Toll-like receptors. Semin Immunol 2007; 19(1):3–10.

172. Barton GM. A calculated response: control of inflammation by the innate immune system. J Clin Invest 2008; 118(2):413–420.

173. Fitzgerald KA, Golenbock DT. Immunology. The shape of things to come. Science 2007; 316(5831):1574–1576.
174. Medzhitov R, Preston-Hurlburt P, Janeway CA Jr. A human homologue of the Drosophila Toll protein signals activation of adaptive immunity. Nature 1997; 388(6640):394–397.
175. Rock FL, Hardiman G, et al. A family of human receptors structurally related to Drosophila Toll. Proc Natl Acad Sci U S A 1998; 95(2): 588–593.
176. Cook DN, Pisetsky DS, et al. Toll-like receptors in the pathogenesis of human disease. Nat Immunol 2004; 5(10):975–979.
177. Decker T. Sepsis: avoiding its deadly toll. J Clin Invest 2004; 113(10):1387–1389.
178. Beutler B, Jiang Z, et al. Genetic analysis of host resistance: toll-like receptor signaling and immunity at large. Annu Rev Immunol 2006; 24:353–389.
179. Zarember KA, Godowski PJ. Tissue expression of human Toll-like receptors and differential regulation of Toll-like receptor mRNAs in leukocytes in response to microbes, their products, and cytokines. J Immunol 2002; 168(2):554–561.
180. Elson G, Dunn-Siegrist I, et al. Contribution of Toll-like receptors to the innate immune response to Gram-negative and Gram-positive bacteria. Blood 2007; 109(4):1574–1583.
181. Plitas G, Burt BM, et al. Toll-like receptor 9 inhibition reduces mortality in polymicrobial sepsis. J Exp Med 2008; 205(6):1277–1283.
182. Kanzler H, Barrat FJ, Hessel EM, et al. Therapeutic targeting of innate immunity with Toll-like receptor agonists and antagonists. Nat Med 2007; 13(5)552–559.
183. Arbour NC, Lorenz E, Schutte BC, et al. TLR4 mutations are associated with endotoxin hyporesponsiveness in humans. Nat Genet 2000; 25(2):187–191.
184. Trinchieri G, Sher A. Cooperation of Toll-like receptor signals in innate immune defence. Nat Rev Immunol 2007; 7(3):179–190.
185. Spiller S, Elson G, Ferstl R, et al. LTR4-induced IFN-gamma production increases TLR2 sensitivity and drives Gram-negative sepsis in mice. J Exp Med 2008; 205(8)1747–1754.
186. Ozinsky A, Underhill MD, Fontenot JD, et al. The repertoire for pattern recognition of pathogens by the innate immune system is defined by cooperation between toll-like receptors. Proc Natl Acad Sci USA 2000; 97(25):13766–13771.
187. Knapp S, von Aulock S, et al. Lipoteichoic acid-induced lung inflammation depends on TLR2 and the concerted action of TLR4 and the platelet-activating factor receptor. J Immunol 2008; 180(5):3478–3484.
188. Ulevitch RJ. New therapeutic targets revealed through investigations of innate immunity. Crit Care Med 2001; 29(Suppl. 7):S8–S12.
189. Kitchens RL, Thompson PA, et al. Plasma CD14 decreases monocyte responses to LPS by transferring cell-bound LPS to plasma lipoproteins. J Clin Invest 2001; 108(3):485–493.
190. Zhang G, Ghosh S. Toll-like receptor-mediated NF-kappaB activation: a phylogenetically conserved paradigm in innate immunity. J Clin Invest 2001; 107(1):13–19.
191. Martin TR. Recognition of bacterial endotoxin in the lungs. Am J Respir Cell Mol Biol 2000; 23(2):128–132.
192. Blackwell TS, Christman JW. Defining the lung's response to endotoxin. Am J Respir Crit Care Med 2001; 163(7):1516–1517.
193. O'Grady NP, Preas HL, et al. Local inflammatory responses following bronchial endotoxin instillation in humans. Am J Respir Crit Care Med 2001; 163(7):1591–1598.
194. Jeyaseelan S, Chu HW, Young SK, et al. Transcriptional profiling of lipopolysaccharide-induced acute lung injury. Infect Immun 2004; 72(12):7247–7256.
195. Abraham E. Effects of recombinant human activated protein C in human models of endotoxin administration. Proc Am Thorac Soc 2005; 2(3):243–247.
196. Menezes SL, Bozza PT, et al. Pulmonary and extrapulmonary acute lung injury: inflammatory and ultrastructural analyses. J Appl Physiol 2005; 98(5):1777–1783.

197. Knapp S, Florquin S, Golenbock DT, et al. Pulmonary lipopolysaccharide (LPS)-binding protein inhibits the LPS-induced lung inflammation in vivo. J Immunol 2006; 176(5):3189–3195.

198. Togbe D, Schnyder-Candrian S, Schnyder B, et al. Toll-like receptor and tumour necrosis factor dependent endotoxin-induced acute lung injury. Int J Exp Path 2007; 88(6):387–391.

199. Hoogerwerf JJ, de Vos AF, et al. Lung inflammation induced by lipoteichoic acid or lipopolysaccharide in humans. Am J Respir Crit Care Med 2008; 178(1):34–41.

200. Held HD, Boettcher S, et al. Ventilation-induced chemokine and cytokine release is associated with activation of nuclear factor-kappaB and is blocked by steroids. Am J Respir Crit Care Med 2001; 163(3, pt 1):711–716.

201. Andonegui G, Bonder CS, Green F, et al. Endothelium-derived Toll-like receptor-4 is the key molecule in LPS-induced neutrophil sequestration into lungs. J Clin Invest 2003; 111(7):1011–1020.

202. Togbe D, Schnyder-Candrian S, Schnyder B, et al. TLR4 gene dosage contributes to endotoxin-induced acute respiratory inflammation. J Leukoc Biol 2006; 80(3):451–457.

203. Tasaka S, Ishizaka A, et al. Effect of CD14 blockade on endotoxin-induced acute lung injury in mice. Am J Respir Cell Mol Biol 2003; 29(2):252–258.

204. Imai Y, Kuba K, Rao S, et al. Angiotensin-converting enzyme 2 protects from severe acute lung failure. Nature 2005; 436(7047):112–116.

205. Didierlaurent A, Goulding J, Patel S, et al. Sustained desensitization to bacterial Toll-like receptor ligands after resolution of respiratory influenza infection. J Exp Med 2008; 205(2):323–329.

206. Meylan E, Tschopp J, et al. Intracellular pattern recognition receptors in the host response. Nature 2006; 442(7098):39–44.

207. Imaizumi T, Aratani S, et al. Retinoic acid-inducible gene-I is induced in endothelial cells by LPS and regulates expression of COX-2. Biochem Biophys Res Commun 2002; 292(1):274–279.

208. Thimmulappa RK, Lee H, Rangasamy T, et al. Nrf2 is a critical regulator of the innate immune response and survival during experimental sepsis. J Clin Invest 2006; 116(4):984–985.

209. Khor CC, Chapman SJ, Vannberg FO, et al. A Mal functional variant is associated with protection against invasive pneumococcal disease, bacteremia, malaria and tuberculosis. Nat Genet 2007; 39(4):523–528.

210. von Bernuth H, Picard C, Jin Z, et al. Pyogenic bacterial infections in humans with MyD88 deficiency. Science 2008; 321(5889):691–696.

211. van 't Veer C, van den Pangaart PS, van Zoelen MA, et al. Induction of IRAK-M is associated with lipopolysaccharide tolerance in a human endotoxemia model. J Immunol 2007; 179(10):7110–7120.

212. Faure E, Thomas L, Xu H, et al. Bacterial lipopolysaccharide and IFN-gamma induce Toll-like receptor 2 and Toll-like receptor 4 expression in human endothelial cells: role of NF-kappa B activation. J Immunol 2001; 166(3):2018–2024.

213. Sato S, Sugiyama M, Yamamoto M, et al. Toll/IL-1 receptor domain-containing adaptor inducing IFN-beta (TRIF) associates with TNF receptor-associated factor 6 and TANK-binding kinase 1, and activates two distinct transcription factors, NF-kappa B and IFN-regulatory factor-3, in the Toll-like receptor signaling. J Immunol 2003; 171(8):4304–4310.

214. O'Neill LA. 'Fine tuning' TLR signaling. Nat Immunol 2008; 9(5):459–461.

215. Imai Y, Kuba K, Neely GG, et al. Identification of oxidative stress and Toll-like receptor 4 signaling as a key pathway of acute lung injury. Cell 2008; 133(2):235–249.

216. Suzuki T, Hashimoto S, et al. Comprehensive gene expression profile of LPS-stimulated human monocytes by SAGE. Blood 2000; 96(7):2584–2591.

217. Wang ZM, Liu C, et al. Chemokines are the main proinflammatory mediators in human monocytes activated by Staphylococcus aureus, peptidoglycan, and endotoxin. J Biol Chem 2000; 275(27):20260–20267.
218. Bozza FA, Salluh JI, et al. Cytokine profiles as markers of disease severity in sepsis: a multiplex analysis. Crit Care 2007; 11(2):R49.
219. Maelfait J, Vercammen E, et al. Stimulation of Toll-like receptor 3 and 4 induces interleukin-1beta maturation by caspase-8. J Exp Med 2008; 205(9):1967–1973.
220. Saleh M, Vaillancourt JP, Graham RK, et al. Differential modulation of endotoxin responsiveness by human caspase-12 polymorphisms. Nature 2004; 429(6987):75–79.
221. Saleh M, Mathison JC, Wolinski MK, et al. Enhanced bacterial clearance and sepsis resistance in caspase-12-deficient mice. Nature 2006; 440(7087):1064–1068.
222. Sarkar A, Hall MW, et al. Caspase-1 regulates Escherichia coli sepsis and splenic B cell apoptosis independently of interleukin-1beta and interleukin-18. Am J Respir Crit Care Med 2006; 174(9):1003–1010.
223. Mastronardi C, Whelan F, Yildiz OA, et al. Caspase 1 deficiency reduces inflammation-induced brain transcription. Proc Natl Acad Sci USA 2007; 104(17):7205–7210.
224. Ware LB, Camerer E, et al. Bench to bedside: targeting coagulation and fibrinolysis in acute lung injury. Am J Physiol Lung Cell Mol Physiol 2006; 291(3):L307–L311.
225. Gomes RN, Figueiredo RT, Bozza FA, et al. Increased susceptibility to septic and endotoxic shock in monocyte chemoattractant protein 1/cc chemokine ligand 2-deficient mice correlates with reduced interleukin 10 and enhanced macrophage migration inhibitory factor production. Shock 2006; 26(25):457–463.
226. Feldmann M, Maini RN. Lasker Clinical Medical Research Award. TNF defined as a therapeutic target for rheumatoid arthritis and other autoimmune diseases. Nat Med 2003; 9(10):1245–1250.
227. Messmer D, Yang H, Telusma G, et al. High mobility group box protein 1: an endogenous signal for dendritic cell maturation and Th1 polarization. J Immunol 2004; 173(1):307–313.
228. Park JS, Svetkauskaite D, He Q, et al. Involvement of toll-like receptors 2 and 4 in cellular activation by high mobility group box 1 protein. J Biol Chem 2004; 279(9):7370–7377.
229. Uchida T, Shirasawa M, Ware LB, et al. Receptor for advanced glycation end-products is a marker of type I cell injury in acute lung injury. Am J Respir Crit Care Med 2006; 173(9):1008–1015.
230. Tsung A, Klune JR, Zhang X, et al. HMGB1 release induced by liver ischemia involves Toll-like receptor 4 dependent reactive oxygen species production and calcium-mediated signaling. J Exp Med 2007; 204(12):2913–2923.
231. Qin S, Wang H, Yuan R, et al. Role of HMGB1 in apoptosis-mediated sepsis lethality. J Exp Med 2006; 203(7):1637–1642.
232. Sundén-Cullberg J, Norrby-Teglund A, Rouhiainen A, et al. Persistent elevation of high mobility group box-1 protein (HMGB1) in patients with severe sepsis and septic shock. Crit Care Med 2005; 33(3):682–683.
233. Ueno H, Matsuda T, Hashimoto S, et al. Contributions of high mobility group box protein in experimental and clinical acute lung injury. Am J Respir Crit Care Med 2004; 170(12):1310–1316.
234. Yang H, Ochani M, Li J, et al. Reversing established sepsis with antagonists of endogenous high-mobility group box 1. Proc Natl Acad Sci USA 2004; 101(1):296–301.
235. Abeyama K, Stern DM, Ito Y, et al. The N-terminal domain of thrombomodulin sequesters high-mobility group-B1 protein, a novel antiinflammatory mechanism. J Clin Invest 2005; 115(5):1267–1274.
236. Esmon C. Do-all receptor takes on coagulation, inflammation. Nat Med 2005; 11(5):475–477.
237. Schofield L. Intravascular infiltrates and organ-specific inflammation in malaria pathogenesis. Immunol Cell Biol 2007; 85(2):130–137.

238. Bozza M, Satoskar AR, et al. Targeted disruption of migration inhibitory factor gene reveals its critical role in sepsis. J Exp Med 1999; 189(2):341–346.
239. Froidevaux C, Roger T, et al. Macrophage migration inhibitory factor and innate immune responses to bacterial infections. Crit Care Med 2001; 29(Suppl. 7):S13–S15.
240. Bozza FA, Gomes RN, et al. Macrophage migration inhibitory factor levels correlate with fatal outcome in sepsis. Shock 2004; 22(4):309–313.
241. Donnelly SC, Haslett C, et al. Regulatory role for macrophage migration inhibitory factor in acute respiratory distress syndrome. Nat Med 1997; 3(3):320–323.
242. Yan JJ, Jung JS, Lee JE, et al. Therapeutic effects of lysophosphatidylcholine in experimental sepsis. Nat Med 2004; 10(2):161–167.
243. Giebelen IA, Leendertse M, Dessing MC, et al. Endogenous beta-adrenergic receptors inhibit lipopolysaccharide-induced pulmonary cytokine release and coagulation. Am J Respir Cell Mol Biol 2008; 39(3):373–379.
244. Coughlin SR. Thrombin signalling and protease-activated receptors. Nature 2000; 407(6801):258–264.
245. Coughlin SR. Protease-activated receptors in hemostasis, thrombosis and vascular biology. J Thromb Haemost 2005; 3(8):1800–1814.
246. Prescott SM, McIntyre TM, et al. Sol Sherry lecture in thrombosis: molecular events in acute inflammation. Arterioscler Thromb Vasc Biol 2002; 22(5):727–733.
247. McIntyre TM, Zimmerman GA, et al. Biologically active oxidized phospholipids. J Biol Chem 1999; 274(36):25189–25192.
248. Prescott SM, Zimmerman GA, et al. Platelet-activating factor and related lipid mediators. Annu Rev Biochem 2000; 69:419–445.
249. Watanabe J, Marathe GK, Neilsen PO, et al. Endotoxins stimulate neutrophil adhesion followed by synthesis and release of platelet-activating factor in microparticles. J Biol Chem 2003; 278(35):33161–33168.
250. Walton KA, Cole AL, Yeh M, et al. Specific phospholipid oxidation products inhibit ligand activation of toll-like receptors 4 and 2. Arterioscler Thromb Vasc Biol 2003; 23(7):1197–1203.
251. Blüml S, Kirchberger S, Bochkov VN, et al. Oxidized phospholipids negatively regulate dendritic cell maturation induced by TLRs and CD40. J Immunol 2005; 175(1):501–508.
252. Nonas S, Miller I, Kawkitinarong K, et al. Oxidized phospholipids reduce vascular leak and inflammation in rat model of acute lung injury. Am J Respir Crit Care Med 2006; 173(10):1130–1138.
253. Lemjabbar H, Basbaum C. Platelet-activating factor receptor and ADAM10 mediate responses to Staphylococcus aureus in epithelial cells. Nat Med 2002; 8(1):41–46.
254. Han SH, Kim JH, Seo HS, et al. Lipoteichoic acid-induced nitric oxide production depends on the activation of platelet-activating factor receptor and Jak2. J Immunol 2006; 176(1):573–579.
255. Mathiak G, Szewczyk D, et al. Platelet-activating factor (PAF) in experimental and clinical sepsis. Shock 1997; 7(6):391–404.
256. Kuijpers TW, van der Poll T. The role of platelet-activating factor in endotoxin-related disease. In: Brade H, Opal SM, Vogel SN, et al., eds. *Endotoxin* in Health and *Disease*. New York: Marcel Dekker, 1999:449–462.
257. Yost CC, Denis MM, et al. Activated polymorphonuclear leukocytes rapidly synthesize retinoic acid receptor-alpha: a mechanism for translational control of transcriptional events. J Exp Med 2004; 200(5):671–680.
258. Yost CC, Cody MJ, Harris ES, et al. Impaired neutrophil extracellular trap (NET) formation: a novel innate immune deficiency of human neonates. Blood 2009; 113(25):6419–6427.
259. Ishii S, Nagase T, Tashiro F, et al. Bronchial hyperreactivity, increased endotoxin lethality and melanocytic tumorigenesis in transgenic mice overexpressing platelet-activating factor receptor. EMBO J 1997; 16(1):133–142.

260. Wang H, Tan X, Chang H, et al. Regulation of platelet-activating factor receptor gene expression in vivo by endotoxin, platelet-activating factor and endogenous tumour necrosis factor. Biochem J 1997; 322(Pt 2):603–608.

261. Rabinovici R, Esser KM, Lysko PG, et al. Priming by platelet-activating factor of endotoxin-induced lung injury and cardiovascular shock. Circ Res 1991; 69(1):12–25.

262. Chang SW. Endotoxin-induced lung vascular injury: role of platelet activating factor, tumor necrosis factor and neutrophils. Clin Res 1992; 40(3):528–536.

263. Chang SW, Feddersen CO, et al. Platelet-activating factor mediates hemodynamic changes and lung injury in endotoxin-treated rats. J Clin Invest 1987; 79(5):1498–1509.

264. Miotla JM, Jeffery PK, Hellewell PG. Platelet-activating factor plays a pivotal role in the induction of experimental lung injury. Am J Respir Cell Mol Biol 1998; 18(2):197–204.

265. Silliman CC, Voelkel NF, Allard JD, et al. Plasma and lipids from stored packed red blood cells cause acute lung injury in an animal model. J Clin Invest 1998; 101(7):1458–1467.

266. Kim JD, Baker CJ, Roberts RF, et al. Platelet activating factor acetylhydrolase decreases lung reperfusion injury. Ann Thorac Surg 2000; 70(2):423–428.

267. Göggel R, Winoto-Morbach S, Vielhaber G, et al. PAF-mediated pulmonary edema: a new role for acid sphingomyelinase and ceramide. Nat Med 2004; 10(2):155–160.

268. Zimmerman GA, McIntyre TM. PAF, ceramide and pulmonary edema: alveolar flooding and a flood of questions. Trends Mol Med 2004; 10(6):245–248.

269. Dhainaut JF, Tenaillon A, Le Tulzo Y, et al. Platelet-activating factor receptor antagonist BN 52021 in the treatment of severe sepsis: a randomized, double-blind, placebo-controlled, multicenter clinical trial. BN 52021 Sepsis Study Group. Crit Care Med 1994; 22(11):1720–1728.

270. Dhainaut JF, Tenaillon A, Hemmer M, et al. Confirmatory platelet-activating factor receptor antagonist trial in patients with severe gram-negative bacterial sepsis: a phase III, randomized, double-blind, placebo-controlled, multicenter trial. BN 52021 Sepsis Investigator Group. Crit Care Med 1998; 26(12):1963–1971.

271. Poeze M, Froon AH, Ramsay G, et al. Decreased organ failure in patients with severe SIRS and septic shock treated with the platelet-activating factor antagonist TCV-309: a prospective, multicenter, double-blind, randomized phase II trial. TCV-309 Septic Shock Study Group. Shock 2000; 14(4):421–428.

272. Vincent JL, Spapen H, Bakker J, et al. Phase II multicenter clinical study of the platelet-activating factor receptor antagonist BB-882 in the treatment of sepsis. Crit Care Med 2000; 28(3):638–642.

273. Gomes RN, Bozza FA, et al. Exogenous platelet-activating factor acetylhydrolase reduces mortality in mice with systemic inflammatory response syndrome and sepsis. Shock 2006; 26(1):41–49.

274. Schuster DP, Metzler M, Opal S, et al. Recombinant platelet-activating factor acetylhydrolase to prevent acute respiratory distress syndrome and mortality in severe sepsis: Phase IIb, multicenter, randomized, placebo-controlled, clinical trial. Crit Care Med 2003; 31(6):1612–1619.

275. Opal S, Laterre PF, Abraham E, et al. Recombinant human platelet-activating factor acetyl-hydrolase for treatment of severe sepsis: results of a phase III, multicenter, randomized, double-blind, placebo-controlled, clinical trial. Crit Care Med 2004; 32(2):332–341.

276. Minneci PC, Deans KJ, et al. Should we continue to target the platelet-activating factor pathway in septic patients? Crit Care Med 2004; 32(2):585–588.

277. Zimmerman GA. Plasma platelet-activating factor acetylhydrolase is a dynamic variable in critical illness: In the end, is change good for you? Crit Care Med 2005; 33(6):1462–1463.

278. Claus RA, Russwurm S, et al. Plasma platelet-activating factor acetylhydrolase activity in critically ill patients. Crit Care Med 2005; 33(6):1416–1419.

279. Grissom CK, Orme JF Jr, et al. Platelet-activating factor acetylhydrolase is increased in lung lavage fluid from patients with acute respiratory distress syndrome. Crit Care Med 2003; 31(3):770–775.

280. Salluh JI, Pino AV, Silva AR, et al. Lung production of platelet-activating factor acetylhydrolase in oleic acid-induced acute lung injury. Prostaglandins Leukot Essent Fatty Acids 2007; 77(1):1–8.

281. Eichacker PQ, Parent C, et al. Risk and the efficacy of antiinflammatory agents: retrospective and confirmatory studies of sepsis. Am J Respir Crit Care Med 2002; 166(9):1197–1205.

282. Hoffmann JA, Kafatos FC, et al. Phylogenetic perspectives in innate immunity. Science 1999; 284(5418):1313–1318.

283. Munford RS, Pugin J. The crucial role of systemic responses in the innate (non-adaptive) host defense. J Endotoxin Res 2001; 7(4):327–332.

284. Scherfer C, Karlsson C, et al. Isolation and characterization of hemolymph clotting factors in Drosophila melanogaster by a pullout method. Curr Biol 2004; 14(7):625–629.

285. Kambris Z, Brun S, et al. Drosophila immunity: a large-scale in vivo RNAi screen identifies five serine proteases required for Toll activation. Curr Biol 2006; 16(8):808–813.

286. Amaral A, Opal SM, Vincent JL. Coagulation in sepsis. Intensive Care Med 2004; 30(6): 1032–1040.

287. Diehl JL, Borgel D. Sepsis and coagulation. Curr Opin Crit Care 2005; 11(5):454–460.

288. Mackman N, Tilley RE, et al. Role of the extrinsic pathway of blood coagulation in hemostasis and thrombosis. Arterioscler Thromb Vasc Biol 2007; 27(8):1687–1693.

289. Panes O, Matus V, et al. Human platelets synthesize and express functional tissue factor. Blood 2007; 109(12):5242–5250.

290. Lorant D, McIntyre T, et al. Platelet-activating factor: a signaling molecule for leukocyte adhesion. In: Pearson JD, ed. Vascular Adhesion Molecules and Inflammation. Basel: Birkhauser, 1999:81–107.

291. Lindemann S, Tolley ND, Dixon DA, et al. Activated platelets mediate inflammatory signaling by regulated interleukin 1beta synthesis. J Cell Biol 2001; 154(3):485–490.

292. Bernard GR, Vincent JL, et al. Efficacy and safety of recombinant human activated protein C for severe sepsis. N Engl J Med 2001; 344(10):699–709.

293. Li W, Zheng X, Gu J, et al. Overexpressing endothelial cell protein C receptor alters the hemostatic balance and protects mice from endotoxin. J Thromb Haemost 2005; 3(7):1351–1359.

294. Esmon CT. Protein C anticoagulant pathway and its role in controlling microvascular thrombosis and inflammation. Crit Care Med 2001; 29(7 Suppl):S48-S51; discussion 51–52.

295. Stephenson, DA, Toltl LJ, et al. Modulation of monocyte function by activated protein C, a natural anticoagulant. J Immunol 2006; 177(4):2115–2122.

296. Hoffmann JN, Vollmar B, Laschke MW, et al. Microhemodynamic and cellular mechanisms of activated protein C action during endotoxemia. Crit Care Med 2004; 32(4):1011–1017.

297. Nick JA, Coldren CD, Geraci MW, et al. Recombinant human activated protein C reduces human endotoxin-induced pulmonary inflammation via inhibition of neutrophil chemotaxis. Blood 2004; 104(13):3878–3885.

298. Lay AJ, Donahue D, et al. Acute inflammation is exacerbated in mice genetically predisposed to a severe protein C deficiency. Blood 2007; 109(5):1984–1991.

299. Kerschen EJ, Fernandez JA, Cooley BC, et al. Endotoxemia and sepsis mortality reduction by non-anticoagulant activated protein C. J Exp Med 2007; 204(10):2439–2448.

300. Neyrinck AP, Liu KD, Howard JP, et al. Protective mechanisms of activated protein C in severe inflammatory disorders. British Journal of Pharmacology 2009, in press.

301. Looney MR, Matthay MA. Bench-to-bedside review: the role of activated protein C in maintaining endothelial tight junction function and its relationship to organ injury. Crit Care 2006; 10(6):239.

302. Ruf W. Protease-activated receptor signaling in the regulation of inflammation. Crit Care Med 2004; 32(5 Suppl):S287–S292.

303. Feistritzer C, Riewald M. Endothelial barrier protection by activated protein C through PAR1-dependent sphingosine 1-phosphate receptor-1 crossactivation. Blood 2005; 105(8):3178–3184.

304. Finigan JH, Dudek SM, Singleton PA, et al. Activated protein C mediates novel lung endothelial barrier enhancement: role of sphingosine 1-phosphate receptor transactivation. J Biol Chem 2005; 280(17):17286–17293.

305. Ware LB, Matthay MA. Measuring microvascular blood flow in sepsis—a continuing challenge. Lancet 2002; 360(9341):1187–1188.

306. Richardson MA, Gupta A, et al. Treatment of sepsis-induced acquired protein C deficiency reverses Angiotensin-converting enzyme-2 inhibition and decreases pulmonary inflammatory response. J Pharmacol Exp Ther 2008; 325(1):17–26.

307. Faust SN, Levin M, Harrison OB, et al. Dysfunction of endothelial protein C activation in severe meningococcal sepsis. N Engl J Med 2001; 345(6):408–416.

308. Abraham E. Coagulation abnormalities in acute lung injury and sepsis. Am J Respir Cell Mol Biol 2000; 22(4):401–404.

309. Idell S. Anticoagulants for acute respiratory distress syndrome: can they work? Am J Respir Crit Care Med 2001; 164(4):517–520.

310. Abraham E. Coagulation abnormalities in acute lung injury and sepsis. Am J Respir Cell Mol Biol 2000; 22(4):401–404.

311. Welty-Wolf KE, Carraway MS, et al. Antibody to intercellular adhesion molecule 1 (CD54) decreases survival and not lung injury in baboons with sepsis. Am J Respir Crit Care Med 2001; 163(3, pt 1):665–673.

312. Welty-Wolf KE, Carraway MS, Ortel TL, et al. Blockade of tissue factor-factor X binding attenuates sepsis-induced respiratory and renal failure. Am J Physiol Lung Cell Mol Physiol 2006; 290(1):L21–L31.

313. Fan J, Kapus A, et al. Priming for enhanced alveolar fibrin deposition after hemorrhagic shock: role of tumor necrosis factor. Am J Respir Cell Mol Biol 2000; 22(4):412–421.

314. Fan J, Li Y, et al. Hemorrhagic shock-activated neutrophils augment TLR4 signaling-induced TLR2 upregulation in alveolar macrophages: role in hemorrhage-primed lung inflammation. Am J Physiol Lung Cell Mol Physiol 2006; 290(4):L738–L746.

315. Matthay MA, Zimmerman GA, et al. Future research directions in acute lung injury: summary of a National Heart, Lung, and Blood Institute working group. Am J Respir Crit Care Med 2003; 167(7):1027–1035.

316. Bachofen M, Weibel ER. Alterations of the gas exchange apparatus in adult respiratory insufficiency associated with septicemia. Am Rev Respir Dis 1977; 116(4):589–615.

317. Bachofen M, Weibel ER. Structural alterations of lung parenchyma in the adult respiratory distress syndrome. Clin Chest Med 1982; 3(1):35–56.

318. McFeely JE, Hudson LD. Sepsis, multi-organ dysfunction syndrome, and adult respiratory distress syndrome in humans. In: Brigham KL, ed. Endotoxin and the Lungs. New York: Marcel Dekker, Inc., 1994:321–350.

319. Brun-Buisson C, Doyon F, et al. Incidence, risk factors, and outcome of severe sepsis and septic shock in adults. A multicenter prospective study in intensive care units. French ICU Group for Severe Sepsis. JAMA 1995; 274(12):968–974.

320. Fein AM, Lippmann M, et al. The risk factors, incidence, and prognosis of ARDS following septicemia. Chest 1983; 83(1):40–42.

321. Nuckton TJ, Alonso JA, et al. Pulmonary dead-space fraction as a risk factor for death in the acute respiratory distress syndrome. N Engl J Med 2002; 346(17):1281–1286.

322. Powe JE, Short A, et al. Pulmonary accumulation of polymorphonuclear leukocytes in the adult respiratory distress syndrome. Crit Care Med 1982; 10(11):712–718.

323. Elliott CG, Zimmerman GA, et al. Granulocyte aggregation in adult respiratory distress syndrome (ARDS)—serial histologic and physiologic observations. Am J Med Sci 1985; 289(2):70–74.
324. Warshawski FJ, Sibbald WJ, et al. Abnormal neutrophil-pulmonary interaction in the adult respiratory distress syndrome. Qualitative and quantitative assessment of pulmonary neutrophil kinetics in humans with in vivo 111indium neutrophil scintigraphy. Am Rev Respir Dis 1986; 133(5):797–804.
325. Zimmerman GA, Renzetti AD, et al. Granulocyte adherence in pulmonary and systemic arterial blood samples from patients with adult respiratory distress syndrome. Am Rev Respir Dis 1984; 129(5):798–804.
326. Schuster DP. The opportunities and challenges of developing imaging biomarkers to study lung function and disease. Am J Respir Crit Care Med 2007; 176(3):224–230.
327. Rodrigues RS, Miller PR, Bozza FA, et al. FDG-PET in patients at risk for acute respiratory distress syndrome: a preliminary report. Intensive Care Med 2008; 34(12):2273–2278.
328. Albertine K. Histopathology of pulmonary edema and the acute respiratory distress syndrome. In: Matthay M, Ingbar DH, eds. Pulmonary Edema. New York: Marcel Dekker, Inc., 1998: 37–83.
329. Imaizumi T, Albertine KH, et al. Human endothelial cells synthesize ENA-78: relationship to IL-8 and to signaling of PMN adhesion. Am J Respir Cell Mol Biol 1997; 17(2):181–192.
330. Dalldorf FG, Carney CN, et al. Pulmonary capillary thrombosis in septicemia due to gram-positive bacteria. JAMA 1968; 206(3):583–586.
331. Tomashefski JF Jr. Pulmonary pathology of acute respiratory distress syndrome. Clin Chest Med 2000; 21(3):435–466.
332. Parsons PE, Gillespie MM, et al. Neutrophil response to endotoxin in the adult respiratory distress syndrome: role of CD14. Am J Respir Cell Mol Biol 1995; 13(2):152–160.
333. Doerschuk CM Mechanisms of leukocyte sequestration in inflamed lungs. Microcirculation 2001; 8(2):71–88.
334. Steinberg KP, Milberg JA, et al. Evolution of bronchoalveolar cell populations in the adult respiratory distress syndrome. Am J Respir Crit Care Med 1994; 150(1):113–122.
335. Rosseau S, Hammerl P, et al. Phenotypic characterization of alveolar monocyte recruitment in acute respiratory distress syndrome. Am J Physiol Lung Cell Mol Physiol 2000; 279(1):L25–L35.
336. Mendez JL, Hubmayr RD. New insights into the pathology of acute respiratory failure. Curr Opin Crit Care 2005; 11(1):29–36.
337. Coalson JJ, Hinshaw LB, et al. The pulmonary ultrastructure in septic shock. Exp Mol Pathol 1970; 12(1):84–103.
338. Dormehl IC, Maree M, et al. Investigation by scintigraphic methods of neutrophil kinetics under normal and septic shock conditions in the experimental baboon model. Eur J Nucl Med 1990; 16(8–10):643–647.
339. Albertine KH, Soulier MF, Wang Z, et al. Fas and fas ligand are up-regulated in pulmonary edema fluid and lung tissue of patients with acute lung injury and the acute respiratory distress syndrome. Am J Pathol 2002; 161(5):1783–1796.
340. Gupta N, Su X, et al. Intrapulmonary delivery of bone marrow-derived mesenchymal stem cells improves survival and attenuates endotoxin-induced acute lung injury in mice. J Immunol 2007; 179(3):1855–1863.
341. Zapol WM, Jones R. Vascular components of ARDS. Clinical pulmonary hemodynamics and morphology. Am Rev Respir Dis 1987; 136(2):471–474.
342. Bertozzi P, Astedt B, et al. Depressed bronchoalveolar urokinase activity in patients with adult respiratory distress syndrome. N Engl J Med 1990; 322(13):890–897.
343. Wang L, Bastarache JA, et al. Novel role of the human alveolar epithelium in regulating intra-alveolar coagulation. Am J Respir Cell Mol Biol 2007; 36(4):497–503.

344. Ware LB, Fang X, et al. Protein C and thrombomodulin in human acute lung injury. Am J Physiol Lung Cell Mol Physiol 2003; 285(3):L514–L521.

345. Abraham E, Laterre PF, Garg R, et al. Drotrecogin alfa (activated) for adults with severe sepsis and a low risk of death. N Engl J Med 2005; 353(13):1332–1341.

346. Parsons PE. Mediators and mechanisms of acute lung injury. Clin Chest Med 2000; 21(3):467–476.

347. Ware LB, Conner ER, et al. von Willebrand factor antigen is an independent marker of poor outcome in patients with early acute lung injury. Crit Care Med 2001; 29(12):2325–2331.

348. Harbarth S, Holeckova K, et al. Diagnostic value of procalcitonin, interleukin-6, and interleukin-8 in critically ill patients admitted with suspected sepsis. Am J Respir Crit Care Med 2001; 164(3):396–402.

349. Claeys R, Vinken S, et al. Plasma procalcitonin and C-reactive protein in acute septic shock: clinical and biological correlates. Crit Care Med 2002; 30(4):757–762.

350. Pettila V. How successful is the intensive care of patients with multiple organ dysfunction?]. Duodecim 2002; 118(16):1663–1670.

351. Reinhart K, Bayer O, et al. Markers of endothelial damage in organ dysfunction and sepsis. Crit Care Med 2002; 30(Suppl. 5):S302–S312.

352. Bajwa EK, Boyce PD, et al. Biomarker evidence of myocardial cell injury is associated with mortality in acute respiratory distress syndrome. Crit Care Med 2007; 35(11):2484–2490.

353. Nobre V, Harbarth S, Graf JD, et al. Use of procalcitonin to shorten antibiotic treatment duration in septic patients: a randomized trial. Am J Respir Crit Care Med 2008; 177(5):498–505.

354. Mestas J, Hughes CC. Of mice and not men: differences between mouse and human immunology. J Immunol 2004; 172(5):2731–2738.

355. Acosta-Rodriguez EV, Napolitani G, Lanzavecchia A, et al. Interleukins 1beta and 6 but not transforming growth factor-beta are essential for the differentiation of interleukin 17-producing human T helper cells. Nat Immunol 2007; 8(9):942–949.

356. Mizgerd JP, Skerrett SJ. Animal models of human pneumonia. Am J Physiol Lung Cell Mol Physiol 2008; 294(3):L387–L398.

357. Lowry SF. Human endotoxemia: a model for mechanistic insight and therapeutic targeting. Shock 2005; 24(Suppl. 1):94–100.

21
Cell-Based Therapy for Acute Lung Injury and Acute Respiratory Distress Syndrome

NAVEEN GUPTA
Department of Medicine, Division of Pulmonary and Critical Care, University of Pittsburgh School of Medicine, Pittsburgh, Pennsylvania, U.S.A.

JAE-WOO LEE
Department of Anesthesiology, University of California, San Francisco, California, U.S.A.

MICHAEL A. MATTHAY
Pulmonary and Critical Care Medicine and Cardiovascular Research Institute, University of California, San Francisco, California, U.S.A.

I. Introduction

Stem cell research has received increasing attention over the past decade with much of the focus centered on the potential tissue regenerative properties these cells possess. While most of the scientific and public attention has focused on the promise of embryonic stem cells (ESCs), given their totipotent potential, there has been a growing movement to investigate the therapeutic potential of adult stem cells. Adult stem cells are tissue specific cells present in organs that have retained the ability to differentiate into a variety of cell lineages thereby making them multipotent. Although adult stem cells do not possess the full range of plasticity that ESCs do, they offer practical advantages such as ease of isolation and propagation, and they are not associated with the political controversy that surrounds ESCs research. One class of adult stem cells that has been of particular interest is mesenchymal stem cells (MSCs). MSCs, also called marrow stromal stem cells, were first discovered in 1968 by Friedenstein (1) who discovered bone marrow stromal cells that were plastic adherent, clonogenic, and fibroblastic in appearance. Since the initial discovery 40 years ago, MSCs have been identified as a unique class of adult stem cells that possess several immune properties that make them a viable candidate for cell-based therapy for a variety of disease processes. This chapter will focus on first describing the basic biology of MSCs, the rationale for using these cells in acute respiratory distress syndrome (ARDS), and then the existing experimental literature that has tested the use of MSCs in models of acute lung injury (ALI) and ARDS. We will conclude with a review of recent attempts to translate the experimental findings with MSCs to patients with ARDS, as well as with a discussion of needed future research directions.

II. Mesenchymal Stem Cell Biology

MSCs can be isolated from a variety of tissues in the postnatal organism, however, this chapter will focus primarily on bone marrow-derived MSCs. MSCs are found near the sinusoids of the bone marrow and function as support cells for hematopoietic stem cells.

Although MSCs comprise less than 0.1% of all bone marrow cells, they can be isolated from whole bone marrow samples and subsequently propagated in culture. One of the limiting factors in isolating a pure population of MSCs has been the lack of an identified cell surface marker specific for MSCs. As a result, studies using MSCs have varied significantly in the type of cell population identified as MSCs. To begin to standardize MSCs research, a recent consensus conference was convened in 2006 to define criteria for MSCs (2). The criteria consisted of three principal components: (a) MSCs must be plastic adherent under standard tissue culture conditions; (b) MSCs should express certain cell surface markers such as CD105, CD90, and CD73, but must not express other markers including CD45, CD34, CD14, or CD11b; and (c) MSCs must differentiate into mesenchymal lineages including osteoblasts, adipocytes, and chrondoblasts under in vitro conditions.

Despite the difficulty in defining a population of MSCs, interest in using these cells as a therapeutic agent for a variety of diseases has grown considerably over the past decade. This interest stems, in part, from three basic properties of MSCs: (1) their low immunogenicity, (2) their immunomodulatory effects, and (3) their ability to secrete epithelial and endothelial growth factors.

The low immunogenicity of MSCs refers to the prevailing thought that allogeneic MSCs are able to evade clearance by the host immune system through a variety of mechanisms including low expression of the MHC (major histocompatibility complex) I and II proteins as well as lack of the T cell costimulatory molecules, CD80 and CD86 (3,4). This property could make MSCs ideal for cell-based therapy since they could be administered to patients without HLA matching, a situation that is more likely to be clinically practical than having to use autologous cells or human leukocyte antigen (HLA) matched cells. However, recent literature has shown that MSCs can express higher levels of the MHC class proteins than originally thought. Specifically, at low levels of IFN-γ, MSCs upregulate expression of MHC II and can have certain immunostimulatory properties (5–7). In addition, recent studies have demonstrated that infusion of allogeneic MSCs can elicit a host response and lead to graft rejection (8). Therefore, it is becoming increasingly apparent that the original belief that MSCs have low immunogenicity is not entirely correct, and that these cells have complex interactions with the innate and adaptive immune systems.

The defining characteristic of MSCs identified over the past decade of research has been the immunomodulatory property that the cells possess. Multiple studies have demonstrated that MSCs possess potent immunosuppressive effects by inhibiting the activity of both innate and adaptive immune cells (9–12). This immunosuppression has been shown to involve both cell contact dependent and independent mechanisms through the release of soluble factors. The list of candidate mediators released or induced by MSCs is growing and includes proteins such as TGF-β, PGE$_2$, IDO, IL-10, and IL-1ra among others (Fig. 1). The relative importance of these various factors is unknown as is the precise molecular mechanism involved in the immunosuppressive effect of MSCs. Several studies have utilized MSCs as cell-based therapy in organ injury models characterized by inflammation and have achieved positive results that have been attributed to their immunosuppressive effects (13–18). These studies will be discussed in greater detail later in this chapter.

Despite the well-documented immunosuppressive effects of MSCs, there has been recent literature describing a dual role for MSCs as an immunostimulatory cell, too (7). As mentioned previously, some studies have reported that MSCs can upregulate expression of MHC II when exposed to low levels of inflammation and function as

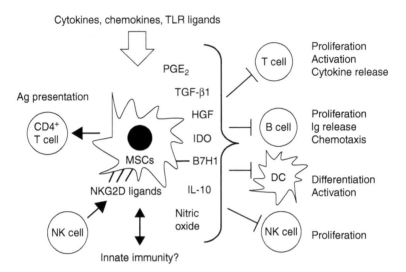

Figure 1 Mechanisms involved in MSCs immunomodulation. MSCs have been demonstrated to have immunosuppressive effects on both the innate and adaptive immune system. Both cell contact dependent and independent mechanisms have been shown to be involved. Several soluble factors have been identified as important mediators in the immunosuppressive effects of MSCs including prostaglandin E_2 (PGE_2), transforming growth factor-$\beta 1$ (TGF-$\beta 1$), hepatocyte growth factor (HGF), indoleamine 2,3-dioxygenase (IDO), interleukin-10 (IL-10), and nitric oxide. These effects are enhanced in the presence of certain stimulatory cytokines. MSCs have also been shown to possess immunostimulatory effects and can process proteins and present antigens on MHC class II molecules to $CD4^+$ T cells. *Source*: From Ref. 7.

antigen-presenting cells stimulating the adaptive immune system (5,6). Recent evidence has also shown that MSCs secrete IL-6 and induce production of IgG by B lymphocytes in an in vitro setting (19). In addition, MSCs have been shown to prevent neutrophil apoptosis and degranulation in culture without inhibiting their phagocytic or chemotactic capabilities (20). Therefore, emerging literature has demonstrated that MSCs have more complex effects on the immune system than their classical role as immune suppressor cells. Understanding the mechanisms responsible for these apparently paradoxical roles that MSCs play in the immune response will be important in developing cell-based therapy for clinical use.

Another property of MSCs that has generated enthusiasm for their potential therapeutic use is their ability to secrete multiple epithelial and endothelial growth factors (21,22). MSCs have proven to be a rich source of hepatocyte growth factor (HGF) and keratinocyte growth factor (KGF) that have known trophic effects on epithelial cells (23,24). KGF, in particular, has been previously studied as a therapeutic agent in lung injury models with beneficial effects seen when given prior to or concurrent with the injurious stimuli (25,26). Also, MSCs secrete vascular endothelial growth factor and angiopoietin 1 (Ang 1) that have protective effects on endothelial cells (27–29). This production of both epithelial and endothelial growth factors makes MSCs ideal for diseases such as ARDS that are characterized by injury to both the epithelial and endothelial surfaces.

III. Initial Studies of MSCs in Experimental Models of Organ Injury

The last decade has witnessed a substantial increase in the number of studies utilizing MSCs as a therapeutic agent for organ injury models. Prior to studies of cell-based therapy for lung disease, several reports had already investigated the potential therapeutic role of MSCs in cardiac and renal injury. Starting with the study by Tomita and coworkers (30), the therapeutic potential of MSCs in cardiac injury models has been described by many research groups. Most of the studies have focused on testing the effects of MSCs in experimental models of myocardial infarction. The bulk of these studies have yielded positive results with MSCs treatment reducing infarct size and improving cardiac function (31). These results have been achieved despite very low levels of MSCs engraftment into the heart, and have been largely attributed to their paracrine effects, particularly their ability to secrete reparative growth factors and induce the production of anti-inflammatory cytokines. Paralleling the cardiac literature has been the investigation of MSCs as a therapy for renal injury, particularly acute ischemic renal failure. Togel and coworkers (18) were one of the first to report that treatment with MSCs ameliorated experimental ischemic acute renal failure. This study further demonstrated that engraftment of MSCs into the kidney was very low and that the beneficial effect of MSCs was likely through paracrine mechanisms, similar to the cardiac studies. Subsequently, several reports have demonstrated protective effects of MSCs in rodent models of toxin and ischemia-induced acute kidney injury (32). Given the positive results obtained with MSCs treatment in both the cardiac and renal fields, clinical trials have already been undertaken to investigate the potential of cell-based therapy in patients with myocardial infarction and acute kidney injury. These trials will be discussed in more detail later in this chapter.

With the field of MSCs therapy already established in other organ injury models, interest in investigating the effects of MSCs gradually grew within the pulmonary community as well. Much of the initial interest stemmed, in part, from the findings of Krause and coworkers (33) who found that a single bone marrow-derived cell could give rise to cells of multiple different organs including the lung. This gave rise to intensive investigation into the possibility that bone marrow-derived stem cells, MSCs specifically, may be able to regenerate the lung epithelium and/or endothelium. However, several publications reported that engraftment of MSCs into the architecture of the lung was an exceedingly rare event with most reporting rates of <1% (13,14,34–36). Despite the low engraftment levels that were observed, beneficial effects with MSCs administration were noted in these initial reports that used the bleomycin model of lung injury (13,14). This finding suggested that the cells may be decreasing bleomycin-induced lung injury in a manner unrelated to engraftment and lung regeneration, a theme similar to that previously described in the renal and cardiac literature. The mechanisms invoked to explain the beneficial effects of MSCs included a reduction in the proinflammatory response to bleomycin, suppression of matrix metalloproteinases, and augmentation of the growth factors G-CSF and GM-CSF (13,14). A more recent study by Ortiz and coworkers (37) identified another potential mechanism of MSCs benefit, the production of interleukin 1 receptor antagonist (IL-1ra) by a subpopulation of MSCs. The authors were able to demonstrate that this subpopulation of IL-1ra expressing MSCs can suppress the proinflammatory response of activated macrophages in an in vitro setting as well as the proinflammatory response to bleomycin in vivo. Although important in establishing the potential for MSC-based therapy for fibrotic lung injury, these studies were somewhat limited in their assessment of the effect of the cells on functional and survival parameters in non-bone marrow suppressed mice. Also, the studies found a benefit with MSCs when the cells were given concurrently with or shortly after the administration of bleomycin, and therefore the applicability to a treatment modality was limited as well.

IV. Experimental Studies of MSCs in ALI/ARDS

The field of cell-based therapy for ALI/ARDS is in its infancy with most of the experimental literature being published within the last year. Nonetheless, there has been compelling evidence to suggest that MSC-based therapy may be a promising, novel therapeutic for clinical ALI/ARDS. The first study to investigate bone marrow-derived MSCs in a model of ALI was by Xu and coworkers (15). In this study, the authors established a sepsis-like syndrome by the intraperitoneal administration of endotoxin and found that systemically administered MSCs, given one hour after endotoxin, suppressed the proinflammatory response to endotoxin and prevented lung inflammation and injury. The authors also used an in vitro system to demonstrate that suppression of the proinflammatory response by MSCs occurred by both cell–cell contact dependent and independent mechanisms. As with the previous studies using bleomycin-induced lung injury, the level of MSCs engraftment into the lung was minimal, further supporting the concept that the cells are acting in a differentiation-independent manner to prevent lung injury.

Another recent study published by our group (16) tested the effects of the intratracheal (local) delivery of MSCs in a mouse model of endotoxin-induced ALI. In these experiments, ALI was induced by administering a large dose of endotoxin (5 mg/kg) intratracheally (IT), and then MSCs were delivered IT four hours later to determine the potential therapeutic value of MSCs in this model. Mice that had received MSCs had both improved survival at 48 and 72 hours after injury and reduced lung injury. Also, there was a reduction in the proinflammatory response to endotoxin and an upregulation of certain anti-inflammatory cytokines such as IL-10. Similar to studies by Ortiz and coworkers (37) and Xu and coworkers (15), an in vitro coculture system demonstrated that MSCs could downregulate the proinflammatory response of activated macrophages by a cell contact-independent mechanism. This study also reported a survival benefit with MSCs in nonbone marrow-suppressed mice with the IT route of delivery (Fig. 2).

Most recently, a study by Mei and coworkers (17) tested the effects of MSCs as well as MSCs transfected with Ang 1, a factor with protective effects on vascular endothelial cells. Similar to the prior two studies, the authors utilized an endotoxin model of ALI using a sublethal dose delivered IT. Thirty minutes after instilling endotoxin, the authors then intravenously injected MSCs with or without the Ang 1 containing plasmid. Using this experimental design, the authors were able to demonstrate that MSCs alone partially reduced lung inflammation, permeability and injury, but that MSCs transfected with Ang 1 nearly completely prevented lung inflammation and permeability. Also, of note, the percentage of MSCs retained in the lungs was somewhat higher than in prior studies with approximately 5–10% of injected MSCs still present three days after injury. This study substantiated the protective effect of MSCs in endotoxin-induced ALI, and was the first to combine both cell and gene-based therapy for ALI and show a synergistic effect between the two approaches (Fig. 3).

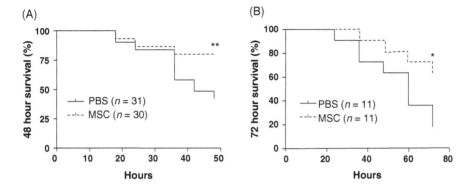

Figure 2 Intratracheal (IT) treatment with MSC improved survival at 48 and 72 hours in an endotoxin model of ALI in mice. MSC (750,000 cells/30 μl) or PBS (30 μl) was administered intratracheally four hours after IT instillation of endotoxin (5 mg/kg). Forty-eight-hour survival was 80% in MSC group versus 42% in phosphate buffered saline (PBS) group ($n = 30$ for MSC group, $n = 31$ for PBS group, $**p < 0.01$ using a log-rank test) (**A**). At 72 hours, survival was 64% in the MSC group versus 18% in the PBS group ($n = 11$ per group, $*p < 0.05$ using a log-rank test) (**B**). *Source*: From Ref. 16.

V. Translating MSC-Based Therapy to Clinical ALI/ARDS

Although the number of experimental studies testing MSC-based therapy for ALI/ARDS is small, the evidence for potential benefit is compelling and has therefore raised the possibility of translating cell-based therapy to patients with ALI/ARDS. One method that has been employed to translate the findings with MSCs in rodent models of ALI to humans is the use of an ex vivo perfused human lung model of ALI/ARDS (38). In this preparation, human lungs rejected for transplantation are perfused with a blood-based solution and given endotoxin IT to induce lung injury. Then, one hour after endotoxin injury, allogeneic human MSCs obtained from a NIH repository at Tulane University (Dr. Prockop, Center for Gene Therapy) are delivered IT. Using this model, Lee and coworkers (38) from our research group has demonstrated that human MSCs reduce endotoxin-induced lung injury and inflammation in the human lung. Furthermore, this study showed that MSCs treatment augmented alveolar fluid clearance compared to controls, and that this effect was dependent on the production of the epithelial growth factor KGF. Although the ex vivo perfused human lung does not allow for the testing of human MSCs in an intact organism, it does provide a novel mechanism for the preclinical testing of cell-based therapy, and the preliminary results obtained to date further raise the possibility of testing MSCs in a clinical trial of patients with ALI/ARDS.

While there have been no clinical trials of MSCs for patients with ALI/ARDS yet, trials of MSC-based therapies for several other diseases are already underway. This is most notably the case in the cardiac field with the emergence of multiple small phase I and II trials of bone marrow-derived cells in patients with myocardial infarction (39). Most of these trials have reported modest improvements in cardiac function and infarct size with cell-based therapy. A more recent trial that was presented in abstract form (American College of Cardiology 2007) demonstrated a significant beneficial effect with

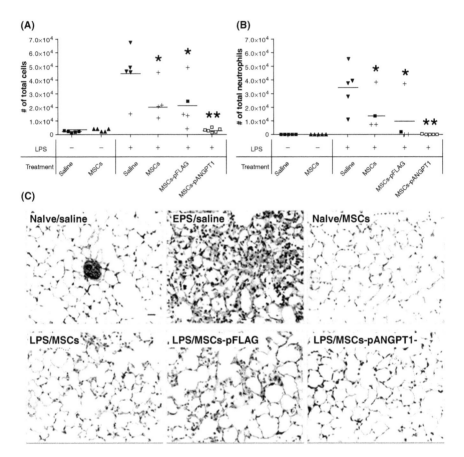

Figure 3 Therapeutic potential of MSCs combined with angiopoietin 1 (Ang 1) in experimental ALI. MSCs administration was associated with a reduction in alveolar inflammation as measured by bronchoalveolar lavage (BAL) total cell count (**A**) and neutrophil count (**B**). This effect was augmented in mice given MSCs transfected with Ang 1. Histology of the lungs of mice treated with MSCs also demonstrated significantly less lung injury and inflammation than control mice (**C**). Again, this protective effect was even more pronounced in mice receiving MSCs transfected with Ang 1. *Source*: From Ref. 17.

the intravenous delivery of MSCs in patients with acute myocardial infarction (MI). Interestingly, MSCs treatment was also associated with an improvement in pulmonary function. In addition to the cardiac field, MSC-based therapy is being planned for a clinical trial for patients with acute kidney injury. This study will enroll cardiac surgery patients at high risk for developing acute kidney injury and randomize them to treatment with allogeneic MSCs or control (32). There are also phase III clinical trials underway for investigating the therapeutic potential of MSCs in other diseases including graft versus host disease and Crohn's Disease (Osiris Therapeutics, Columbia, MD). The initial results from these clinical trials appear promising and demonstrate a good safety record for cell-based therapy. Furthermore, these human studies can provide valuable practical knowledge in developing MSC-based therapy for trials in patients with ALI/ARDS.

VI. Future Directions

The field of cell based, specifically MSCs based, therapy for ALI has stimulated a high level of enthusiasm for the potential development of a novel therapeutic modality for patients with ALI/ARDS. Experimental data have been published demonstrating significant functional and survival benefits of MSCs in rodent models of ALI (15–17). New studies have also been presented using human MSCs in a novel ex vivo perfused human lung model of ALI/ARDS and have reported beneficial effects (38). While the evidence for MSCs is compelling, there are still several unanswered questions that will need to be addressed before cell-based therapy can safely move toward a clinical application.

One of the major areas of research that is needed is a more precise understanding of the cellular and molecular mechanisms involved in the beneficial effects observed with MSC therapy. While most investigators have invoked both the immunomodulatory and growth factor production properties of MSCs to explain the protective effects, the exact mechanisms responsible for these effects remain unclear. For example, MSCs secrete or induce production of a variety of soluble factors such as IL-10, PGE_2, TGF-β, KGF and others, but it is not known which of these factors is essential in the protection provided by MSCs. A corollary question is whether the protective effects seen with MSCs can be replicated with a mixture of these factors or with MSCs-conditioned medium. Furthermore, it is now known that MSCs possess more complex immunoregulatory functions than initially thought, and understanding what molecular mechanisms control their net effect on the immune system will be important to achieving the desired clinical effect in patients.

Concurrent with efforts to understand the mechanistic effects of MSCs, investigators will need to address several practical questions to make cell-based therapy a reality for patients with ALI/ARDS. First, the procurement, isolation, and propagation of MSCs will need to be standardized so that it can be ensured that the same cell population is administered to different patients. This is particularly important since MSCs lack a specific cell surface marker to allow for the isolation of a pure population of MSCs. Also, investigators will need to determine how to ensure that MSCs retain their fundamental biological properties while being grown and passaged in culture and at what point they lose these characteristics. The development of a potency assay to measure a biochemical or functional output of the cells is a potential manner in which this question can be addressed. Furthermore, the implementation of good manufacturing practice protocols for isolating and propagating MSCs will need to be enforced in order to ensure that cells used for clinical trials are free of infectious or chemical contaminants (40).

In addition to basic issues related to MSCs isolation and culturing, there are also several questions regarding their delivery to patients. Specifically, the optimal dose and route of cell delivery remain to be determined. The experimental literature has utilized doses ranging from 5×10^5 to 10^6 cells per animal, which have been predominantly mice. However, dose response analyses have not been reported in the experimental literature so the optimal dose in mice is unknown as well. Recently presented data using the ex vivo perfused human lung provide some help in selecting a dose, since in this study 5×10^6 human MSCs were instilled into an injured lobe of the right human lung (38). However, further studies will need to be done to determine the optimal dose in this model. Prior clinical trials using human MSCs can also provide a guide for the dose of cells to use, though this is complicated by the fact that these investigators were targeting different organs and diseases. A question related to the optimal dose of MSCs is the issue of what is the most effective route of delivery. The experimental literature has utilized both intravenous and intratracheal routes of delivery with reported beneficial effects (15–17). However, a comparison or even combination of these two routes has not been studied. There are potential advantages to each route including relative ease of delivery using the intratracheal route, since this could likely be accomplished with a fiberoptic bronchoscope and could specifically target affected areas of the lung. On the other hand, the intravenous route may offer greater systemic benefit and help alleviate the multiple organ dysfunction that often accompanies ALI/ARDS. Nonetheless, this is an important practical issue that must be resolved before moving forward with clinical trials.

Once the above mentioned questions are answered, there is still the issue of which patients would be selected for a clinical trial with MSCs. Given the potential short- and long-term adverse effects of cell-based therapy, which will be discussed below, the risk–benefit ratio would seem to be most optimal for patients with severe, nonresolving ARDS. These patients have a poor prognosis with the current available interventions for ARDS and have traditionally been the population targeted for novel therapies. Further, practical issues such as the optimal timing of cell delivery and which endpoints to use to assess efficacy will then need to be determined.

The final area of future research for MSC-based therapy that will be considered is safety. Since MSCs are multipotent stem cells with the capability of differentiating into cells of various lineages and of self-renewal, one of the primary concerns with administering MSCs to patients is the potential for the cells to undergo malignant transformation. While human MSCs have not been shown to cause malignancy, mouse MSCs have been shown to cause malignant tumors in mice (41,42). Also, there have been reports of MSCs enhancing the metastatic potential of solid tumors such as breast cancer in mouse models (43,44). Furthermore, there is concern that MSCs may transform after repeated passage in vitro since studies have demonstrated that some of the cells develop abnormal karyotypes that predispose the cells to malignant transformation (41,42,45). Ironically, the fact that MSCs may have greater immunogenicity than first thought may prove to be beneficial with respect to the concerns of malignancy, since their eventual recognition and clearance by the host immune system would make the development of tumors less likely.

Another safety concern with MSC-based therapy, particularly in treating ARDS, is their effect on host defense against bacterial infection. Bacterial pneumonia and sepsis from a nonpulmonary cause are two of the most common etiologies of ARDS (46). Given the preponderance of literature that describes the immunosuppressive effect of MSCs, there is concern that this effect may impede the host's ability to clear an infection. However, as mentioned previously, there is emerging literature describing a dual role for MSCs in regulating the immune system and their immunostimulatory effects (5–7). Furthermore, there has been a recent report demonstrating a protective effect of systemically administered MSCs in a mouse model of bacterial sepsis and ventilator-induced ALI (47). Additional work is clearly needed to better define the effects of MSCs in the setting of a bacterial infection before MSC-based therapy can be used in patients with ALI/ARDS.

VII. Summary

ALI and the ARDS are the most common causes of hypoxemic respiratory failure among critically ill patients, and are associated with high morbidity and mortality. Current treatment for ALI/ARDS is primarily supportive and new treatments are needed. MSCs are adult stem cells most commonly isolated from the bone marrow that possess unique immunomodulatory and paracrine properties that make them attractive for cell-based therapy. There has been rapidly emerging literature demonstrating the therapeutic potential of MSCs in various organ injury models including myocardial infarction and acute kidney injury. Recently, investigators have also reported that MSCs have beneficial effects in experimental models of ALI. Efforts to translate these findings to clinical ALI/ARDS have included testing the effects of human MSCs in an ex vivo perfused human lung model of ALI/ARDS. Given the promising initial results obtained with the use of MSCs in experimental models of ALI/ARDS, there has been a high level of enthusiasm to advance cell-based therapy to patients with ALI/ARDS. While clinical trials of MSC-based therapy have started in patients with cardiac, renal, and autoimmune diseases, there are several important questions that need to be addressed before cell-based therapy can be safely applied to patients with ALI/ARDS. Future research in this field should continue to focus on elucidating the basic mechanisms responsible for the beneficial effects of MSCs, as well as determining the practical issues involved in producing a cell-based therapy for patients. In the process, a novel therapy for ALI/ARDS may emerge as a reality, and as importantly, investigators will learn more about the biology of lung injury and repair.

References

1. Friedenstein AJ, Petrakova KV, Kurolesova AI, et al. Heterotropic transplants of bone marrow: analysis of precursor cells for osteogenic and hematopoietic tissues. Transplantation 1968; 6:230–247.
2. Dominici M, Le Blanc K, Mueller I, et al. Minimal criteria for defining multipotent mesenchymal stromal cells. The International Society for Cellular Therapy position statement. Cytotherapy 2006; 8:315–317.
3. Patel SA, Sherman L, Munoz J, et al. Immunological properties of mesenchymal stem cells and clinical implications. Arch Immunol Ther Exp 2008; 56:1–8.
4. Barry FP, Murphy JM, English K, et al. Immunogenicity of adult mesenchymal stem cells: lessons from the fetal allograft. Stem Cells Dev 2005; 14:252–265.
5. Chan JL, Tang KC, Patel AP, et al. Antigen-presenting property of mesenchymal stem cells occurs during a narrow window at low levels of interferon-γ. Blood 2006; 107:4284–7184.
6. Stagg J, Pommey S, Eliopoulos N, et al. Interferon-γ-stimulated marrow stromal cells: a new type of nonhematopoietic antigen-presenting cell. Blood 2006; 107:2570–2577.
7. Stagg J. Immune regulation by mesenchymal stem cells: two sides to the coin. Tissue Antigens 2006; 69:1–9.
8. Nauta AJ, Westerhuis G, Kruisselbrink AB, et al. Donor-derived mesenchymal stem cells are immunogenic in an allogeneic host and stimulate donor graft rejection in a nonmyeloablative setting. Blood 2006; 108:2114–2120.
9. Aggarwal S, Pittenger MF. Human mesenchymal stem cells modulate allogeneic immune cell responses. Blood 2005; 105:1815–1822.
10. Beyth S, Borovsky Z, Mevorach D, et al. Human mesenchymal stem cells alter antigen-presenting cell maturation and induce T-cell unresponsiveness. Blood 2005; 105:2214–2219.
11. Corcione A, Benvenuto F, Ferretti E, et al. Human mesenchymal stem cells modulate B-cell functions. Blood 2006; 107:367–372.

12. Glennie S, Soeiro I, Dyson PJ, et al. Bone marrow mesenchymal stem cells induce division arrest anergy of activated T cells. Blood 2005; 105:2821–2827.
13. Ortiz LA, Gambelli F, McBride C, et al. Mesenchymal stem cell engraftment in lung is enhanced in response to bleomycin exposure and ameliorates its fibrotic effects. Proc Natl Acad Sci U S A 2003; 100:8407–8411.
14. Rojas M, Jianguo X, Woods CR, et al. Bone marrow derived mesenchymal stem cells in repair of the injured lung. Am J Respir Cell Mol Biol 2005; 33:145–152.
15. Xu J, Woods CR, Mora AL, et al. Prevention of endotoxin-induced systemic response by bone marrow derived mesenchymal stem cells in mice. Am J Physiol Lung Cell Mol Physiol 2007; 293:L131–L141.
16. Gupta N, Su X, Popov B, et al. Intrapulmonary delivery of bone marrow-derived mesenchymal stem cells improves survival and attenuates endotoxin-induced acute lung injury in mice. J Immunol 2007; 179:1855–1863.
17. Mei SH, McCarter SD, Deng Y, et al. Prevention of LPS-induced acute lung injury in mice by mesenchymal stem cells overexpressing angiopoietin 1. PLoS Med 2007; 4:e269.
18. Togel F, Hu Z, Weiss K, et al. Administered mesenchymal stem cells protect against ischemic acute renal failure through differentiation-independent mechanisms. Am J Physiol Renal Physiol 2005; 289:F31–F42.
19. Rasmusson I, Le Blanc K, Sundberg B, et al. Mesenchymal stem cells stimulate antibody secretion in human B-cells. Scand J Immunol 2007; 65:336–343.
20. Raffaghello L, Bianchi G, Bertolotto M, et al. Human mesenchymal stem cells inhibit neutrophil apoptosis: a model for neutrophil preservation in the bone marrow nice. Stem Cells 2008; 26:151–162.
21. Togel F, Weiss K, Yang Y, et al. Vasculotropic, paracrine actions of infused mesenchymal stem cells are important to the recovery from acute kidney injury. Am J Physiol Renal Physiol 2007; 292:F1626–F1635.
22. Miyahara Y, Nagaya N, Kataoka M, et al. Monolayered mesenchymal stem cells repair scarred myocardium after myocardial infarction. Nat Med 2006; 12:459–465.
23. Adamson IY, Bakowska J. Relationship of keratinocyte growth factor and hepatocyte growth factor levels in rat lung lavage fluid to epithelial cell regeneration after bleomycin. Am J Pathol 1999; 155:949–954.
24. Mason RJ, McCormick-Shannon K, Rubin JS, et al. Hepatocyte growth factor is a mitogen for alveolar type II Cells in rat lavage fluid. Am J Physiol 1996; 271:L46–L53.
25. Panos RJ, Bak PM, Simone WS, et al. Intratracheal instillation of keratinocyte growth factor decreases hyperoxia-induced mortality in rats. J Clin Invest 1995; 96:2026–2033.
26. Ware LB, Matthay MA. Keratinocyte and hepatocyte growth factors in the lung: roles in lung development, inflammation, and repair. Am J Physiol Lung Cell Mol Physiol 2002; 282:L924–L940.
27. Chen L, Tredget EE, Wu PY, et al. Paracrine factors of mesenchymal stem cells recruit macrophages and endothelial lineage cells and enhance wound healing. PLoS One 2008; 3:e1886.
28. Schinkothe T, Bloch W, Schmidt A. In vitro secreting profile of human mesenchymal stem cells. Stem Cells Dev 2008; 17:199–206.
29. Wu Y, Chen L, Scott PG, et al. Mesenchymal stem cells enhance wound healing through differentiation and angiogenesis. Stem Cells 2007; 25:2648–2659.
30. Tomita S, Li RK, Weisel RD, et al. Autologous transplantation of bone marrow cells improves damaged heart function. Circulation 1999; 100:II247–II256.
31. Pittenger MF, Martin BJ. Mesenchymal stem cells and their potential as cardiac therapeutics. Circ Res 2004; 95:9–20.
32. Humphreys BD, Bonventre JV. Mesenchymal stem cells in acute kidney injury. Annu Rev Med 2008; 59:311–325.

33. Krause DS, Theise ND, Collector MI, et al. Multi-organ, multi-lineage engraftment by a single bone marrow-derived stem cell. Cell 2001; 105:369–377.

34. Kotton DN, Ma BY, Cardoso WY. Bone marrow-derived cells as progenitors of lung alveolar epithelium. Development 2001; 128:5181–5188.

35. Kotton DN, Fabian AJ, Mulligan RC. Failure of bone marrow to reconstitute lung epithelium. Am J Respir Cell Mol Biol 2005; 33:328–334.

36. Loi R, Beckett T, Goncz KK, et al. Limited restoration of cystic fibrosis lung epithelium in vivo with adult bone marrow-derived cells. Am J Respir Crit Care Med 2006; 173:171–179.

37. Ortiz LA, Dutreil M, Fattman C, et al. Interleukin 1 receptor antagonist mediates the anti-inflammatory and antifibrotic effect of mesenchymal stem cells during lung injury. Proc Natl Acad Sci U S A 2007; 104:11002–11007.

38. Lee JW, Fang X, Gupta N, et al. Allogenic human mesenchymal stem cells for treatment of E. coli-induced acute lung injury in the ex vivo perfused human lung. Proc Natl Acad Sci USA 2009, epub.

39. Abdel-Latif A, Bolli R, Tleyjeh IM, et al. Adult bone marrow-derived cells for cardiac repair: a systematic review and meta-analysis. Arch Intern Med 2007; 167:989–997.

40. Bluestone JA, Thomson AW, Shevach EM, et al. What does the future hold for cell-based tolerogenic therapy? Nat Rev Immunol 2007; 7:650–654.

41. Aguilar S, Nye E, Chan J, et al. Murine but not human mesenchymal stem cells generate osteosarcoma-like lesions in the lung. Stem Cells 2007; 25:1586–1594.

42. Tolar J, Nauta AJ, Osborn MJ, et al. Sarcoma derived from cultured mesenchymal stem cells. Stem Cells 2007; 25:371–379.

43. Karnoub AE, Dash AB, Vo AP, et al. Mesenchymal stem cells within tumour stroma promote breast cancer metastasis. Nature 2007; 449:557–563.

44. Corcoran KE, Trzaska KA, Fernandes H, et al. Mesenchymal stem cells in early entry of breast cancer into bone marrow. PLoS One 2008; 3:e2563.

45. Izadpanah R, Kaushal D, Kriedt C, et al. Long-term in vitro expansion alters the biology of adult mesenchymal stem cells. Cancer Res 68:4229–4238.

46. LB Ware, Matthay MA. The acute respiratory distress syndrome. N Engl J Med 2000; 342:1334–1349.

47. Mei SH, Haitsma JJ, James D, et al. Efficacy of mesenchymal stem cells in a mouse model of sepsis-induced acute lung injury. Am J Respir Crit Care Med 2008; 177:A327.

22
Chemokines and Cytokines in ARDS

MICHAEL P. KEANE, EMER KELLY, and ROBERT M. STRIETER
Department of Medicine, St Vincent's University Hospital and University College Dublin, Dublin, Ireland and Department of Medicine, University of Virginia, Charlottesville, Virginia, U.S.A.

I. Introduction

Many clinical entities, including trauma, pneumonia/sepsis, ischemia–reperfusion injury, as well as ARDS, are characterized by varying degrees of acute pulmonary inflammation. This inflammatory response is initiated, maintained, resolves, and depends upon a complex yet coordinated intercellular interaction between immune and nonimmune cells. For example, the host response to bacterial pneumonia is characterized by acute inflammation and once the inciting microbe is cleared the inflammatory reaction resolves and normal repair and tissue remodeling occurs. This re-establishes normal lung function without the sequela of chronic inflammation and pulmonary fibrosis. In contrast, the acute inflammatory response associated with ARDS may culminate in severe lung injury, ultimately impairing lung function and impacting on host survival.

While these events are often accomplished through direct cell-to-cell adhesive interaction via specific cellular adhesion molecules, cells also signal each other through soluble mediators, such as cytokines. Cytokines display concentration-dependent effects, being expressed in low concentrations during normal homeostasis, with modest increases exerting local effects, and still greater elevations resulting in systemic effects. Individual subpopulations of immune cells possess different capacities to elaborate and secrete specific cytokines in response to particular stimuli. Nonimmune cells, including endothelial cells, fibroblasts, and epithelial cells also demonstrate particular responses to specific signals resulting in the production of other cytokines. Furthermore, cell populations vary in their expression of receptors for individual cytokines, and, as a result, differ in their capacity to respond to specific cytokine signals.

II. Early Response Cytokines
A. Interleukin-1 Family of Cytokines

The interleukin-1 family of cytokines consists of two agonists, interleukin-1 alpha (IL-1α) and interleukin-1 beta (IL-1β), and one antagonist, interleukin-1 receptor antagonist (IL-1ra) (1). The interleukin-1 agonists are pleiotropic cytokines that exist as two distinct genes, for IL-1α and IL-1β, respectively (1). These two forms of IL-1 are also distinguished by whether they are found predominantly membrane associated (IL-1α) or secreted (IL-1β) (1). Both isoforms of IL-1 are produced by a variety of cells, and bind to the type I IL-1 receptor on target cells with similar biologic function (1–3). Alpha and beta forms of IL-1 share approximately 26% amino acid sequence homology (1).

IL-1 ligand binding to the IL-1 type I receptor and the IL-1 receptor-associated protein recruits an intracellular adapter molecule, MyD88, which in turn recruits IL-1 receptor-associated kinase (IRAK). IRAK recruits the adapter molecule, tumor necrosis factor (TNF) receptor-associated factor 6 (TRAF6), which recruits the NF-κB-inducing kinase (NIK). NIK activates the IκB kinase complex that phosphorylates IκBα leading to ubiquitination and release of NF-κB for translocation to the nucleus and subsequent transactivation of a number of genes (i.e., cyclooxygenase, adhesion molecules, NO synthase, acute phase proteins, cytokines, and chemokines) (4,5). Interestingly, the signal coupling of IL-1 and the IL-1 type I receptor is identical to signaling coupling of lipopolysaccharide (LPS) on TLR4 (6–8). These two divergent ligand-receptor pairs ultimately signal through the same cytoplasmic pathway leading to NF-κB activation, nuclear translocation, and transactivation of several genes critical to the amplification of the inflammatory and innate host response. This exemplifies that an exogenous factor such as LPS may be the initial triggering event on specific cells that express the complex of CD14/TLR4/MD-2, however, host endogenous ligands, such as IL-1 can further amplify this response. The presence of IL-1 receptors on essentially all immune and nonimmune cells affords the ability of IL-1 to bind to the IL-1 type I receptor, activate, and engage all of these cells as participants of the inflammatory/innate host response. In addition to the IL-1 type I receptor, IL-1 also binds to an IL-1 type II or decoy receptor that does not signal (9,10). Binding of IL-1 to the IL-1 type II receptor may be a mechanism to sequester IL-1 from interacting with the IL-1 type I receptor (9,10).

In contrast to the two IL-1 agonists, IL-1ra is the only known naturally occurring cytokine with specific antagonistic activity. The discovery of the IL-1ra led to an appreciation of a dynamic balance between IL-1 agonists and IL-1ra in the maintenance of IL-1-dependent homeostasis and inflammation (1,11). IL-1Ra is produced in response to a variety of agents, the most potent being adherent IgG, LPS, GM-CSF, and IL-4 (12). Investigations have demonstrated that IL-1ra acts as a pure antagonist of either IL-1α or IL-1β and, when present in sufficient quantities, can attenuate a variety of IL-1 actions in both in vitro and in vivo model systems (13). These studies have led to an appreciation that IL-1ra normally modulates IL-1-dependent activity and speculation that it may play a role in the resolution of the pulmonary inflammatory cascade necessary for the lung to return to homeostasis.

IL-1 and IL-1Ra have been implicated in the pathogenesis of ARDS (14). In ARDS, low levels of the anti-inflammatory cytokines, IL-10 and IL-1Ra, in the BAL of patients with early disease correlated with a poor prognosis (14). When LPS, IL-1, or TNF are intratracheally injected, these inflammatory mediators induce an intra-alveolar inflammatory response composed of predominately of neutrophils, followed later by a mononuclear cell infiltrate (15). However, IL-1 is more potent than TNF in this response. In addition, LPS is capable of inducing both TNF and IL-1 gene expression in the lung that is important for its effect in amplifying the inflammatory response. In fact, IL-1ra has been found to reduce the inflammatory response to LPS in the lungs (15). These findings suggest that IL-1ra has an important immunomodulating influence on IL-1, and its production by mononuclear phagocytes and other cells in the lung may impact on the pathogenesis of the innate response.

Various models of lung injury have shown an important role for IL-1. Piguet and coworkers have shown that exogenous IL-1ra can inhibit bleomycin- or silica-induced lung injury (16). The importance of IL-1β and IL-1ra has been confirmed by Gasse and coworkers who have shown that IL-1R1 and MyD88 and the inflammasome are essential in pulmonary inflammation and subsequent fibrosis in the bleomycin model (13). Kolb and coworkers have demonstrated that transient expression of IL-1β using an adenoviral vector can lead to progressive fibrosis long after the IL-1β levels have declined and the acute inflammatory response has resolved (17). There was an early increase in levels of the proinflammatory cytokines IL-6 and TNF and the profibrotic cytokine platelet derived growth factor (PDGF), followed by a sustained increase in levels of TGF-β1 (17).

However, genetic approaches have led to findings that are less impressive for IL-1 in the innate immune response. For example, IL-1α−/− and IL-1β−/− animals display no phenotype at birth and appear similar to their wild-type littermates (+/+) (18). When doubly deficient knockout animals (IL-1α−/− /IL-1β−/− mice), were injected with a nonspecific inducer of inflammation (i.e., turpentine), as compared to IL-1α−/−, IL-1β−/−, and IL-ra−/− mice fever was suppressed in IL-1β−/− as well as IL-1α/β−/− mice, whereas IL-1α−/− mice displayed no abnormal response. In contrast IL-1ra−/− mice showed an elevated febrile response (18). In response to LPS, IL-1β−/− mice behave very similarly to IL-1β+/+ mice in regard to generation of IL-1α, IL-6, and TNF-α, and were equally sensitive to the lethal effects of LPS (19,20). However, in response to influenza infection, IL-1β−/− mice demonstrated a higher mortality rate, as compared to IL-1β+/+ mice (21). These studies suggest disparate roles for IL-1 in mediating inflammation depending on the initial insult or alternatively may reflect redundancy that may have occurred during embryogenesis in the genetically modified mice.

B. Tumor Necrosis Factor-alpha (TNF)

TNF is a mononuclear phagocyte-derived cytokine, which has been increasingly recognized for its pleiotropic effects on numerous inflammatory and immunological responses. It is one of 10 known members of a family of ligands that activate a corresponding family of receptors (22). TNF is produced primarily by monocytes/macrophages, and has many overlapping biologic activities with IL-1. In solution, TNF is a homotrimer and binds to two different cell surface receptors, p55 and p75 (22,23). The p55 receptor and the Fas receptor contain a 60 amino-acid domain known as the "death domain" that is essential for signal transduction of an apoptotic signal (22).

Elevated levels of TNF have been implicated in the pathogenesis of a number of disease states, including septic shock/sepsis syndrome (23), ARDS (24), and hepatic ischemia/reperfusion injury (25). TNF exhibits a variety of inflammatory effects, including: induction of neutrophil- and mononuclear cell-endothelial cell adhesion and transendothelial migration via expression of adhesion molecules and chemokines and acting as an early response cytokine in the promotion of a proinflammatory/fibrotic cytokine cascade. It leads to enhancement of a procoagulant environment by upregulating the expression of tissue factor and plasminogen activator inhibitor, and suppressing the protein C pathway.

Although the pathogenesis of septic shock and the development of acute lung injury are multifactorial, the role of TNF and IL-1 in mediating septic shock and ARDS has been clearly demonstrated in a number of studies. Waage and coworkers (26) examined sera from patients suffering from meningococcal septicemia with acute lung injury. They found a significant correlation between serum TNF levels and mortality. In a similar study of 55 patients with a clinical diagnosis of sepsis and purpura fulminans due to meningococcemia, serum levels of both TNF and IL-1 correlated with mortality (27). In another study of patients with septic shock (28), serum levels of TNF were detected in 33% of the patients with septic shock. TNF levels were elevated with equal frequency in patients with shock due to either gram-positive or negative bacteria. The magnitude of TNF measured also correlated with a higher incidence and severity of ARDS and mortality. The ratio of TNF to the anti-inflammatory cytokine IL-10, in BAL fluid, has been shown to be significantly higher in ARDS patients than in at risk patients; however, there was no difference in the ability of alveolar macrophages to produce IL-10 in response to endotoxin (29). In several animal studies, systemically administered TNF induced similar pathophysiological effects as compared to either endotoxin or infusion of live gram-negative bacteria (30). In other studies, the concomitant administration of both TNF and IL-1 has been found to be synergistic in mediating similar pathophysiological effects (31).

While these animal studies demonstrate an important role for TNF in inflammation, inhibition of TNF in human studies has been disappointing (32,33). However, one study has suggested that there may be subgroups of patients that may derive benefit (34). Therapy with anti-TNF antibodies is however fraught with difficulty. First, anti-TNF antibodies do not prevent lymphotoxin from signaling at the TNF receptors. Second, formation of immune complexes may lead to the activation of complement with potentially harmful effects. Third, murine monoclonal antibodies, and even humanized monoclonal antibodies, are antigenic that may preclude long-term therapy. Attempts to overcome these obstacles led to the development of chimeric inhibitor molecules that are minimally antigenic and highly specific and neutralize all ligands for the TNF receptor including lymphotoxin-α (35). The two molecules available to target TNF activity are a chimeric IgG1 antibody, infliximab, and a 75 kD fusion protein etanercept (36). These chimeric inhibitors have demonstrated efficacy in the treatment of rheumatoid arthritis, ankylosing spondylitis, Crohn's disease, and psoriatic arthritis (36–39). These beneficial effects, however, may be at the expense of increased risk for infectious complications. In animal models of both neutropenic and non-neutropenic Aspergillus infection, there is increased mortality following depletion of TNF (40). Furthermore, an increased incidence of tuberculosis has been reported in a large cohort of patients that were treated with anti-TNF therapy (infliximab) (41).

III. Chemotactic Cytokines
A. The Chemokines

The salient feature of chronic inflammation is the association of leukocyte infiltration. The maintenance of leukocyte recruitment during inflammation requires intercellular communication between infiltrating leukocytes and the endothelium, resident stromal and parenchymal cells. These events are mediated via the generation of early response cytokines, for example, IL-1 and TNF, the expression of cell-surface adhesion molecules, and the production of chemotactic molecules, such as chemokines.

The human CXC, CC, C, and CXXXC chemokine families of chemotactic cytokines are four closely related polypeptide families that behave, in general, as potent chemotactic factors for neutrophils, eosinophils, basophils, monocytes, mast cells, dendritic cells, NK cells, T- and B-lymphocytes (Table 1). These cytokines in their monomeric form range from 7 to 10 kD and are characteristically basic heparin-binding proteins. The

Table 1   The Human C, CC, CXC, and CXXXC Chemokine Families of Chemotactic Cytokines

The C chemokines	
XCL1	Lymphotactin
XCL2	SCM-1 β
The CC chemokines	
CCL1	I-309
CCL2	Monocyte chemotactic protein-1 (MCP-1)
CCL3	Macrophage inflammatory protein-1 alpha (MIP-1α)
CCL4	Macrophage inflammatory protein-1 beta (MIP-1β)
CCL5	Regulated on activation normal T-cell expressed and secreted (RANTES)
CCL7	Monocyte chemotactic protein-3 (MCP-3)
CCL8	Monocyte chemotactic protein-2 (MCP-2)
CCL9	Macrophage inflammatory protein-1 delta (MIP-1δ)
CCL11	Eotaxin
CCL13	Monocyte chemotactic protein-4 (MCP-4)
CCL14	HCC-1
CCL15	HCC-2
CCL16	HCC-4
CCL17	Thymus and activation-regulated chemokine (TARC)
CCL18	DC-CK-1
CCL19	Macrophage inflammatory protein-3 beta (MIP-3β)
CCL20	Macrophage inflammatory protein-3 alpha (MIP-3α)
CCL21	6Ckine
CCL22	MDC
CCL23	MPIF-1
CCL24	MPIF-2
CCL25	TECK
CCL26	Eotaxin-3
CCL27	CTACK
CCL28	MEC
The CXC chemokines	
CXCL1	Growth-related oncogene alpha (GRO-α)
CXCL2	Growth-related oncogene beta (GRO-β)
CXCL3	Growth-related oncogene gamma (GRO-γ)
CXCL4	Platelet factor-4 (PF4)
CXCL5	Epithelial neutrophil activating protein-78 (ENA-78)
CXCL6	Granulocyte chemotactic protein-2 (GCP-2)
CXCL7	Neutrophil activating protein-2 (NAP-2)
CXCL8	Interleukin-8 (IL-8)
CXCL9	Monokine induced by interferon-γ (MIG)
CXCL10	Interferon-γ-inducible protein (IP-10)
CXCL11	Interferon-inducible T Cell alpha chemoattractant (ITAC)
CXCL12	Stromal cell-derived factor-1 (SDF-1)
CXCL13	B cell-attracting chemokine-1 (BCA-1)
CXCL14	BRAK
CXCL16	SR-PSOX
The CXXXC chemokine	
CXC3CL1	Fractalkine

CCL6 and CXCL15 have been described only in the mouse.

chemokines display highly conserved cysteine amino acid residues. The CXC chemokine family has the first two NH_2-terminal cysteines separated by one nonconserved amino acid residue, the CXC cysteine motif. The CC chemokine family has the first two NH_2-terminal cysteines in juxtaposition, the CC cysteine motif. The C chemokine has one lone NH_2-terminal cysteine amino acid, the C cysteine motif; and the CXXXC chemokine has the first two NH_2-terminal cysteines separated by three nonconserved amino acid residues. There is approximately 20% to 40% homology between the members of the four chemokine families.

Chemokines have been found to be produced by an array of cells including monocytes, alveolar macrophages, neutrophils, platelets, eosinophils, mast cells, T- and B-lymphocytes, NK cells, keratinocytes, mesangial cells, epithelial cells, hepatocytes, fibroblasts, smooth muscle cells, mesothelial cells, and endothelial cells. These cells can produce chemokines in response to a variety of factors, including viruses, bacterial products, IL-1, TNF, C5a, LTB4, and IFNs. The production of chemokines by both immune and nonimmune cells supports the contention that these cytokines may play a pivotal role in orchestrating chronic inflammation. We will focus our discussion on the role of the CXC and CC chemokine families.

B. The CXC Chemokines

The CXC chemokines can be further divided into two groups on the basis of a structure/function domain consisting of the presence or absence of three amino acid residues (Glu-Leu-Arg; "ELR" motif) that precedes the first cysteine amino acid residue in the primary structure of these cytokines (42–44). The ELR^+ CXC chemokines are chemoattractants for neutrophils and act as potent angiogenic factors (45). In contrast, the ELR^- CXC chemokines are chemoattractants for mononuclear cells and are potent inhibitors of angiogenesis (Table 2) (45,46).

Based on the structural/functional difference, the members of the CXC chemokine family are unique cytokines in their ability to behave in a disparate manner in the regulation of angiogenesis. The angiogenic members include CXCL1, 2, 3, 5, 6, 7, and 8. CXCL1, 2, and 3 are closely related CXC chemokines, with CXCL1 originally described for its

Table 2 The CXC Chemokines That Display Disparate Angiogenic Activity

Angiogenic CXC chemokines containing the ELR motif	
CXCL1	Growth-related oncogene alpha (GRO-α)
CXCL2	Growth-related oncogene beta (GRO-β)
CXCL3	Growth-related oncogene gamma (GRO-γ)
CXCL5	Epithelial neutrophil activating protein-78 (ENA-78)
CXCL6	Granulocyte chemotactic protein-2 (GCP-2)
CXCL7	Neutrophil activating protein-2 (NAP-2)
CXCL8	Interleukin-8 (IL-8)
Angiostatic CXC chemokines that lack the ELR motif	
CXCL4	Platelet factor-4 (PF4)
CXCL9	Monokine induced by interferon-γ (MIG)
CXCL10	Interferon-γ-inducible protein (IP-10)
CXCL11	Interferon-inducible T cell alpha chemoattractant (ITAC)
CXCL12	Stromal cell-derived factor-1 (SDF-1)

melanoma growth stimulatory activity (Table 2). CXCL5, CXCL6, and CXCL8 were all initially identified on the basis of neutrophil activation and chemotaxis. The angiostatic (ELR$^-$) members of the CXC chemokine family include CXCL4, which was originally described for its ability to bind heparin and inactivate heparin's anticoagulation function. Other angiostatic ELR$^-$ CXC chemokines include CXCL9, CXCL10, and CXCL11 (Table 2). CXCL12 is a member of the CXC chemokine family, and has been found to recruit CD34$^+$ hematopoietic progenitor cells, megakaryocytes, B- and T-cells, and fibrocytes (47). CXCL12 binds to the CXC chemokine receptor, CXCR4. CXCR4 was originally discovered as the coreceptor for lymphotropic strains of HIV, and CXCL12 is its lone CXC chemokine ligand.

C. CXC Chemokine Receptors

Chemokine activities are mediated through G-protein-coupled receptors. Seven CXC chemokine receptors have been identified (Table 3) (48). The ELR$^+$ chemokines bind to CXCR1 and CXCR2 receptors that are found on neutrophils, T-lymphocytes, monocytes/ macrophages, eosinophils, basophils, keratinocytes and mast cells, and endothelial cells (49,50). The intracellular COOH-terminus of these receptors is rich in serine and threonine amino acid residues that may be important in phosphorylation and signal coupling via G-proteins (51,52).

The receptor for CXCL9, CXCL10, and CXCL11 is CXCR3 and is expressed on activated T-lymphocytes in the presence of IL-2; however, it is not significantly present on resting T- and B-lymphocytes, monocytes or neutrophils. CXCR4 is the specific receptor for CXCL12 and is the cofactor for lymphotropic HIV-1. CXCL12 is a potent inhibitor of HIV entry into T-lymphocytes. In contrast to CXCR3, CXCR4 appears to be expressed on resting T-lymphocytes. These findings suggest that ELR$^-$ CXC chemokines and their receptors are important in regulating mononuclear cell function. CXCR1, CXCR2, and CXCR4 are expressed on human umbilical vein endothelial cells (HUVEC) and the spontaneously transformed HUVEC cell line, ECV304 (53). CXCR2 is expressed on human microvascular endothelial cells (HUMVEC) and it mediates the angiogenic effects of ELR$^+$ chemokines (50). CXCR3 is also expressed on HUMVEC in a cell cycle-dependent fashion (54).

CXCR5 is the receptor for B cell-attracting chemokine-1 (BCA-1)/CXCL13 (55). CXCL13 and CXCR5 are necessary for the homing of B-lymphocytes and proper development of the B cell-rich regions of lymphoid organs (56). CXCR6 is a receptor for CXCL16 and was initially described as an orphan receptor that could serve as a coreceptor

Table 3 The CXC Chemokine Receptors

Receptor	Ligand
CXCR1	CXCL6, CXCL8
CXCR2	CXCL1, CXCL2, CXCL3, CXCL5, CXCL6, CXCL7, CXCL8
CXCR3	CXCL9, CXCL10, CXCL11
CXCR4	CXCL12
CXCR5	CXCL13
CXCR6	CXCL16
CXCR7	CXCL11, CXCL12

for HIV (57,58). CXCR6 is downregulated upon T cell activation and is predominantly expressed on type 1 polarized T cells suggesting it may have a role in type 1-mediated processes (59,60). CXCR7 has recently been described as a receptor for CXCL11 and CXCL12 and is expressed on endothelial cells, tumor cells, and fetal liver cells (61).

Two other chemokine receptors have been identified that bind chemokines without a subsequent signal-coupling event. The duffy antigen receptor for chemokines (DARC) demonstrates a seven transmembrane-spanning receptor motif, similar to other chemokine receptors and demonstrates promiscuity in that it binds both CXC and CC chemokines without apparent signal coupling (62). This receptor was originally found on human erythrocytes and felt to represent a "sink" for chemokines. In addition to binding of the chemokine family, this receptor has been found to be shared by the malarial parasites, Plasmodium vivax and knowlesi, and may allow their invasion into erythrocytes. The second nonsignaling chemokine receptor is the D6 receptor that has significant homology to CC chemokine receptors and binds several CC chemokines with high affinity, including CCL2, CCL4, CCL5, and CCL7 (63). D6 is only weakly expressed on circulating cells but is highly expressed in the placenta and on lymphatic endothelium and may function to aid in clearing of CC chemokines and prevent excessive diffusion to lymph nodes (63). Further studies are required to examine the functional nature of these receptors.

D. CXC Chemokines in Lung Injury

CXC chemokines have also been found to play a significant role in mediating neutrophil infiltration in the lung parenchyma and pleural space in response to endotoxin and bacterial challenge. Frevert and coworkers (64) have passively immunized rats with neutralizing CXCL1 antibodies prior to intratracheal LPS, and found a 71% reduction in neutrophil accumulation within the lung. Broaddus and coworkers (65,66) have found that passive immunization with neutralizing CXCL8 antibodies blocked 77% of endotoxin-induced neutrophil influx in the pleura of rabbits. However, in the context of microorganism invasion, depletion of a CXC chemokine and reduction of infiltrating neutrophils may have a major impact on the host.

ELR^+ CXC chemokines have been implicated in mediating neutrophil sequestration in the lungs of patients with pneumonia. CXCL8 has been found in the bronchoalveolar lavage of patients with community-acquired pneumonia and nosocomial pneumonia following trauma (67,68). In animal models of pneumonia, ELR^+ CXC chemokines have been found in a number of murine models including *Klebsiella pneumoniae, Pseudomonas aeruginosa, Nocardia asteroides*, and *Aspergillus fumigatus* pneumonia (40,69–74). In a model of *A. fumigatus* pneumonia, neutralization of TNF resulted in marked attenuation of the expression of murine CXCL1 and CXCL2/3 that was paralleled by a reduction in the infiltration of neutrophils and associated with increased mortality (71,75). Interestingly, Cole has demonstrated that similar to defensins, ELR^- CXC chemokines have direct antimicrobial properties (76) against *Escherichia coli and Listeria monocytogenes*.

Several studies have demonstrated that CXCL8 levels correlates with the development and mortality of the acute respiratory distress syndrome (77,78). Of particular interest is the study of Donnelly and coworkers (78), which correlated early increases in CXCL8 in bronchoalveolar lavage fluid with an increased risk of subsequent development of ARDS, and also demonstrated that alveolar macrophages were an important source of CXCL8 prior to neutrophil influx. High concentrations of CXCL8 were found in bronchoalveolar lavage fluid from trauma patients, some within one hour of injury and prior to any evidence of significant neutrophil influx. Patients who progressed to ARDS had significantly greater bronchoalveolar lavage fluid levels of CXCL8 than those who failed to develop this condition. Levels of CXCL8 in plasma, as opposed to lavage, were not found to be significantly different between patients who did or did not develop ARDS (78). More recently it has been suggested that anti-CXCL8 autoantibody: CXCL8 complexes may have a role in the pathogenesis of ALI/ARDS (79–81). Furthermore, there is an imbalance in the expression of ELR$^+$ (CXCL1, CXCL5, CXCL8) as compared to ELR$^-$ CXC (CXCL10, CXCL11) chemokines from bronchoalveolar lavage fluid (BALF) of patients with ARDS as compared to controls (82). This imbalance correlated with angiogenic activity and both procollagen I and procollagen III levels in BALF (82). These findings suggest that CXC chemokines have an important role in the fibroproliferative phase of ARDS via the regulation of angiogenesis.

CXCL8 significantly contributed to reperfusion lung injury in a rabbit model of lung ischemia–reperfusion injury (83). Reperfusion of the ischemic lung resulted in the production of CXCL8, which correlated with maximal pulmonary neutrophil infiltration. Passive immunization of the animals with neutralizing antibodies to CXCL8 prior to reperfusion of the ischemic lung prevented neutrophil extravasation and tissue injury, suggesting a causal role for CXCL8 in this model. Ventilator-induced lung injury in a murine model is associated with increased expression of CXCL1 and CXCL2 that parallels lung injury and neutrophil recruitment (84). Furthermore, these levels correlated with NF-κB activation (84). CXCR2−/− mice were protected from ventilator-induced lung injury (84). These findings support the notion that ventilator-induced lung injury is secondary to stretch-induced NF-κB activation and chemokine release with a subsequent inflammatory response and neutrophil recruitment (84). In other studies, Colletti and coworkers (85) have demonstrated that hepatic ischemia–reperfusion injury and the generation of TNF can result in pulmonary-derived CXCL5, showing the importance of cytokine networks between the liver and the lung. The production of CXCL5 in the lung was correlated with the presence of neutrophil-dependent lung injury, and passive immunization with neutralizing CXCL5 antibodies resulted in significant attenuation of lung injury (85).

E.   The CC Chemokines

The CC chemokines (Table 1) are chemoattractants for monocyte, T- and B-lymphocytes, NK cells, dendritic cells, basophils, mast cells, and eosinophils. The CC chemokines have been found to be produced by an array of cells including monocytes, alveolar macrophages, neutrophils, platelets, eosinophils, mast cells, T-cell, B-cells, NK cells, keratinocytes, mesangial cells, epithelial cells, hepatocytes, fibroblasts, smooth muscle cells, mesothelial cells, and endothelial cells. These cells can produce CC chemokines in response to a variety of factors, including viruses, bacterial products, IL-1, TNF, C5a, LTB4, and IFNs and appear to be significantly susceptible to suppression by IL-10. The CC chemokines lack a conserved NH$_2$-terminal sequence analogous to the ELR motif of the CXC chemokine family. NH$_2$-terminal processing of CC chemokines by CD26/dipeptidyl peptidase IV can alter receptor selectivity and chemotactic activity (86,87).

F.   CC Chemokine Receptors

CC Chemokine activities are mediated by seven-transmembrane domain, G-protein-coupled receptors. The CC chemokine receptors are structurally homologous. Currently

Table 4 The CC Chemokine Receptors

Receptor	Ligand
CCR1	CCL3, CCL5, CCL7, CCL14, CCL15, CCL16, CCL23
CCR2	CCL2, CCL7, CCL13,
CCR3	CCL5, CCL7, CCL11, CCL11, CCL15, CCL26
CCR4	CCL17, CCL22
CCR5	CCL3, CCL4, CCL5
CCR6	CCL20
CCR7	CCL19
CCR8	CCL1
CCR9	CCL25, CCL28
CCR10	CCL27, CCL28

at least 10 cellular CC chemokine receptors have been cloned, expressed, and identified to have specific ligand-binding profiles (Table 4) (49).

The expression of specific CCRs may be restricted to a state of cellular activation (i.e., resting or activated) and differentiation. Mononuclear phagocytes stimulated with IL-2 express CCR2, whereas, CCL2 itself has no effect in regulating expression of CCR2 on these cells (88). IL-2 induces the expression of CCR1 and CCR2 on CD45RO+ T cells, the primary receptors for CCL5 and CCL2, respectively (89). Combined activation of TCR/CD3 complex with CD28 antigen caused rapid downregulation of CCR1 and CCR2 expression. This effect was paralleled by a decline in chemotactic response to either CCL5 or CCL2, even in the presence of IL-2 (89). These findings support the notion that IL-2, by induction of specific CCRs, in conjunction with specific CC chemokine ligand production can have a significant impact on the recruitment of mononuclear cells.

G. CC Chemokines in Lung Injury

The CC chemokines, CCL2, CCL3, CCL4, CCL5, have been implicated in mediating the innate host defense in animal models of *Influenza* A virus, *Paramyxovirus* pneumonia virus, *A. fumigatus*, and *Cryptococcus neoformans* pneumonias (90). The host response to *Influenza* A virus is characterized by an influx of mononuclear cells into the lungs that is associated with the increased expression of CC chemokine ligands (90). Dawson and coworkers have used a genetic approach to determine the role of CC chemokines in mediating the innate response to this virus (90). Using a mouse adapted strain of *Influenza* A infected in CCR5−/− and CCR2−/− mice, as compared to control +/+ mice, these investigators demonstrated that CCR5−/− mice displayed increased mortality related to severe pneumonitis, whereas CCR2−/− mice were protected from the severe pneumonitis due to defective macrophage recruitment. The delay in macrophage accumulation in CCR2−/− mice was correlated with high pulmonary viral titers (90). These studies support the potential of different roles that CC chemokine ligand/receptor biology plays in influenza infection. In addition, this study also demonstrates the importance of macrophage recruitment during the innate response is critical to the development of adaptive immunity to this microbe. Domachowske and coworkers (91) have examined the role of CC chemokine ligands (i.e., CCL3 and CCL5) that bind to the CC chemokine receptor CCR1 in response to *Paramyxovirus* pneumonia virus infection in mice. This infection is associated with predominant neutrophil and eosinophil infiltration into the lung that is accompanied by expression of CCR1 ligands (91). However, in CCR1$-$/$-$ mice infected with *Paramyxovirus* pneumonia virus, the inflammatory response was found to be minimal, the clearance of virus from lung tissue was reduced, and mortality was markedly increased (91). These results indicate that CC chemokine-dependent innate responses limited the rate of virus replication in vivo and played an important role in reducing mortality.

IV. Conclusions

Inflammation, injury, and repair are a sequence of events that occur in response to a variety of insults that affect the lungs and other organs. At times, despite considerable injury, tissue remodeling and repair occur with resolution and return of normal function to the involved lung. At other times, the injury results in tissue destruction and ongoing inflammation that fail to resolve and culminate in end-stage fibrosis. As illustrated in this chapter, the mechanisms and mediators involved in these processes are complex. There are numerous animal studies showing that neutralization of individual mediators can attenuate injury. Experience from sepsis trials in humans suggest that this is unlikely to be the case in both acute and chronic lung injury in humans and that novel treatments will involve "cocktail" interventional therapy consisting of monoclonal antibodies and specific inhibitors of several inflammatory mediators. Furthermore, attenuation of the inflammatory response is not always beneficial in the setting of infection. Future directions may include systemic or local intrapulmonary gene therapy, which may either attenuate or augment the expression of some of the inflammatory mediators at specific time points.

References

1. Dinarello CA. Biologic basis for interleukin-1 in disease. Blood 1996; 87:2095–2147.
2. Vigers GPA, Anderson LJ, Caffes P, et al. Crystal structure of the type-I interleukin-1 receptor complexed with interleukin-1b. Nature 1997; 386:190–194.
3. Schreuder H, Tardif C, Trump-Kallmeyer S, et al. A new cytokine-receptor binding mode revealed by the crystal structure of the IL-1 receptor with an antagonist. Nature 1997; 386: 194–200.
4. Murphy JE, Robert C, Kupper TS. Interleukin-1 and cutaneous inflammation: a crucial link between innate and acquired immunity. J Invest Dermatol 2000; 114(3):602–608.
5. Ghosh S, May MJ, Kopp EB. NF-kappa B and Rel proteins: evolutionarily conserved mediators of immune responses. Annu Rev Immunol 1998; 16:225–260.
6. Medzhitov R, Janeway C Jr. Innate immunity. N Engl J Med 2000; 343(5):338–344.
7. Strieter RM, Belperio JA, Keane MP. Cytokines in innate host defense in the lung. J Clin Invest 2002; 109(6):699–705.
8. Strieter RM, Belperio JA, Keane MP. Host innate defenses in the lung: the role of cytokines. Curr Opin Infect Dis 2003; 16(3):193–198.
9. Mantovani A, Muzio M, Ghezzi P, et al. Regulation of inhibitory pathways of the interleukin-1 system. Ann N Y Acad Sci 1998; 840:338–351.
10. Dinarello CA. Interleukin-1 beta, interleukin-18, and the interleukin-1 beta converting enzyme. Ann N Y Acad Sci 1998; 856:1–11.
11. Dinarello CA. Interleukin-1 and interleukin-1 antagonism. Blood 1991; 77:1627–1635.
12. Arend WP, Malyak M, Guthridge CJ, et al. Interleukin-1 receptor antagonist: role in biology. Annu Rev Immunol 1998; 16:27–55.

13. Gasse P, Mary C, Guenon I, et al. IL-1R1/MyD88 signaling and the inflammasome are essential in pulmonary inflammation and fibrosis in mice. J Clin Invest 2007; 117(12):3786–3799.
14. Donnelly SC, Strieter RM, Reid PT, et al. The association between mortality rates and decreased concentrations of interleukin-10 and interleukin-1 receptor antagonist in the lung fluids of patients with the adult respiratory distress syndrome. Ann Intern Med 1996; 125(3): 191–196.
15. Ulich TR, Watson LR, Yin SM, et al. The intratracheal administration of endotoxin and cytokines. I. Characterization of LPS-induced inflammatory infiltrate. A J Pathol 1991; 138(6):1485–1496.
16. Piguet P, Vesin C, Grau G, et al. Interleukin 1 receptor anatgonist (IL-1ra) prevents or cures pulmonary fibrosis elicited in mice by bleomycin or silica. Cytokine 1993; 5(1):57–61.
17. Kolb M, Margetts PJ, Anthony DC, et al. Transient expression of IL-1beta induces acute lung injury and chronic repair leading to pulmonary fibrosis. J Clin Invest 2001; 107(12): 1529–1536.
18. Horai R, Asano M, Sudo K, et al. Production of mice deficient in genes for interleukin (IL)-1alpha, IL-1beta, IL-1alpha/beta, and IL-1 receptor antagonist shows that IL-1beta is crucial in turpentine-induced fever development and glucocorticoid secretion. J Exp Med 1998; 187(9):1463–1475.
19. Fantuzzi G, Dinarello CA. The inflammatory response in interleukin-1 beta-deficient mice: comparison with other cytokine-related knock-out mice. J Leukoc Biol 1996; 59(4): 489–493.
20. Fantuzzi G, Zheng H, Faggioni R, et al. Effect of endotoxin in IL-1 beta-deficient mice. J Immunol 1996; 157(1):291–296.
21. Kozak W, Zheng H, Conn CA, et al. Thermal and behavioral effects of lipopolysaccharide and influenza in interleukin-1 beta-deficient mice. Am J Physiol 1995; 269(5, pt 2):R969–R977.
22. Bazzoni F, Beutler B. The tumor necrosis factor ligand and receptor families. N Engl J Med 1996; 334(26):1717–1725.
23. Strieter RM, Kunkel SL, Bone RC. Role of tumor necrosis factor-alpha in disease states and inflammation. Crit Care Med 1993; 21:S447–S463.
24. Millar AB, Foley NM, Singer M, et al. TNF in bronchopulmonary secretions of patients with adult respiratory distress syndrome. Lancet 1989; 2(8665):712–714.
25. Colletti LM, Remick DG, Burtch GD, et al. Role of tumor necrosis factor-alpha in the patho-physiologic alterations after hepatic ischemia/reperfusion injury in the rat. J Clin Invest 1990; 85(6):1936–1943.
26. Waage A, Halstensen A, Espevik T. Association between tumor necrosis factor in serum and fatal outcome in patients with meningococcal disease. Lancet 1987; 1:355–357.
27. Girardin E, Grau GE, Dayer JM, et al. Tumor necrosis factor and interleukin-1 in the serum of children with severe infectious purpura. N Engl J Med 1988; 319:397–400.
28. Marks JD, Marks CB, Luce JM, et al. Plasma tumor necrosis in patients with septic shock: mortality rate, incidence of adult respiratory distress syndrome. Am Rev Respir Dis 1990; 141:94–97.
29. Armstrong L, Millar AB. Relative production of tumour necrosis factor alpha and interleukin 10 in adult respiratory distress syndrome. Thorax 1997; 52(5):442–446.
30. Tracey KJ, Beutler B, Lowry SF, et al. Shock and tissue injury induced by recombinant human cachectin. Science 1986; 234(4775):470–474.
31. Dinarello CA. Interleukin-1 and its biologically related cytokines. Adv Immunol 1989; 44:153–205.
32. Wherry JC, Pennington JE, Wenzel RP. Tumor necrosis factor and the therapeutic potential of anti-tumor necrosis factor antibodies. Crit Care Med 1993; 21(Suppl. 10):S436–S440.
33. Abraham E, Wunderink R, Silverman H, et al. Efficacy and safety of monoclonal antibody to human tumor necrosis factor alpha in patients with sepsis syndrome. A randomized, controlled,

double-blind, multicenter clinical trial. TNF-alpha MAb Sepsis Study Group. JAMA 1995; 273(12):934–941.

34. Abraham E, Glauser MP, Butler T, et al. p55 Tumor necrosis factor receptor fusion protein in the treatment of patients with severe sepsis and septic shock. A randomized controlled multicenter trial. Ro 45–2081 Study Group. JAMA 1997; 277(19):1531–1538.

35. Peppel K, Crawford D, Beutler B. A tumor necrosis factor (TNF) receptor-IgG heavy chain chimeric protein as a bivalent antagonist of TNF activity. J Exp Med 1991; 174(6):1483–1489.

36. Braun J, de Keyser F, Brandt J, et al. New treatment options in spondyloarthropathies: increasing evidence for significant efficacy of anti-tumor necrosis factor therapy. Curr Opin Rheumatol 2001; 13(4):245–249.

37. Maini R, St Clair EW, Breedveld F, et al. Infliximab (chimeric anti-tumour necrosis factor alpha monoclonal antibody) versus placebo in rheumatoid arthritis patients receiving concomitant methotrexate: a randomised phase III trial. ATTRACT Study Group. Lancet 1999; 354(9194):1932–1939.

38. Mease PJ, Goffe BS, Metz J, et al. Etanercept in the treatment of psoriatic arthritis and psoriasis: a randomised trial. Lancet 2000; 356(9227):385–390.

39. Brandt J, Haibel H, Cornely D, et al. Successful treatment of active ankylosing spondylitis with the anti-tumor necrosis factor alpha monoclonal antibody infliximab. Arthritis Rheum 2000; 43(6):1346–1352.

40. Mehrad B, Strieter RM, Standiford TJ. Role of TNF-alpha in pulmonary host defense in murine invasive aspergillosis. J Immunol 1999; 162(3):1633–1640.

41. Keane J, Gershon S, Wise RP, et al. Tuberculosis associated with infliximab, a tumor necrosis factor alpha- neutralizing agent. N Engl J Med 2001; 345(15):1098–1104.

42. Strieter RM, Lukacs NW, Standiford TJ, et al. Cytokines and lung inflammation. Thorax 1993; 48:765–769.

43. Koch AE, Strieter RM. Chemokines in Disease. Austin, TX: R.G. Landes, Co., Biomedical Publishers, 1996.

44. Strieter RM, Kunkel SL. Chemokines in the lung. In: Crystal R, West J, Weibel E, et al., eds. Lung: Scientific Foundations, 2nd ed. New York: Raven Press, 1997:155–186.

45. Strieter RM, Polverini PJ, Kunkel SL, et al. The functional role of the 'ELR' motif in CXC chemokine-mediated angiogenesis. J Biol Chem 1995; 270(45):27348–27357.

46. Luster AD, Greenberg SM, Leder P. The IP-10 chemokine binds to a specific cell surface heparan sulfate shared with platelet factor 4 and inhibits endothelial cell proliferation. J Exp Med 1995; 182:219–232.

47. Phillips RJ, Burdick MD, Hong K, et al. Circulating fibrocytes traffic to the lungs in response to CXCL12 and mediate fibrosis. J Clin Invest 2004; 114(3):438–446.

48. Thelen M, Thelen S. CXCR7, CXCR4 and CXCL12: an eccentric trio? J Neuroimmunol 2008; 198(1–2):9–13.

49. Lukacs NW, Miller AL, Hogaboam CM. Chemokine receptors in asthma: searching for the correct immune targets. J Immunol 2003; 171(1):11–15.

50. Addison CL, Daniel TO, Burdick MD, et al. The CXC chemokine receptor 2, CXCR2, is the putative receptor for ELR(+) CXC chemokine-induced angiogenic activity [In Process Citation]. J Immunol 2000; 165(9):5269–5277.

51. Rollins BJ. Chemokines. Blood 1997; 90(3):909–928.

52. Luster AD. Chemokines–chemotactic cytokines that mediate inflammation. N Engl J Med 1998; 338(7):436–445.

53. Murdoch C, Monk PN, Finn A. Cxc chemokine receptor expression on human endothelial cells. Cytokine 1999; 11(9):704–712.

54. Romagnani P, Annunziato F, Lasagni L, et al. Cell cycle-dependent expression of CXC chemokine receptor 3 by endothelial cells mediates angiostatic activity. J Clin Invest 2001; 107(1):53–63.

55. Legler DF, Loetscher M, Roos RS, et al. B cell-attracting chemokine 1, a human CXC chemokine expressed in lymphoid tissues, selectively attracts B lymphocytes via BLR1/CXCR5. J Exp Med 1998; 187(4):655–660.

56. Forster R, Mattis AE, Kremmer E, et al. A putative chemokine receptor, BLR1, directs B cell migration to defined lymphoid organs and specific anatomic compartments of the spleen. Cell 1996; 87(6):1037–1047.

57. Liao F, Alkhatib G, Peden KW, et al. STRL33, a novel chemokine receptor-like protein, functions as a fusion cofactor for both macrophage-tropic and T cell line-tropic HIV-1. J Exp Med 1997; 185(11):2015–2023.

58. Deng HK, Unutmaz D, KewalRamani VN, et al. Expression cloning of new receptors used by simian and human immunodeficiency viruses. Nature 1997; 388(6639):296–300.

59. Koprak S, Matheravidathu S, Springer M, et al. Down-regulation of cell surface CXCR6 expression during T cell activation is predominantly mediated by calcineurin. Cell Immunol 2003; 223(1):1–12.

60. Kim CH, Kunkel EJ, Boisvert J, et al. Bonzo/CXCR6 expression defines type 1-polarized T-cell subsets with extralymphoid tissue homing potential. J Clin Invest 2001; 107(5):595–601.

61. Burns JM, Summers BC, Wang Y, et al. A novel chemokine receptor for SDF-1 and I-TAC involved in cell survival, cell adhesion, and tumor development. J Exp Med 2006; 203(9):2201–2213.

62. Premack BA, Schall TJ. Chemokine receptors: gateways to inflammation and infection. Nat Med 1996; 2:1174–1178.

63. Fra AM, Locati M, Otero K, et al. Cutting edge: scavenging of inflammatory CC chemokines by the promiscuous putatively silent chemokine receptor D6. J Immunol 2003; 170(5):2279–2282.

64. Frevert CW, Huang S, Danaee H, et al. Functional characterization of the rat chemokine KC and its importance in neutrophil recruitment in a rat model of pulmonary inflammation. J Immunol 1995; 154(1):335–344.

65. Boylan AM, Hebert CA, Sadick M, et al. Interleukin-8 is a major component of pleural liquid chemotactic activity in a rabbit model of endotoxin pleurisy. Am J Physiol 1994; 267(2, pt 1):L137–L144.

66. Broaddus VC, Boylan AM, Hoeffel JM, et al. Neutralization of IL-8 inhibits neutrophil influx in a rabbit model of endotoxin-induced pleurisy. J Immunol 1994; 152(6):2960–2967.

67. Boutten A, Dehoux MS, Seta N, et al. Compartmentalized IL-8 and elastase release within the human lung in unilateral pneumonia. Am J Respir Crit Care Med 1996; 153(1):336–342.

68. Rodriguez JL, Miller CG, DeForge LE, et al. Local production of interleukin-8 is associated with nosocomial pneumonia. J Trauma 1992; 33(1):74–81; discussion 81–82.

69. Greenberger MJ, Strieter RM, Kunkel SL, et al. Neutralization of macrophage inflammatory protein-2 attenuates neutrophil recruitment and bacterial clearance in murine Klebsiella pneumonia. J Infect Dis 1996; 173(1):159–165.

70. Standiford TJ, Kunkel SL, Greenberger MJ, et al. Expression and regulation of chemokines in bacterial pneumonia. J Leukoc Biol 1996; 59(1):24–28.

71. Mehrad B, Strieter RM, Moore TA, et al. CXC chemokine receptor-2 ligands are necessary components of neutrophil-mediated host defense in invasive pulmonary aspergillosis. J Immunol 1999; 163(11):6086–6094.

72. Tsai WC, Strieter RM, Mehrad B, et al. CXC chemokine receptor CXCR2 is essential for protective innate host response in murine Pseudomonas aeruginosa pneumonia. Infect Immun 2000; 68(7):4289–4296.

73. Tsai WC, Strieter RM, Wilkowski JM, et al. Lung-specific transgenic expression of KC enhances resistance to Klebsiella pneumoniae in mice. J Immunol 1998; 161(5):2435–2440.

74. Moore TA, Newstead MW, Strieter RM, et al. Bacterial clearance and survival are dependent on CXC chemokine receptor-2 ligands in a murine model of pulmonary Nocardia asteroides infection. J Immunol 2000; 164(2):908–915.
75. Mehrad B, Standiford TJ. Role of cytokines in pulmonary antimicrobial host defense. Immunol Res 1999; 20(1):15–27.
76. Cole AM, Ganz T, Liese AM, et al. Cutting edge: IFN-inducible ELR⁻ CXC chemokines display defensin-like antimicrobial activity. J Immunol 2001; 167(2):623–627.
77. Chollet-Martin S, Montravers P, Gibert C, et al. High levels of interleukin-8 in the blood and alveolar spaces of patients with pneumonia and adult respiratory distress syndrome. Infect Immun 1993; 61(11):4553–4559.
78. Donnelly SC, Strieter RM, Kunkel SL, et al. Interleukin-8 and development of adult respiratory distress syndrome in at-risk patient groups. Lancet 1993; 341:643–647.
79. Allen TC, Fudala R, Nash SE, et al. Anti-interleukin 8 autoantibody:Interleukin 8 immune complexes visualized by laser confocal microscopy in injured lung. Arch Pathol Lab Med 2007; 131(3):452–456.
80. Fudala R, Krupa A, Matthay MA, et al. Anti-IL-8 autoantibody: IL-8 immune complexes suppress spontaneous apoptosis of neutrophils. Am J Physiol Lung Cell Mol Physiol 2007; 293(2):L364–L374.
81. Fudala R, Krupa A, Stankowska D, et al. Anti-interleukin-8 autoantibody: interleukin-8 immune complexes in acute lung injury/acute respiratory distress syndrome. Clin Sci (Lond) 2008; 114(6):403–412.
82. Keane MP, Donnelly SC, Belperio JA, et al. Imbalance in the expression of CXC chemokines correlates with bronchoalveolar lavage fluid angiogenic activity and procollagen levels in acute respiratory distress syndrome. J Immunol 2002; 169(11):6515–6521.
83. Sekido N, Mukaida N, Harada A, et al. Prevention of lung reperfusion injury in rabbits by a monoclonal antibody against interleukin-8. Nature 1993; 365(6447):654–657.
84. Belperio JA, Keane MP, Burdick MD, et al. Critical role for CXCR2 and CXCR2 ligands during the pathogenesis of ventilator-induced lung injury. J Clin Invest 2002; 110(11):1703–1716.
85. Colletti LM, Kunkel SL, Walz A, et al. Chemokine expression during hepatic ischemia/reperfusion-induced lung injury in the rat. The role of epithelial neutrophil activating protein. J Clin Invest 1995; 95(1):134–141.
86. Proost P, De Meester I, Schols D, et al. Amino-terminal truncation of chemokines by CD26/dipeptidyl-peptidase IV. Conversion of RANTES into a potent inhibitor of monocyte chemotaxis and HIV-1-infection. J Biol Chem 1998; 273(13):7222–7227.
87. De Meester I, Korom S, Van Damme J, et al. CD26, let it cut or cut it down. Immunol Today 1999; 20(8):367–375.
88. Sica A, Saccani A, Borsatti A, et al. Bacterial lipopolysaccharide rapidly inhibits expression of C-C chemokine receptors in human monocytes. J Exp Med 1997; 185(5):969–974.
89. Loetscher P, Seitz M, Baggiolini M, et al. Interleukin-2 regulates CC chemokine receptor expression and chemotactic responsiveness in T lymphocytes [see comments]. J Exp Med 1996; 184(2):569–577.
90. Dawson TC, Beck MA, Kuziel WA, et al. Contrasting effects of CCR5 and CCR2 deficiency in the pulmonary inflammatory response to influenza A virus. Am J Pathol 2000; 156(6):1951–1959.
91. Domachowske JB, Bonville CA, Gao JL, et al. The chemokine macrophage-inflammatory protein-1 alpha and its receptor CCR1 control pulmonary inflammation and antiviral host defense in paramyxovirus infection. J Immunol 2000; 165(5):2677–2682.

Index

ACE. *See* Angiotensin converting enzyme
ACM. *See* Alveolar-capillary membrane
Actin and myosin microfilaments, 265–68, 266–67t
Activated protein C (APC), 156, 395
Acute cor-pulmonale, 322, 343
Acute exacerbation (AE), of idiopathic pulmonary fibrosis (IPF), 55
Acute interstitial pneumonia, 55
Acute lung injury/Acute respiratory distress syndrome (ALI/ARDS), genetic epidemiology of, 196
  biomarkers detection in, 221
  candidate gene studies, 197
    gene selection, 197, 198f, 199–200
    genotyping and analyses, 200–201
    power, Type I error, and replication, 213–14
    study design, 201, 202–209f, 210–213
  future directions, 214–15
  pathogenesis understanding, gene expression profiles for, 231–33
  study using microarrays, 221–22
Acute Physiology and Chronic Health Evaluation (APACHE), 23
Acute respiratory distress syndrome (ARDS), definition of, 1, 12
Acute respiratory failure (ARF), 20, 21, 23
Adenosine triphosphate (ATP), 277
Adherens junctions (AJs), 271
Adult stem cells, 420
AECC diagnostic criteria, for ARDS, 5–6
AFC. *See* Alveolar fluid clearance
Age factor associated with mortality, from ARDS, 10
Age-specific mortality and incidence rates, of ALI, 26
Aging population, effect of, 26–27
AII. *See* Angiotensin II
Airspace edema clearance, in VILI, 117–18

Airway pressure release ventilation (APRV), 348
AJs. *See* Adherens junctions
Alcohol, 9
Alveolar-capillary membrane (ACM)
  alveolar unit, 76
  disruption of
    increased permeability, 60–63
    lung inflammation, development of, 63
    surfactant dysfunction, 63–65
  endothelium, 77
  epithelium, 77–79
  extracellular matrix, 79
Alveolar edema, resolution of, 237
  alveolar epithelial fluid absorption, mechanisms of, 237–38
    cultured alveolar epithelial cells, sodium transport in, 240–41
    distal pulmonary epithelia, structure of, 238–39
    fluid transport in lung, 239–40
  alveolar fluid transport under pathological conditions, 246
    clinical studies, 246–47
    hyperoxia, experimental studies of, 249–50
    hypovolemic shock, experimental studies of, 247–48
    infection, experimental studies of, 248–49
  epithelial fluid transport regulation, 241
    cAMP-mediated upregulated fluid transport, CFTR in, 242–43
    catecholamine-dependent mechanisms, upregulation by, 241–42
    catecholamine-lndependent regulation, 243–44
  vectorial fluid transport impairment, mechanisms of, 244
    anesthetics, 244–45
    hypoxia, 244
    reactive oxygen and nitrogen species, 245

Note: Page numbers followed by "f" indicate figure and page numbers followed by "t" indicate table.

Alveolar epithelial type II cells, 78
Alveolar epithelium, 50, 77, 78, 239
Alveolar fluid, 74, 240, 401
Alveolar fluid clearance (AFC), 78, 240, 243, 244
Alveolar inflation, 111
Alveolar macrophages, 54–55, 101, 400, 439
Alveolar type II epithelial cells, 185, 288
Alveolar wall tension, 111, 112f
Alveoli, rupture of, 35
Alveolus, during ALI, 85
American Association of Blood Banks, 180
American-European Consensus Conference
    (AECC), on ARDS, 3–4
Angiopoietin, 275
Angiotensin converting enzyme (ACE), 199
Angiotensin II (AII), 99, 274
Antifibrinolytic (PAI-1) protein, 83
APACHE II score, 156, 325, 348
APACHE III score, 302
APACHE. *See* Acute Physiology and Chronic
    Health Evaluation
APC. *See* Activated protein C
Apoptosis in pathogenesis/resolution, of ALI, 93,
    102–104
    endothelial cell apoptosis, 101–102
    epithelial cell apoptosis, 98–101
    neutrophil apoptosis, 94–98
APRV. *See* Airway pressure release ventilation
ARDSNet trial, 11, 79, 80, 82
ARF. *See* Acute respiratory failure
Aspergillus fumigatus, 439, 441
ATP. *See* Adenosine triphosphate
Attributable morbidity, for ALI, 21, 24
    on functional status, 25
    long-term mortality, 23–24
    on psychiatric outcomes and quality of life, 25
    short term mortality, 22–23
Autopsy, 76

B cell-attracting chemokine-1 (BCA-1), 438
Bacteremia, 147
Barotraumas, 35–38
BCA-1. *See* B cell-attracting chemokine-1
BCL-2, 53
BCL-3, 379
β-agonists, 78
Bilevel ventilation, 348
Biochemical marker, for ARDS, 7
Bioinformatics, 220

Black patients
    with ALI, 22
    with ARDS, 11
BLES. *See* Bovine lipid extract surfactant
Blood transfusions and ALI/ARDS, 173
    observational studies, 173
    randomized clinical trials, 173
    specific donor characteristics, 174
BMI. *See* Body mass index
Body mass index (BMI), 151
Bolus instillation, 300, 305
Bound integrins, 120f
Bovine lipid extract surfactant (BLES), 296–97,
    305
BRCA1 gene, 210
Broad-spectrum antibiotic therapy, 153
Bronchoalveolar lavage (BAL) fluid, 63, 72–74,
    94, 129, 184, 189, 190, 288, 295
    in DAD, 54–55
Bronchoscopic instillation, of surfactant, 300

C-1543T alleles, 210
Caldesmon, 267, 267t
Calfactant, 304, 305
Canadian Consensus Conference, 171, 172, 174,
    175
Canadian Critical Care Network, 173
Captopril, 274
Carbohydrate recognition domain (CRD), 289
Catheter-related bloodstream infections, 148t
Catheter-related complications, 362t
CC chemokines, 440
    in lung injury, 441–42
    receptors, 440–41
Cell–cell interactions, in sepsis and septic ALI,
    380–82
Cell-based therapy, for ALI and ARDS
    mesenchymal stem cell (MSCs)
        in ALI/ARDS, experimental studies of,
        424–25
        biology, 420–22
        in experimental models of organ injury,
        423–24
        future directions, 427–28
        MSC-based therapy to clinical ALI/ARDS,
        425–27
Central venous catheters (CVC), 35, 151
CFTR. *See* Cystic fibrosis transmembrane
    regulator

Chemokines and cytokines, in ARDS, 432
  chemotactic cytokines
    CC chemokine receptors, 440–41
    CXC chemokine receptors, 438–39
    CXC chemokines, 437–38
    CXC chemokines, in lung injury, 439–40
    lung injury, CC chemokines in, 441–42
  early response cytokines
    interleukin-1 family of cytokines, 432–34
    tumor necrosis factor-alpha (TNF)-α, 434–35
Chest radiography, 6, 32–34, 43
CHF. *See* Congestive heart failure
Chronic alcohol abuse, 82, 175
Cirrhosis, and mortality from ARDS, 10, 11
Clara Cell Secretory Protein promoter, 66
Class discovery, 223, 227–229
Class prediction, 223–26
  for biomarkers uncovering, 226–29
Clinical risk factors, for mortality from ARDS,
    10–12
Coagulation pathway, 82–83
Cofilin, 267, 276
Collagenase, 295
"Common variant/multiple disease" hypothesis,
    199
Comorbidity, of ARDS, 9–10
Complications, of ARDS, 41
  barotrauma, 35–38
  pneumonia, 38–39
  support lines, 34–35
Computational biology, 220–21
Computed tomography (CT) and ARDS, 40–42
Congestive heart failure (CHF), 7, 63
Continuous diaphragm sign, 37
Convertase, 291
CRD. *See* Carbohydrate recognition domain
Criteria, for ALI and ARDS, 4
Cross validation, 224
Cryptococcus neoformans, 441
Curosurf®, 302
CVC. *See* Central venous catheters
CXC chemokines, 437–38
  in lung injury, 439–40
  CXC chemokine receptors, 438–39
Cystic fibrosis transmembrane regulator (CFTR),
    239, 242–43
Cytokines
  of ALI, 80–81
  and chemokines, in sepsis, 386–89

DAD with organizing pneumonia (DAD-OP), 53
DAD. *See* Diffuse alveolar damage
Damage-associated molecular pattern (DAMP)
    recognition, 83–84
DARC. *See* Duffy antigen receptor for chemokines
Dead-space fraction, 11
Death, cause of
  for patients with ARDS, 10
Deep sulcus sign, 38
Deep venous thrombosis (DVT), 157, 158
Delphi definition, of ARDS, 4–5
Demographics, of ARDS, 9–10
Desmosine, 79
DETANONOate, 245
Development of ARDS, clinical risk factors
    for, 7
  comorbidity, demographics, and incidence,
    9–10
Diabetes mellitus, 9, 84
Diagnostic criteria, of ARDS, 1, 2, 3, 4, 6, 7–8, 12,
    31
DIC. *See* Disseminated intravascular coagulation
Diffuse alveolar damage (DAD), 46
  acute interstitial pneumonia, 55
  bronchoalveolar lavage in, 54–55
  exudative phase, 47–49
  fibrotic phase, 51–52
  history and overview, 46–47
  open lung biopsy role, in ARDS, 54
  pathogenesis, 52–54
  proliferative phase, 49–51
  superimposed on interstitial lung disease, 55
Dipalmitoylphosphatidylcholine (DPPC), 289,
    302
Diperoxovanadate, 265
Direct lung injury, 9, 60, 62, 63
Disseminated intravascular coagulation (DIC),
    156, 377
Distal lung epithelial cells (DLECs), 100f
Distal pulmonary epithelia, structure of, 238–39
Diuretic therapy, 179
DLECs. *See* Distal lung epithelial cells
Dobutamine, 154
Dopamine, 154, 243
Dose–response relationship, 173
DPPC. *See* Dipalmitoylphosphatidylcholine
Drosophila, 382, 392
Drotrecogin alfa (activated), 156–57
Dual-radionuclide method, 42

Duffy antigen receptor for chemokines (DARC), 439
DVT. *See* Deep venous thrombosis

EBC-pH, 79
ECM. *See* Extracellular matrix
ECs. *See* Endothelial cells
ED-1. *See* Ethidium homodimer-1
Elastase, 295
Electrical impedance tomography, 75
ELR$^+$CXC chemokines, 437, 439
ELR$^-$CXC chemokines, 437, 439
Embryonic stem cells (ESCs), 420
EMMPRIN. *See* Extracellular matrix
    metalloproteinase inducer
EMT. *See* Epithelial-mesenchymal transition
Endothelial cell (EC) cytoskeleton components, 264–65
    actin and myosin microfilaments, 265–68, 266–67f
    intermediate filaments, 269–70
    microtubules, 268–69
Endothelial cells (ECs)
    apoptosis in ALI, 101–102
    in sepsis, 375–77
    in VILI, 125
Endothelial injury, 49
Endothelin-1 (ET-1), 77, 191
Endothelium, lung microvascular, 77
Endotoxin. *See* Lipopolysaccharide
Endotracheal (ET) intubation, 34
Enhanceosomes, 68
Enoxaparin, 157
Enterobacteriaceae, 38
Epidemiology, of ALI, 17
    aging population, effect of, 26–27
    attributable morbidity, 21, 24
        on functional status, 25
        long-term mortality, 23–24
        on psychiatric outcomes and quality of life, 25
        short term mortality, 22–23
    incidence, 18–21
    pediatrics, 27
Epithelial cell apoptosis, 98–101
Epithelial injury and repair, 187–88
Epithelial-mesenchymal transition (EMT), 188
Epithelium, alveolar, 77–79
ERK. *See* Extracellular signal-regulated kinase

Erythropoietin, 159
Escherichia coli, 396, 439
ESCs. *See* Embryonic stem cells
ET tube balloon cuff, 34
ET-1. *See* Endothelin-1
Ethidium homodimer-1 (ED-1), 121, 122
EVLW. *See* Extravascular lung water
Exhaled breath condensate (EBC), 74–75
Exosurf, 302
Expiratory pressure (Express), 124
Express. *See* Expiratory pressure
External validation, 225
Extracellular matrix (ECM), 79
Extracellular matrix metalloproteinase inducer (EMMPRIN), 121
Extracellular signal-regulated kinase (ERK), 126
Extracorporeal gas exchange, 347
Extrapulmonary ARDS, 60
Extravascular lung water (EVLW), 75–76, 78
Extravascular lung water accumulation, in ARDS
    patients, 7
Exudative phase, 32
    of ARDS, 185
    of DAD, 47–49

F-18 fluorodeoxyglucose PET/CT, 43
FACs. *See* Focal adhesion complexes
Factor V Leiden (FVL) mutation, 83
FACTT. *See* Fluid and Catheter Treatment Trial
FAKs. *See* Focal adhesion kinases
Fas/FasL system, 98–99, 100, 101
Femoral insertions, 151
FFP. *See* Fresh frozen plasma
Fibrin deposition, in alveolar space, 82–83
Fibrinolysis, 83
Fibroblasts, 102, 188–190
Fibroproliferation, in ALI, 184
    markers as predictors, of outcome/mortality, 191–92
    pathological features, 185
        epithelial injury and repair, 187–88
        fibroblast, 188–190
        tissue remodeling mediators, 190–91
Fibroproliferative phase, 184
    histological features, 186f
Fibrosing alveolitis, 184
Fibrotic phase, of DAD, 51–52
Fibrotid phase, 32
Fio$_2$, 155, 302, 323, 351

Fluid and Catheter Treatment Trial (FACTT), 359
  limitations of, 365–66
  pulmonary outcomes in, 364t
Fluid therapy
  and hemodynamic monitoring, in ALI, 359, 361–62
    design of trial, 359–60
    FACTT trial, limitations of, 365–66
    fluid strategies, 362–64
    relevance of trial to clinical practice, 364–65, 366f
Focal adhesion complexes (FACs), 114, 126, 131
Focal adhesion kinases (FAKs), 114, 120f
Focal ARDS, 342–43
FRC. *See* functional residual capacity
Fresh frozen plasma (FFP), 174, 175
Functional residual capacity (FRC), 112, 315
Future directions, of ARDS, 7

G-CSF. *See* Granulocyte-stimulating factor
G-protein-coupled receptors (GPCRs), 389
Gadolinium, 119
"Gain of function" studies, 66
Gallium-67 pulmonary leak index, 42
Gallium-68–labeled transferring, 43
Gallium-transferrin, 75
Gastric stress ulcer prophylaxis, 158
Gender differences, in ARDS mortality, 11
Gene expression, alteration of
  changes in expression
    of individual genes in vitro, 66–68
    of many genes, 68
    of single genes in vivo, 66
Gene expression profiling and biomarkers, in ARDS, 220
  additional high-throughput methods for biomarkers identification, 229–231
  biomarker detection, 221
  class prediction, 223–26
  genomic and proteomic markers identification, 222–23
  microarrays, use of, 221–22
  pathogenesis understanding, gene expression profiles for, 231–33
  uncover biomarkers, using class prediction to, 226–29
Genome-wide association studies (GWASs), 214–15

Genomic and proteomic markers identification, for ARDS, 222–23
Glycemia and glycated proteins, 84
GM-CSF. *See* Granulocytemacrophage colony-stimulating factor
GPCRs. *See* G-protein-coupled receptors
Granulocyte-stimulating factor (G-CSF), 94
Granulocytemacrophage colony-stimulating factor (GM-CSF), 94
Gravitational pleural pressure gradient, 317
GWASs. *See* Genome-wide association studies

Hamman–Rich syndrome, 55
Heat–moisture exchange devices (HMEs), 149
Heat shock protein 47, 70, 53
Heme oxygenase (HO)-1, 82
Hemodialysis, 159, 361
Hemodynamic monitoring, 361–62
  and fluid therapy, in ALI, 359
    design of trial, 359–360
    FACTT trial, limitations of, 365–66
    fluid strategies, 362–64
    relevance of trial to clinical practice, 364–65, 366f
Hemorrhagic shock, 396
Heparin, 157
Hepatocyte growth factor (HGF), 187, 191, 276–77, 422
HFOV. *See* High-frequency oscillatory ventilation
HFV. *See* High frequency ventilation
HGF. *See* Hepatocyte growth factor
High frequency ventilation (HFV), 346–47
High Mobility Group A1 (HMGA1) protein, 68
High tidal volume ventilation
  and ECM constituents, 121
  endothelial permeability with, 118–19
  epithelial permeability with, 119, 121
  and pulmonary edema, 115–17
High-frequency oscillatory ventilation (HFOV), 124
High-mobility group box 1 protein (HMGB1), 84, 386, 387, 388
High-throughput methods, for biomarkers identification, 229–231
Hispanic patients, with ALI, 11, 22
HMEs. *See* Heat–moisture exchange devices
HMGB1. *See* High-mobility group box 1 protein
HPE. *See* hydrostatic pulmonary edema
Human ARDS, pathologic hallmarks of, 60

Human microvascular endothelial cells
　　(HUMVEC), 438
Human umbilical vein endothelial cells (HUVEC),
　　438
HUMVEC. *See* Human microvascular endothelial
　　cells
HUVEC. *See* Human umbilical vein endothelial
　　cells
Hyaline membranes, 46, 47–48, 80
Hydrostatic pulmonary edema (HPE), 77, 179,
　　246, 325, 326
Hypercapnia, effects of, 128
Hyperoxia, 47
Hyperoxic pulmonary injury, 47
Hypovolemic shock, experimental studies of,
　　247–48
Hypoxemia, 1, 11
　　criteria for ARDS, 6

ICD-9 diagnostic codes, 24
ICU organizational model, 12
Idiopathic pulmonary fibrosis (IPE), 187
　　acute exacerbation (AE) of, 55
IGF-I, 191
IGFBP-3. *See* Insulin-like growth factor binding
　　protein
IL-1, 433
IL-1α. *See* Interleukin-1 alpha
IL-1β. *See* Interleukin-1 beta
IL-6 gene, 76
IL-10, 424
IL1-β receptor agonist, 81
Incidence figures, for ALI, 18–21
Incidence, of ARDS, 9–10
Indirect lung injury, 9, 60, 62, 63
Inflammation, coagulation, and thrombosis, in
　　sepsis, 392–96
Influenza A virus, 441
Inspiratory plateau pressure (Pplat)
　　safe upper limit for, 336–38
Insulin-like growth factor binding protein
　　(IGFBP-3), 190
Interleukin (IL)-6, 80–81
Interleukin (IL)-8, 80–81
Interleukin-1 alpha (IL-1α), 432
Interleukin-1 beta (IL-1β), 379, 432
Interleukin-1 family of cytokines, 432–34
Intermediate filaments (IFs), 269–270
Intra-alveolar fibrosis, 50

Intratracheal (IT) treatment, with MSC, 425f
Intratracheal bolus instillation, 299–300
Intravenous catheters, 150–151
Iron, 82

Keratinocyte growth factor (KGF), 187–88, 422
KGF. *See* Keratinocyte growth factor
Klebsiella pneumoniae, 439
Krebs van den Lungen 6 antigen (KL-6), 78

LAP. *See* Latency-associated peptide
Laryngotracheal stenosis, 34
Latency-associated peptide (LAP), 190
LBP. *See* LPS-binding protein
Leave-one-outcross validation (LOOCV), 226
Leukocyte integrins. *See* Neutrophil β₂ integrins
Leukocytes, in sepsis, 372, 374–75
Lidocaine, 245
Limulus, 392
Lipopolysaccharide (LPS), 53, 369, 378, 379, 383,
　　396
Listeria monocytogenes, 439
LOOCV. *See* Leave-one-outcross validation
Look-back studies, 174
"Loss of function" studies, 66
LOV. *See* Lung Open Ventilation
Low lung volume ventilation, injury from, 122
　　experimental studies, 124
　　protective ventilation, clinical studies of,
　　　123–24
Low tidal volume ventilation, 10, 115, 128
LPS-binding protein (LBP), 384
LPS. *See* Lipopolysaccharide
Lung and Blood Institute Acute Respiratory
　　Distress Syndrome Network, 359
Lung biopsy, 76
Lung endothelial cell barrier regulation, 262–64
Lung inflammation, development of, 63
Lung injury score, 3t
Lung microvascular endothelium, 77
Lung Open Ventilation (LOV), 124
Lung surfactant fraction, 288
Lung ultrasound, 75
Lung vascular dysfunction and repair, 262
　　bioactive agonists that increase lung vascular
　　　permeability
　　　angiopoietin, 275
　　　angiotensin II, 274
　　　PBEF, 273

thrombin and TNF-α, 272–73
VEGF, 274
EC cytoskeleton components, 264–65
actin and myosin microfilaments, 265–68,
266–67f
intermediate filaments, 269–270
microtubules, 268–69
endothelial barrier, structural and junctional
elements of, 271–72
lung endothelial cell barrier regulation, 262–64
mechanical stress and EC barrier regulation,
270–271
vascular barrier integrity
hepatocyte growth factor (HGF), 276–77
MLCK inhibitors, 275
simvastatin and ATP, 277
sphingosine 1-phosphate, 275–76
Lyso-PCs, 177

Macrophage migration inhibitory factor (MIF),
389
Magnetic resonance imaging (MRI), 43
MAL (MyD88-adaptor-like), 385
MALDI. *See* Matrix-assisted laser
desorption/ionization
Mammalian TLRs, 382
Marrow stromal stem cells. *See* Mesenchymal
stem cell (MSCs)
Matrix metalloproteases, 121, 191
Matrix-assisted laser desorption/ionization
(MALDI), 229
Mayo Clinic, 175
Mechanical stress, 120f, 125
Mechanical ventilation (MV), in ARDS, 335
extracorporeal gas exchange, 347
high frequency ventilation (HFV), 346–47
noninvasive ventilation (NIV), 347–48
recommendations, for clinical use of MV in
ALI/ARDS, 349
NIV, 349–350
PEEP and Fio$_2$, 351
recruitment maneuvers, 351
tidal volumes and inspiratory pressures,
350
ventilator mode, 350
spontaneous ventilation vs. neuromuscular
blockade, 348–49
VILI, from high volumes and pressures during
inspiration, 335

inspiratory plateau pressure (Pplat), safe
upper limit for, 336–38
tidal volume adjustment, 338–39
volume-and-pressure limited MV, in patients
without ALI/ARDS, 339
VILI, from low volumes and pressures during
expiration, 339
higher PEEP in ALI/ARDS, clinical trials of
MV, 340–41
higher PEEP, patients more vulnerable to
adverse effects of, 342–43
nonresponders, receiving PEEP by, 343
recruitment maneuvers, 345–46
responders and nonresponders, identification
of, 341–42
setting PEEP, methods for, 343–45
Mechanotransduction, in VILI, 125
endothelial cells, 125
indirect mechanical signaling, 127
signaling pathways, 125–26
Mediastinal weight, on lung parenchyma, 317–21
Mesenchymal stem cell (MSCs)
in ALI/ARDS, experimental studies of, 424–25
biology, 420–22
in experimental models of organ injury,
423–24
future directions, 427–28
MSC-based therapy to clinical ALI/ARDS,
425–27
Messenger RNAs (mRNAs), 376
Microarray technology, 68, 221
Microtubules, 268–69
MIF. *See* Macrophage migration inhibitory factor
Mild hypoxemia, 343
Mini-B, 298
MLCK gene, 211
MLCK inhibitors, 275
MLCK. *See* Myosin light chain kinase
MODS. *See* Multiple organ dysfunction syndrome
Monocytes, 374, 398f
Mortality rates. *See* Attributable mortality, for ALI
Mouse models, of ARDS, 59, 60, 62
MRI. *See* Magnetic resonance imaging
mRNAs. *See* Messenger RNAs
MSC-based therapy to clinical ALI/ARDS,
425–27
MSCs immunomodulation, mechanisms involved
in, 422f
MSCs. *See* Mesenchymal stem cell

Multiple-hit hypothesis, 174
Multiple organ dysfunction syndrome (MODS), 115, 132–33
Multivariate analysis, 329
Murray lung injury score, 2–3
MyD88, 385, 386, 433
Myeloid leukocytes, 374
Myofibroblasts, 189
Myosin light chain kinase (MLCK), 119, 120f, 125, 199, 265
Myosin microfilaments, 265

N-nitroso-*N*-methylurethane (NNMU), 127
NAECC. *See* North American/European Consensus Conference Committee
National Blood Service, 180
National Center for Health Statistics, 17
National Heart, Lung, and Blood Institute (NHLBI), 171, 172
Negative pressure ventilation, 117
NETs. *See* Neutrophil extracellular traps
Neuromuscular blockade vs. spontaneous ventilation, 348–49
Neutropenia, 79
Neutrophil apoptosis, 80, 94–98, 104
Neutrophil deformability study, 80
Neutrophil elastase, 295
Neutrophil extracellular traps (NETs), 375
Neutrophil β_2 integrins, 374
Neutrophils, 49, 79–80, 177, 374, 398f,
NFκB. *See* Nuclear factor κB
NHLBI. *See* National Heart, Lung, and Blood Institute
Nick-end labeling (TUNEL), 101
Nitrate, 82
Nitric oxide (NO), 75, 82
Nitrite, 82
NIV. *See* Noninvasive ventilation
NNMU. *See* *N*-nitroso-*N*-methylurethane
Nocadozole, 268
Nocardia asteroids, 439
Nondiabetic patients and ARDS, 9
Noninvasive ventilation (NIV), 347–48, 349–50
Nonprotein-containing preparations, 298
Nonresponders, receiving PEEP by, 343
Norepinephrine, 154, 155
North American/European Consensus Conference Committee (NAECC), 31
Nosocomial pneumonia, 38

Nuclear factor κB (NFκB), 80
Nuclear medicine, 42–43

Obesity and ARDS, 11
Open lung biopsy role, in ARDS, 54, 56
Organizing phase, of ARDS, 40
OX-PLs. *See* Oxidatively modified phospholipids
Oxidatively modified phospholipids (OX-PLs), 390

P53, 53
P-selectin glycoprotein ligand 1 (PSGL-1), 394
PAC. *See* Pulmonary artery catheter
PAF acetylhydrolases, 390
PAF-like lipids, 389
PAF receptor, 389
PAFR. *See* PAF receptor
Palmitoyloleoylphosphatidylglycerol (POPG), 302
PAMPs. *See* Pathogen-associated molecular patterns
Pao_2/Fio_2 ratio, 304, 323, 325–26, 328, 329, 330, 351
Paramyxovirus, 441, 442
Pathogen-associated molecular patterns (PAMPs), 382
Pathogenesis, of ALI, 59
  alveolar-capillary membrane
    alveolar unit, 76
    endothelium, 77
    epithelium, 77–79
    extracellular matrix, 79
  alveolar-capillary membrane, disruption of
    increased permeability, 60–63
    lung inflammation, development of, 63
    surfactant dysfunction, 63–65
  changes in expression
    of individual genes in vitro, 66–68
    of many genes, 68
    of single genes in vivo, 66
  future directions, 84–85
  inflammatory cells, pathways, and mediators
    coagulation pathway, 82–83
    cytokines, 80–81
    damage-associated molecular pattern (DAMP) recognition, 83–84
    glycemia and glycated proteins, 84
    neutrophils, 79–80
    pro-oxidant/antioxidant balance, 81–82
    uncharacterized mechanisms, 84

lung injury, 59–60
  resolution, 65–66
  methodologies, 72
    autopsy and lung biopsy, 76
    bronchoalveolar lavage, 72–74
    exhaled gas and breath condensate, 74–75
    genetic analysis, 76
    imaging, 75
    physiological measurements, 75–76
    pulmonary edema fluid and pulmonary
      epithelial lining fluid, 74
    urine, 75
Pathologic fibrin deposition, 401
PBEF. *See* Pre-B cell colony-enhancing factor
PC. *See* Phosphatidylcholine
Pediatrics, ALI in, 27
PEEP. *See* Positive end-expiratory pressure
Peroxynitrite, 245
PET. *See* Positron emission tomography
PG. *See* Phosphatidylglycerol
Phosphatidylcholine (PC), 289, 292
Phosphatidylglycerol (PG), 289, 292
Phospholipase A$_2$, 295
Physiological dead space, 11
Physiological derangements of acute lung injury
  (ALI), 17
PIE. *See* Pulmonary interstitial emphysema
PKA. *See* Protein kinase A
PKC. *See* Protein kinase C
Plasma membrane disruption (PMD), 120f, 122
Platelet–leukocyte interactions, 380, 382
PMD. *See* Plasma membrane disruption
PMN apoptosis, 374–75
PMNs. *See* Polymorphonuclear leukocytes
Pneumocystis carinii, 295
Pneumomediastinum, 37
Pneumonia, 38–39, 147–150
Pneumopericardium, 37
Pneumothorax, 35, 37, 38, 39
Polymorphonuclear leukocytes (PMNs), 94, 97, 98
POPG. *See* Palmitoyloleoylphosphatidylglycerol
Porcine liver carboxylesterase, 291
Positive end-expiratory pressure (PEEP), 6, 35,
    116, 116f, 117, 121, 123, 124, 128, 147,
    155, 156, 326
Positive-pressure ventilation, 111–14
Positron emission tomography (PET), 7, 43
Posthoc analysis, 327
Post-transfusion acute pulmonary edema., 178f

Post-traumatic stress disorder (PTSD), 26
Pre-B cell colony-enhancing factor (PBEF), 199,
  273
Pre-existing medical conditions, on mortality from
  ARDS, 10
Procoagulant activity, in ALI patients, 83
Procoagulant protein, 83
Proliferative phase
  of ARDS, 32
  of DAD, 49–51
Prone position, in ARDS, 313
  effects, 315–17
  mediastinal weight on lung parenchyma,
    317–21
  pathophysiology in, 313–15
  prone ventilation
    in ARDS, 322–30
    on heart, 322
  ventilator-induced lung injury, 321–22
Pro-oxidant and antioxidant activity, in lung,
  81–82
Protein C, 83, 395
  plasma levels, 396
Protein kinase A (PKA), 120f
Protein kinase C (PKC), 119, 120f
Protein S, plasma levels of, 396
Protein-containing preparations, 298
Pseudomonas aeruginosa, 38, 389, 439
Pseudomonas pneumonia, 33
PSGL-1. *See* P-selectin glycoprotein ligand 1
PTCER. *See* Pulmonary transcapillary escape rate
PTSD. *See* Post-traumatic stress disorder
Pulmonary ARDS, 60
Pulmonary artery catheter (PAC), 35, 153, 154
Pulmonary dead space, 11
Pulmonary edema and high tidal volume
  ventilation, 115–17
Pulmonary edema fluid, 74
Pulmonary embolism, 158
Pulmonary epithelial lining fluid, 74
Pulmonary hypertension, 274
Pulmonary interstitial emphysema (PIE), 35–36,
  41
Pulmonary pathology, of ARDS. *See* Diffuse
  alveolar damage (DAD)
Pulmonary resection surgery, 8
Pulmonary transcapillary escape rate (PTCER), 43
Pulmonary vascular permeability (PVP), in ARDS
  patients, 7

Quality of life measures, in ALI survivors, 25

Racial differences, in ARDS mortality, 11
Radiographic findings, of ARDS, 31
  chest radiography, 32–34
  complications
    barotrauma, 35–38
    pneumonia, 38–39
    support lines, 34–35
  computed tomography (CT), 40–42
  MRI, 43
  nuclear medicine, 42–43
  pathophysiology, 32
RAGE. *See* Receptor for advanced glycation end
    products
RDS. *See* Respiratory distress syndrome
Receptor for advanced glycated end-products
    (RAGE), 84, 387
Recombinant human activated protein C (rhAPC),
    83
Recombinant plasma PAF acetylhydrolase (rPAF
    AH), 391, 392
Recruitment maneuvers, 345–346, 351
Regional computer tomography analysis, 314
Regional ventilation/perfusion (VE/Q) ratio,
    317
Renal-replacement therapy, 158–59
"Respirator lung syndrome", 46
Respiratory distress syndrome (RDS), 297
Responders and nonresponders, identification of,
    341–42
rhAPC. *See* Recombinant human activated protein
    C
Rho, 120f
Rho kinase, 268
Risk factors, for ARDS, 32
Rodent "two-hit" model, 396
rPAF AH. *See* Recombinant plasma PAF
    acetylhydrolase

S1P. *See* Sphingosine 1-phosphate
Salbutamol, 78
Saline lavage model, 296
Salmonella, 374
SELDI. *See* Surface-enhanced laser
    desorption/ionization
Sepsis, in ARDS
  ALI and ARDS, preventing infection in
    intravenous catheters, 150–51

    pneumonia, 147–150
    urinary tract infection, 151–52
  ALI and sepsis
    pathophysiological similarities between,
      146–47
    relationship between, 146
  as complication of ALI, 147
  severe sepsis treatment, in ALI and ARDS
    antibiotics and infection source control,
      152–53
    circulatory support, 153–55
    drotrecogin alfa (activated), 156–57
    nutrition and metabolism, 157–58
    supportive therapies, 158–59
    ventilatory support, 155–56
Sepsis and sepsis-induced ALI, pathogenesis of,
    369
  cellular effectors, 370f
  definitions, 371–72
  pathophysiology of, 372, 373f
    cell–cell interactions, 380–82
    cytokines and chemokines, 386–89
    endothelial function, in sepsis, 375–77
    inflammation, coagulation, and thrombosis in
      sepsis and complications, 392–96
    leukocytes, in sepsis, 372, 374–75
    platelets, 377–80
    TLRs, 382–86, 389–92
  research in, 402–403
  septic ALI/ARDS in critically III patients,
    features of, 397–402
Sepsis-induced ARDS, 10
Septic shock, 371
Septic transfusion reactions, 178
Severe sepsis treatment, in ALI and ARDS
  antibiotics and infection source control, 152–53
  circulatory support, 153–55
  drotrecogin alfa (activated), 156–57
  nutrition and metabolism, 157–58
  supportive therapies, 158–59
  ventilatory support, 155–56
SFasL. *See* Soluble FasL
SFTPB. *See* Surfactant protein-B
Shear stress, 111, 120f, 125, 126
Simvastatin, 277
Single nucleotide polymorphisms (SNPs), 200
SIRS. *See* Systemic inflammatory response
    syndrome
SNPs. *See* Single nucleotide polymorphisms

Soluble FasL (sFasL), 99, 101
SP-A. *See* Surfactant protein A
SP-B, 289, 291, 292, 293, 298
SP-C. *See* Surfactant protein C
SP-C33, 298
SP-D. *See* Surfactant protein D
Sphingosine 1-phosphate (S1P), 275–76
Spontaneous ventilation vs. neuromuscular
    blockade, 348–49
Staphylococcus aureus, 38
Subglottic suctioning, 149
Subpulmonic pneumothorax, 38
Sucralfate, 158
Surface-enhanced laser desorption/ionization
    (SELDI), 229
Surfactant alterations associated, with ALI,
    292–95
Surfactant dysfunction, 63–65
Surfactant protein A (SP-A), 78, 99, 289, 291, 293
Surfactant protein-B (SFTPB), 199, 212
Surfactant protein C (SP-C), 289, 292, 298
Surfactant protein D (SP-D), 78, 289, 291, 293
Surfactant replacement, clinical trials of, 297
    surfactant treatment, of ARDS patients, 298
      mode of administration, 299–300
      results, 302–305
      surfactant dose and dose volume, 300–301
      surfactant preparations, 298–99
      timing of surfactant administration, 301–302
Surfactant system, of mature lung, 287
Surfactant therapy, in ARDS, 287
    preclinical observations, 295–97
    surfactant alterations associated, with ALI,
      292–95
    surfactant replacement, clinical trials of,
      297–305
    surfactant system, of mature lung, 287–92
      composition and biophysical function,
      288–91
      host defense properties, 291–92
Survanta®, 302
Surveillance, Epidemiology, and End Results
    (SEER) Program, 18
Systemic inflammatory response syndrome
    (SIRS), 371

TACO. *See* Transfusion-associated circulatory
    overload
TGF-β. *See* Transforming growth factor-beta

TGF-β$_1$. *See* Transforming growth factor-β$_1$
Thrombin, 272, 273f, 395
Thrombocytopenia, 53
TICAM1. *See* TIR-domain-containing molecule 1
Tidal volumes
    adjustment, 338–39
    and inspiratory pressures, 350
Tight junctions, 271, 272
TIR-associated protein (TIRAP), 385
TIR-domain-containing adaptor protein-inducing
    IFN-β (TRIF), 385
TIR-domain-containing molecule 1 (TICAM1),
    385
TIRAP. *See* TIR-associated protein
Tissue factor (TF), 83
Tissue inhibitor of metalloproteinases, 80
Tissue inhibitors of metalloproteases, 191
Tissue remodeling mediators, in lung injury,
    190–91
TLR2 gene, 383
TLR4 gene, 383
TLRs. *See* Toll-like receptors
TNF-α. *See* Tumor necrosis factor receptor-α
TNFR. *See* Tumor necrosis factor receptor
Toll-like receptors (TLRs), 374, 382–85
    in gene expression pathways, 385–86
    inflammatory mediators, synthesis of, 385–86
    in intracellular signaling, 385–86
TRALI. *See* Transfusion-related acute lung injury
TRAM. *See* TRIF-related adaptor molecule
Transforming growth factor-beta (TGF-β), 190,
    191, 244
Transforming growth factor-β$_1$ (TGF-β$_1$), 184
Transfusion-associated circulatory overload
    (TACO), 172, 178
Transfusion-related acute lung injury (TRALI),
    10
    blood transfusions and ALI/ARDS, 173
      observational studies, 173
      randomized clinical trials, 173
      specific donor characteristics, 174
    clinical definition, presentation, and incidence,
      171–72
    clinical pathogenesis, 174–76
    diagnosis, 177–79
    experimental studies, 176–77
    future directions, 180
    historical perspective, 171
    treatment and prevention, 179–180

Transfusion-related lung injury, 84
Transpulmonary pressure, 115
Transpulmonary thermodilution technique, 75
Trauma patients, with ARDS, 10
TRIF-related adaptor molecule (TRAM), 385
TRIF. *See* TIR-domain-containing adaptor
protein-inducing IFN-β
Tumor necrosis factor alpha (TNF)-α, 60, 78,
81, 199, 243, 272–73, 273f, 387,
434–35
Tumor necrosis factor receptor (TNFR), 120f
TUNEL. *See* Nick-end labeling
Type I epithelial cells, 187
Type I error, 213
Type I pneumocytes, 187
Type II epithelial cells, 187
Type II pneumocytes, 48, 50, 54, 187

UIP. *See* Usual interstitial pneumonia
Upper gastrointestinal bleeding, 158
Urinary markers, analysis of, 75
Urinary tract infection, 148t, 151–52
Urine NO levels, 82
Usual interstitial pneumonia (UIP), 55

VALI. *See* Ventilator-associated lung injury
VAP. *See* Ventilator-associated pneumonia
Variants T-1001G, 210
Vascular catheter-related infections, 147
Vascular endothelial growth factor (VEGF), 274,
377
Vasopressin, 155
Vectorial fluid transport impairment, mechanisms
of, 244
anesthetics, 244–45
hypoxia, 244
reactive oxygen and nitrogen species, 245
VEGF. *See* Vascular endothelial growth factor
Venticute®, 303
Ventilator mode, 350
Ventilator-associated lung injury (VALI), 76, 84,
110

Ventilator-associated pneumonia (VAP), 147,
148t, 149, 150
Ventilator-free days (VFDs), 303, 305
Ventilator-induced lung injury (VILI), 109,
321–22
hypercapnia, effects of, 128
low lung volume ventilation, injury from, 122
experimental studies, 124
protective ventilation, clinical studies of,
123–24
mechanical ventilation, 110–111
and MODS, 132–33
mechanotransduction, 125
endothelial cells, 125
indirect mechanical signaling, 127
signaling pathways, 125–26
from overdistension, 114
excessive lung volume, in clinical studies,
115
experimental models, 115–121
mechanical strain in vitro, 121–22
positive-pressure ventilation, 111–14
surfactant secretion and function, 127–28
ventilator-induced pulmonary and systemic
inflammation, 128
biomarkers of inflammation, 128–29
mediators of inflammation, 129–131
strain-induced inflammatory response,
131–32
Ventilator-induced pulmonary edema, 116, 116f,
118
VFDs. *See* Ventilator-free days
VILI. *See* Ventilator-induced lung injury
Vimentin, 269–270
Visceral pleura, rupture of, 35
Volume-and-pressure limited MV, in patients
without ALI/ARDS, 339
Von Willebrand factor (VWF), 77
VWF. *See* Von Willebrand factor

White patients, with ALI, 22
White patients, with ARDS, 11
Whole-lung CT, 42

Milton Keynes UK
Ingram Content Group UK Ltd.
UKHW022053141024
449569UK00031B/1620